AF746057

The Shoulder Made Easy

Charalambos Panayiotou Charalambous

The Shoulder Made Easy

Springer

Charalambos Panayiotou Charalambous
Blackpool Teaching Hospitals NHS Foundation Trust
and School of Medicine
University of Central Lancashire
Blackpool, Lancashire
UK

ISBN 978-3-319-98907-5 ISBN 978-3-319-98908-2 (eBook)
https://doi.org/10.1007/978-3-319-98908-2

Library of Congress Control Number: 2019934462

© Springer Nature Switzerland AG 2019
This work is subject to copyright. All rights are reserved by the Publisher, whether the whole or part of the material is concerned, specifically the rights of translation, reprinting, reuse of illustrations, recitation, broadcasting, reproduction on microfilms or in any other physical way, and transmission or information storage and retrieval, electronic adaptation, computer software, or by similar or dissimilar methodology now known or hereafter developed.
The use of general descriptive names, registered names, trademarks, service marks, etc. in this publication does not imply, even in the absence of a specific statement, that such names are exempt from the relevant protective laws and regulations and therefore free for general use.
The publisher, the authors, and the editors are safe to assume that the advice and information in this book are believed to be true and accurate at the date of publication. Neither the publisher nor the authors or the editors give a warranty, express or implied, with respect to the material contained herein or for any errors or omissions that may have been made. The publisher remains neutral with regard to jurisdictional claims in published maps and institutional affiliations.

The sketches included in this book were drawn by Robert Brownlow and the figures by Chrysanthos Therapontos, commissioned by CP Charalambous. The copyright is held by CP Charalambous.

This Springer imprint is published by the registered company Springer Nature Switzerland AG
The registered company address is: Gewerbestrasse 11, 6330 Cham, Switzerland

I dedicate this book to my parents and to all my special teachers and trainers.

Preface

This book aims to provide the reader with a basic understanding of commonly encountered shoulder conditions and guide as to how these may be managed. It is directed to a wide audience ranging from undergraduate students to those in postgraduate training or in full practice. I hope that medical professionals (medical students, general practitioners, orthopaedic surgeons) as well as allied health professionals (physiotherapists) will find this book of use. It aims to transmit knowledge that one may call upon in day-to-day clinical practice but also help prepare those with upcoming exams (undergraduate medical, MRCS, FRCS (Orth)).

This book attempts to present information in an easily read, succinct way and break down a vast complex subject into small, manageable sections. In particular, this book tries to unpick and explain those concepts of shoulder surgery that may be difficult to understand. An attempt is made to provide the reader with knowledge and information, but also stimulate lateral thinking.

I would like to thank Liz Pope, Associate Editor at Springer UK, for supporting the concept of this book, as well as Julia Squarr, Associate Editor at Springer UK, and Vignesh Iyyadurai, Project Coordinator for Springer Nature, for their support in seeing through the project to its completion. Gratitude is paid to colleagues for their constructive feedback in preparation of this book, particularly Dr. Wael Mati, Consultant Radiologist at Blackpool Victoria Hospital.

My special thanks to Chrysanthos Therapontos for communicating through illustrations many of the book's concepts and Tariq Kwaees for helping to demonstrate clinical examination techniques.

Blackpool, UK Charalambos Panayiotou Charalambous

Contents

Chapter 1
Introduction

When setting out to understand and manage disorders of the shoulder, it is essential to recognise the normal structure and function of this joint. Hence, the clinical anatomy of the shoulder is initially presented along with a description of the healthy shoulder joint's biomechanics and function.

The first step in the successful management of shoulder disorders is the acquisition of a thorough clinical history. Such a clinical history elicits the presenting symptoms, their onset, progress and severity but also determines the patient's overall condition, functional demands, personal circumstances and expectations. Although in obtaining a clinical history one aims to mainly utilise open-ended questions, the use of direct, specific questioning may help to get a better grasp of the presenting problem and assist in formulating potential diagnoses. A structured approach for obtaining a clinical history for shoulder complaints is presented in the fourth chapter.

Clinical examination aims to elicit signs that can supplement the clinical history and prove or disprove the working diagnosis that the clinician is already considering by having listened to the patient's troubles. The fifth chapter guides as how to perform a structured clinical examination with an emphasis on some of the many special tests described in shoulder assessment. Such a structured approach may ensure that important signs are not overlooked.

In combination, clinical history and clinical examination help to guide as to the most likely diagnosis, as well as to potential alternative diagnoses. Once the likely origin of the patient's symptoms is determined, one aims to investigate this further, to confirm or dispute the working diagnosis. The sixth chapter gives an overview of the potential radiological and neurophysiological tests that are available in the diagnosis of shoulder conditions, helping to guide the reader as to what information these may provide. The value of diagnostic local anaesthetic injections is also discussed.

When managing shoulder conditions, a wide spectrum of potential interventions are available, and it is a skill to decide when and how to intervene. The next chapter introduces some of the challenges faced in treating shoulder disorders and discusses

© Springer Nature Switzerland AG 2019
C. Panayiotou Charalambous, *The Shoulder Made Easy*,
https://doi.org/10.1007/978-3-319-98908-2_1

the role of the management ladder for shoulder conditions. The next two chapters discuss the principles and techniques of injection and needling therapy as well as common surgical procedures employed in the management of the troublesome shoulder.

Physiotherapy has a huge role to play in the management of shoulder conditions either in isolation or in combination with non-invasive or invasive interventions. Although a detailed description of physiotherapy modalities utilised in shoulder conditions is beyond the scope of this book, the subsequent chapter introduces the reader to some physiotherapy principles considered from a surgeon's perspective.

Patients don't present with a clinical diagnosis but with symptoms such as pain, stiffness, weakness or instability. Although common symptoms have common causes, a thorough consideration of what could be accounting for such symptoms may ensure that unusual pathologies are not overlooked. Hence, the subsequent chapters describe a structured consideration of potential causes of common presenting shoulder symptoms and advice on how such symptoms may be further investigated and managed.

The rest of the book reverts to the usual approach of describing specific shoulder conditions rather than symptoms. These chapters present in greater detail common conditions that may be encountered in clinical practice, their pathogenesis, demographics, clinical symptoms and signs and guide as to the investigation and management for each.

Reaching a clinical diagnosis relies on knowledge but also on the ability to structure the clinical thought process, to stay open minded, to identify what is vital and to eliminate the unnecessary, skills that this book aims to help develop. Similarly, when it comes to clinical management, this book tries to highlight that one solution does not fit all but the specifics of the patient and their personal circumstances must be carefully considered. Shared decision-making between clinician and patient has a vital role in choosing amongst of many management options. Surgery for many shoulder conditions may be seen as the last resort and one to be approached with careful consideration and caution.

As a consultant surgeon in trauma and orthopaedics who has done all my undergraduate and postgraduate training in the United Kingdom, the guidance presented in this book originates from personal experiences but also the teachings and "wisdoms" of my senior trainers, peers and colleagues. Much of what is presented is commonly available knowledge, and every attempt has been made to acknowledge and reference its original sources as warranted. Some may not fully agree with what is presented, some may have opposite views but that is understandable and acceptable. Nevertheless, I hope the reader will gain and benefit from what is said and incorporate some of the advice given in their clinical practice.

Chapter 2
Shoulder Anatomy

This chapter describes the normal anatomy of the shoulder considering the bones, ligaments, muscles, tendons, arterial and nerve supply. The clinical relevance of these structures is also described.

2.1 Shoulder: Anatomical Structures

We may explore the anatomy of the shoulder [1–3] in layers, starting from the deepest and moving onto the most superficial:

- Bones
- Joint capsule and ligaments
- Muscles and their tendons
- Subcutaneous tissue and skin

When considering the shoulder, the bones to describe are the:

- Scapula
- Humerus
- Clavicle
- Thoracic wall
- Sternum

The joints these bones form between them are the:

- Glenohumeral joint
- Acromio-clavicular joint (ACJt)
- Scapulo-thoracic articulation
- Sterno-clavicular joint

© Springer Nature Switzerland AG 2019

C. Panayiotou Charalambous, *The Shoulder Made Easy*,
https://doi.org/10.1007/978-3-319-98908-2_2

Shoulder bones – anterior view

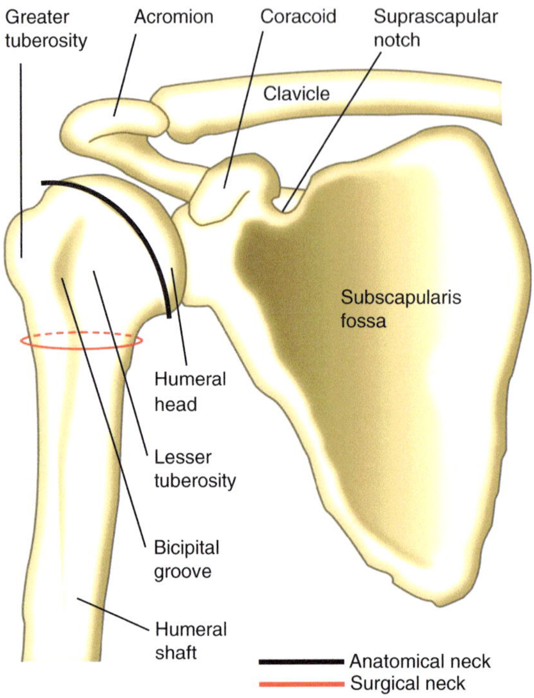

Shoulder bones – posterior view

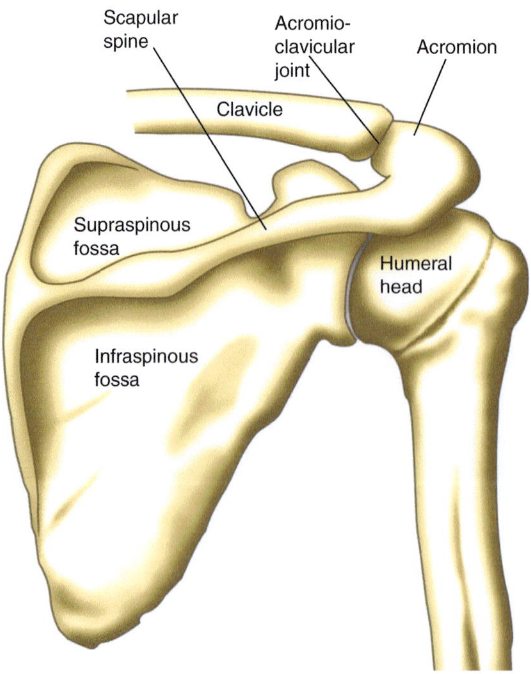

Scapula side view

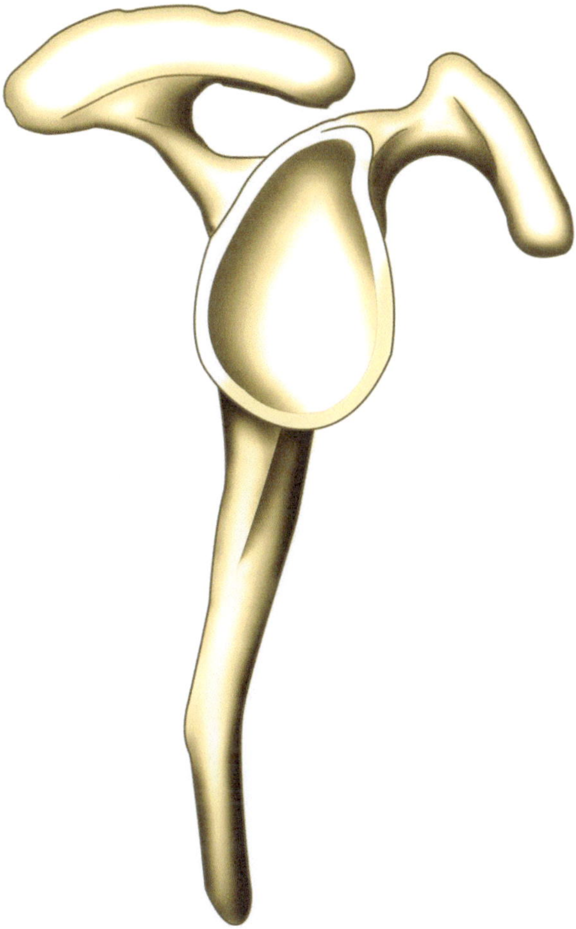

2.1.1 *Scapula*

This is a large triangular bone located just lateral to the vertebral column on the posterior part of the thoracic wall. It consists of the main part, the body, that laterally gives rise to the scapular neck, glenoid and coracoid process.

The body has medial, superior and inferior borders. The anterior surface of the body of the scapula is flat. The posterior surface gives rise to the spine of the scapula which passes laterally, curves forwards and flattens to form the acromion. The posterior surface of the scapula superior to its spine is known as the supraspinous fossa, and that inferior to the spine as the infraspinous fossa.

The coracoid process arises from the anterior part of the scapula, arches upwards and then hooks down, like the beak of a "coracas" (Greek for crow) from which it gets its name.

Medial to the coracoid process, the superior scapular border forms a notch, the suprascapular notch, through which the suprascapular nerve and veins pass.

The glenoid forms the "socket" part of the glenohumeral joint, which is the main shoulder joint. The glenoid is pear shaped and is covered with articular (hyaline) cartilage.

2.1.2 Humerus

This is the arm bone. It consists of the:

- Upper part – the humeral head
- Middle part – the shaft
- Lower part – gives rise to the humeral condyles that articulate at the elbow joint with the radius and ulna

The humeral head is shaped like a ball, and its medial surface is covered with articular cartilage. The humeral head articulates with the glenoid at the glenohumeral joint.

Just lateral to the articular cartilage are two bony prominences, the lesser and the greater tuberosities, separated by a groove, the bicipital groove.

Two humeral necks are described:

1. Anatomical neck – marks the junction of the articular part of the humeral head with the surrounding bone
2. Surgical neck – located more inferiorly and marks the junction between the humeral neck and the humeral shaft

2.1.3 Clavicle

This is a flat-shaped bone. Its medial border articulates with the sternum at the sterno-clavicular joint, whereas its lateral end articulates with the acromion at the acromio-clavicular joint.

2.1.4 *Glenohumeral Joint*

The humerus articulates with the scapula at the glenohumeral joint. This is the main joint of the shoulder. It is a ball and socket joint, with the articular surfaces covered by hyaline cartilage.

Arthroscopic view of the humeral head articulating with the glenoid

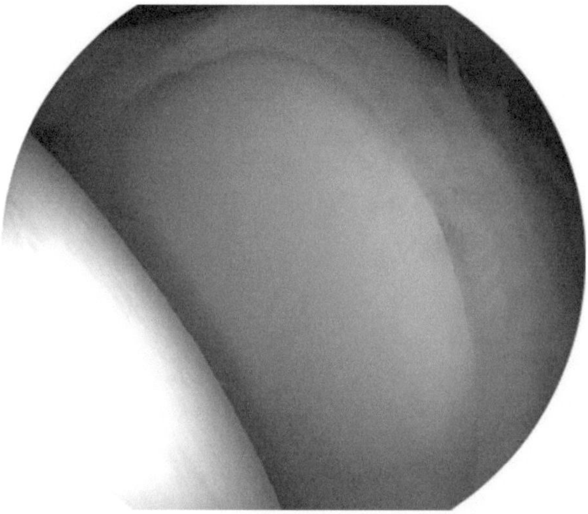

The articular surface of the humeral head makes a superiorly pointing angle of 130–150° in relation to the long axis of the humeral shaft. It is also retroverted (pointing backwards) in relation to the humeral shaft. Retroversion is commonly defined in relation to the trans-epicondylar axis (the axis of the distal humerus around which elbow flexion occurs) and varies between 18 and 22°.

The glenoid fossa is shaped like a pear. The vertical and transverse diameters of the glenoid are much smaller than those of the humeral head. Hence, the surface area of the glenoid is much less than that of the humeral head (about 1/3–1/4). In most shoulders the glenoid fossa is also retroverted (pointing backwards) by about 7° in relation to the long horizontal axis of the scapula.

The edge of the glenoid is lined by a fibrocartilaginous fold, the labrum. The inner surface of the labrum is covered with synovium, and the outer surface attaches to the joint's capsule [1, 2].

Face view of glenoid, with intact labrum and long head of biceps tendon insertion

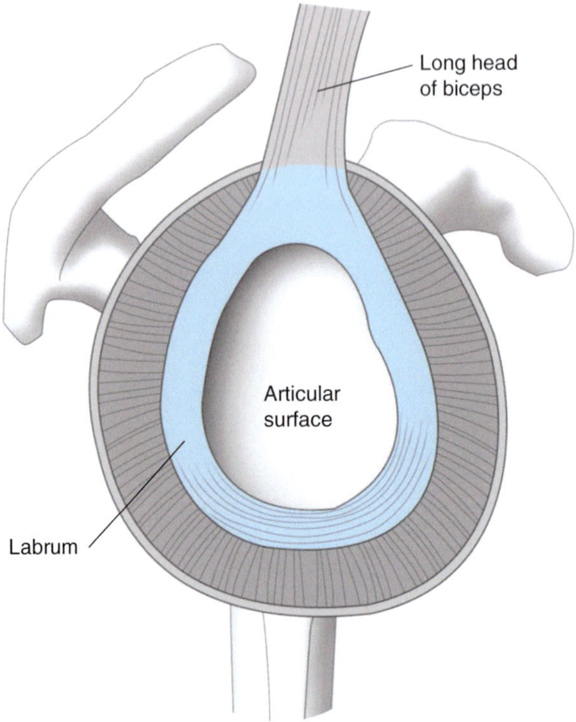

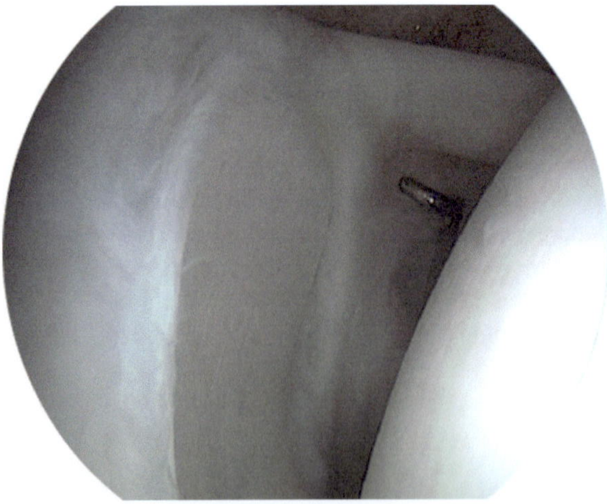

The labrum has several functions:

- Increases the depth of the glenoid
- Increases the articulating surface of the glenoid

- Provides attachment for the glenohumeral ligaments
- Provides attachment to the long head of the biceps tendon

In most shoulders the labrum encircles the glenoid edge and is firmly attached to it. However, in some shoulders there are normal anatomical variants of this [4]. Three such anatomical variants are:

- Sub-labrum recess – the superior labrum is not firmly attached to the glenoid, but there is a space between the two
- Anterior labrum recess – the anterior-superior labrum is not firmly attached to the glenoid, but there is a space between the two
- Buford complex – the anterior-superior labrum is absent, and the middle gleno-humeral ligament is thickened and looks like a vertically orientated cord that originates from the superior labrum distal to the biceps insertion

Arthroscopic view of Buford complex

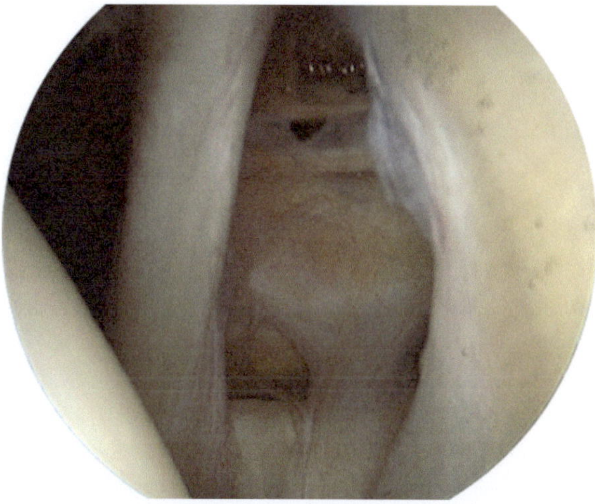

MRI showing Buford complex (red arrows) with space between the anterior-superior labrum and anterior glenoid rim and cord-like middle glenohumeral ligament (green arrow)

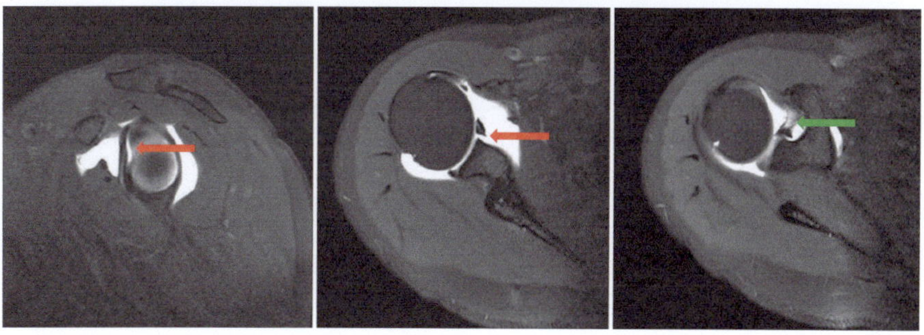

The importance of such anatomic variants is that they may be mistaken for detachments of the labrum either during magnetic resonance imaging (MRI) or arthroscopic surgery. Hence, labrum recesses and holes should be treated with caution when involving the superior or anterior-superior labrum. However, lesions involving the rest of the labrum are often pathological.

The glenohumeral joint is enclosed by the capsule. This is a fibrous layer that passes from the edges of the glenoid to insert onto the humeral head at the edge of the articular cartilage, to which it is firmly attached. Superiorly, the capsule is apposed to the undersurface of the rotator cuff tendons [5]; hence full-thickness rotator cuff tears also involve a tear of the capsule. Inferiorly, the capsule is loose and forms a capsular fold. Anteriorly, the capsule has several thickenings forming distinct ligaments, known as the glenohumeral ligaments (superior, middle and inferior). Disruption of these ligaments and capsule is associated with glenohumeral instability. In contrast, thickening and contracture of these ligaments and capsule are associated with shoulder stiffness, such as adhesive capsulitis. The loose, inferior capsular fold is characteristically reduced in adhesive capsulitis.

MRI arthrogram showing spacious inferior capsular fold (green arrow)

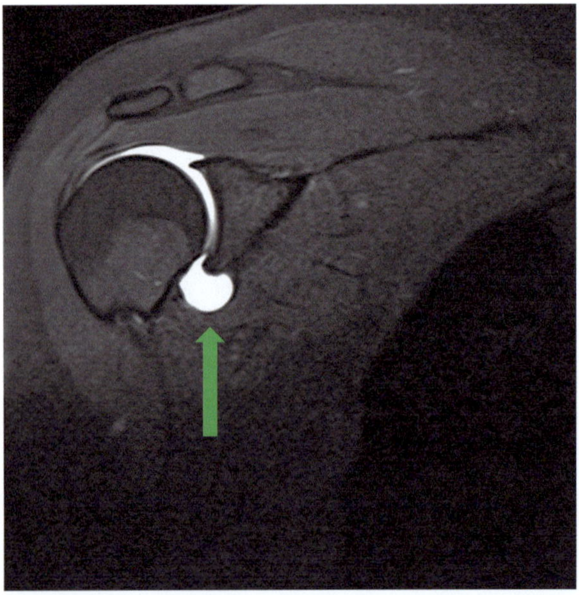

MRI showing thickened inferior capsule in adhesive capsulitis (red arrow)

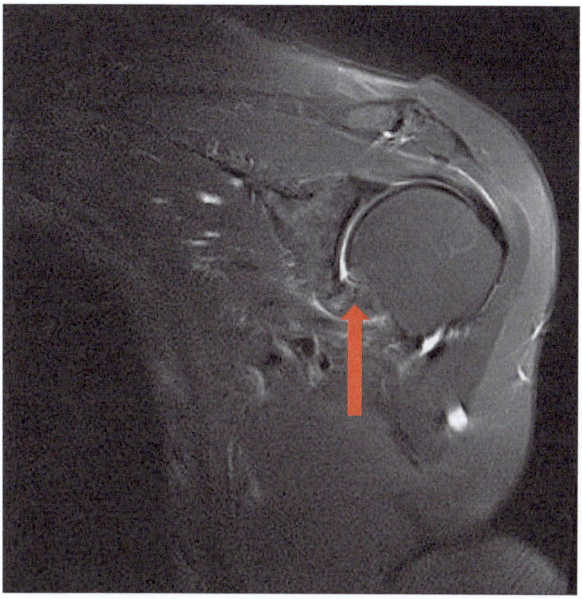

The internal surface of the capsule is lined by synovium; hence the glenohumeral joint is a synovial joint. Hence, it may be affected by the various disorders of synovial origin, including inflammatory arthropathy. The synovium also forms a sheath around the tendon of the long head of the biceps and extends into the bicipital groove covering this tendon.

2.1.5 Acromio-Clavicular Joint

This is the joint between the medial edge of the acromion and the lateral pat of the clavicle, the surfaces of which are covered by fibrocartilage. The capsule attaches to the articular margins and encloses the joint. The inner surface of the capsule is lined by synovium. An intra-articular disc made of fibrocartilage may be present, originating from the upper part of the capsule. Three types of ACJt have been described based on the presence and extent of this articular disc [6]:

- Type 1: disc divides the joint completely (4%)
- Type 2: disc is incomplete and divides the joint incompletely (25%)
- Type 3: disc is absent (71%)

2.1.6 *Sterno-clavicular Joint*

This is the joint between the medial end of the clavicle and the superior part of the sternum (the manubrium) and the costal cartilage of the first rib. A capsule attaches to the articular margins and encloses the joint [7].

The medial end of the clavicle is much larger than the corresponding articulating part of the manubrium. It is shaped convex vertically and concave anterior-posteriorly; hence the articulation with the manubrium is saddle shaped. The articular surfaces are covered with fibrocartilage.

A vertical intra-articular disc may split the joint into two (completely or incompletely) and is attached to the anterior and posterior part of the capsule. The ligaments providing stability to this joint are the:

- Costo-clavicular ligament
- Inter-clavicular ligament

Front view of the sterno-clavicular joints and associated ligaments

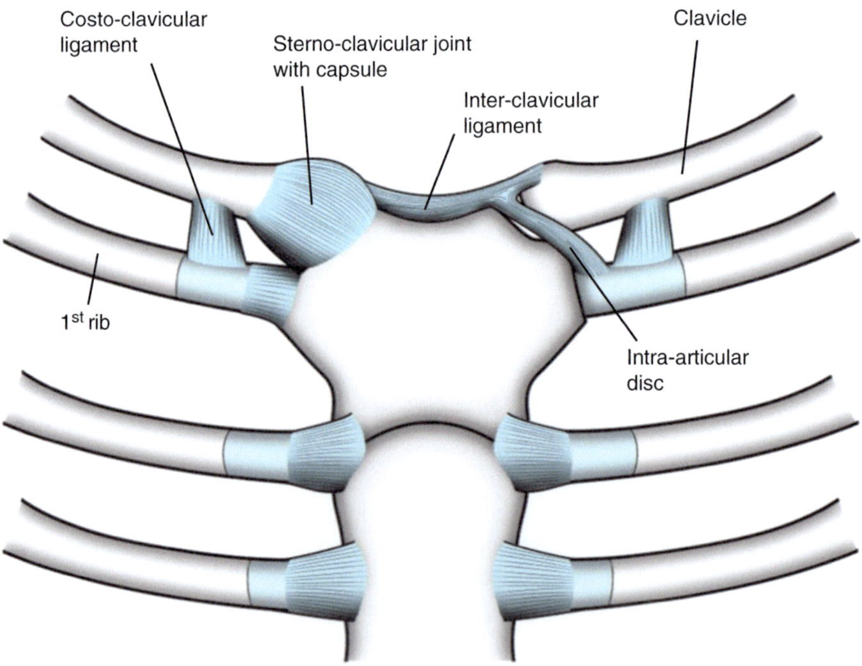

2.1.7 *Scapulo-thoracic Articulation*

The scapulo-thoracic articulation is not a true joint; instead this refers to the contact of the anterior surface of the scapula with the outer posterior surface of the chest wall. The anterior surface of the scapula is concave and corresponds to the convex shape of the posterior chest wall.

2.2 Anatomy Overview

Consider the axial skeleton as consisting of the vertebral column at the back, the sternum at the front, with the rib cage in between. Lower down, the vertebral column articulates via the sacrum to the pelvis. The scapula is connected to the trunk via:

- The clavicle which articulates with the acromion at the ACJt and with the sternum at the sterno-clavicular joint
- Muscles that pass between the scapula and the vertebral column, the rib cage and pelvis

Apart from its attachments through the ACJt and sterno-clavicular joint, the scapula is without any other bony or ligamentous attachments to the axial skeleton. Hence, the scapula and, indirectly, the upper limb hang from the lateral end of the clavicle.

The scapula is held against the chest wall by muscles that pass from the axial skeleton to the scapula including the trapezius, serratus anterior, rhomboids (major and minor) and levator scapulae.

2.2.1 Orientation of the Shoulder Bones in Space

Looking at the scapula from above, at rest, its long horizontal axis is not in line with the coronal plane of the trunk but is pointing about 30–45° forwards in relation to that. This plane at which the long axis of the scapula lies is referred to as the scapular plane. When examining the shoulder, we often place the arm forwards so it is in line with the scapular plane rather than the coronal plane.

Scapular plane in relation to coronal plane

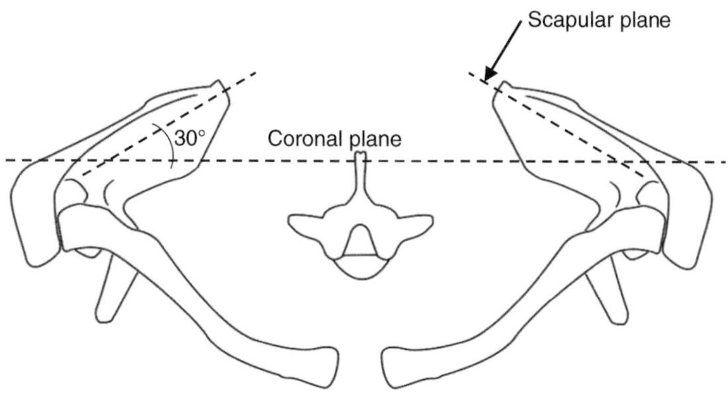

Movements of the humerus in relation to the glenoid fossa can be described in relation to the frontal and coronal planes or in relation to the scapular plane. The glenohumeral structures (such as the capsule, rotator cuff tendons, deltoid) are in optimal alignment when shoulder movement occurs in the scapular plane [8].

2.3 Ligaments

Ligaments are fibrous structures that connect two bones. The following ligaments are to be considered in the shoulder region:

Glenohumeral ligaments – The capsule of the glenohumeral joint has several thickenings on its anterior aspect, forming distinct ligaments that contribute to the stability of the glenohumeral joint [1, 2, 9]. These are the:

- Superior glenohumeral ligament – originates from the upper part of the glenoid labrum and the base of the coracoid and inserts onto the upper part of the humerus (between the lesser tuberosity and anatomical neck). It limits downward displacement of the humeral head. The inferior sulcus sign may be related to dysfunction of this ligament
- Middle glenohumeral ligament – originates from the anterior part of the glenoid labrum (up to the junction of the middle and inferior thirds of the glenoid) and passes laterally to insert on the anterior aspect of the anatomical neck of the humerus. The middle glenohumeral ligament limits external rotation of the humeral head and provides anterior stability
- Inferior glenohumeral ligament – originates from the anterior, inferior and posterior margins of the glenoid labrum and passes laterally to the inferior aspect of the anatomical and surgical necks of the humerus. It is a broad, thick ligament that acts like a hammock and supports the anterior and inferior aspects of the humeral head

Arthroscopic view of the middle glenohumeral ligament attached to the labrum and descending to its humeral insertion, crossing subscapularis

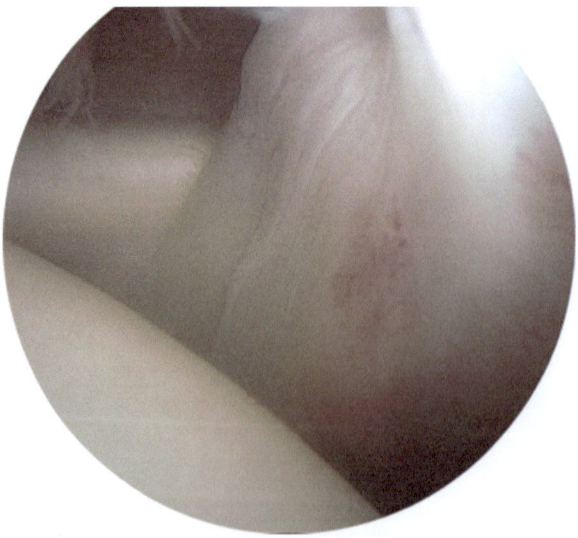

Arthroscopic view of the inferior glenohumeral ligament inserting onto the proximal humerus

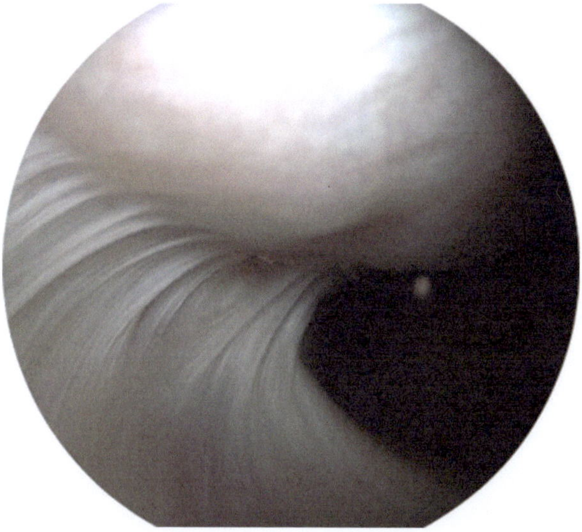

Coraco-acromial ligament – passes from the lateral part of the coracoid to insert onto the anterior-inferior border of the acromion. It forms part of the roof of the subacromial arch which can cause external impingement on the underlying supraspinatus and long head of the biceps tendon. This ligament also limits superior/anterior translation of the humeral head, a role that becomes important in the presence of massive rotator cuff tears. Hence, in performing arthroscopic subacromial debridement/decompression in the presence of massive non-repairable rotator cuff tears, the integrity of the coraco-acromial ligament needs to be preserved, to prevent anterior escape of the humeral head.

Coraco-humeral ligament – passes from the lateral part of the coracoid to the greater tuberosity of the humerus. It is the ligament implicated in the pathogenesis of adhesive capsulitis as its contraction limits external rotation and forward elevation of the humeral head.

Transverse humeral ligament – passes from the lesser to the greater tuberosity overlying the long head of the biceps tendon.

Suprascapular ligament – lines the superior free edge of the suprascapular notch. In this way a tunnel is formed bounded superior by a thick ligament and inferiorly by the bone through which the suprascapular nerve passes [10].

Spino-glenoid ligament – passes from the lateral part of the base of the scapular spine to the superior/posterior part of the glenoid rim. The suprascapular nerve passes under this ligament [11].

Costo-clavicular ligament – passes from the inferior surface of the medial part of the clavicle to the medial end of the first rib and first costal cartilage.

Anterior sterno-clavicular ligament – passes from the anterior part of the medial end of the clavicle to the anterior part of the sternum, covering the anterior surface of the sterno-clavicular joint.

Posterior sterno-clavicular ligament – passes from the posterior part of the medial end of the clavicle to the posterior part of the sternum covering the posterior surface of the sterno-clavicular joint.

Inter-clavicular ligament – passes from the posterior-superior part of the medial clavicle and superior part of the capsule of the right sterno-clavicular joint to the posterior-superior part of the medial clavicle and superior part of the capsule of the left sterno-clavicular joint [7].

Coraco-clavicular ligaments (conoid and trapezoid) – pass from the superior surface of the base of the coracoid to the inferior surface of the lateral end of the clavicle. They provide vertical stability limiting upward displacement of the clavicle in relation to the acromion [12, 13].

Superior and inferior acromio-clavicular ligaments – pass between the acromion and lateral end of the clavicle, covering the superior and inferior surfaces of the ACJt. They provide anterior-posterior stability of the clavicle in relation to the acromion [14, 15].

Shoulder capsule and ligaments – anterior view

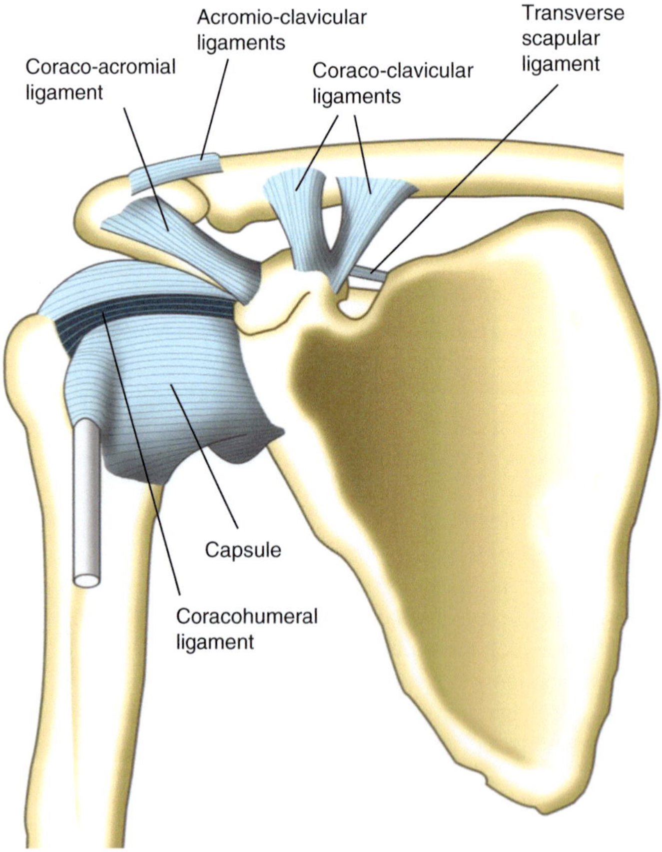

Shoulder capsule and ligaments – posterior view

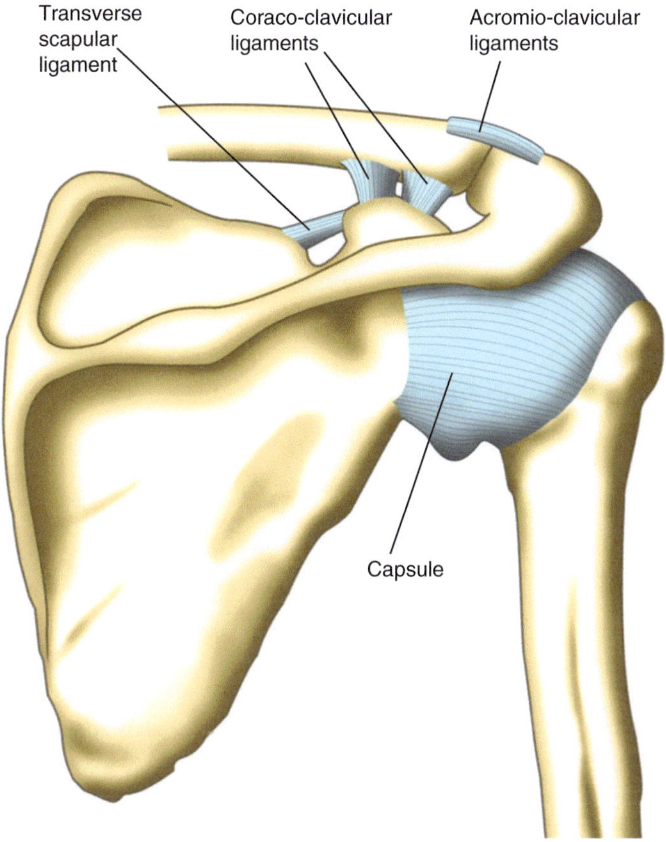

2.4 Muscles

The muscles around the shoulder may be described as:

1. Muscles that connect the scapula to the humerus
2. Muscles that connect the trunk to the scapula
3. Muscles that connect the trunk to the humerus

2.4.1 Muscles Connecting the Scapula to the Humerus

Rotator Cuff Muscles

The rotator cuff muscles are four muscles whose main function is to move and stabilise the glenohumeral joint. They consist of:

Supraspinatus – originates from the supraspinous fossa and passes laterally to insert onto the most anterior area of the greater tuberosity of the humeral head. The anterior part of the supraspinatus is thicker, whilst the posterior is thinner. It has a long area of insertion (footprint) with an average maximum medial-to-lateral thickness of about 7 mm and an average maximum anteroposterior length of about 13 mm [16]. It is supplied by the suprascapular nerve.

Arthroscopic view of the insertion of supraspinatus onto the humeral head-articular view

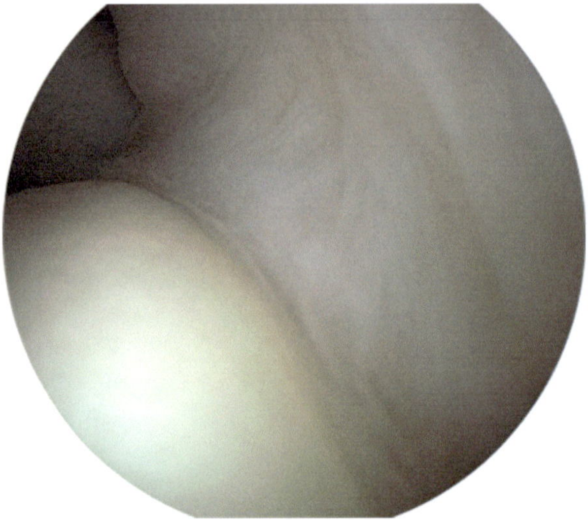

Infraspinatus – originates from the infraspinous fossa and passes laterally to insert onto the posterior facet of the greater tuberosity of the humeral head but may also extend forwards to insert onto the anterior part of the greater tuberosity. It has a long insertion footprint with an average maximum medial-to-lateral thickness of about 10 mm and an average maximum anteroposterior length of about 33 mm [16]. It is supplied by the suprascapular nerve.

Arthroscopic view of the insertion of infraspinatus onto the humeral head-articular view

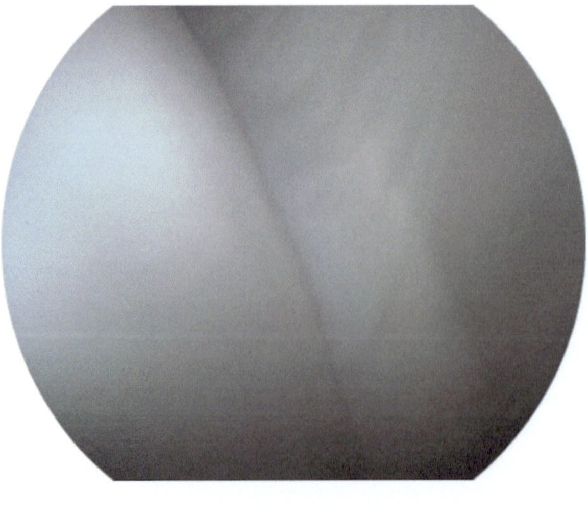

Subscapularis – originates from the anterior surface of the body of the scapula and passes laterally to insert onto the lesser tuberosity of the humeral head. It has an extensive insertion footprint. The superior inferior length of the footprint is about 25 mm. The medial-to-lateral thickness of the footprint is trapezoidal with the superior part being wider than the inferior part (18 vs. 3 mm, respectively) [17]. It is supplied by the subscapular nerves.

Arthroscopic view of the superior edge of the subscapularis tendon passing horizontally to its insertion onto the humeral head

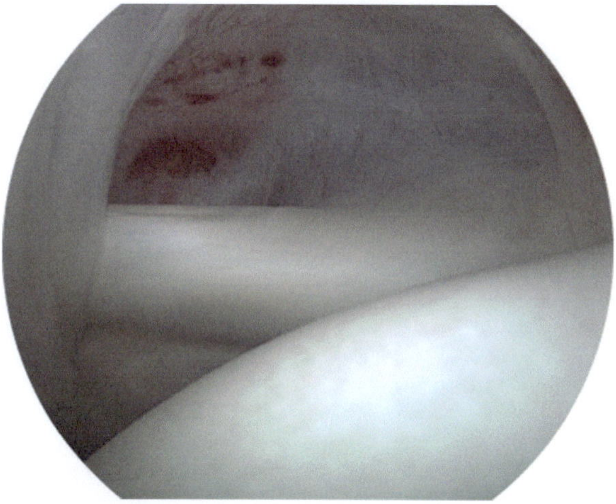

MRI showing normal appearance of supraspinatus (yellow arrow), infraspinatus (green arrow) and subscapularis (blue arrow) tendons

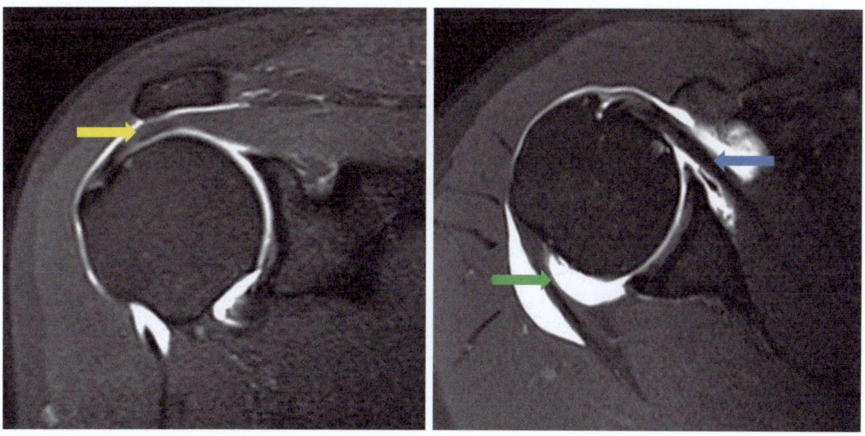

Teres minor – originates from the posterior surface of the scapula, inferior to the infraspinatus, and attaches onto the inferior part (facet) of the greater tuberosity of the humeral head. It is supplied by the axillary nerve.

The tendons of the rotator cuff muscles are flat tendons rather than tubular, hence their broad area of attachment. The tendons of the individual muscles blend to form a common insertion. The common tendon consists of multiple layers of fibres which mainly pass in line with the long axis of the tendon but also transverse fibres found mainly in the deep part of the tendon and which hold the individual tendons together [17]. In addition to having a broad insertion to the bone, the rotator cuff tendons also have a thick insertion. Hence, it is possible that only part of this thick insertion is detached from the bone giving rise to a partial thickness (as compared to a full thickness) tear. This may be likened to a thick pillar of bricks, whereby some bricks may be lost without the pillar collapsing.

Arch, the pillars of which are made of multiple layers of bricks. Some bricks may be lost (equivalent to a partial thickness tendon tear) without the pillar collapsing

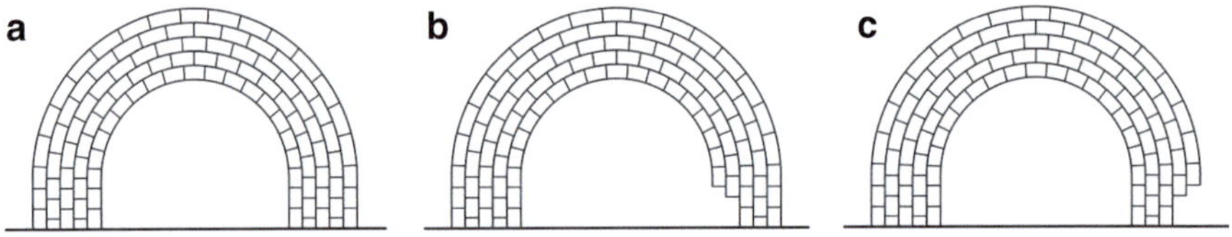

Supraspinatus tendon front view: (a) intact tendon, (b) partial thickness articular side tear, (c) partial thickness bursal side tear

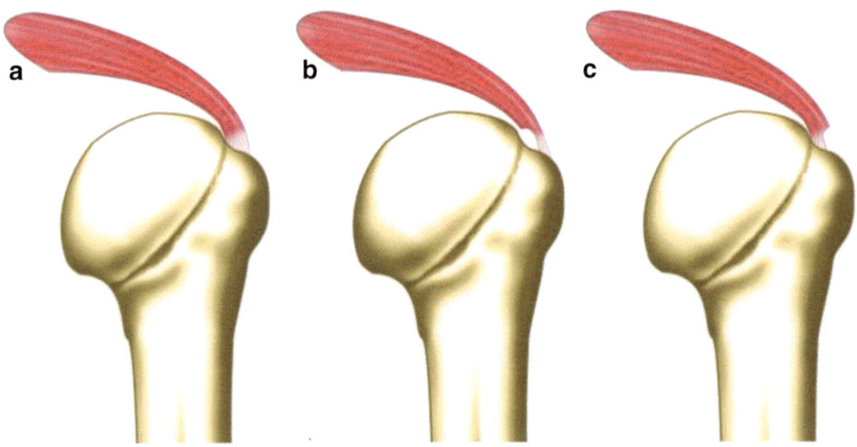

Intact (a) and torn (b) supraspinatus tendon, top view. A partial length but full thickness tear is demonstrated

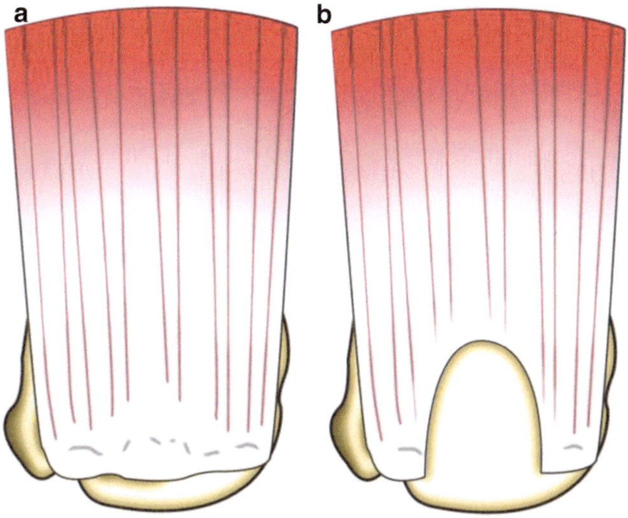

Teres major – originates from the lower part of the posterior surface of the scapula and passes laterally to attach to the medial lip of the bicipital groove. It is supplied by the lower subscapular nerve. On the anterior aspect of the humerus, the latissimus dorsi tendon overlies the teres major [18].

Shoulder muscles – anterior view

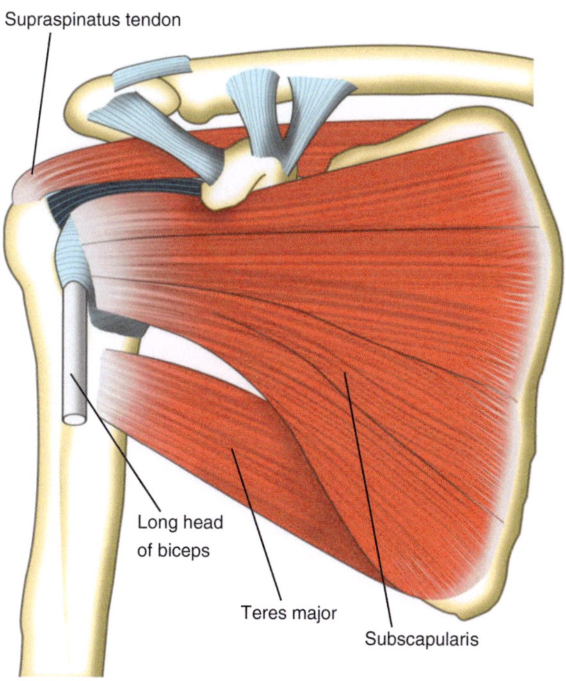

Shoulder muscles – posterior view

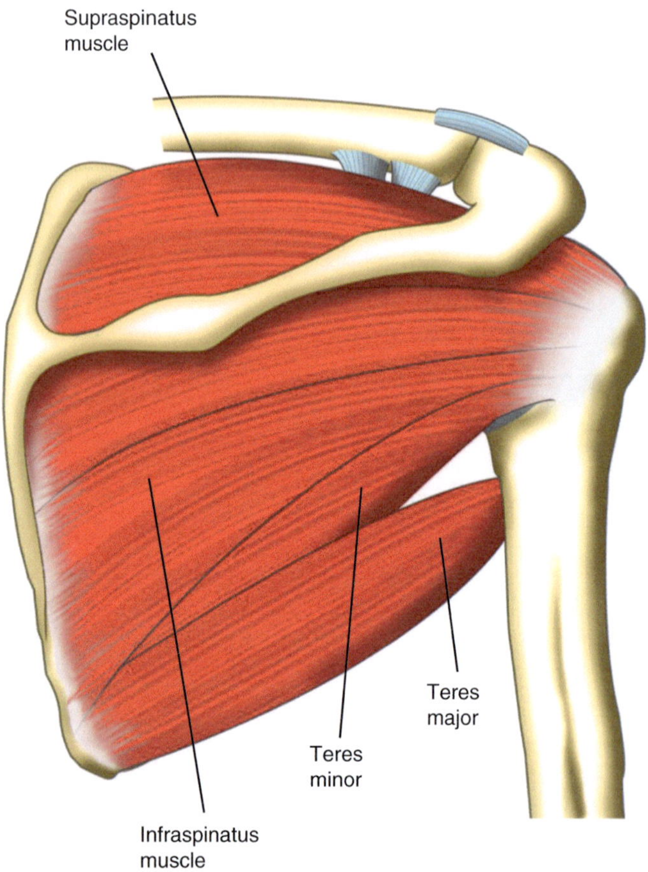

Biceps – this muscle has two muscular heads (the long head and short head) which at its distal end give rise to the distal biceps tendon that crosses in front of the elbow joint and inserts onto the radial tuberosity. At the top end, the long head of the biceps muscle attaches via a tendon to the superior labrum and the supraglenoid tubercle (a bony prominence on the superior aspect of the glenoid, located about 7 mm medial to the glenoid face) [19]. This long head of the biceps tendon runs in the bicipital groove where it is crossed by the transverse humeral ligament and the pectoralis major tendon. It is lined in a synovial sheath in the shoulder joint which continues to cover the tendon in the bicipital groove. The length of the long head of the biceps tendon is about 10 cm, whilst its diameter is 5–6 mm. Its intra-articular part tends to be wide and flat, whereas its extra-articular part is round and narrow [19]. The short head of the biceps muscle attaches to the coracoid process. This attachment is not via a true tubular tendon but instead through a combination of muscle fibres and a flattened tendinous aponeurosis [20].

Insertion of the long and short heads of biceps tendons

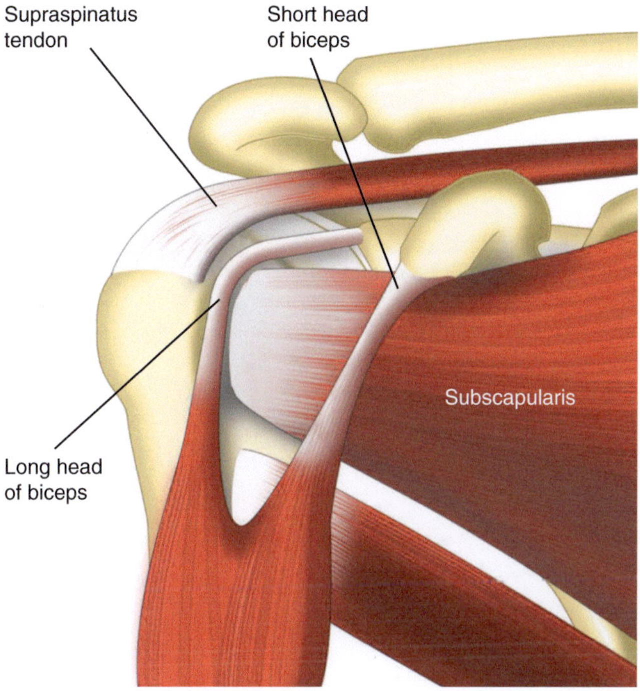

The biceps pulley or "sling" is a U-shaped ligamentous structure that acts to stabilise the long head of the biceps tendon in the bicipital groove. It is formed by fibres from the capsule of the glenohumeral joint, the coraco-humeral ligament, the superior glenohumeral ligament as well as the supraspinatus and subscapularis tendons. It is located within the rotator interval between the anterior edge of the supraspinatus tendon and the superior edge of the subscapularis tendon. Pulley lesions (tears) are associated with supraspinatus and subscapularis tears as well as superior labrum and long head of the biceps tendon tears [21–23]. Pulley tears may lead to instability of the long head of the biceps tendon, which displaces out of the bicipital groove.

Arthroscopic view of the long head of biceps inserting onto the superior labrum (a) and held in position by the biceps pulley (b–d)

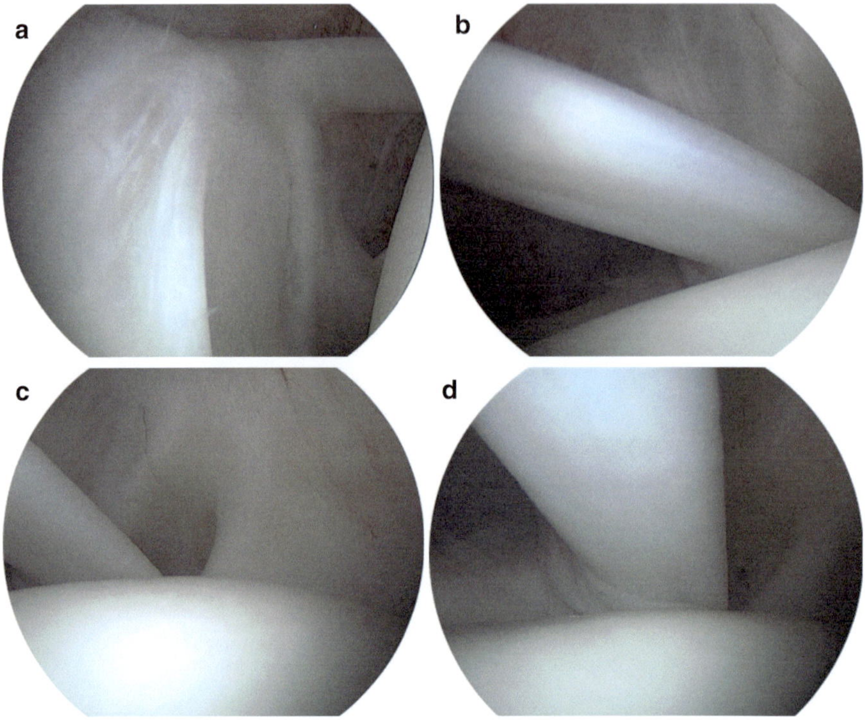

The bicipital tunnel is an extra-articular, fibro-osseous structure that encloses the long head of the biceps tendon. It is a closed space that has three zones [24]:

1. Zone 1 – passes from the articular margin of the humeral head to the distal margin of the subscapularis tendon
2. Zone 2 – passes from the distal margin of the subscapularis tendon to the proximal margin of the pectoralis major tendon
3. Zone 3 – the subpectoral region

Zones 1 and 2 are enclosed by a dense connective tissue sheath and are lined by synovium. Zone 3 is more capacious than zones 1 and 2; hence a bottleneck occurs between zones 2 and 3.

Triceps – located at the posterior aspect of the arm. It has three muscle heads:

- Long head – originates from the infra-glenoid tubercle of the scapula
- Lateral head – originates from the posterior surface of the humerus proximal to the spiral (radial) groove
- Medial head – originates from the posterior surface of the humerus distal to the spiral groove

Distally the three heads merge to give rise to a common tendon (the triceps tendon) that crosses the elbow joint and inserts onto the olecranon of the ulna. Dysfunction of the triceps may lead to weakness of elbow extension.

Coracobrachialis (a) and biceps (b) muscles

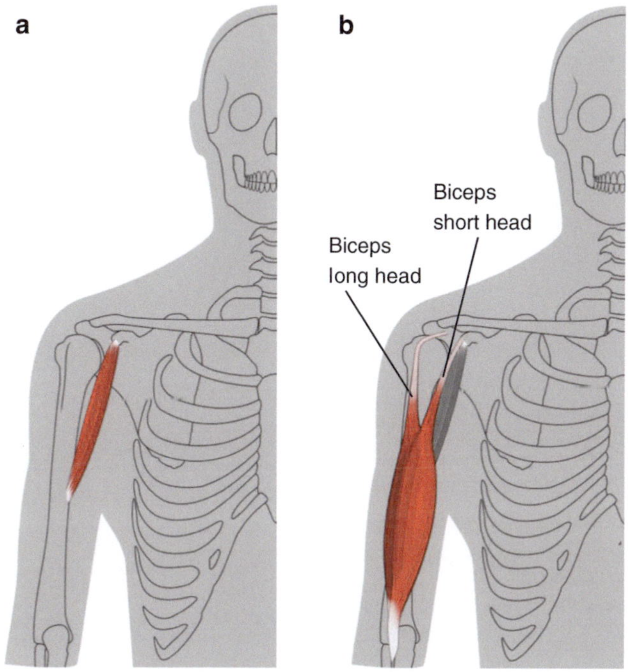

Serratus anterior (a) and pectoralis minor (b) muscles

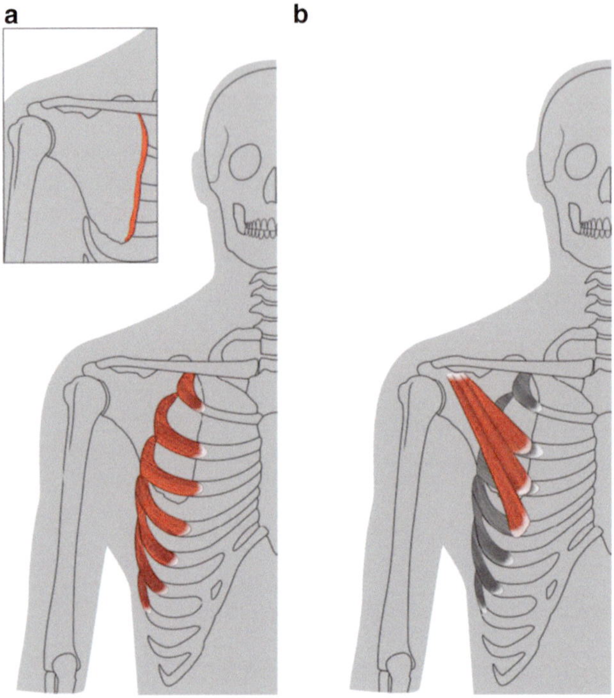

Pectoralis major (a) and deltoid (b) muscles

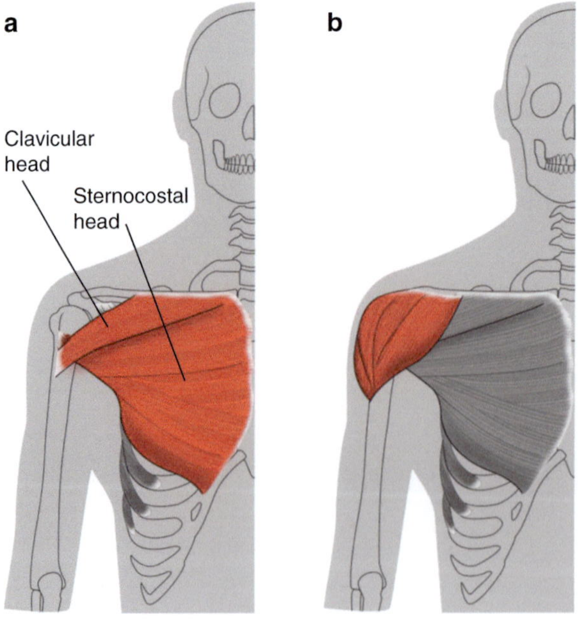

Latissimus dorsi (a), rhomboids and levator scapulae (b) muscles

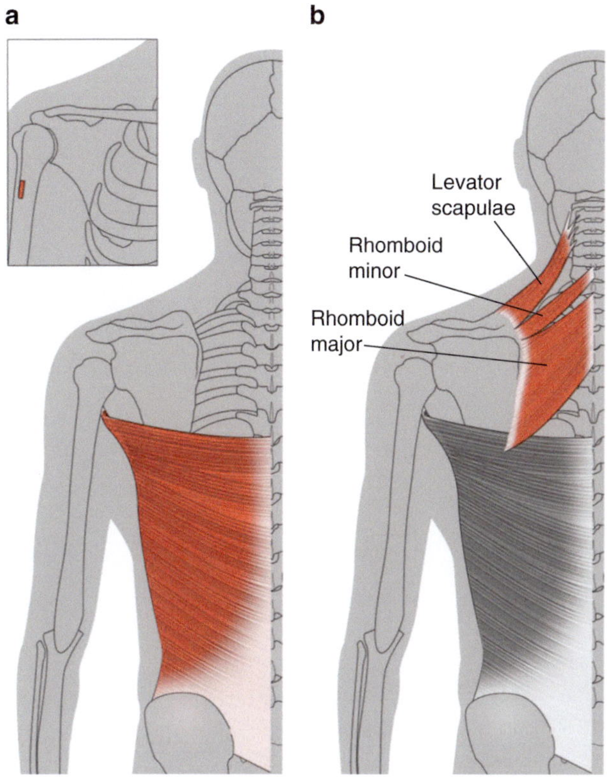

Trapezius, latissimus dorsi (a) and triceps (b) muscles

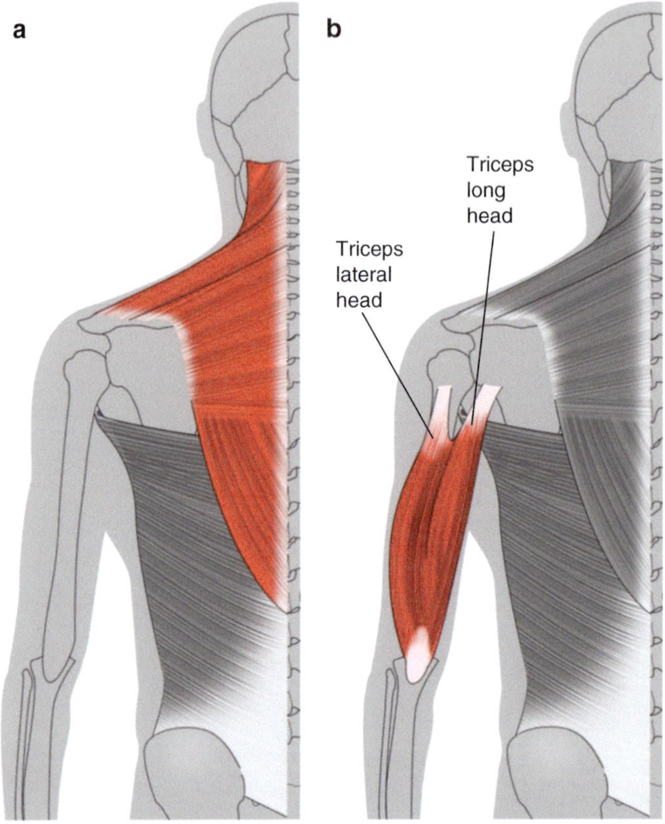

2.4.2 *Muscles Connecting the Trunk to the Scapula*

Trapezius – this is a large superficial muscle which lies on the posterior aspect of the neck and the superior part of the thorax. Its origin is extensive from the base of the skull and the cervical spinous processes and passes laterally to insert onto the spine of the scapula and the acromion. The trapezius is supplied by the accessory nerve which crosses the posterior triangle of the neck. Its dysfunction may lead to scapular winging.

Rhomboids – the rhomboids (minor and major) originate from the spinous processes of the lower cervical and upper thoracic vertebrae and attach to the medial border of the scapula. They are supplied by the dorsal scapular nerve which arises from the brachial plexus (C5). Their dysfunction may lead to scapular winging.

Serratus anterior – lies between the scapula and the rib cage. It originates from the upper eight ribs and attaches to the anterior medial border of the scapula. It is supplied by the long thoracic nerve. Its dysfunction may lead to scapular winging.

Pectoralis minor – originates from anterior aspect of the third to fifth ribs and inserts onto the medial pat of the coracoid process.

Deltoid – originates from the lateral third of the clavicle, the acromion and the spine of the scapula and attaches onto the deltoid tuberosity (found halfway down the lateral surface of the shaft of the humerus). It is supplied by the axillary nerve and is one of the main movers of the glenohumeral joint. Its dysfunction may lead to substantial shoulder weakness.

2.4.3 Muscles Connecting the Trunk to the Humerus

Pectoralis major – this is a large muscle located on the anterior part of the chest wall. It has two parts:

1. Clavicular head that originates from the anterior surface of the medial part of the clavicle
2. Sternocostal head that originates from the sternum and costal cartilage of ribs 2–7 as well as the aponeurosis of the external oblique muscle

The two muscular heads give rise to flat tendons that pass laterally to inert onto the anterior surface of the humerus just lateral to the bicipital groove. The tendon of the sternocostal head passes deep to the tendon of the clavicular head and inserts more proximally than the latter. It is supplied by the pectoral nerves. Injuries to the pectoralis major tendon often involve avulsion of the humeral insertion of its tendon.

Latissimus dorsi – this is a large muscle that overlies most of the posterior aspect of the trunk. It originates from the:

- Spinous processes of the thoracic vertebra T7–T12
- Inferior angle of the scapula
- Posterior part of the iliac crest
- 9–12th ribs
- Sacrum
- Thoracolumbar fascia and the fascia overlying the gluteus medius muscle

Its fibres come together to form a tendon which winds around the lower border of teres major to attach onto the medial edge of the bicipital groove of the humerus. It is supplied by the thoracodorsal nerve.

Front view of the shoulder demonstrating insertion of latissimus dorsi

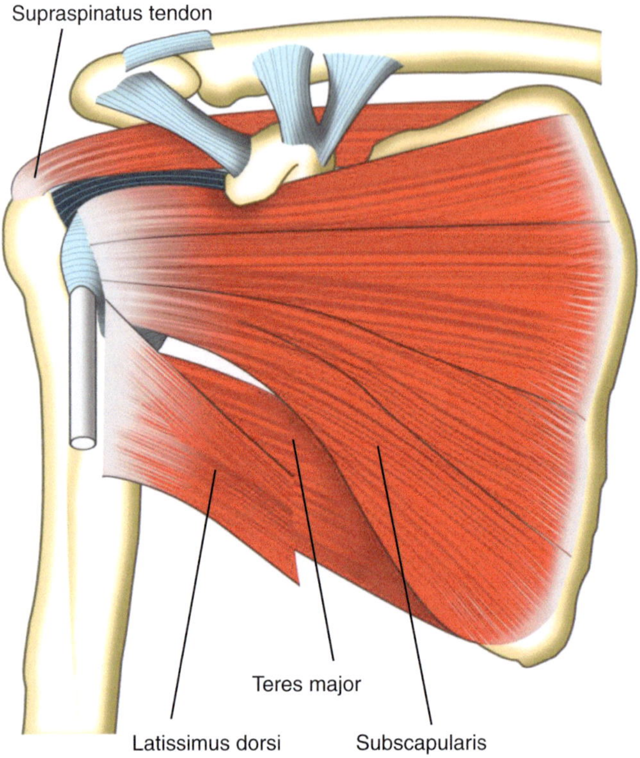

2.5 Rotator Interval

The rotator interval is a triangular-shaped area of the anterior part of the glenohumeral joint. It is located between the anterior-inferior border of the supraspinatus tendon and the superior border of the subscapularis tendon [25, 26]. It is well recognised during arthroscopic examination of the shoulder. Its contents include the:

- Coraco-humeral ligament
- Superior glenohumeral ligament
- Joint capsule
- Long head of the biceps tendon
- Biceps pulley

Inflammation and contraction of the rotator interval are seen in adhesive capsulitis.

Intact (a) and inflamed (b) rotator internal arthroscopic view

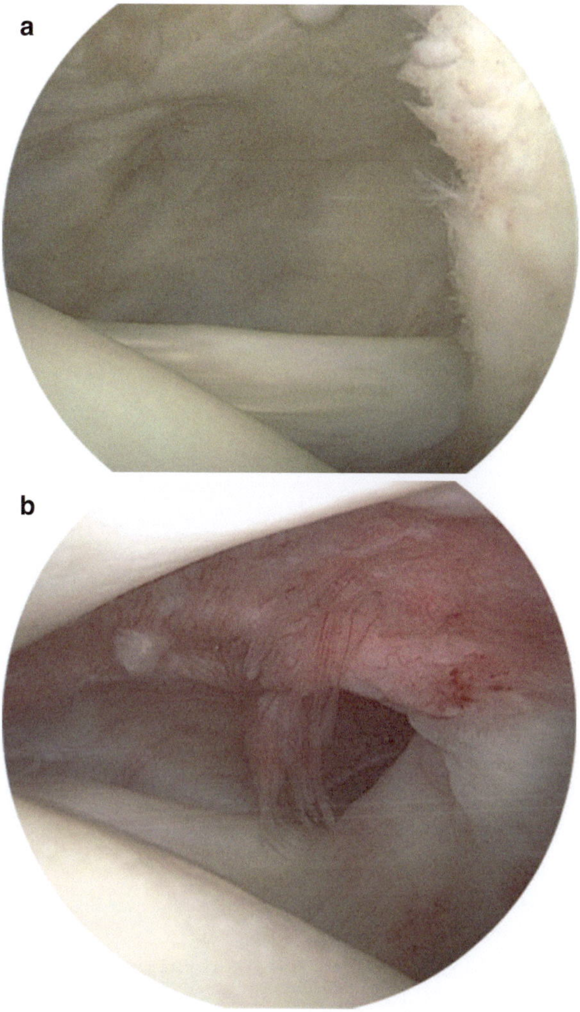

2.6 Bursae

Several bursae are found in the shoulder region. These are cyst-like synovial sacs that facilitate smooth motion between layers of soft tissue, improving gliding and reducing friction. They are found where motion is required between adjacent structures, such as between muscles, or between tendons and bony or ligamentous structures. Their clinical significance is that they may become inflamed or irritated causing pain. Some of the bursae encountered are [27–29] the:

- Subacromial bursa – located between the acromion and the coraco-acromial ligament superiorly, the supraspinatus tendon inferiorly and the deltoid muscle anteriorly and laterally. Inflammation of this bursa is one of the causes of subacromial pain syndrome

Subacromial bursa location – anterior view

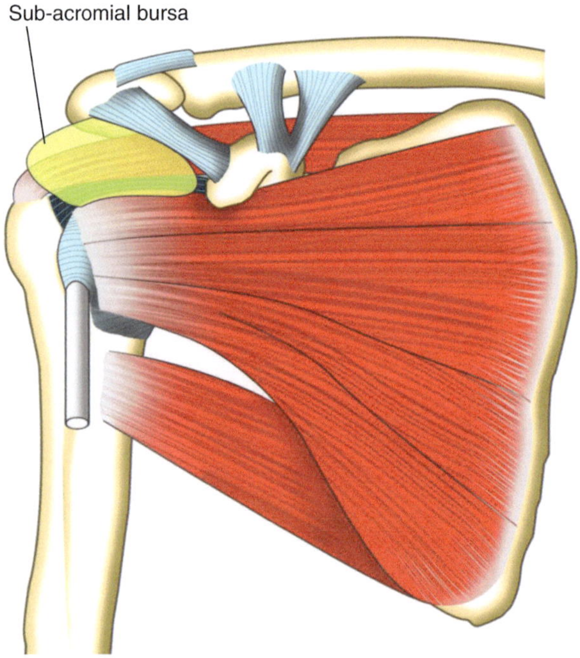

- Subscapular bursa – located between the subscapularis tendon and the neck of the scapula. It protects this tendon where it passes under the base of the coracoid process and over the neck of the scapula
- Infraserratus bursa – located anterior to the serratus anterior muscle, between the muscle and the chest wall
- Supraserratus bursa – located between the subscapularis muscle and the serratus anterior muscle
- Scapular minor bursae – several of these have been described but are not consistently present. These include bursae located at the:
  - Inferior angle of the scapula
  - Inferior medial border of the scapula deep or superficial to the serratus anterior
  - Deep to the trapezius muscle at the medial base of the spine of the scapula
  - Superior medial border of the scapula

Of the scapular bursae, those located along the superior medial border and the inferior angle of the scapula are the ones which are most commonly symptomatic.

2.7 Blood Supply

Consideration of the blood supply of the humeral head is important as its disruption may lead to bone necrosis. Similarly, consideration of the blood supply of the rotator cuff and long head of the biceps tendon is essential as areas of hypo-vascularity may predispose to tendon degeneration and rupture. The border of two adjacent vascular territories may provide an area of poor perfusion, known as a watershed area. Disruption of perfusion may be, amongst others, due to the ageing process and due to pathological conditions or may occur secondary to trauma or surgery.

The blood supply to the humeral head is provided by the:

- Anterolateral branch of the anterior humeral circumflex artery
- Posterior humeral circumflex artery

Arterial supply of the humeral head

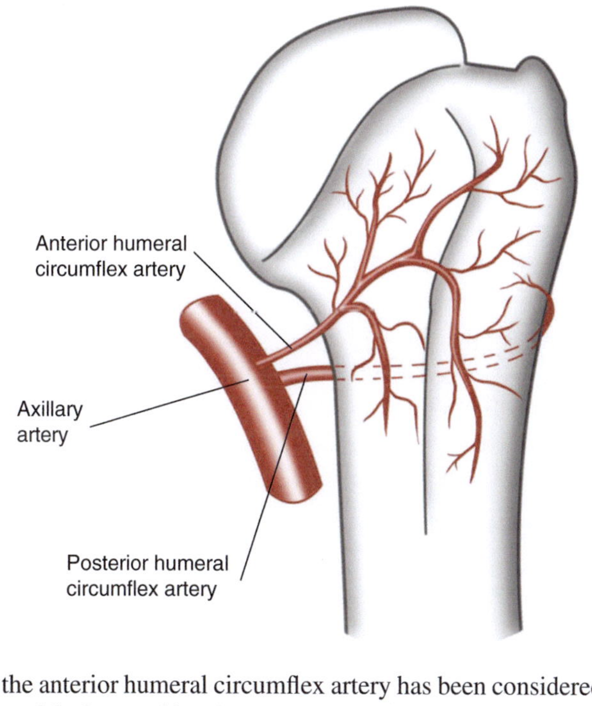

Although the anterior humeral circumflex artery has been considered as the main arterial supply of the humeral head, more recent evidence suggests that the posterior humeral circumflex artery has a more important role to play. It is estimated that the posterior humeral circumflex artery provides about 65% of the blood supply to the humeral head, whereas the anterior humeral circumflex artery supplies about 35% [30, 31].

The blood supply to the rotator cuff comes from multiple sites:

- Infraspinatus and teres minor – posterior humeral circumflex, suprascapular arteries
- Supraspinatus and subscapularis – thoraco-acromial, anterior humeral circumflex artery, subscapular arteries

Earlier studies have suggested that there may be a critical area of hypo-vascularity close to the edge of the supraspinatus tendon (involving its last 10–15 mm), but more recent studies have questioned this [32–35].

The blood supply of the long head of the biceps originates from the thoraco-acromial and brachial arteries. There may be a hypovascular area in the LHB tendon 1–3 cm from the proximal tendon attachment (extending from the glenohumeral joint to the top end of the bicipital groove), which may account for the susceptibility of this area to rupture [36].

2.8 Nerve Supply

The shoulder region has a rich nerve supply that comes from multiple nerves. Its innervation pattern is variable, and the territories of the involved nerves often overlap.

The upper limb and hence the shoulder are innervated by the third to eighth cervical spinal nerve roots (C3–C8) and the top two thoracic spinal roots (T1 and T2). The C3 to C8 and T1 nerve roots come together to form the brachial plexus, which gives rise to peripheral nerves that innervate the upper limb. The brachial plexus is located in the thoracic outlet that is described below.

Brachial plexus

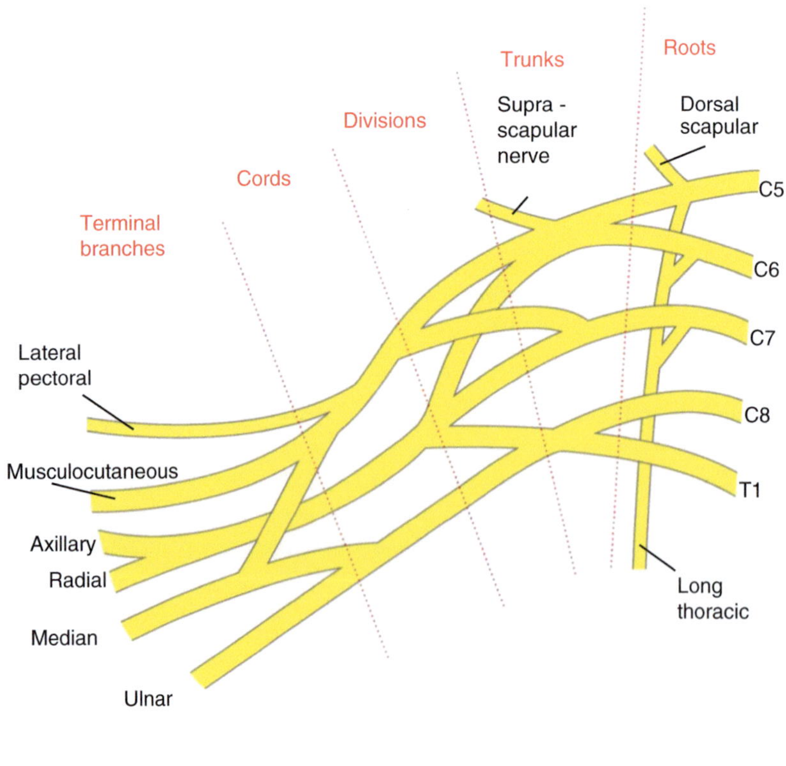

2.8.1 *Sensory Supply*

2.8.1.1 Cutaneous

Sensory supply may be described in terms of:

- Dermatomes – the part of the skin innervated mainly by a specific spinal nerve root
- Peripheral nerve sensory territory – the part of the skin supplied by a specific peripheral nerve that may have contributions from nerve fibres originating in multiple nerve roots

Dermatomal sensory innervation of the upper limb

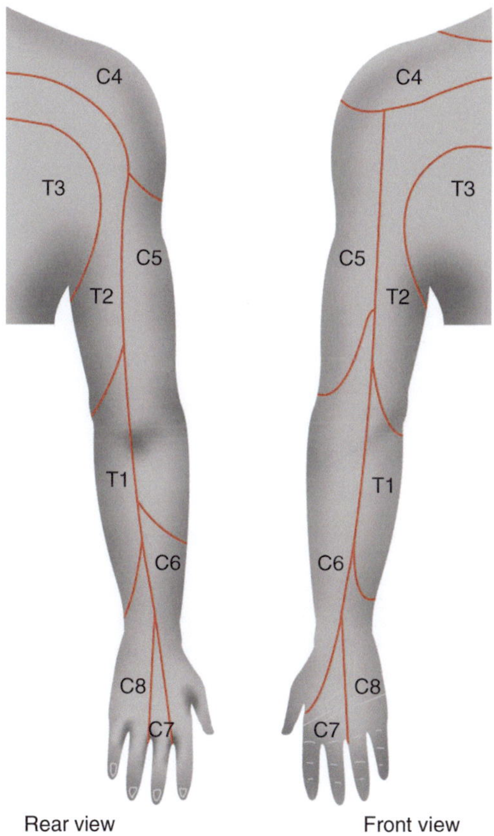

Distribution of peripheral sensory nerves of the upper limb

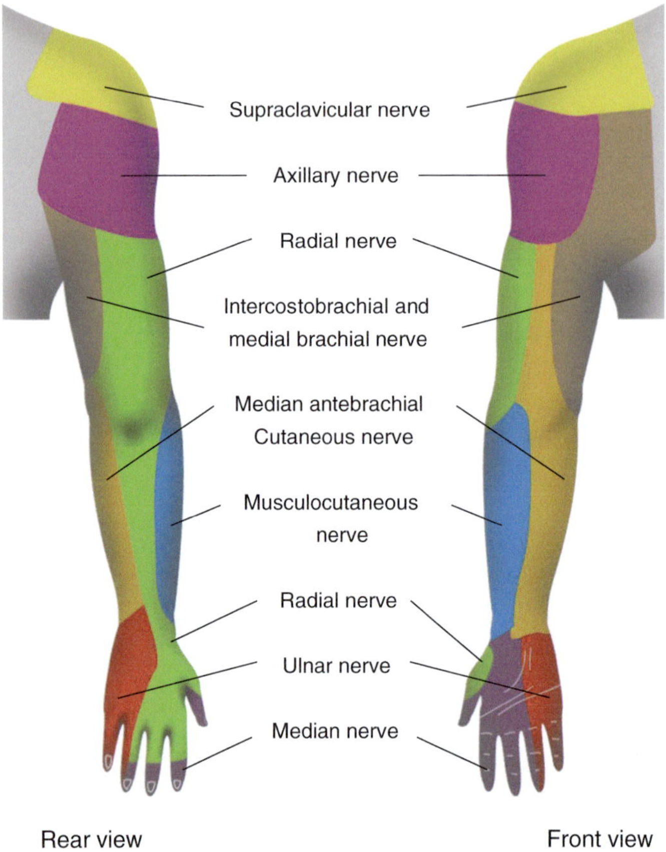

The main peripheral nerves involved in the cutaneous nerve supply of the shoulder are the:

- Supraclavicular nerves (C3 and C4) – anterior, posterior and superior part of the shoulder
- Posterior branch of the axillary nerve – lateral part of the shoulder

2.8.1.2 Deep Sensory

Extensive nerve supply of the ligaments, capsule and synovium is provided by the following nerves:

- Axillary
- Suprascapular
- Subscapular

- Musculocutaneous
- Long thoracic
- Dorsal scapular
- Spinal accessory

2.8.2 Motor Supply

Motor supply may be described in terms of:

- Myotomes – those muscles innervated primarily by a specific spinal nerve root
- Peripheral nerve motor territory – those muscles innervated by a specific peripheral nerve

Several peripheral nerves need special consideration as they supply important muscles around the shoulder area and their dysfunction may lead to specific shoulder symptoms.

2.8.3 Suprascapular Nerve

Arises from the brachial plexus and passes deep to the trapezius muscle to reach the suprascapular notch. It passes through the notch, under the transverse scapular ligament, and supplies supraspinatus. The suprascapular artery passes superficial to the ligament, whereas the suprascapular veins usually pass with the nerve under the ligament. The nerve then passes under the spino-glenoid ligament and supplies infraspinatus. The nerve may be trapped under the suprascapular or spino-glenoid ligaments or may be compressed by mass lesions such as paralabrum cysts.

The nerve gives sensory branches to the coraco-humeral and coraco-acromial ligaments and the glenohumeral joint. It may also have a cutaneous sensory branch supplying the posterior part of the shoulder, and hence patients with suprascapular palsy may complain of sensory disturbance around the shoulder. This sensory branch may split from the main nerve proximal, inferior or distal to the superior transverse scapular ligament. Due to this variable origin, the area of sensory disturbance may vary when the suprascapular nerve is trapped at the suprascapular notch [37–39].

Course of the suprascapular nerve and vessels

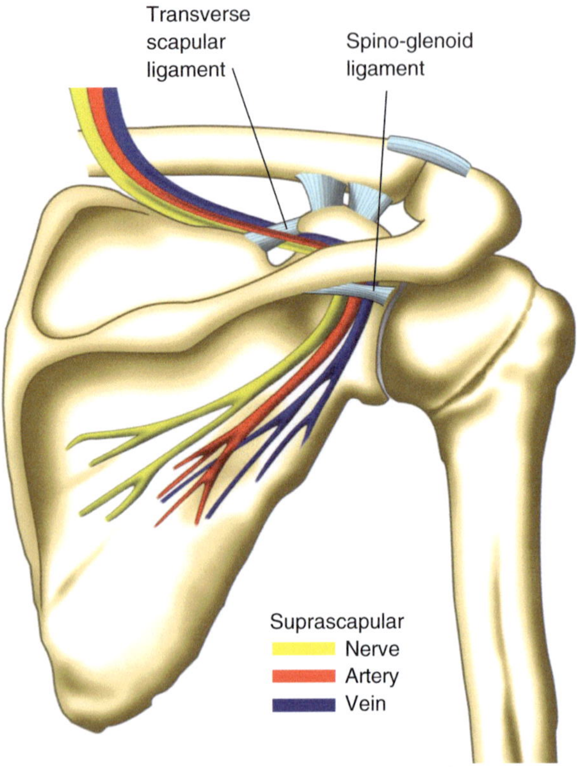

2.8.4 *Axillary Nerve*

Arises from the posterior cord of the brachial plexus and passes along the inferior border of subscapularis, through the quadrilateral space (an anatomical space bounded by the teres major inferiorly, the long head of the biceps medially, subscapularis superiorly and the surgical neck of humerus laterally) and curves round the surgical neck of the humerus and then anteriorly under the deltoid muscle. The axillary nerve is thus prone to injury by dislocations of the glenohumeral joint and by surgical approaches that involve mobilisation of subscapularis.

It divides into anterior and posterior branches, either in the quadrilateral space (90%) or under the deltoid muscle (10%). The anterior branch of the axillary nerve is accompanied by the posterior circumflex humeral artery.

The anterior part of the deltoid is supplied by the anterior branch of the axillary nerve, the posterior part of the deltoid mainly by the posterior branch and the middle part of the deltoid either by the anterior or a combination of both branches. Teres minor is supplied by the posterior branch of the axillary nerve.

The posterior branch gives rise to the superior-lateral brachial cutaneous nerve. This is the nerve tested as the regimental patch on the upper lateral part of the arm and gives an indication as to the integrity of the axillary nerve.

Course of the axillary nerve. The regimental batch area (R) is tested for sensation

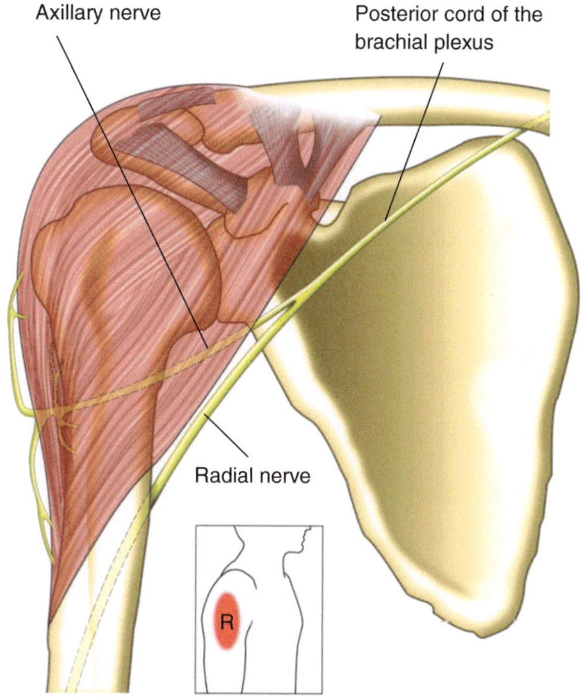

It is important to appreciate that the axillary nerve runs on the deep surface of the deltoid rather than being closely apposed to the humerus and hence vertical splitting of the deltoid during surgery without identification of the axillary nerve may cause nerve damage [40, 41].

2.8.5 *Subscapular Nerves*

Upper and lower subscapular nerves are described. They arise from the posterior division of the brachial plexus. They innervate subscapularis and teres major.

2.8.6 *Thoracodorsal Nerve*

Arises from the posterior cord of the brachial plexus and innervates latissimus dorsi.

2.8.7 Long Thoracic Nerve

Arises from the C5, C6 and C7 nerve roots and innervates serratus anterior.

2.8.8 Dorsal Scapular Nerve

Arises from C5 and innervates the rhomboid muscles.

2.8.9 Musculocutaneous Nerve

Arises from the lateral cord of the brachial plexus (C5,6,7). It innervates biceps and other muscles of the anterior part of the arm (coracobrachialis, brachialis) and may be damaged in Latarjet procedures either directly or due to extensive traction [42, 43].

2.8.10 Spinal Accessory Nerve

Arises from lower motor neurons in the upper part of the spinal cord to the C6 level, enters the skull through the foramen magnum and exits the skull through the jugular foramen. It crosses the internal jugular vein in the neck to reach sternocleidomastoid and trapezius which it innervates and may be damaged by surgery to the neck.

2.9 Thoracic Outlet

This is a canal-like space that extends from the cervical spine to the inferior border of the pectoralis minor muscle. It consists of three distinct components [44–46]:

- Inter-scalene triangle – located behind the sternocleidomastoid muscle in the lateral part of the neck and bounded by the:
  - Anterior scalene muscle anteriorly (which arises from the transverse processes of C3 to C6 cervical vertebrae to insert onto the superior surface of the first rib)
  - Middle scalene muscle posteriorly (which arises from the transverse processes of C2 to C7 cervical vertebrae to insert onto the superior surface of the first rib)
  - First rib inferiorly

- Costo-clavicular space – bounded by the:
  - Middle third of the clavicle anteriorly and subclavius muscle (which passes from the inferior surface of the clavicle to the first rib) medially
  - First rib and the insertions of the anterior and middle scalene muscles posterior-medially
  - Upper border of the scapula posterior-laterally
- Retro-pectoralis minor space bounded by the:
  - Coracoid process superiorly
  - Pectoralis minor muscle anteriorly
  - Rib cage posteriorly

Thoracic outlet

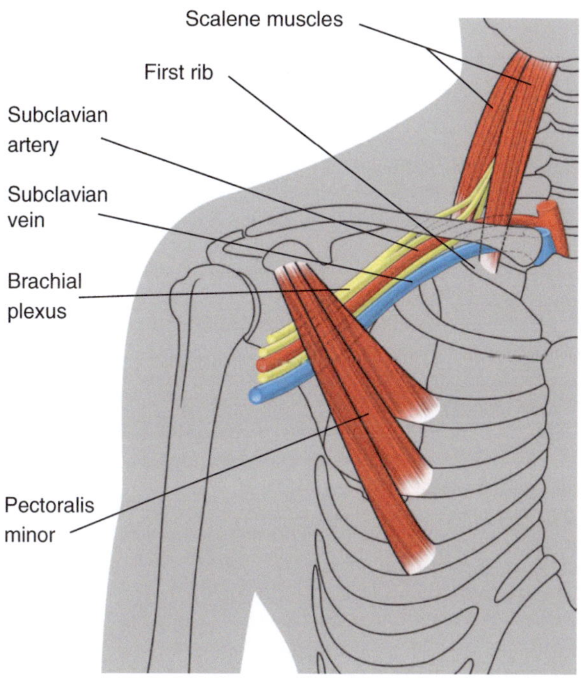

Contents of the thoracic outlet include the:

- C5 to T1 nerve roots and brachial plexus
- Subclavian artery
- Subclavian vein

The C5–C8 nerve roots, trunks of brachial plexus and the subclavian artery pass between the anterior and middle scalene muscles.

The subclavian vein passes anterior to the anterior scalene muscle.

The T1 nerve root arches upwards and joins the C8 nerve root prior to passing between the scalene muscles.

The inter-scalene triangle is the most common site for compression in true neurogenic thoracic outlet syndrome (TOS).

The lower trunk formed by T1 and C8 nerve roots has limited mobility, as it is tethered inferiorly by the T1 root. Hence, the lower trunk is most commonly involved in true TOS.

References

1. Culham E, Peat M. Functional anatomy of the shoulder complex. J Orthop Sports Phys Ther. 1993;18(1):342–50.
2. Terry GC, Chopp TM. Functional anatomy of the shoulder. J Athl Train. 2000;35(3):248–55.
3. Sinnatamby CS. FRCS Last's Anatomy: Regional and Applied. London: Churchill Livingstone Elsevier; 2011. p. 12e.
4. Dunham KS, Bencardino JT, Rokito AS. Anatomic variants and pitfalls of the labrum, glenoid cartilage, and glenohumeral ligaments. Magn Reson Imaging Clin N Am. 2012;20(2):213–28.
5. Nimura A, Kato A, Yamaguchi K, Mochizuki T, Okawa A, Sugaya H, Akita K. The superior capsule of the shoulder joint complements the insertion of the rotator cuff. J Shoulder Elb Surg. 2012;21(7):867–72.
6. Emura K, Arakawa T, Miki A, Terashima T. Anatomical observations of the human acromioclavicular joint. Clin Anat. 2014;27(7):1046–52.
7. van Tongel A, MacDonald P, Leiter J, Pouliart N, Peeler J. A cadaveric study of the structural anatomy of the sternoclavicular joint. Clin Anat. 2012;25(7):903–10.
8. Flatow EL. The biomechanics of the acromioclavicular, sternoclavicular, and scapulothoracic joints. Instr Course Lect. 1993;42:237–45.
9. Pouliart N, Gagey OJ. The arthroscopic view of the glenohumeral ligaments compared with anatomy: fold or fact? J Shoulder Elb Surg. 2005;14(3):324–8.
10. Polguj M, Jędrzejewski K, Podgórski M, Majos A, Topol M. A proposal for classification of the superior transverse scapular ligament: variable morphology and its potential influence on suprascapular nerve entrapment. J Shoulder Elb Surg. 2013;22(9):1265–73.
11. Won HJ, Won HS, Oh CS, Han SH, Chung IH, Yoon YC. Morphological study of the inferior transverse scapular ligament. Clin Anat. 2014;27(5):707–11.
12. Fukuda K, Craig EV, An KN, Cofield RH, Chao EY. Biomechanical study of the ligamentous system of the acromioclavicular joint. J Bone Joint Surg Am. 1986;68:434–40.
13. Klimkiewicz JJ, Williams GR, Sher JS, Karduna A, Des Jardins J, Iannotti JP. The acromioclavicular capsule as a restraint to posterior translation of the clavicle: a biomechanical analysis. J Shoulder Elb Surg. 1999;8:119–24.
14. Rockwood C, Williams GR, Young D. Disorders of the acromioclavicular joint. Rockwood Greens Fract Adults. 1996;2(Ed 4):1341–3.
15. Lee KW, Debski RE, Chen CH, Woo SL, Fu FH. Functional evaluation of the ligaments at the acromioclavicular joint during anteroposterior and superoinferior translation. Am J Sports Med. 1997;25:858–62.
16. Mochizuki T, Sugaya H, Uomizu M, Maeda K, Matsuki K, Sekiya I, Muneta T, Akita K. Humeral insertion of the supraspinatus and infraspinatus. New anatomical findings regarding the footprint of the rotator cuff. J Bone Joint Surg Am. 2008;90(5):962–9.
17. Richards DP, Burkhart SS, Tehrany AM, Wirth MA. The subscapularis footprint: an anatomic description of its insertion site. Arthroscopy. 2007;23(3):251–4.

18. Mochizuki T, Sugaya H, Uomizu M, Maeda K, Matsuki K, Sekiya I, Muneta T, Akita K. Humeral insertion of the supraspinatus and infraspinatus. New anatomical findings regarding the footprint of the rotator cuff. J Bone Joint Surg Am. 2008;90(5):962–9.
19. Denard PJ, Dai X, Hanypsiak BT, Burkhart SS. Anatomy of the biceps tendon: implications for restoring physiological length-tension relation during biceps tenodesis with interference screw fixation. Arthroscopy. 2012;28(10):1352–8.
20. Crichton JC, Funk L. The anatomy of the short head of biceps - not a tendon. Int J Shoulder Surg. 2009;3(4):75–9.
21. Nakata W, Katou S, Fujita A, Nakata M, Lefor AT, Sugimoto H. Biceps pulley: normal anatomy and associated lesions at MR arthrography. Radiographics. 2011;31(3):791–810.
22. Werner A, Mueller T, Boehm D, Gohlke F. The stabilizing sling for the long head of the biceps tendon in the rotator cuff interval: a histoanatomic study. Am J Sports Med. 2000;28(1):28–31.
23. Braun S, Horan MP, Elser F, Millett PJ. Lesions of the biceps pulley. Am J Sports Med. 2011;39(4):790–5.
24. Taylor SA, Fabricant PD, Bansal M, Khair MM, McLawhorn A, DiCarlo EF, Shorey M, O'Brien SJ. The anatomy and histology of the bicipital tunnel of the shoulder. J Shoulder Elb Surg. 2015;24(4):511–9.
25. Wilson WR, Magnussen RA, Irribarra LA, Taylor DC. Variability of the capsular anatomy in the rotator interval region of the shoulder. J Shoulder Elb Surg. 2013;22(6):856–61.
26. Hunt SA, Kwon YW, Zuckerman JD. The rotator interval: anatomy, pathology, and strategies for treatment. J Am Acad Orthop Surg. 2007;15(4):218–27.
27. Kennedy MS, Nicholson HD, Woodley SJ. Clinical anatomy of the subacromial and related shoulder bursae: A review of the literature. Clin Anat. 2017;30(2):213–26.
28. Merolla G, Cerciello S, Paladini P, Porcellini G. Snapping scapula syndrome: current concepts review in conservative and surgical treatment. Muscles Ligaments Tendons J. 2013;3(2):80–90.
29. Gaskill T, Millett PJ. Snapping scapula syndrome: diagnosis and management. J Am Acad Orthop Surg. 2013;21(4):214–24.
30. Gerber C, Schneeberger AG, Vinh TS. The arterial vascularization of the humeral head. An anatomical study. J Bone Joint Surg Am. 1990;72(10):1486–94
31. Hettrich CM, Boraiah S, Dyke JP, Neviaser A, Helfet DL, Lorich DG. Quantitative assessment of the vascularity of the proximal part of the humerus. J Bone Joint Surg Am. 2010;92(4):943–8.
32. Brooks CH, Revell WJ, Heatley FW. A quantitative histological study of the vascularity of the rotator cuff tendon. J Bone Joint Surg Br. 1992;74(1):151–3.
33. Ling SC, Chen CF, Wan RX. A study on the vascular supply of the supraspinatus tendon. Surg Radiol Anat. 1990;12(3):161–5.
34. Lohr JF, Uhthoff HK. The microvascular pattern of the supraspinatus tendon. Clin Orthop Relat Res. 1990;254:35–8.
35. Hegedus EJ, Cook C, Brennan M, Wyland D, Garrison JC, Driesner D. Vascularity and tendon pathology in the rotator cuff: a review of literature and implications for rehabilitation and surgery. Br J Sports Med. 2010;44(12):838–47.
36. Cheng NM, Pan WR, Vally F, Le Roux CM, Richardson MD. The arterial supply of the long head of biceps tendon: Anatomical study with implications for tendon rupture. Clin Anat. 2010;23(6):683–92.
37. Vorster W, Lange CP, Briët RJ, Labuschagne BC, du Toit DF, Muller CJ, de Beer JF. The sensory branch distribution of the suprascapular nerve: an anatomic study. J Shoulder Elb Surg. 2008;17(3):500–2.
38. Polguj M, Rożniecki J, Sibiński M, Grzegorzewski A, Majos A, Topol M. The variable morphology of suprascapular nerve and vessels at suprascapular notch: a proposal for classification and its potential clinical implications. Knee Surg Sports Traumatol Arthrosc. 2015;23(5):1542–8.
39. Oizumi N, Suenaga N, Funakoshi T, Yamaguchi H, Minami A. Recovery of sensory disturbance after arthroscopic decompression of the suprascapular nerve. J Shoulder Elb Surg. 2012;21(6):759–64.

40. Gurushantappa PK, Kuppasad S. Anatomy of axillary nerve and its clinical importance: a cadaveric study. J Clin Diagn Res. 2015;9(3):AC13–7.
41. Traver JL, Guzman MA, Cannada LK, Kaar SG. Is the axillary nerve at risk during a deltoid-splitting approach for proximal humerus fractures? J Orthop Trauma. 2016;30(5):240–4.
42. Southam JD, Greis PE. Delayed, transient musculocutaneous nerve palsy after the Latarjet procedure. J Shoulder Elb Surg. 2012;21(5):e8–11. https://doi.org/10.1016/j.jse.2011.09.025.
43. Shah AA, Butler RB, Romanowski J, Goel D, Karadagli D, Warner JJ. Short-term complications of the Latarjet procedure. J Bone Joint Surg Am. 2012;94(6):495–501.
44. Ferrante MA, Ferrante ND. The thoracic outlet syndromes: part 1. Overview of the thoracic outlet syndromes and review of true neurogenic thoracic outlet syndrome. Muscle Nerve. 2017;55(6):782–93.
45. Ferrante MA, Ferrante ND. The thoracic outlet syndromes: Part 2. The arterial, venous, neurovascular, and disputed thoracic outlet syndromes. Muscle Nerve. 2017;56(4):663–73.
46. Klaassen Z, Sorenson E, Tubbs RS, Arya R, Meloy P, Shah R, Shirk S, Loukas M. Thoracic outlet syndrome: a neurological and vascular disorder. Clin Anat. 2014;27(5):724–32.

Chapter 3
Shoulder Biomechanics

This chapter describes the direction and components of shoulder motion as well as the muscles acting upon the shoulder to achieve that motion. In addition, it explores the forces acting on the shoulder joint with particular reference to the muscle force couples that exist across the glenohumeral and scapulo-thoracic joints. Furthermore, it describes the various structures contributing to stability of the glenohumeral, sterno-clavicular and acromio-clavicular joints.

3.1 Shoulder Movement

The shoulder shows a large amount of movement in multiple planes. Its main function is to position the upper limb and thus the hand, in space for efficient function. Most upper extremity functions are performed with the hand placed in front of the body rather than on the side; hence, the shoulder is put more frequently in forward elevation rather than lateral elevation (abduction).

Motion of the shoulder is a combination of individual movements occurring at the following articulations:

- Glenohumeral
- Scapulo-thoracic
- Sterno-clavicular
- Acromio-clavicular (ACJt)

© Springer Nature Switzerland AG 2019

C. Panayiotou Charalambous, *The Shoulder Made Easy*,
https://doi.org/10.1007/978-3-319-98908-2_3

3.1.1 Glenohumeral Joint Movements

The humeral head rolls, slides and rotates on the glenoid allowing [1, 2]:

- Flexion-extension
- Abduction-adduction
- Internal-external rotation
- Circumduction

3.1.2 Scapular Movements

The scapulo-thoracic articulation is not a true joint. Instead, this articulation refers to the contact of the concave anterior surface of the scapula on the convex postero-lateral part of the thoracic wall. The anterior surface of the scapula is covered by subscapularis and the corresponding part of the chest wall by serratus anterior, which glide over each other during scapular movements.

The scapula exhibits the following movements [3, 4]:

- Upwards and downwards rotation:
  - Upwards – glenoid facing upwards
  - Downwards – glenoid facing downwards
- Upwards and downwards translation (elevation-depression) – this is equivalent to shrugging up the shoulders and returning them to the resting position
- Medial and lateral translation following the curvature of the chest wall:
  - Protraction – medial border of the scapula moves away from the vertebral column (as in crossing the arms forwards)
  - Retraction – medial border of the scapula moves towards the vertebral column (as in pulling scapulae towards each other)
- Anterior and posterior tilt:
  - Anterior tilt – medial border of the scapula moves anteriorly (closer to the chest wall)
  - Posterior tilt – medial border of the scapula moves posteriorly (away from the chest wall)

Direction of possible scapular movements: (a) upwards/downwards, (b) medial/lateral, (c, d) anterior/posterior

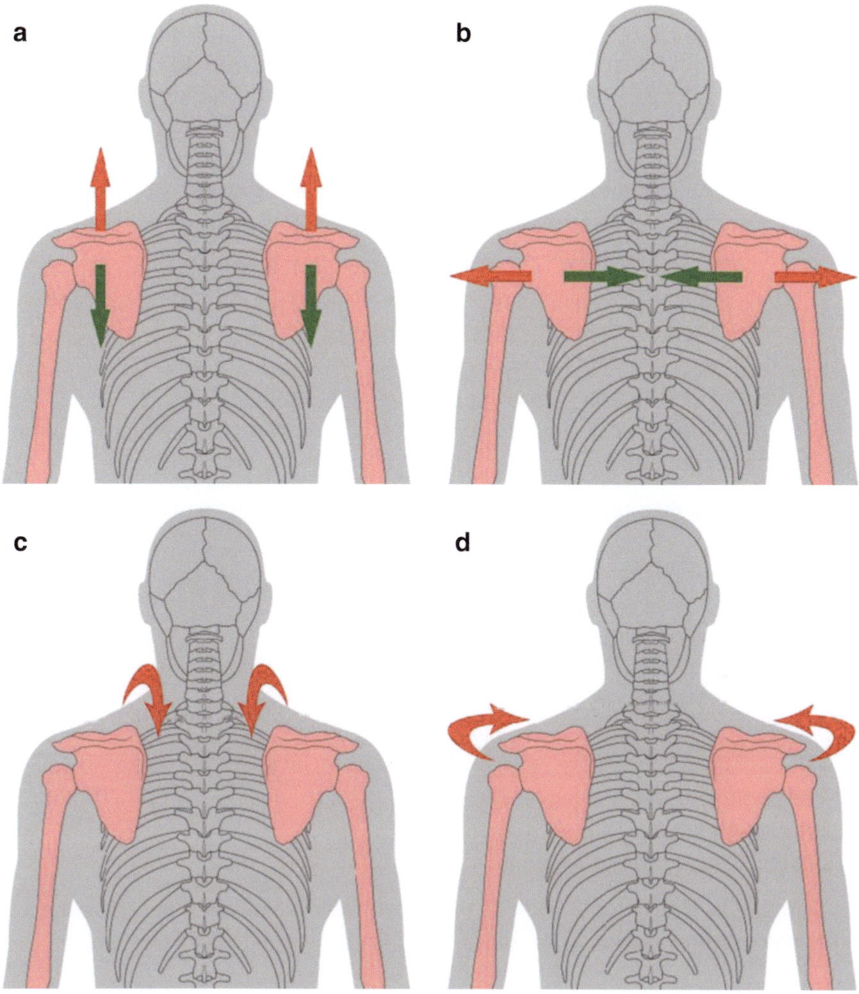

There is controversy as to the relation between the scapulo-thoracic and glenohumeral movements during forward elevation or abduction of the arm. Two of the various patterns of scapular movements that have been proposed are the following [5]:

1. In up to 90° of arm forward elevation or abduction, motion occurs at the glenohumeral joint with further elevation occurring by rotation of the scapula at the scapulo-thoracic articulation
2. The first 30–60° of arm elevation occur at the glenohumeral joint, during which the scapula remains fixed or moves side to side on the chest wall (setting phase). Further shoulder movement occurs at a ratio of 2:1 of glenohumeral to scapulothoracic motion (i.e. for every 30° of forward elevation or abduction, 20° occurs at the glenohumeral and 10° at the scapulo-thoracic articulation)

It is of note that variable patterns of scapular rhythm have been described in addition to the above [6, 7]. Furthermore, although patterns of combinations of glenohumeral and scapula-thoracic movements may be recognised, it is appreciated that the exact combination may vary amongst individuals. Hence, when evaluating unilateral shoulder disease, comparing the affected side with the opposite side in a particular individual is preferable, rather than simply comparing to a predetermined "norm".

Motion of the scapula has several functions [8]:

1. It contributes to shoulder movement through its rotation on the chest wall, allowing greater range of motion than what is possible solely at the glenohumeral joint
2. By rotating in coordination with the humeral head it:
   - Stops the humeral head impinging on the undersurface of the acromion during abduction or forward elevation of the arm
   - Allows the glenoid to follow and keep facing the humeral head throughout the range of arm motion improving glenohumeral stability
   - Avoids kinking or twisting of the rotator cuff muscles and tendons facilitating optimum function

Movement of the scapula requires motion at the sterno-clavicular joint and ACJt [8–10].

3.1.3 Sterno-Clavicular Joint Movements

Motion at the sterno-clavicular joint is described in terms of the clavicle in relation to the sternum. These are:

- Elevation/depression about an anterior-posterior axis – about 35° of elevation
- Protraction/retraction about a vertical axis
- Anterior/posterior rotation about a horizontal axis – about 50° of rotation

During arm abduction or forward elevation, there is increased elevation, retraction and posterior rotation of the clavicle at the sterno-clavicular joint.

3.1.4 ACJt Movements

Motion at the ACJt joint is described in terms of the scapula in relation to the clavicle. It has been shown that during arm abduction in the scapular plane, the following movements occur at the ACjoint:

- Upwards rotation – about 15° about an axis perpendicular to the scapular plane
- Internal rotation – about 4° about a vertical axis
- Posterior tilting – about 7° about an axis directed from medial to lateral direction

3.2 Range of Motion at the Shoulder

Range of motion may be described as the theoretically possible range of motion that can occur in a particular direction (anatomic range of motion) [11]:

- Forward elevation – about 170°
- Extension – about 60°
- Abduction – about 180°
- External rotation with arm abducted at 90° – about 100°

However, it is important to recognise that in real life a great variation may exist in the amount of motion that can be achieved between individuals with healthy shoulders, due to anatomical and other factors. Hence, comparing a diseased shoulder with the opposite healthy shoulder of the same individual may provide more meaningful information, rather than simply comparing it to the general population.

Range of motion may also be described in terms of functional range of motion. This is defined as the minimum range of motion necessary to perform activities of daily living in a comfortable and effective fashion, and it often much less than the anatomic range of motion [12]:

- Forward elevation – about 120°
- Extension – about 45°
- Abduction – about 130°
- External rotation with arm abducted – about 60°
- Internal rotation – about 100°

Hence, although attaining full motion is a reasonable goal of shoulder interventions, it should be recognised that a smaller range of motion is required to perform many of the daily activities of life and achieve efficient function. It should be remembered, however, that the functional range will depend on the individual with their specific circumstances and functional demands. Certain individuals may need much greater levels of mobility than the average "norm" due to occupational or recreational (sports) reasons.

3.3 Muscles Bringing About Motion

Muscles attach via their tendons to bones. Upon contraction, they exert forces in a direction influenced by the site of muscle origin, muscle fibre orientation and site of tendon insertion. Through contraction a muscle may:

- Move a body segment in line with the direction of its pull:
  - In arm elevation, the supraspinatus contracts, rotating the humeral head upwards and pulling it medially

- Slow down a body segment motion occurring in a direction opposite to its pull:
  - In bringing the arm down from an elevated position, supraspinatus contracts opposing the effect of gravity and preventing an uncontrolled arm drop
- Oppose a muscle acting in an opposite direction and hence stabilise a body segment in a particular position
- Stabilise a body segment so that it rotates rather than translates under the action of another muscle. This is equivalent to a force acting on a wheel. If the force is unopposed, it will cause the wheel to rotate but also translate in the direction of the applied force. However, if an opposite force is applied to the wheel at the same time, it can stabilise the wheel so that it simply rotates rather than translate. This force may be applied in an opposite direction to the distracting force, causing the wheel to translate, or in any other direction (such as perpendicular to the distracting force)

A force applied to a wheel may rotate and displace the wheel (a). An opposing force applied at opposite (b) or other directions (c) may limit displacement allowing the wheel to spin in place

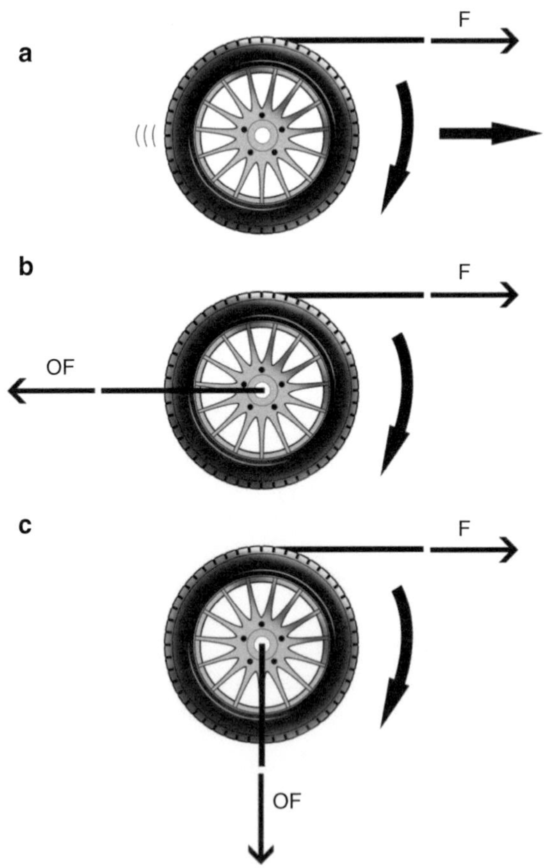

By recognising the anatomic origin and insertion of muscles, and the joints across which they act, one may thus determine the movement they can achieve upon contraction. This can form the basis of assessing strength of these muscles and formulating a diagnosis when shoulder motion or shoulder stability is impaired.

In considering shoulder motion, it is important to appreciate that although a muscle may be described as having a major function:

- Different parts of the muscle may have different effects with regard to moving or stabilising a body segment (such as the anterior vs. middle vs. posterior deltoid, upper trapezius vs. lower trapezius)
- A muscle can exert different effects depending on arm position (deltoid may act as both an internal rotator and external rotator of the glenohumeral joint with the exact effect influenced by the degree of humeral abduction and rotation) [13, 14]

The above may help explain at least partly:

- The variability that may be observed in the detrimental effect of tendon tears between individuals
- The variability in strength improvement achieved by exercises targeting specific muscles between individuals

3.4 Muscles Controlling Glenohumeral Joint Motion

Several muscles bring about motion at the glenohumeral joint [15–17] as below:

- Forward elevation: deltoid (anterior part), pectoralis major, biceps, coracobrachialis
- Abduction: deltoid (middle part), supraspinatus
- External rotation: infraspinatus, teres minor, deltoid (posterior part)
- Internal rotation: subscapularis, pectoralis major, latissimus dorsi, deltoid
- Adduction: pectoralis major, latissimus dorsi, teres major, teres minor
- Extension: deltoid (posterior part), latissimus dorsi, teres major

3.5 Initiation of Shoulder Abduction

It is commonly stated that supraspinatus initiates abduction. However, this has not been consistently demonstrated in electromyography studies. Instead, both supraspinatus and deltoid have been shown to have similar activation times during shoulder abduction in the coronal and scapular planes suggesting an equal role of both muscles in achieving this action [18–22].

3.6 Muscles Controlling Scapular Motion

Scapular motion is very complex. However, in a simplified version, one may consider the effect of muscles inserted onto the scapula. Their effect may be worked out if the exact attachment of these muscles, as described in the anatomy chapter, is considered.

All muscles that connect the scapula to the axial skeleton (except the upper part of trapezius and pectoralis minor muscles) are inserted near or on the medial border of the scapula. These muscles include serratus anterior, levator scapulae muscle, rhomboids and the lower part of trapezius [15–17]. Given their origin and attachment, their effect is demonstrable:

- Elevation: upper part of trapezius, rhomboids
- Retraction: upper part of trapezius, rhomboids
- Protraction: serratus anterior
- Upwards rotation: upper part of trapezius, serratus anterior
- Downwards rotation: lower part of trapezius, rhomboids

Hence, the effect of dysfunction of any one of the above muscles is often predictable.

3.7 Forces Transmitted by the Shoulder

The shoulder is often described as a non-weight bearing joint, unlike the hip and knee which are weight bearing. However, this is a misconception as huge amounts of forces may be transmitted through the glenohumeral joint.

The forces transmitted across a joint are the result of [23–25]:

- Transmitted weight – weight of the arm and weight carried by the arm
- Forces generated by the surrounding muscles which contract in order to maintain position of the limb in space and also achieve joint stability
- Friction force between the articular surfaces
- Compressive (exerted by the rotator cuff) and shear forces (exerted by the anterior and middle deltoid) operating at the glenohumeral joint

Analysis of the forces acting on the glenohumeral joint [23] has suggested that:

- The weight of the arm is about 5% of the body weight
- At 90° of arm abduction, the resultant force acting at the glenohumeral joint could be as high as 0.9 times the total body weight
- Holding a 1 kg weight in the hand may increase the resultant force by up to 60%

Hence, huge forces are transmitted through the glenohumeral joint during normal activities [23–25].

3.8 Shoulder Instability

Instability of a joint describes an abnormal translation of one articular surface in relation to the other. This can vary from dislocation where there is complete loss of contact between the articular surfaces, to subluxation where some contact between the articular surfaces is maintained.

Instability must be distinguished from laxity. In instability, the patient has symptoms, related to the abnormal translation between the articular surfaces. In contrast, laxity refers to abnormal translation evident on examination (usually by the application of a force by the examiner) but which is not symptomatic.

3.8.1 Joint Stability

In considering stability of a joint, one may look at static and dynamic stabilisers [25–40].

Static stabilisers: Those factors that are constant in shape and size and parameters that cannot be altered according to the need of stability. These include:

- Shape of the articular surfaces
  - Conforming surfaces – ball in a cup
  - Nonconforming surfaces – flat on flat surface, ball on a flat surface
- Negative intra-articular pressure providing a suction force of one articular surface on the other
- Ligaments

Ligaments are fibrous structures that connect two bones. Ligaments are static stabilisers as they cannot actively change their shape or size to limit motion. Instead, when a force is applied, all they can do is stretch from a resting lax state to a taut state. Ligaments may provide stability in two ways:

1. Check-rein effect – the ligament allows motion between two bones in a direction along the line of the ligament, until it stretches to its maximum length at which no further movement is allowed
2. Buttress effect – the ligament acts like a fence, limiting motion in a direction perpendicular to the ligament

The mode in which a ligament exerts its effect may be influenced by the way in which a ligament is applied (its origin and insertion). These functions may be explained by the analogy of the rope used to anchor a boat onto the dock cleat:

- A rope passing from the cleat to the boat will allow some movement up to the point it becomes taut. However, such a rope may not stop the boat from moving sideways at an angle and colliding with neighbour boats!
- A rope passing on either side of the boat and also round its back may stop it from drifting into the open sea but in addition limit the extent to which it can slide side to side

A rope (like a ligament) (a) becomes taut once stretched out to length (b)

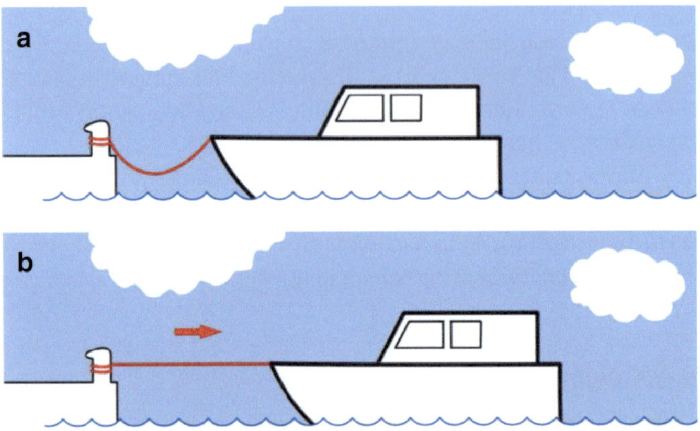

A rope (like a ligament) passing from the cleat to the boat (a) may provide a check-rein effect but no buttress effect depending on its insertion (b, c)

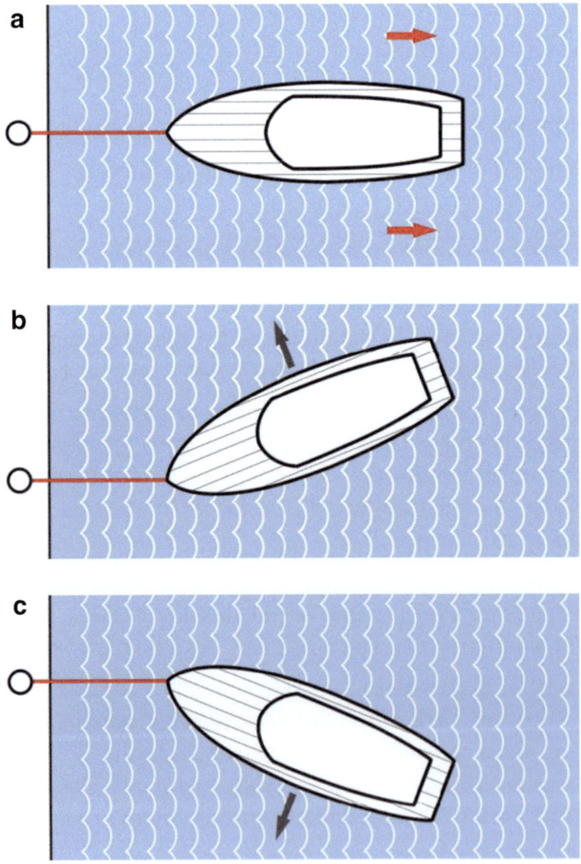

A rope (like a ligament) may provide a buttress effect in addition to check-rein effect depending on its insertion (a, b)

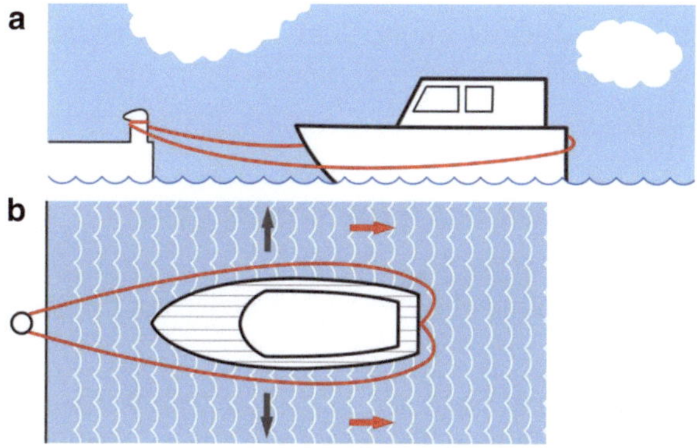

Dynamic stabilisers: Those factors that can alter the force they exert across a joint as the situation demands. This refers to muscles acting across a joint in order to:

1. Compress the articular surfaces together
2. Oppose a distracting force

Muscles can contract adjusting the force applied to bones, hence adjusting joint stability as a situation dictates. This may be likened to a person pulling on the rope, anchoring the boat (controlling how lax or taut the rope is).

Unlike ligaments which are static, muscles can adjust the force applied and hence provide dynamic stability, equivalent to modifying the pull on a rope (a, b)

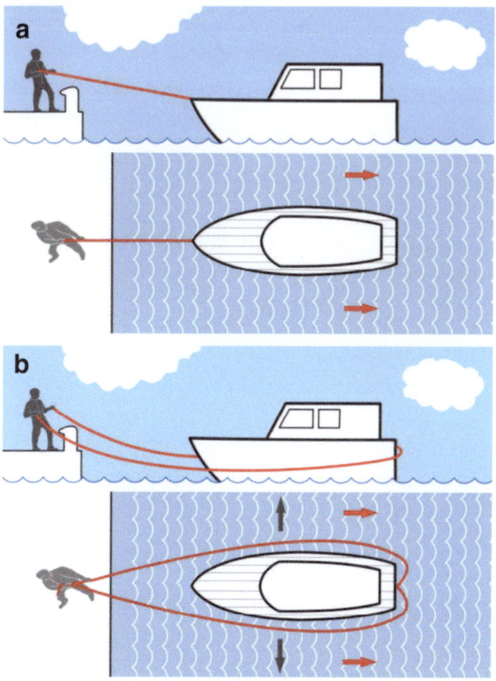

Muscles are considered the main stabilisers of joints. This would explain why joints whose main ligaments are torn can continue to be stable allowing return to normal activities. In addition, by strengthening certain muscles, a greater stabilising force may be exerted across a joint. Similarly, by getting the muscles to work in a more balanced and coordinated way, joint stability may be improved.

3.8.2 Static Glenohumeral Joint Stabilisers

If we examine the potential stabilisers described above, for the glenohumeral joint, we can see that:

- The glenohumeral joint is a ball and socket joint, but the shape of the humeral head and glenoid does not confer substantial inherent stability. The glenohumeral joint involves a ball articulating with a flat surface which makes it inherently unstable. This is in contrast to the hip joint which is also ball and socket joint, but the acetabulum is a deep socket. The glenohumeral joint is analogous to a ball of ice cream sitting at the top of a cone, whilst the hip joint is analogous to an ice cream ball sitting in a plastic cup; one can easily appreciate which of the two would be more likely to slip off. Hence, the glenohumeral joint is inherently unstable because the glenoid fossa is shallow

The glenohumeral joint is equivalent to an ice cream scoop on top of a cone (a). The hip joint is more like a scoop of ice cream in a cup (b)

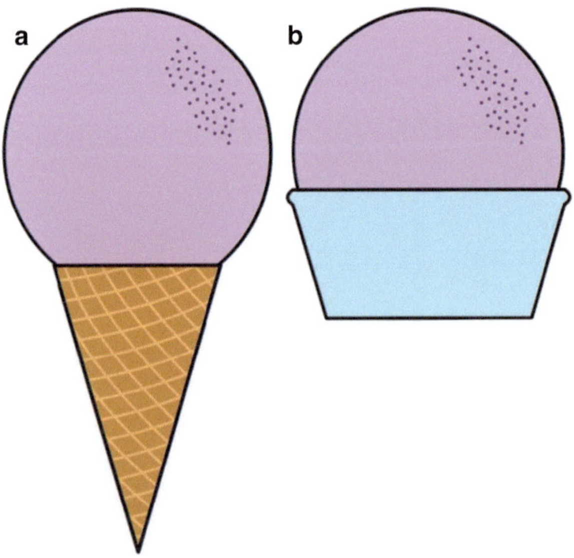

- The glenoid labrum increases glenoid depth, concavity and surface area. It is also a stable anchor for the glenohumeral ligaments and capsule. The labrum attempts to deepen the glenoid, to improve stability, but with minimal effect
- The posterior tilt of the glenoid fossa and the posterior tilt of the humeral head counteract the tendency towards anterior instability
- There is a suction effect of the negative intra-articular pressure found in the glenohumeral joint, but this is a minor contributor to joint stability
- The long head of the biceps tendon may act as humeral head stabiliser in an anterior and superior direction. The long head of the biceps tendon is considered a passive superior stabiliser of the glenohumeral joint exerting a buttress-like effect
- The glenohumeral joint capsule is thin and loose fitting, especially at its inferior part. However, the joint capsule is reinforced by ligaments which contribute to stability
  - The anterior band of the inferior glenohumeral ligament resists anterior translation and external rotation in the abducted position
  - The posterior band of the inferior glenohumeral ligament resists posterior translation
  - The superior glenohumeral ligament resists inferior translation

The role of the glenohumeral ligaments in supporting the humeral head and providing stability is analogous to that of two ropes supporting a person sitting on the seat of a frame swing. As long as both ropes are taut and balanced, one can happily swing along. However, one cannot swing happily if one rope:

- Pulls off the swing frame and floats in free space (analogous to a glenoid avulsion of the glenohumeral ligaments)
- Pulls off and reattaches lower down the frame (analogous to an avulsion of the glenohumeral ligaments from the glenoid and healing to a more medial position on the glenoid neck, effectively lengthening the glenohumeral ligaments which thus become lax)
- Pulls off the swing seat (analogous to an avulsion of the glenohumeral ligament from its insertion on the humerus – HAGL lesion)
- Snaps halfway down its length (analogous to a mid-substance glenohumeral ligament tear)
- Stretches out (analogous to the glenohumeral ligaments or capsule stretching and lengthening, which thus become lax)

Support on a swing relies on its supporting taut ropes (a), as stability of the humeral head on the glenoid relies on taut glenohumeral ligaments. If one rope pulls off (b, d) and reattaches further down (c), snaps (e) or stretches (f), support cannot be maintained and instability ensues

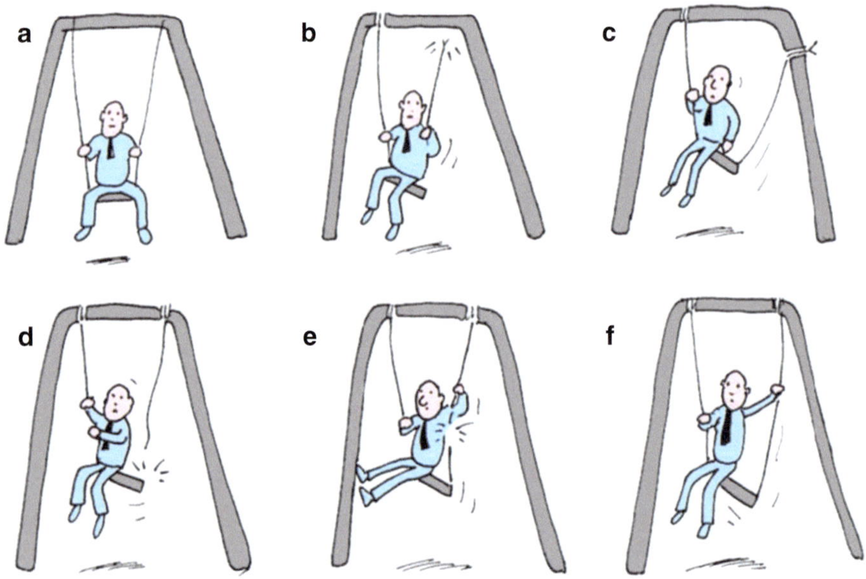

3.8.3 *Dynamic Glenohumeral Joint Stabilisers*

Most of the stability of the glenohumeral joint is brought about by the contraction of the rotator cuff muscles. These work to stabilise the humeral head on the glenoid [26, 31, 41–47]. They form force couples that limit:

- Upwards translation of the humeral head
- Translation of the humeral head anteriorly or posteriorly

3.8.3.1 Force Couples Limiting Upward Humeral Head Translation

When the arm is on the side of the body, contraction of the deltoid muscle causes abduction at the glenohumeral joint but also pulls the humeral head upwards away from the glenoid. In contrast, supraspinatus causes abduction at the glenohumeral joint but also compresses the humeral head against the glenoid. Hence, supraspinatus works with deltoid to bring about abduction but opposes the superior distracting effect of the deltoid.

In addition, deltoid forms a force couple in the coronal plane with infraspinatus, subscapularis, latissimus dorsi and teres minor and major:

- Deltoid contracts pulling the humeral head upwards
- Infraspinatus, teres minor, subscapularis, latissimus dorsi and teres major contract pulling the humeral head downwards, thus opposing the deltoid

Force couple acting at the glenohumeral joint in the coronal plane

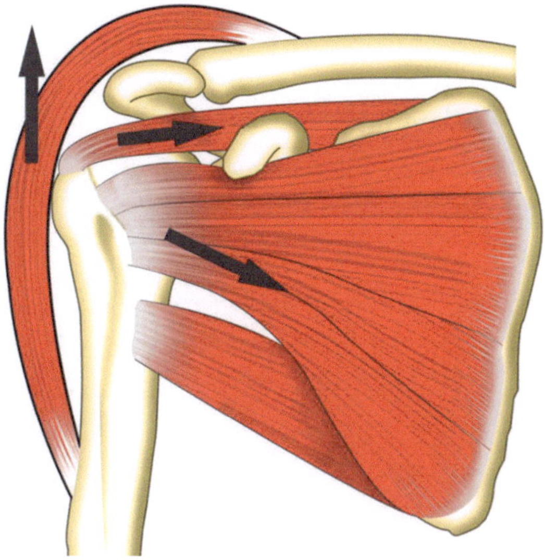

As a result of these force couples, when deltoid contracts the arm abducts rather than pulling the head upwards.

Another couple exists in the horizontal plane between infraspinatus and subscapularis:

- Infraspinatus contracts pulling the humeral head medially and posteriorly
- Subscapularis contracts pulling the humeral head medially and anteriorly

Force couple applied at the glenohumeral joint in the horizontal plane, with subscapularis anterior and infraspinatus posterior

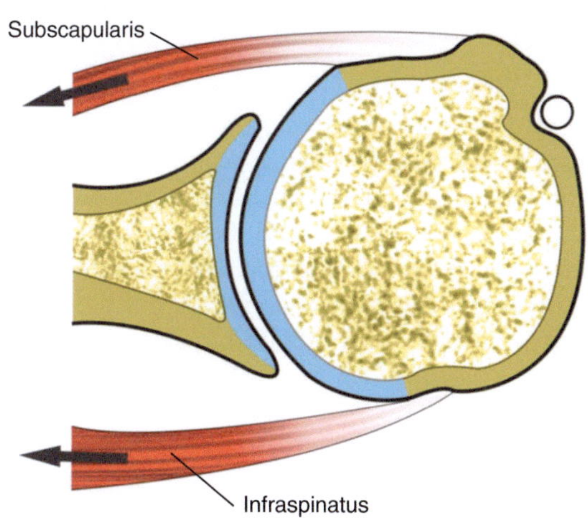

This couple may also oppose the upward translating effect of deltoid. Infraspinatus and subscapularis co-contract upon elevation of the arm to ensure that the humeral head is centred on the glenoid. This resists the superior translation of the humeral head upon deltoid activation. It is of note that these muscles prevent the humeral head from sliding upwards by opposing a force (that of deltoid) that is at right angles to their line of pull. This is almost analogous to the anchoring ropes of a tent. If the tent is anchored on either side, the ropes can resist the wind blowing at a direction that is not in line with their pull. However, if one of the ropes snaps, then the tent will no longer be stable and will be lifted up by the wind.

Side ropes may hold a tent in place against the wind blowing in a direction perpendicular to that of the ropes (a). If one rope snaps, the tent can no longer be supported and is lifted off the ground by the wind (b)

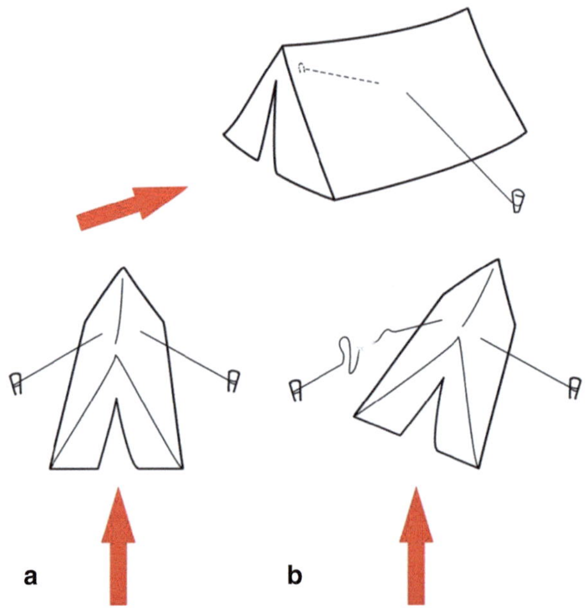

The above may help explain the variability in superior translation of the humeral head associated with supraspinatus tears. In some massive supraspinatus tears, the humeral head migrates upwards in relation to the glenoid, whereas in some cases, it remains well centred on the glenoid. Supraspinatus tears would lead to loss of the medial compression pull that supraspinatus exerts. However, the effects of the downward action of infraspinatus, latissimus dorsi, subscapularis, teres minor and major as well as the medial compression force couple between infraspinatus and subscapularis may still be sufficient to oppose a superior migration. However, supraspinatus tears that are associated with infraspinatus or subscapularis tears may impair this force couple that opposes deltoid, leading to upward translation of the humeral head upon deltoid contraction, which in turn leads to loss of arm elevation. The above may also suggest that in rotator cuff repair surgery, there is a need to repair infraspinatus and subscapularis, whenever possible, rather than simply addressing supraspinatus [28, 48, 49].

Complete rupture of the supraspinatus tendon, but with an intact subscapularis and infraspinatus - arthroscopic view

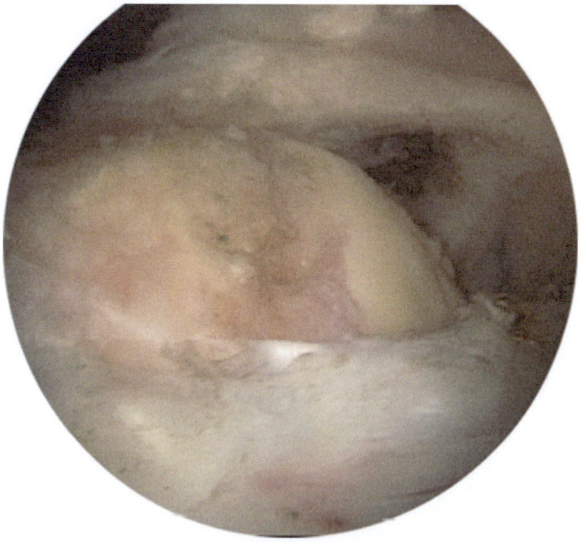

MRI showing massive supraspinatus tear retracted to the level of the glenoid (red arrow) (a). Despite this, the humeral head has not migrated superiorly and is centred on the glenoid (b) likely due to an effective horizontal force couple

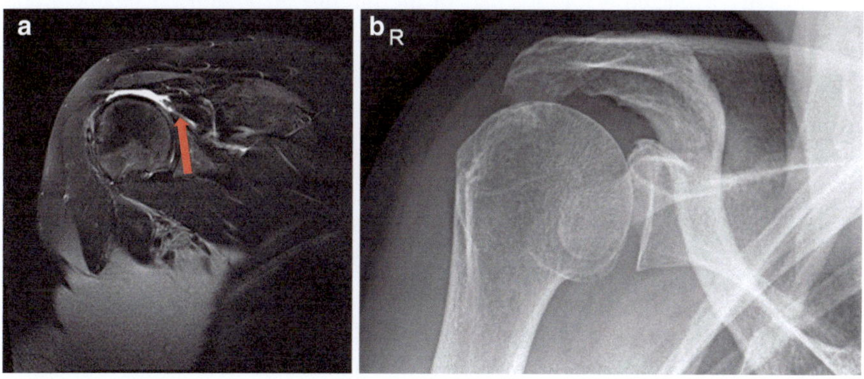

3.8.3.2 Force Couples Limiting Anterior or Posterior Humeral Head Translation

Muscles that exert their force in an opposite direction may balance out and provide stability. The anterior part of the rotator cuff (subscapularis) and the posterior part of the rotator cuff (infraspinatus, teres minor) form a horizontal force couple:

- Infraspinatus pulls the humeral head backwards and medially
- Subscapularis pulls the humeral head anteriorly and medially

Acting together, they stop the humeral head sliding backwards or forwards in relation to the glenoid. However, if one of these muscle tendons is torn, the head can be pulled forwards or backwards by the remaining intact muscle. A similar effect may be seen if there is relative overactivity or underactivity of one component of the force couple allowing an inbalanced force in the anterior or posterior direction.

3.8.4 Variation in Glenohumeral Joint Stabilisers with Arm Position

Different structures are responsible for providing most of the stability of the glenohumeral joint at different arm positions. The main stabilisers in an anterior-inferior direction are considered to be:

- Arm hanging by the side – supraspinatus, superior glenohumeral ligament
- Arm abducted at 90° – subscapularis, middle and inferior glenohumeral ligaments
- Arm fully abducted – inferior part of the inferior glenohumeral ligament and inferior capsule

3.8.5 Core Control and Glenohumeral Joint Stability

In considering glenohumeral stability, it is vital to recognise that we do not simply have a mobile humeral head that moves on a fixed glenoid. Instead:

- The humeral head articulates with the glenoid which is part of the scapula
- The scapula is mobile and rotates on the chest wall as the arm moves
- The chest wall articulates with the axial skeleton
- The axial skeleton has various components that exhibit mobility relative to each other

Hence, in order to allow coordinated movements of the humeral head on the scapula, there is a need for well-controlled and coordinated movements of the scapula on the chest wall and well-controlled, coordinated movements of the axial skeleton. In this way, the axial skeleton can provide a stable platform for the scapula to rotate upon, and the scapula can provide a stable platform for the humeral head to move in relation to.

Control and coordination of the scapular motion on the chest wall are provided by the various muscles passing from the trunk to the scapula as described above. Control and coordination of the axial skeleton are provided by the core muscles [50–54].

The core has been described as a "box" with the:

- Abdominal muscles at the front
- Paraspinal muscles, thoracolumbar fascia and gluteal muscles at the back
- Diaphragm forms the roof
- Pelvic floor and hip joint muscles (hip adductors, gluteus medius, iliopsoas) form the floor

The core muscles act as a corset that helps to stabilise the vertebral column both at rest and during limb movements (similar to the belt that weight lifters wear to give them more stability during weight lifting). Contraction of the diaphragm increases the intra-abdominal pressure which further helps to stabilise the lumbar spine.

The core provides a stable platform for the extremities and upper spine to work. A stable core allows strong coordinated motion of the upper limbs, especially in overhead activities. A weak core cannot provide the stability necessary for limb motion to occur in a coordinated way to exert sufficient power to achieve its goals. A weak core is analogous to a weight lifter trying to lift a heavy weight bar whilst trying to balance on a wobbly ball.

Efficient motion and power exertion require a stable platform to act upon. (a) stable platform (b) unstable platform

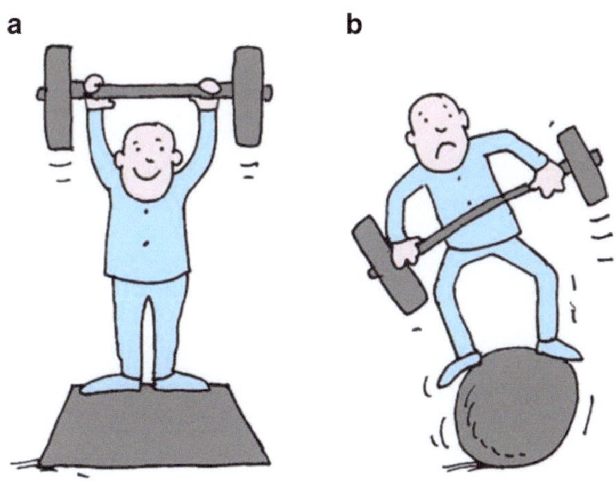

Hence, in improving functional stability of the glenohumeral joint, there is a need to address not only those muscles that pass between the scapula and humerus but also the muscles that give scapular and core stability. This is achieved by improving muscle strength but also muscle endurance. Individuals may be taught to recruit muscles (that have been relatively inactive) either in isolation or as part of a group of muscles. Once a muscle is awakened and recruited, further training can improve its functional abilities.

3.9 Sterno-Clavicular Joint Stability

Only about 50% of the medial clavicle articulates with the manubrium; hence, there is little osseous component to the stability of the sterno-clavicular joint [55, 56].

Stability is mainly provided by ligaments:

- The posterior capsule (posterior sterno-clavicular ligament) is considered to be the main restraint to anterior and posterior translation of the clavicle
- The anterior capsule (anterior sterno-clavicular ligament) acts as an important restraint to anterior-posterior translation
- The costo-clavicular and inter-clavicular ligaments have little role in limiting anterior-posterior translation

3.10 ACJt Stability

This is mainly provided by joint ligaments [55, 57–61]:

- Coraco-clavicular ligaments – provide superior-inferior stability
- Acromio-clavicular ligaments – provide anterior-posterior stability

Learning Pearls

- A muscle-tendon complex can provide a static stabilisation effect in addition to its dynamic stabilisation effect. This may be achieved by providing a:
  - Buttress effect due to its position
  - Check-rein-effect

An example is the subscapularis tendon which:

- Acts as a buttress to anterior translation of the humeral head at the glenohumeral joint
- Acts as a check-rein limiting external rotation of the humeral head at the glenohumeral joint

Disruption of the subscapularis tendon may thus lead to anterior glenohumeral instability.

References

1. Halder AM, Itoi E, An KN. Anatomy and biomechanics of the shoulder. Orthop Clin North Am. 2000;31(2):159–76.
2. An KN, Browne AO, Korinek S, Tanaka S, Morrey BF. Three-dimensional kinematics of glenohumeral elevation. J Orthop Res. 1991;9(1):143–9.
3. Struyf F, Nijs J, Baeyens JP, Mottram S, Meeusen R. Scapular positioning and movement in unimpaired shoulders, shoulder impingement syndrome, and glenohumeral instability. Scand J Med Sci Sports. 2011;21(3):352–8.
4. McClure PW, Michener LA, Sennett BJ, Karduna AR. Direct 3-dimensional measurement of scapular kinematics during dynamic movements in vivo. J Shoulder Elb Surg. 2001;10:269–77.
5. Inman VT, Abbot L, Saunders JB. Observations on the function of the shoulder joint. J Bone Joint Surg. 1944;26(1):1–30.
6. Poppen NK, Walker PS. Normal and abnormal motion of the shoulder. J Bone Joint Surg Am. 1976;58:195–201.
7. Bagg SD, Forrest WJ. A biomechanical analysis of scapular rotation during arm abduction in the scapular plane. Am J Phys Med Rehabil. 1988;67:238–45.
8. Flatow EL. The biomechanics of the acromioclavicular, sternoclavicular, and scapulothoracic joints. Instr Course Lect. 1993;42:237–45.
9. Ludewig PM, Phadke V, Braman JP, Hassett DR, Cieminski CJ, LaPrade RF. Motion of the shoulder complex during multiplanar humeral elevation. J Bone Joint Surg Am. 2009;91(2):378–89.
10. Teece RM, Lunden JB, Lloyd AS, Kaiser AP, Cieminski CJ, Ludewig PM. Three-dimensional acromioclavicular joint motions during elevation of the arm. J Orthop Sports Phys Ther. 2008;38(4):181–90.
11. Greene WB, Heckman JD. The clinical measurement of joint motion. In: Rosemont IL, editor. American Academy of Orthopaedic Surgeons. 1st ed. Rosemont: American Academy of Orthopaedic Surgeons; 1994. p. 15–26.
12. Namdari S, Yagnik G, Ebaugh DD, Nagda S, Ramsey ML, Williams GR Jr, Mehta S. Defining functional shoulder range of motion for activities of daily living. J Shoulder Elb Surg. 2012;21(9):1177–83.
13. Bitter NL, Clisby EF, Jones MA, Magarey ME, Jaberzadeh S, Sandow MJ. Relative contributions of infraspinatus and deltoid during external rotation in healthy shoulders. J Shoulder Elb Surg. 2007;16(5):563–8.
14. Alizadehkhaiyat O, Hawkes DH, Kemp GJ, Frostick SP. Electromyographic Analysis of the Shoulder Girdle Musculature During External Rotation Exercises. Orthop J Sports Med. 2015;3(11):2325967115613988. https://doi.org/10.1177/2325967115613988.
15. Culham E, Peat M. Functional anatomy of the shoulder complex. J Orthop Sports Phys Ther. 1993;18(1):342–50.
16. Sinnatamby CS. FRCS Last's Anatomy: Regional and Applied. London: Churchill Livingstone Elsevier; 2011. p. 12e.
17. Kronberg M, Németh G, Broström LA. Muscle activity and coordination in the normal shoulder. An electromyographic study. Clin Orthop Relat Res. 1990;257:76–85.
18. Werthel JD, Bertelli J, Elhassan BT. Shoulder function in patients with deltoid paralysis and intact rotator cuff. Orthop Traumatol Surg Res. 2017;103(6):869–73.
19. Reed D, Cathers I, Halaki M, Ginn K. Does supraspinatus initiate shoulder abduction? J Electromyogr Kinesiol. 2013;23(2):425–9.
20. Howell SM, Imobersteg AM, Seger DH, Marone PJ. Clarification of the role of the supraspinatus muscle in shoulder function. J Bone Joint Surg Am. 1986;68(3):398–404.
21. Liu J, Hughes RE, Smutz WP, Niebur G, Nan-An K. Roles of deltoid and rotator cuff muscles in shoulder elevation. Clin Biomech (Bristol, Avon). 1997;12(1):32–8.
22. Wickham J, Pizzari T, Stansfeld K, Burnside A, Watson L. Quantifying 'normal' shoulder muscle activity during abduction. J Electromyogr Kinesiol. 2010;20(2):212–22.

23. Poppen NK, Walker PS. Forces at the glenohumeral joint in abduction. Clin Orthop Relat Res. 1978;135:165–70.
24. McMahon PJ, Debski RE, Thompson WO, Warner JJ, Fu FH, Woo SL. Shoulder muscle forces and tendon excursions during glenohumeral abduction in the scapular plane. J Shoulder Elb Surg. 1995;4(3):199–208.
25. Apreleva M, Parsons IM 4th, Warner JJ, Fu FH, Woo SL. Experimental investigation of reaction forces at the glenohumeral joint during active abduction. J Shoulder Elb Surg. 2000;9(5):409–17.
26. Halder AM, Zhao KD, Odriscoll SW, Morrey BF, An KN. Dynamic contributions to superior shoulder stability. J Orthop Res. 2001;19(2):206–12.
27. Pouliart N, Gagey O. The effect of isolated labrum resection on shoulder stability. Knee Surg Sports Traumatol Arthrosc. 2006;14(3):301–8.
28. Lee SB, Kim KJ, O'Driscoll SW, Morrey BF, An KN. Dynamic glenohumeral stability provided by the rotator cuff muscles in the mid-range and end-range of motion. A study in cadavera. J Bone Joint Surg Am. 2000;82(6):849–57.
29. Wuelker N, Korell M, Thren K. Dynamic glenohumeral joint stability. J Shoulder Elb Surg. 1998;7(1):43–52.
30. Ernstbrunner L, Werthel JD, Hatta T, Thoreson AR, Resch H, An KN, Moroder P. Biomechanical analysis of the effect of congruence, depth and radius on the stability ratio of a simplistic 'ball-and-socket' joint model. Bone Joint Res. 2016;5(10):453–60.
31. An KN. Muscle force and its role in joint dynamic stability. Clin Orthop Relat Res. 2002;403(Suppl):S37–42.
32. Lee SB, An KN. Dynamic glenohumeral stability provided by three heads of the deltoid muscle. Clin Orthop Relat Res. 2002;400:40–7.
33. Motzkin NE, Itoi E, Morrey BF, An KN. Contribution of capsuloligamentous structures to passive static inferior glenohumeral stability. Clin Biomech (Bristol, Avon). 1998;13(1):54–6.
34. Halder AM, Halder CG, Zhao KD, O'Driscoll SW, Morrey BF, An KN. Dynamic inferior stabilizers of the shoulder joint. Clin Biomech (Bristol, Avon). 2001;16(2):138–43.
35. Itoi E, Berglund LJ, Grabowski JJ, Naggar L, Morrey BF, An KN. Superior-inferior stability of the shoulder: role of the coracohumeral ligament and the rotator interval capsule. Mayo Clin Proc. 1998;73(6):508–15.
36. Itoi E, Newman SR, Kuechle DK, Morrey BF, An KN. Dynamic anterior stabilisers of the shoulder with the arm in abduction. J Bone Joint Surg (Br). 1994;76(5):834–6.
37. Itoi E, Motzkin NE, Morrey BF, An KN. Stabilizing function of the long head of the biceps in the hanging arm position. J Shoulder Elb Surg. 1994;3(3):135–42.
38. Itoi E, Motzkin NE, Morrey BF, An KN. Scapular inclination and inferior stability of the shoulder. J Shoulder Elb Surg. 1992;1(3):131–9.
39. Itoi E, Motzkin NE, Browne AO, Hoffmeyer P, Morrey BF, An KN. Intraarticular pressure of the shoulder. Arthroscopy. 1993;9(4):406–13.
40. Itoi E, Hsu HC, An KN. Biomechanical investigation of the glenohumeral joint. J Shoulder Elb Surg. 1996;5(5):407–2.
41. Halder AM, Kuhl SG, Zobitz ME, Larson D, An KN. Effects of the glenoid labrum and glenohumeral abduction on stability of the shoulder joint through concavity-compression : an in vitro study. J Bone Joint Surg Am. 2001;83-A(7):1062–9.
42. Sharkey NA, Marder RA, Hanson PB. The entire rotator cuff contributes to elevation of the arm. J Orthop Res. 1994;12(5):699–708.
43. Sharkey NA, Marder RA. The rotator cuff opposes superior translation of the humeral head. Am J Sports Med. 1995;23(3):270–5.
44. Yanagawa T, Goodwin CJ, Shelburne KB, Giphart JE, Torry MR, Pandy MG. Contributions of the individual muscles of the shoulder to glenohumeral joint stability during abduction. J Biomech Eng. 2008;130(2):021024.
45. Thompson WO, Debski RE, Boardman ND 3rd, Taskiran E, Warner JJ, Fu FH, Woo SL. A biomechanical analysis of rotator cuff deficiency in a cadaveric model. Am J Sports Med. 1996;24(3):286–92.

46. Campbell ST, Ecklund KJ, Chu EH, McGarry MH, Gupta R, Lee TQ. The role of pectoralis major and latissimus dorsi muscles in a biomechanical model of massive rotator cuff tear. J Shoulder Elb Surg. 2014;23(8):1136–42.
47. Mura N, O'Driscoll SW, Zobitz ME, Heers G, Jenkyn TR, Chou SM, Halder AM, An KN. The effect of infraspinatus disruption on glenohumeral torque and superior migration of the humeral head: a biomechanical study. J Shoulder Elb Surg. 2003;12(2):179–84.
48. Steenbrink F, de Groot JH, Veeger HE, van der Helm FC, Rozing PM. Glenohumeral stability in simulated rotator cuff tears. J Biomech. 2009;42(11):1740–5.
49. Hsu JE, Reuther KE, Sarver JJ, Lee CS, Thomas SJ, Glaser DL, Soslowsky LJ. Restoration of anterior-posterior rotator cuff force balance improves shoulder function in a rat model of chronic massive tears. J Orthop Res. 2011;29(7):1028–33.
50. Reuther KE, Thomas SJ, Tucker JJ, Sarver JJ, Gray CF, Rooney SI, Glaser DL, Soslowsky LJ. Disruption of the anterior-posterior rotator cuff force balance alters joint function and leads to joint damage in a rat model. J Orthop Res. 2014;32(5):638–44.
51. Huxel Bliven KC, Anderson BE. Core stability training for injury prevention. Sports Health. 2013;5(6):514–22.
52. Willson JD, Dougherty CP, Ireland ML, Davis IM. Core stability and its relationship to lower extremity function and injury. J Am Acad Orthop Surg. 2005;13(5):316–25.
53. Kibler WB, Press J, Sciascia A. The role of core stability in athletic function. Sports Med. 2006;36(3):189–98.
54. Rosemeyer JR, Hayes BT, Switzler CL, Hicks-Little CA. Effects of Core-Musculature Fatigue on Maximal Shoulder Strength. J Sport Rehabil. 2015;24(4):384–90.
55. Radwan A, Francis J, Green A, Kahl E, Maciurzynski D, Quartulli A, Schultheiss J, Strang R, Weiss B. Is there a relation between shoulder dysfunction and core instability? Int J Sports Phys Ther. 2014;9(1):8–13.
56. Renfree KJ, Wright TW. Anatomy and biomechanics of the acromioclavicular and sternoclavicular joints. Clin Sports Med. 2003;22(2):219–37.
57. Spencer EE, Kuhn JE, Huston LJ, Carpenter JE, Hughes RE. Ligamentous restraints to anterior and posterior translation of the sternoclavicular joint. J Shoulder Elb Surg. 2002;11(1):43–7.
58. Fukuda K, Craig EV, An KN, Cofield RH, Chao EY. Biomechanical study of the ligamentous system of the acromioclavicular joint. J Bone Joint Surg Am. 1986;68:434–40.
59. Klimkiewicz JJ, Williams GR, Sher JS, Karduna A, Des Jardins J, Iannotti JP. The acromioclavicular capsule as a restraint to posterior translation of the clavicle: a biomechanical analysis. J Shoulder Elb Surg. 1999;8:119–24.
60. Rockwood C, Williams GR, Young D. Disorders of the acromioclavicular joint. Rockwood Greens Fract Adults. 1996;2(Ed 4):1341–3.
61. Lee KW, Debski RE, Chen CH, Woo SL, Fu FH. Functional evaluation of the ligaments at the acromioclavicular joint during anteroposterior and superoinferior translation. Am J Sports Med. 1997;25:858–62.

Chapter 4
Clinical History for Shoulder Conditions

The first step in making a clinical diagnosis is taking a thorough history of the patient's complaints. This is achieved by using both open questions (where patients are given the opportunity to open up and express the difficulties they face) but also more direct questions that aim to elicit specific facts which the patient may not otherwise volunteer but which can guide the diagnosis.

Clinical history taking for shoulder conditions takes the formal structure of asking about the presenting complaint, events around the onset of the complaint and its effects upon the patient in terms of pain, loss of function or other disturbance. The clinician then tries to determine what treatments have already been tried and what the patient's response has been to those. Furthermore, information is obtained about the overall health of the patient, previous and current medications received and any relevant family history. The personal circumstances of the patient including recreational and occupational activities are also elicited.

This chapter describes some of the enquiries [1–6] that may be made in obtaining a clinical history for the troublesome shoulder.

4.1 Presenting Complaint

The patient may describe one or more complaints, and more information is gathered for each of these. These are described next.

© Springer Nature Switzerland AG 2019

C. Panayiotou Charalambous, *The Shoulder Made Easy*,
https://doi.org/10.1007/978-3-319-98908-2_4

4.1.1 Nature of Complaint

- Pain
  - Location
  - Nature
    - Sharp
    - Dull
    - Burning
  - Severity
    - On a scale of 0 to 10, with 0 being no pain and 10 severe pain
    - Effect on going to sleep/awakening
- Stiffness
  - Global versus a specific direction
- Weakness
  - Global versus specific movement direction
  - Global versus specific arm position
  - In high- versus low-demand activities
  - Severity
    - Absence of power vs. less power than expected vs. early fatigue
- Clicking/clucking
  - Type of noise
  - Heard versus felt
    - By patient or others
  - Location/source
- Paraesthesia
  - Nature
    - Altered sensation
    - Pins and needles
    - Reduced sensation
    - Tingling
    - Numbness
    - "Dead" arm
  - Location
  - Severity
  - Painful versus painless

- Swelling
  - Description
    - Prominence
    - Deformity
    - Asymmetry between sides
    - Something out of place, something sticking out
  - Noticed by patient or others
- Isolated symptom or in combination

4.1.2 *Onset of Complaint*

- Speed of onset
  - Sudden
  - Gradual
- Possible precipitating event
  - Nil obvious
  - Chronic repetitive strain
  - Chronic repetitive loading
  - Change in activities prior to onset of symptoms
  - Onset due to sudden loading
  - Post-injury
  - How did injury happen?
  - What exactly happened to the arm?
    - Traction
    - Forced in a particular direction
    - Direct impact
    - Axial loading (such as holding car steering wheel when crashing, fall on elbow or outstretched arm)

4.1.3 *Progress of Complaint*

- Duration
  - Length
  - Continuous/intermittent

- Change in size or shape (such as of a lump):
  - Bigger/smaller/up and down – intermittently changing size
  - Speed of change – slow, rapid
  - Constant size and shape versus changing with joint movement or position

4.1.4 *Exacerbating and Relieving Factors*

- Arm position
- Rest versus exertion, still versus arm motion
- Arm weight versus additional weight lifting
- Specific activities
  - Reaching upwards (reach a shelf)
  - Lifting weights over the head
  - Combing hair
  - Throwing phase
  - Hand reaching bottom
- Timing – night versus day, morning versus rest of day

4.1.5 *Impact of Presenting Complaint*

Understanding the effect of the presenting complaint on the patient is essential to help a clinician consider the level of intervention necessary and any potential benefits of any such intervention. These include:

- Functional limitations
  - Day-to-day activities of living
  - Occupational limitations
  - Recreational limitations
- What does it stop you from doing that you would like to do?
- Effect on personal/social life
- Effect on psychological well-being

4.1.6 *Up-to-Date Management of Presenting Complaint*

An enquiry is made as to how the complaint has been previously managed. Such information may be obtained from the patient and their close ones or, where relevant, from previous medical or surgical records:

- What has been tried?
  - How?
  - By whom?
  - How many times?
- What has been tried and helped symptoms?
- What has been tried but failed to improve symptoms?

4.2 Previous Musculoskeletal History

In this part of clinical history, information is obtained about any other musculoskeletal problems:

- Symptomatic shoulder/arm
- Opposite shoulder/arm
- Other joints
- Inflammatory or other arthropathy
- Previous injuries – fractures or otherwise

4.3 Previous Medical History

The previous medical history of the patient is examined to identify disorders that may be associated with the development of shoulder symptoms and to determine the overall health of the patient and their ability to undergo surgery or other interventions:

- Diabetes mellitus
  - Association with frozen shoulder
  - Link to perioperative complications
  - Possibly less improvement with surgical interventions
  - Steroid injection therapy and risk of hyperglycaemia
- Cardiovascular and respiratory fitness if considering surgery
- Malignancy – possibility of metastatic cause of symptoms, fitness for surgery
- Infection
- Avascular necrosis
- Conditions associated with steroid use
- Deep venous thrombosis/pulmonary embolism – increased risk in surgery

4.4 Previous Surgical History

Enquiries are made about any previous surgical history both with regard to musculoskeletal and non-musculoskeletal problems, to help determine fitness for surgery and anticipate any surgery/anaesthetic complications the patient may be predisposed to:

- Any previous surgery
- What type of anaesthesia
- Timing of previous surgery
- Development of postsurgical complications

4.5 Drug History

Information is obtained about current and previous medications, details of any allergies as well as alcohol and tobacco use:

- History of steroid use – due to link with avascular necrosis
- Medications that may influence anaesthetic risk or injection therapy
- Other drugs if relevant – anabolic steroids and stimulants
- Allergies:
  - Agent
  - Reaction
  - Alternatives tried and safe?
  - May be associated with predisposition to joint stiffness
- Alcohol use
  - Link with avascular necrosis
  - Compliance with treatment
- Smoking

4.6 Family Musculoskeletal History

Certain musculoskeletal conditions may show a familial association and these are sought:

- Family history of shoulder conditions which may affect knowledge of patient, preconceptions or expectations
- Familial association of frozen shoulder
- Family history of other joint conditions such as inflammatory arthropathy
- Conditions associated with arthropathy such as gout and inflammatory bowel disease

Learning Pearls

- A systematic history taking may ensure that all important information is gathered and that important facts are not overlooked
- Maintain lateral thinking, even when the diagnosis seems very obvious

References

1. Sigman SA, Richmond JC. Office diagnosis of shoulder disorders. Phys Sportsmed. 1995;23(7):25–31.
2. Somerville LE, Willits K, Johnson AM, Litchfield R, LeBel ME, Moro J, Bryant D. Diagnostic validity of patient-reported history for shoulder pathology. Surg J (N Y). 2017;3(2):e79–87.
3. Gray M, Wallace A, Aldridge S. Assessment of shoulder pain for non-specialists. BMJ. 2016;355:i5783.
4. Kennedy DJ, Mattie R, Nguyen Q, Hamilton S, Conrad B. Glenohumeral joint pain referral patterns: a descriptive study. Pain Med. 2015;16(8):1603–9.
5. Minns Lowe CJ, Moser J, Barker K. Living with a symptomatic rotator cuff tear 'bad days, bad nights': a qualitative study. BMC Musculoskelet Disord. 2014;15:228. https://doi.org/10.1186/1471-2474-15-228.
6. Mancuso CA, Altchek DW, Craig EV, Jones EC, Robbins L, Warren RF, Williams-Russo P. Patients' expectations of shoulder surgery. J Shoulder Elb Surg. 2002;11(6):541–9.

Chapter 5
Clinical Examination of the Shoulder

Clinical examination aims to elicit signs that can supplement the clinical symptoms gathered from the clinical history and prove or disprove the working diagnosis.

Examination of any joint in orthopaedics may follow look/feel/move/special tests sequence [1, 2], and this order is also applied to examination of the shoulder. The examiner inspects the patient and their shoulders, palpates the shoulder and scapular areas and then determines the active and passive range of shoulder motion. Individual muscle strength is subsequently examined along with special tests that are guided towards specific underlying conditions. The cervical spine, elbow and other upper limb joints are also examined as indicated.

This chapter presents a structured shoulder clinical examination with special emphasis on some of the many special tests described for shoulder assessment. A structured clinical approach may ensure that any significant findings are not overlooked. A selection of special tests may be utilised according to the working diagnosis.

Clinical examination of the shoulder follows a structured look, feel, move and special tests approach, and this is described next.

5.1 Look

The patient is inspected overall:

- Comfortable at rest or in discomfort?
- The patient is asked to stand and take a few steps to assess the overall posture, balance and mobility of lower and upper limbs
- Ability to walk with or without a walking aid is noted

The patient's upper trunk is exposed, and the patient is asked to stand or sit so that the examiner can move around the patient to inspect the shoulders, scapulae, spine, clavicles and chest wall.

© Springer Nature Switzerland AG 2019

C. Panayiotou Charalambous, *The Shoulder Made Easy*,
https://doi.org/10.1007/978-3-319-98908-2_5

Look at the:

- Front
- Side
- Back

Look – (a) Front, (b) Side, (c) Back

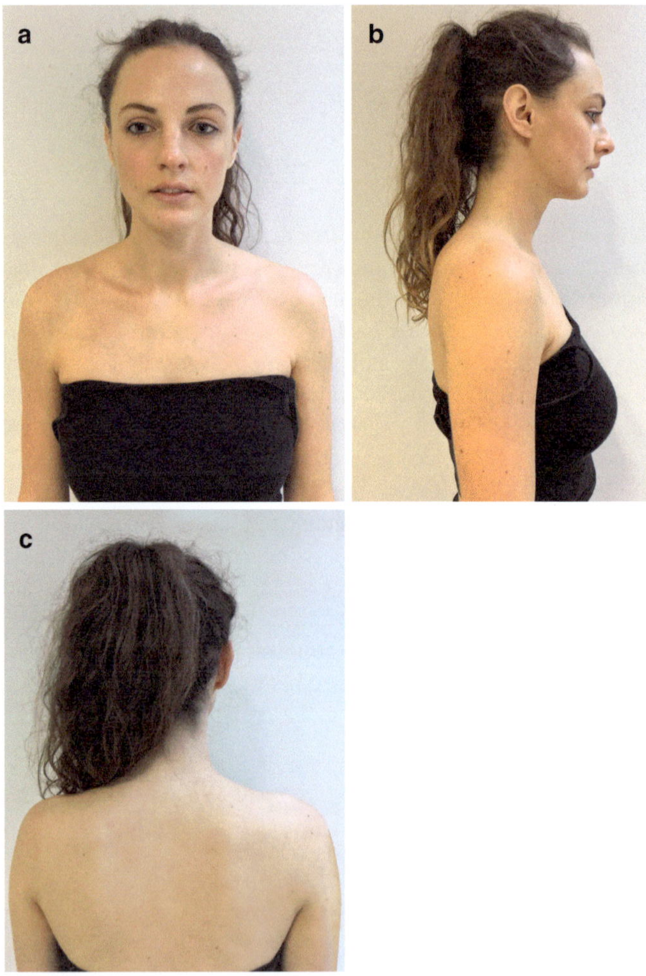

Look for:

- Surgical or traumatic scars
- Lumps or bumps
- Abnormal posture or asymmetry – shoulder and arm, humeral head, scapula, cervical spine and clavicle
- Muscle wasting
- Skin – colour, rash or other cutaneous lesions

Rotator cuff arthropathy – diffuse swelling of the glenohumeral joint with marked wasting of the supra- and infraspinous fossae

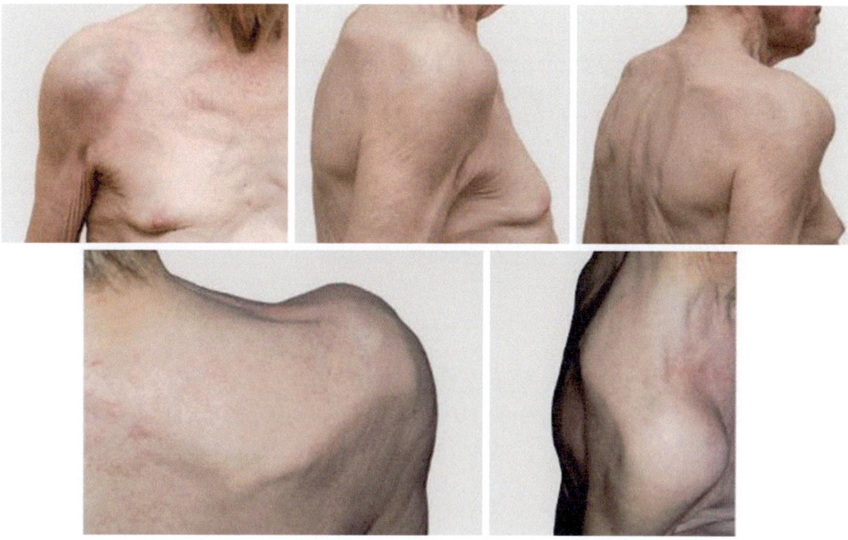

5.2 Feel

Palpate potential sources of pain:

- Cervical and thoracic spine along with paraspinal muscles
- Peri-scapular and shoulder muscles for tender spots
- Sterno-clavicular joint
- Acromio-clavicular joint
- Anterior-lateral part of subacromial space
- Bicipital groove
- Anterior capsule
- Coracoid
- Posterior capsule

5.3 Move

Movement may be described as:

- Active – performed by the patient
- Passive – performed by the examiner

The patient is asked to perform a particular movement, and the extent (range) to which this can be achieved is observed. The examiner then tries to push the arm in the specified direction further, and any additional passive movement is observed.

Under normal conditions most motion will be achievable actively, but in certain disorders the amount of passive motion may exceed the range achieved actively.

In examining active motion, the examiner may:

- Instruct verbally the patient as to what movement to perform
- Instruct verbally and demonstrate to the patient the motion using own arms (preferable)

5.3.1 Shoulder Movements Assessed

- Forward elevation
- Abduction
- External rotation with the elbow flexed 90° and apposed to the trunk
- External rotation with the arm in 90° abduction and the elbow flexed 90°
- Internal rotation

Active forward elevation

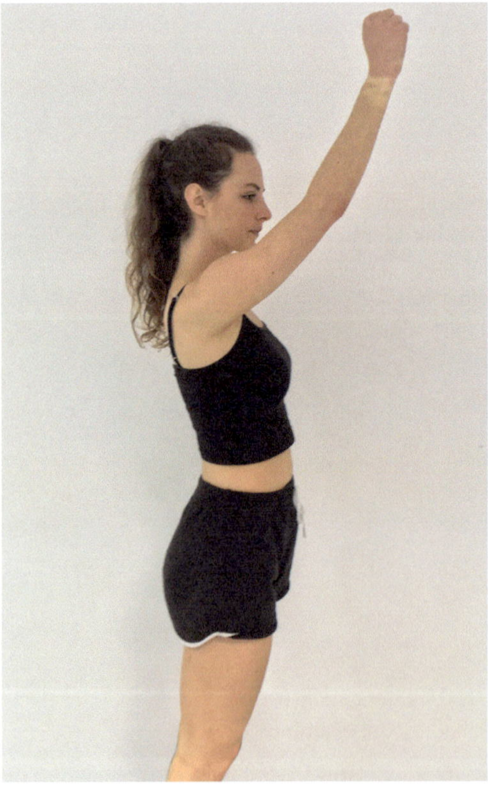

Active abduction

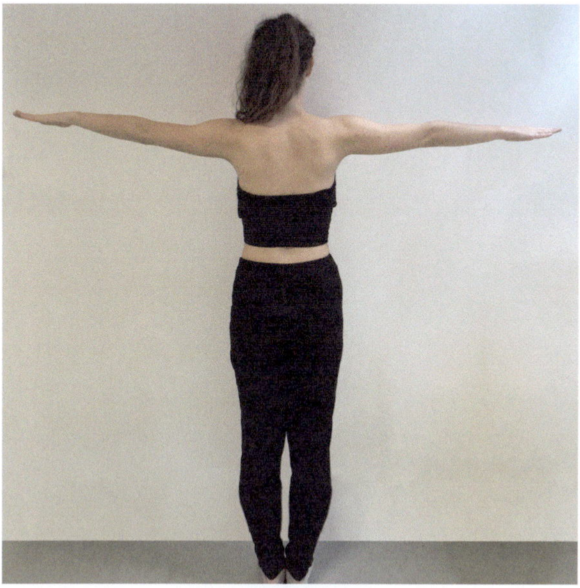

Active external rotation

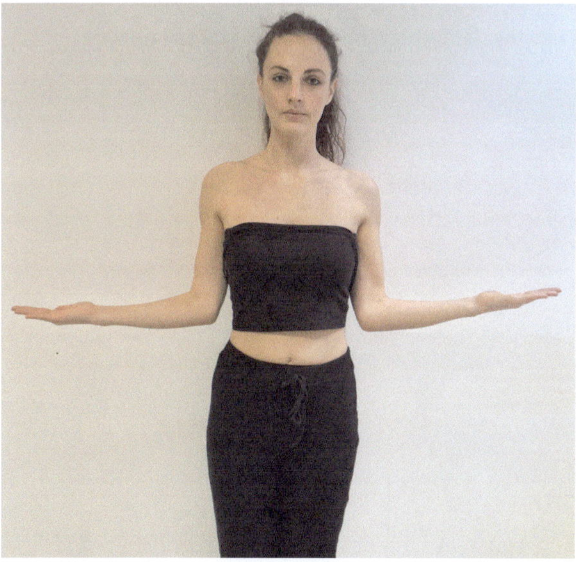

Internal rotation

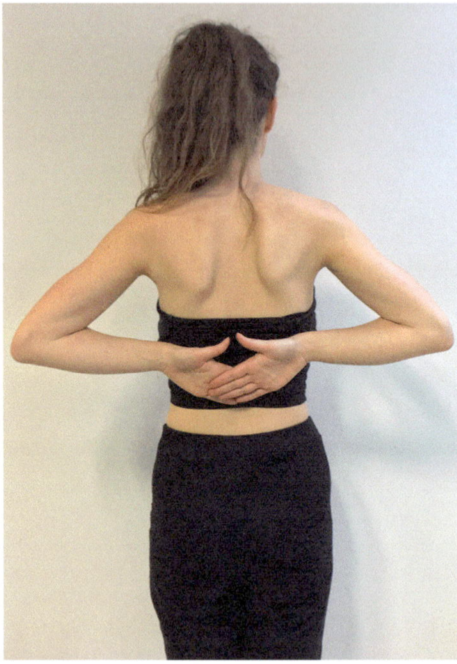

Assessing passive motion (a) forward elevation, (b) external rotation

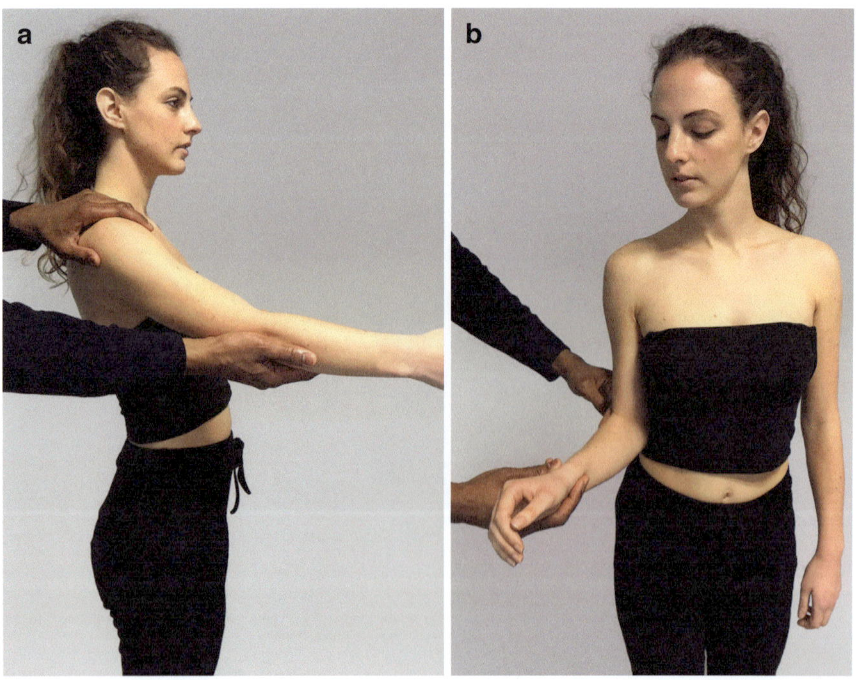

Motion can be described:

- Quantitatively – range in degrees or in the case of internal rotation described as to how far the extended thumb can reach on the patient's back:
  - Side of the thigh
  - Buttock
  - Lower lumbar spine
  - Upper lumbar spine
  - Lower angle of the scapula (normal)
- Qualitatively – smooth, interrupted

Internal rotation — (a) Extended thumb can reach the side of the thigh on the right and the lower angle of the scapula on the left side, (b) Extended thumb can reach the buttock, (c) Extended thumb can reach the lower lumbar spine, (d) Extended thumb can reach upper lumbar spine

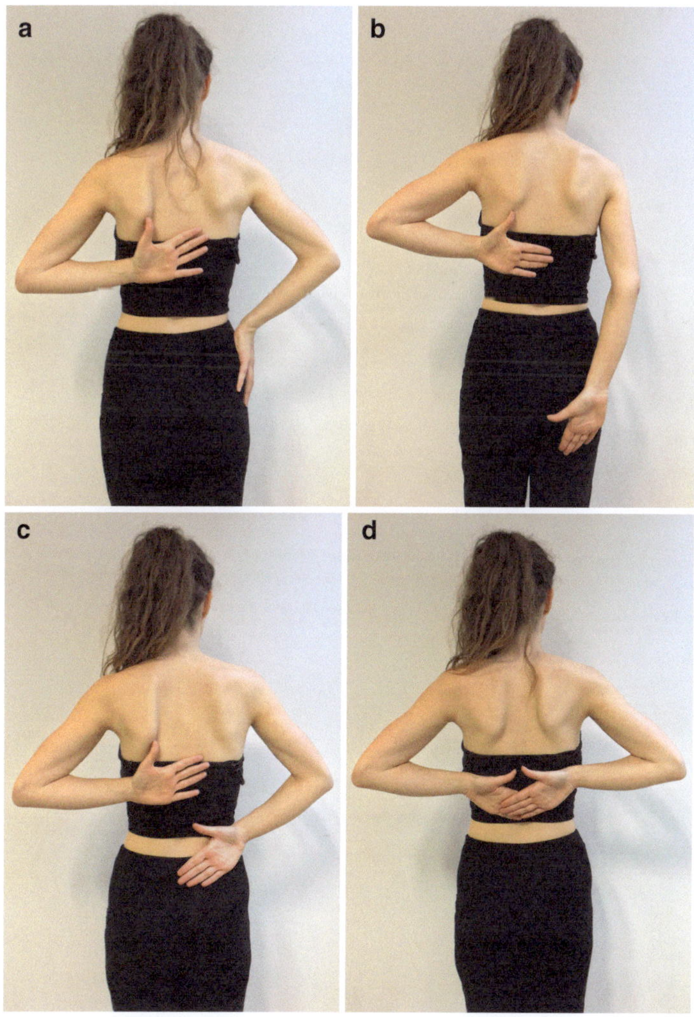

Shoulder motion can be described as total motion (combination of glenohumeral and scapulo-thoracic). Alternatively, it may be described in terms of the individual movements occurring at the glenohumeral and scapulo-thoracic articulations. For the latter the examiner may rest their hands on the scapula to stabilise the scapula and palpate when scapular motion commences.

5.3.2 Cervical Spine Movements Assessed

- Flexion
- Extension
- Lateral rotation
- Lateral flexion

Cervical spine movements (a) Flexion, (b) Extension, (c) Lateral rotation, (d) Lateral flexion

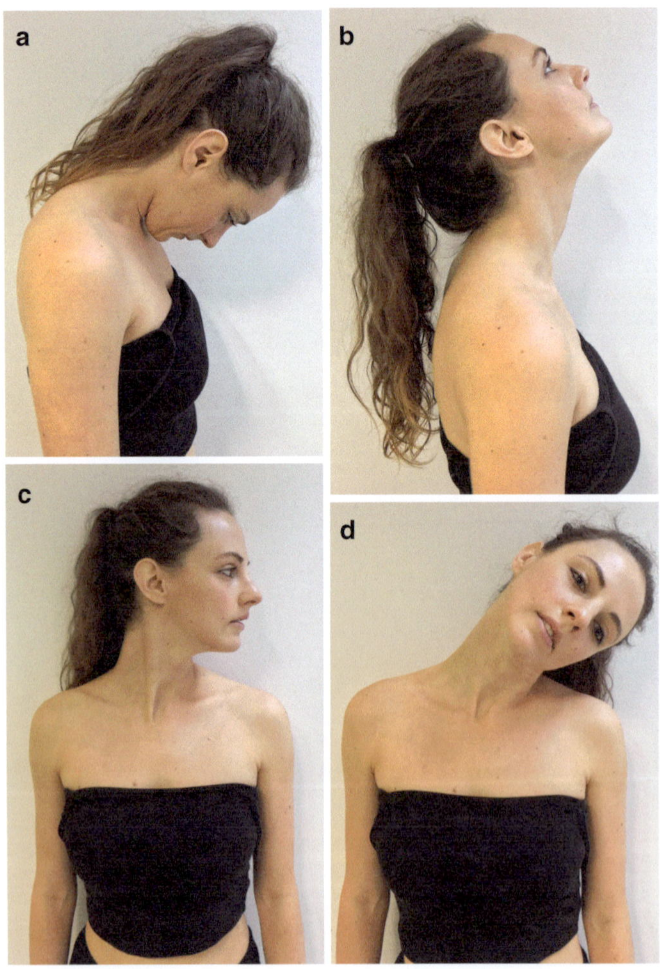

5.4 Special Tests in Shoulder Examination

Special tests are clinical examination manoeuvres that aim to assess the presence of specific disorders or the specific source of an individual's symptoms. Such tests may examine:

- Muscle strength
- Pain provocation
- Apprehension provocation
- Instability provocation
- Other symptom provocation

Special tests aim to isolate and specifically test one structure or group of structures at a time such as:

- One muscle at a time in assessing muscle strength
- One pain source structure at a time in assessing pain provocation
- One process at a time in assessing apprehension
- One group of structures in assessing instability

An ideal special test is one which has high:

- Sensitivity – the ability of a test to correctly identify diseased states
- Specificity – the ability of a test to correctly identify non-diseased states

However, the qualities of commonly used special tests in orthopaedic examinations and specifically in examination of the shoulder have been questioned, as such tests are often not highly sensitive or specific [3–9]. This may be due to:

- Close anatomical relationship of various structures that may make it difficult to isolate and thus test a single structure in order to implicate it in pathology
- Multiple structures can have common origin of innervation, hence causing similar pain upon provocation
- Multiple structures may have similar functions and can compensate for the loss of one of those structures – such as one muscle compensating for the loss of another muscle
- A test may identify the area of origin of symptoms, but not the pathology in that area – such as subacromial pain being the final result of multiple pathological conditions in the subacromial space
- Certain tests may be positive in certain disorders, but the anatomic basis upon which the tests were developed has not been proven by cadaveric studies; hence the reason as to why some tests are positive in some disorders is not fully understood
- The amount of symptoms such as pain reported by individuals upon provocation tests may not be all or none but hugely vary, with no specific cut point as to when a test is considered positive. With clinical experience it may become easier to quantify what is substantial pain, what is exacerbated pain or what is pain out of proportion

- Some tests may be unreliable or cannot be performed in the presence of concomitant pathology, as that pathology may:
  - Prevent the individual to place the arm in the position required in order to perform the special test
  - Cause symptoms similar to the ones that the special test aims to elicit

A systematic review into special shoulder tests has shown that many tests for rotator cuff pathology are inaccurate and may not be useful in clinical practice [3].

These limitations of special tests must be considered in clinical examination. Special tests should thus be used as another piece to the diagnostic jigsaw rather than a process that gives an absolute answer.

A plethora of special tests have been described for shoulder disorders, but a description of all of these is beyond the scope of this book. In addition the use of all the previously described shoulder tests is practically impossible in routine clinical practice. Hence, clinicians often choose and utilise certain tests in their routine examination. Special tests used by the author in clinical examination of the shoulder are presented here.

5.5 Assessing Muscle Strength in Shoulder Examination

Assessing muscle strength is challenging as:

- It is essential to distinguish between true and apparent weakness
- Several muscles may contribute to a motion; hence an attempt is made to isolate the activity of the muscle in question during examination

In grading muscle strength, you may consider the:

Medical Research Council grading system whereby muscle strength is graded 0–5 [10]:

Grade 0 No muscle contraction
Grade 1 Flicker or trace of muscle contraction
Grade 2 Contraction enabling movement with gravity eliminated
Grade 3 Contraction enabling movement against gravity
Grade 4 Active movement against gravity and resistance
Grade 5 Normal motor function

Alternatively, a more simplified grading system may be utilised, whereby three grades of muscle strength are described as:

- Strong
- Weak but can maintain preposition
- Severely weak – cannot maintain preposition

In assessing muscle strength, the following approach may be utilised:

- Ask the patient to perform the motion actively. From this you will get an impression as to whether there is severe weakness or only some weakness
- Then place the arm passively to the position you would expect the patient to achieve, and ask them to maintain it there. In the case of forward elevation, be ready to catch the patient's arm, to stop it from dropping suddenly and causing discomfort. If the patient cannot maintain such a preposition, then this is a lag sign positive, and it indicates a severe weakness (such as due to substantial tendon tear)
- If they can maintain the position, then proceed to further examine the strength, and quantify it or compare it to the opposite healthy shoulder where applicable. This is achieved by asking the patient to maintain the arm in the position, whilst you apply an opposing force

5.6 Testing Muscle Strength: Individual Muscles

5.6.1 Supraspinatus

5.6.1.1 **Drop-Arm Sign** [11]

The patient's arm is elevated by the examiner to about 90° in the scapular plane. The patient is warned that the examiner will let go and is asked to maintain the arm in that position. The examiner lets go but with the examiner's hand staying close in order to catch the arm if the patient cannot maintain this position. Inability to maintain the arm in that position is suggestive of substantial supraspinatus weakness.

5.6.1.2 **Supraspinatus Resistance Strength Test** [12]

With the patient standing, the arm is elevated to 90° in the scapular plane and internally rotated, so the thumb is pointing downwards. The patient is asked to maintain the arm in that position resisting a downward force applied by the examiner. The test is repeated with the arm in external rotation (thumb pointing upwards). It is preferable for the examiner to use one or two fingers to apply force rather than the full hand and also to apply the force proximal to the elbow to minimise the moment arm effect (moment exerted at the joint is the product of the force multiplied by the distance at which this force is applied from the joint). The author prefers to perform this test with the arm in 30° forward elevation, as greater elevation may cause pain.

Supraspinatus strength test with arm in (a) internal rotation and (b) external rotation

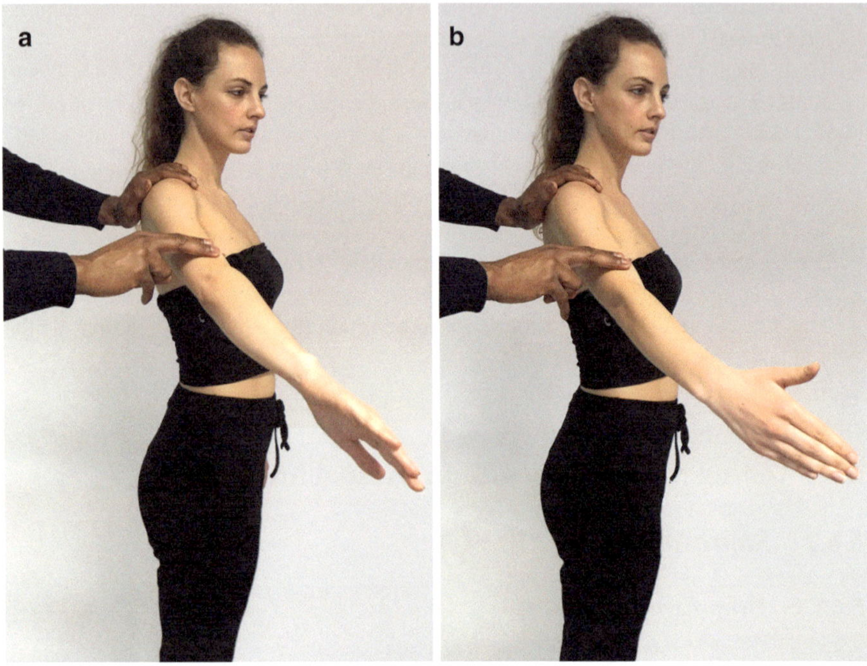

In cases of massive supraspinatus tendon rupture, whereby arm forward elevation or abduction cannot be initiated, if the arm is assisted passively for the first 15–30° of motion, the deltoid may then take over and complete the movement. The patient may be able to demonstrate that they assist their bad arm with the opposite good one in the initiation of motion, or the examiner may assist the patient in this initial stage. Similarly, some patients learn to use their upper body to throw their arm forwards to a degree that the deltoid can take over and further elevate the arm, hence compensating for the loss of supraspinatus.

In cases of supraspinatus dysfunction, the patient may (a) throw the weak arm forwards using their body or (b) may assist the weak arm with the opposite arm in early elevation to facilitate the initiation of further active motion

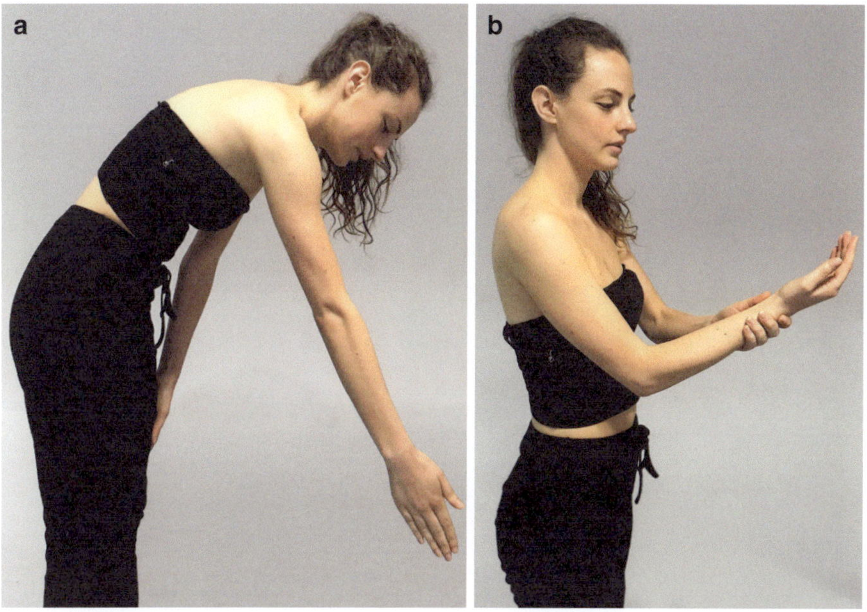

5.6.2 *Infraspinatus and Teres Minor*

5.6.2.1 Infraspinatus External Rotation Lag Sign [11, 13]

With the patient standing, the elbow is flexed at 90°, with the elbow kept by the trunk (or with the arm elevated 20° in the scapular plane). The arm is passively externally rotated to the maximum that can be achieved, and the patient is asked to hold this position once the examiner lets go. The test is positive if the patient is unable to hold the arm in this position, and the arm internally rotates back towards the trunk.

External rotation lag test – the examiner places patient's arm passively in external rotation. When the examiner lets go, the arm cannot stay in the preposition and drifts towards internal rotation

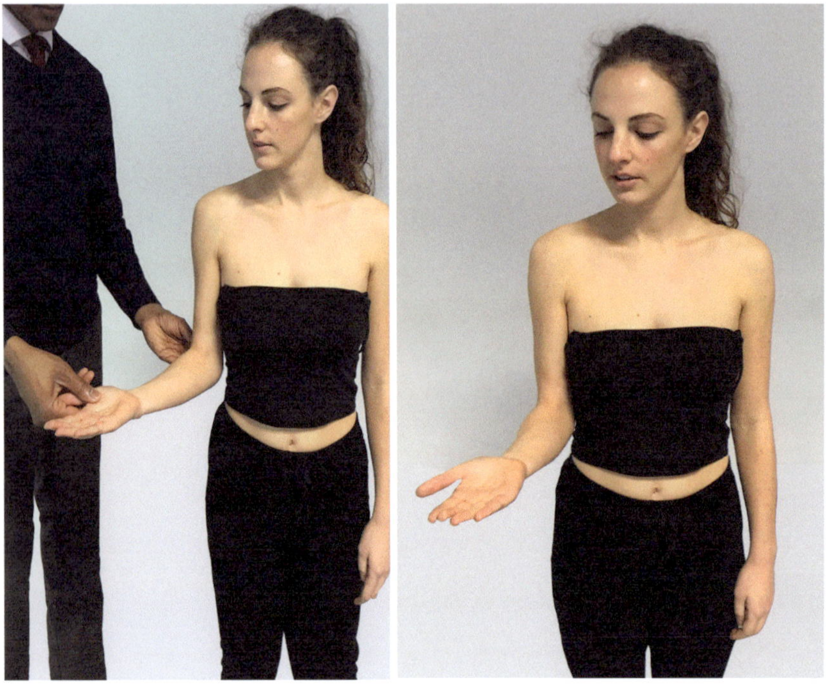

5.6.2.2 Hornblower's Sign [13, 14]

The patient is asked to bring the hand to their mouth, and the examiner observes as to whether this is achieved or how it is achieved. This sign is positive when in order to achieve this motion, the patient abducts the affected arm to raise the elbow to the same or higher than the hand level. This is due to lack of active external rotation of the shoulder. Such an external rotation deficit can hinder or prevent eating and drinking.

Hornblower's sign: (a, b) Patient can bring the hand to mouth on left but not right side, (c) On the right the hand can reach the mouth only by abductive the shoulder

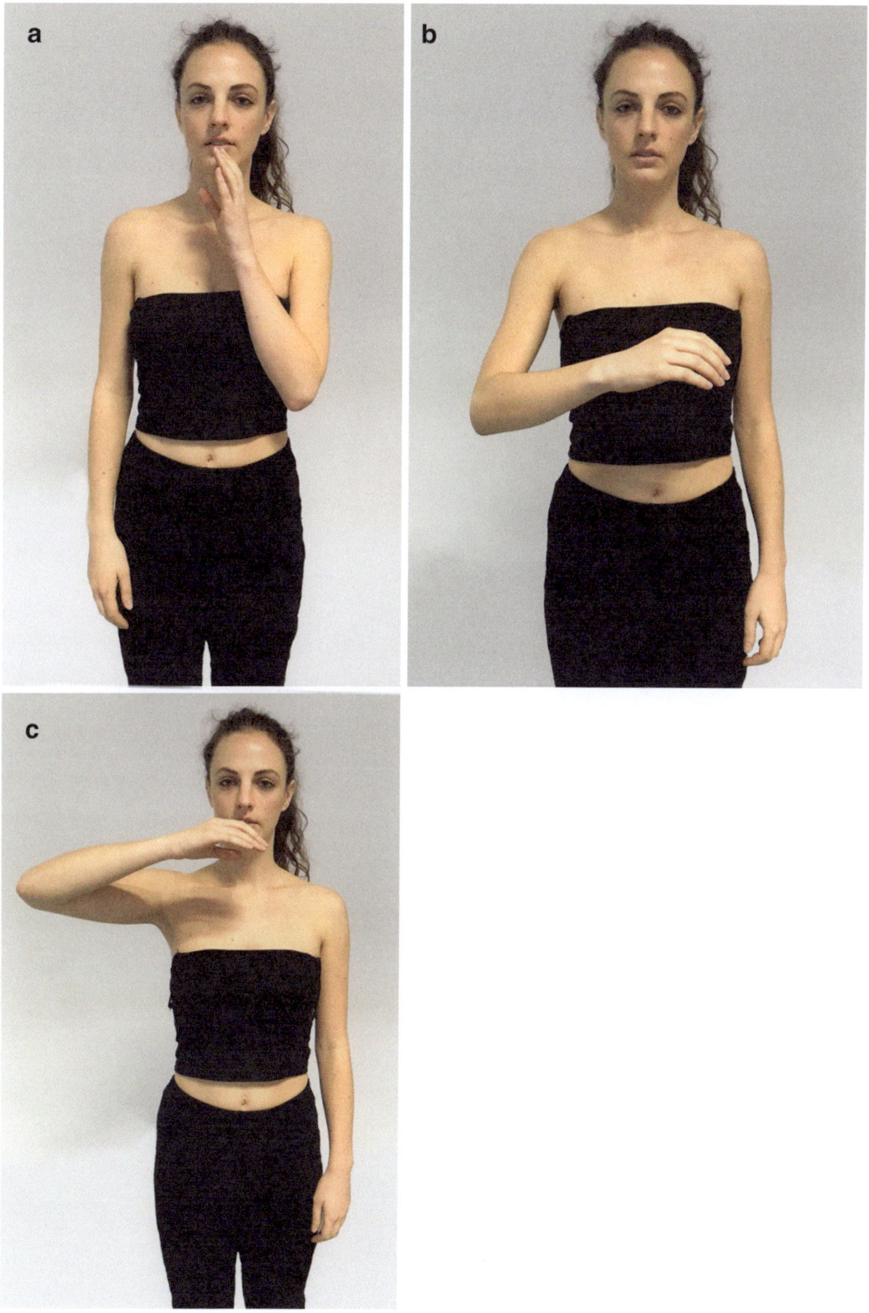

Hornblower's sign on right arm

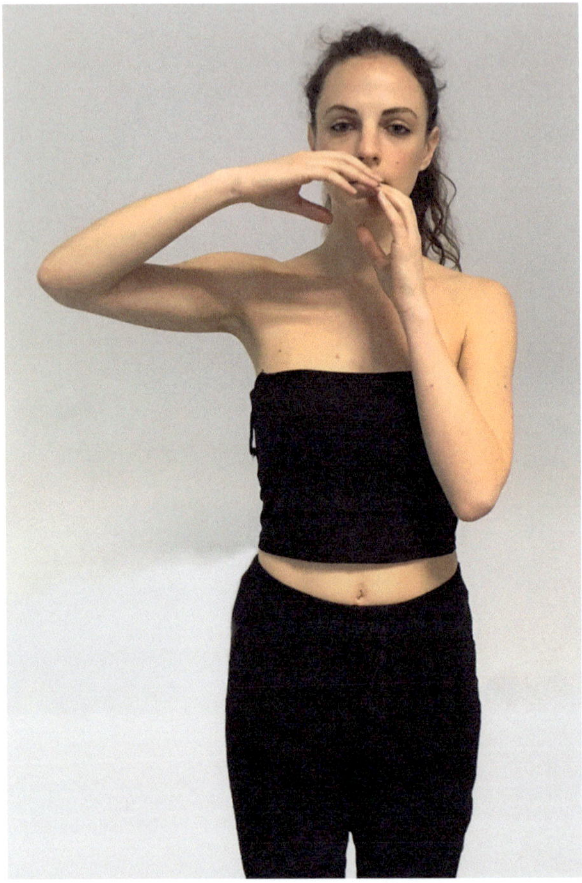

5.6.2.3 Infraspinatus Resistance Strength Test [13]

With the patient standing, the elbow is flexed at 90° and placed by the trunk. The shoulder is externally rotated 45°. The patient is asked to maintain this position, whilst the examiner applies an internal rotation force to the distal forearm.

External rotation resistance strength test for infraspinatus

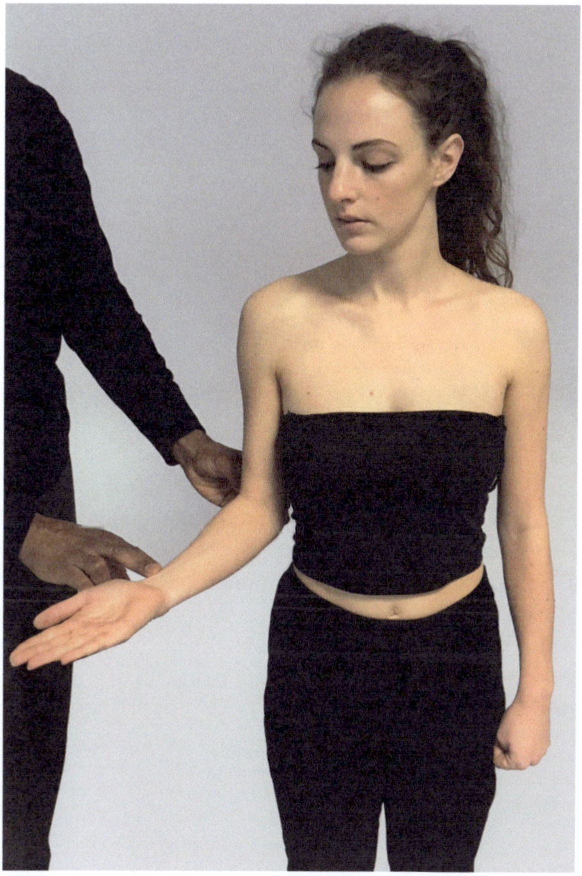

5.6.2.4 External Rotation Strength at 90° of Abduction [13]

The patient's arm is passively elevated to 90° of abduction in the scapular plane. The elbow is then flexed to 90°, and the patient is asked to externally rotate the shoulder. The patient is asked to maintain the arm in external rotation resisting an internal rotation force applied by the examiner.

The main external rotators of the shoulder are the infraspinatus and teres minor. Teres minor may be responsible for up to 45% of the power of external rotation.

Hence, in the presence of a massive infraspinatus tear, an intact teres minor can contribute enough power to external rotation to avoid the Hornblower's sign.

By assessing the external rotation lag sign and Hornblower's sign, the extent of external rotators dysfunction may be determined:

- External rotation lag sign positive – suggestive of substantial tear of infraspinatus
- Hornblower's sign positive – substantial tear of infraspinatus and teres minor

Left arm external rotation weakness and positive Hornblower's sign

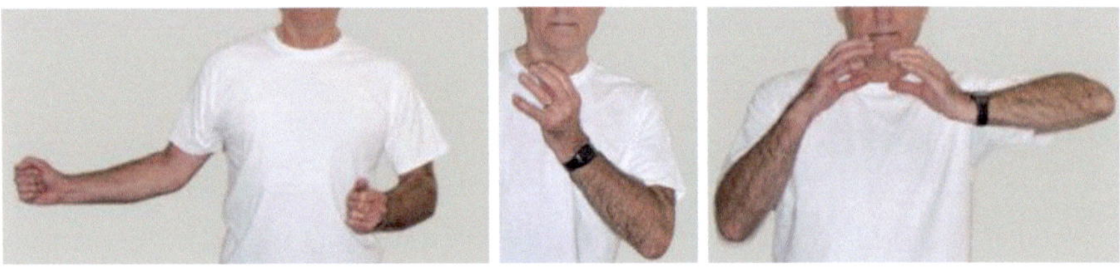

5.6.3 *Subscapularis*

5.6.3.1 **Belly-Off Lag Sign** [15]

The arm of the patient is brought passively into flexion and maximum internal rotation, with the elbow flexed 90°. The elbow of the patient is supported in this position by one hand of the examiner, whilst the examiner's other hand presses the patient's hand on the patient's abdomen. The patient is then asked to maintain that position with the wrist straight as the examiner releases the hand whilst still supporting the elbow. The test is positive if the patient cannot maintain that position and the hand lifts off the abdomen.

5.6.3.2 **Belly Press Test** [16]

The arm is on the side of the body with the elbow flexed 90°. The patient is asked to press their hand against the belly whilst keeping the wrist straight and the elbow forwards and, hence, the forearm at 90° with the trunk. In this position the shoulder is rotated internally. The patient is asked to hold the arm in this position. The test is positive if the patient cannot maintain pressure with the wrist straight and elbow forwards (with arm internally rotated) and if pressure can only be exerted with extension of the shoulder, the elbow dropping backwards and the wrist flexing.

If the patient can achieve and maintain this position, strength is further tested by applying a distracting force. The patient is asked to hold the arm in this position and resist a force applied by the examiner trying to lift the patient's hand off their belly. In this way the pressing force (internal rotation strength) that can be applied by the patient is assessed and compared to the opposite side.

Belly press test for subscapularis

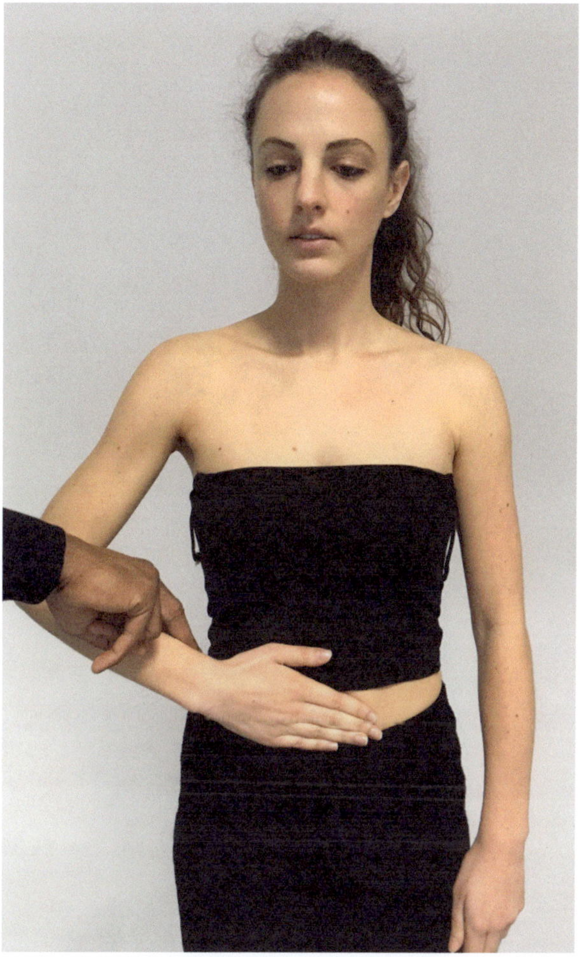

Subscapularis tear of the right shoulder. Patient can only press on the abdomen by arm extension and wrist flexion

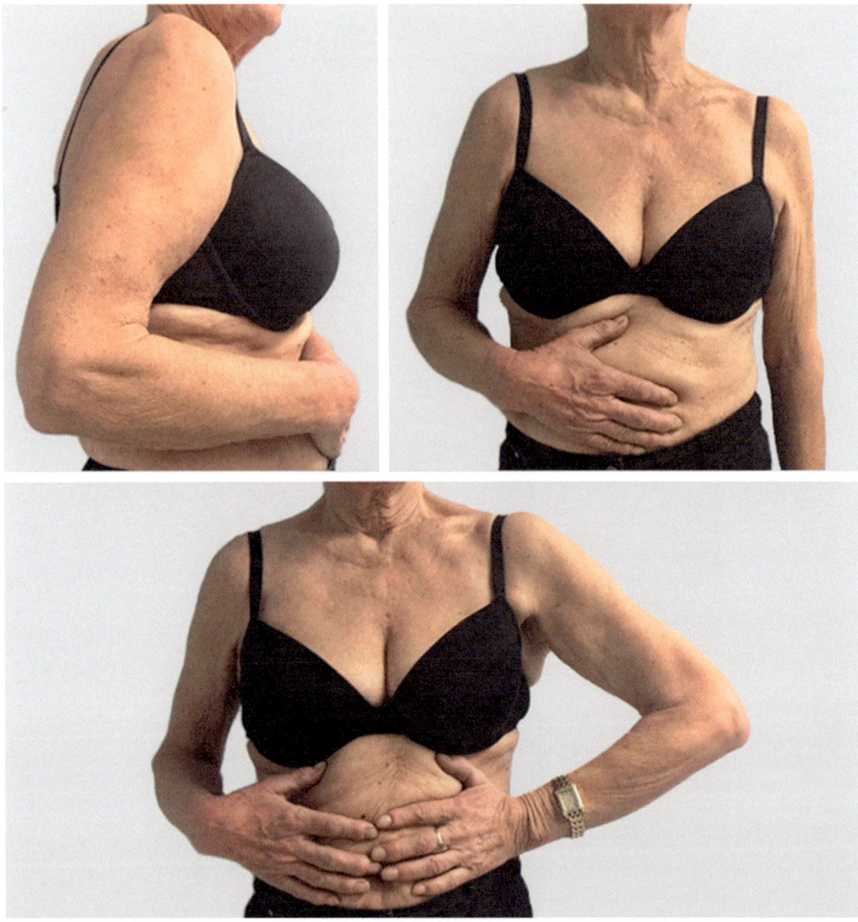

5.6.3.3 Internal Rotation Lag Sign [11]

The patient is asked to put their hand on their lower back with the back of the hand touching the lumbar region. In this position the arm is internally rotated and extended. The hand is passively lifted away from the body, and the patient is asked to maintain this position. The sign is positive when this position cannot be maintained and the hand drops back. In this position the subscapularis is the main internal rotator helping to isolate its effects from those of latissimus dorsi and pectoralis major. If the patient is unable to hold their hand off the back, it is suggestive of subscapularis tear.

5.6.3.4 Lift-Off Test [17]

The patient is asked to put their hand on their lower back with the back of the hand touching the lumbar region. In this position the arm is internally rotated and extended. The patient is then asked to raise the hand off the back. The test is positive if the patient is not able to raise the arm posteriorly off the back. If the patient can lift the hand, the patient is asked to maintain that position whilst the examiner applies an anterior force to the hand, assessing muscle strength.

The internal rotation lag sign and lift-off test may be difficult to perform because of pain on internal rotation of the arm or restricted motion. The belly press test, whereby the arm is placed in internal rotation with the hand in front of the body, may be easier to perform.

Lift-off test for subscapularis

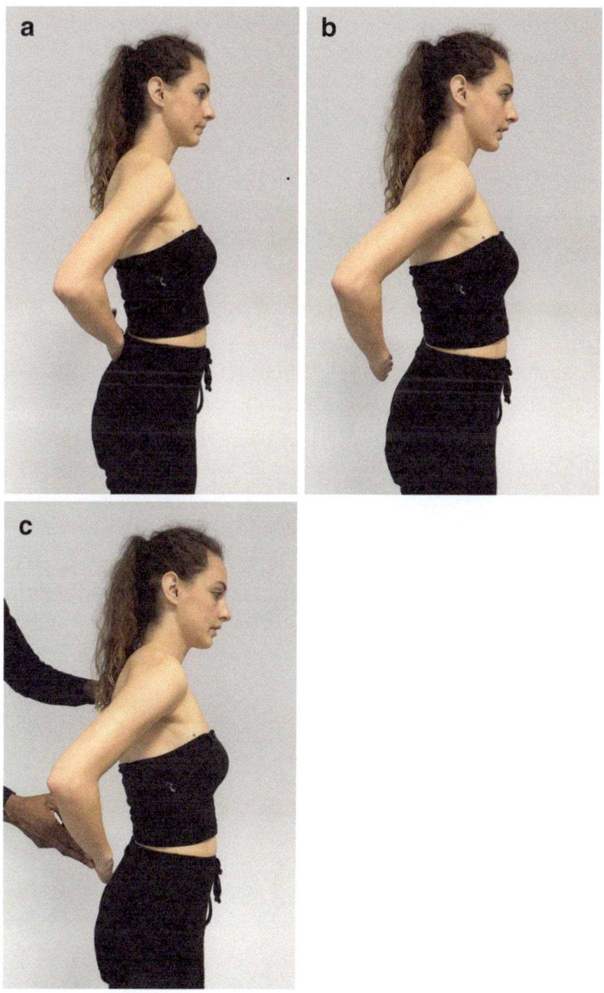

5.6.4 Rhomboids

5.6.4.1 Rhomboids Resistance Test [18]

The patient is facing away from the examiner. The arms are placed in 90° abduction and slight internal rotation with the elbows in 90° flexion. The examiner presses on the patient's posterior aspect of the arm (just above the elbow) and applies an anterior/medial directed force, which the patient is asked to resist.

5.6.5 Trapezius

5.6.5.1 Shrug Test [19]

The patient shrugs their shoulders against a downward force applied by the examiner. This tests the upper trapezius.

5.7 Pain Provoking Tests

5.7.1 Subacromial Pain Provoking Tests

5.7.1.1 Painful Arc Sign [20]

This describes a range of motion which brings on or worsens pain. With the patient standing the patient is asked to actively abduct the arm in the scapular plane up to full elevation and then bring the arm back down. Pain felt on the lateral aspect of the upper arm in the region of the deltoid muscle and its insertion between 60° and 120° of elevation is suggestive of subacromial origin. In contrast, a painful arc from 120° to 180° elevation, felt over the top of the shoulder, is suggestive of ACJt origin. On occasions more pain is experienced during arm descend as compared to ascend. The manoeuvre may be repeated with the arm in external rotation, and then in internal rotation.

Painful arc on arm abduction. Low arc is suggestive of subacromial pain. A high arc is suggestive of ACJt pain

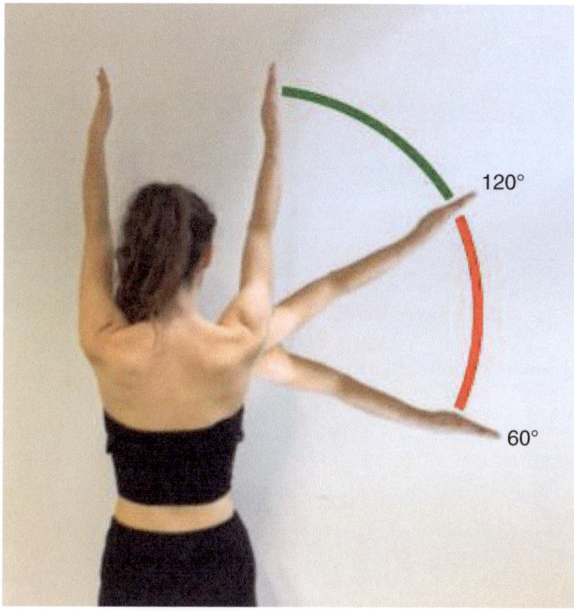

5.7.1.2 Neer Impingement Sign [21]

The patient's arm is placed in the scapular plane with the thumb facing downwards (internal rotation). The examiner stabilises the patient's scapula and then passively elevates the patient's arm in the scapular plane until the patient reports new or worse pain or until full elevation is achieved. The test is considered positive if pain is reported in the anterior or lateral part of the shoulder typically occurring between 60° and 120° of elevation. The same manoeuvre is then repeated with the patient's arm in external rotation (thumb facing upwards) which is expected to cause less pain.

Subacromial impingement test with the arm in internal (a) and external (b) rotation

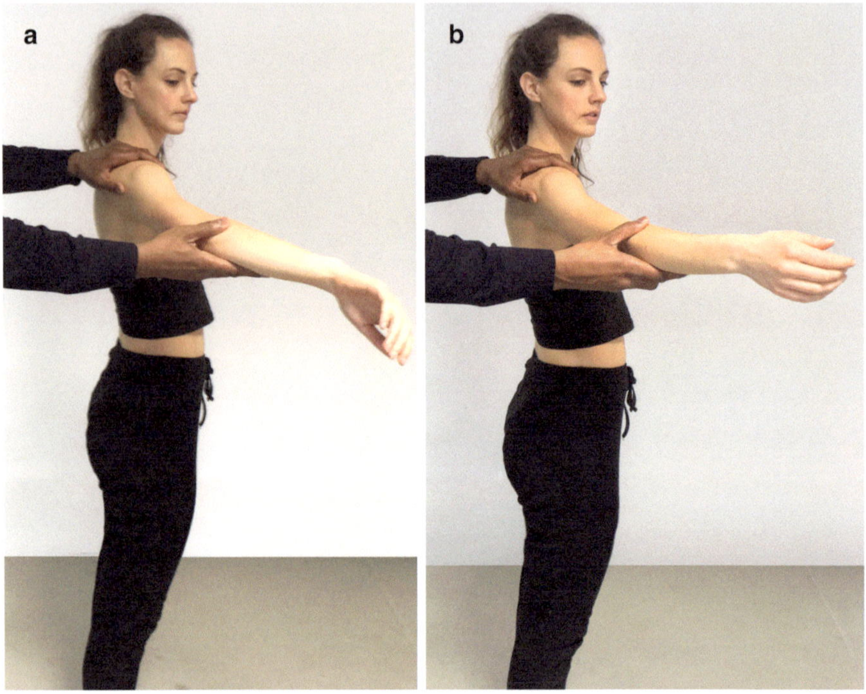

Injection of local anaesthetic (such as lignocaine) in the subacromial space may improve or eliminate this pain during the above manoeuvre. This is known as the Neer impingement test which further helps to confirm the subacromial origin of the pain.

5.7.1.3 Hawkins-Kennedy Impingement Test [22]

The arm is passively elevated forwards to 90°, and with the elbow flexed 90°, the arm is placed into internal rotation. The test is positive if such internal rotation causes pain. The test may be repeated in various positions of the arm from 90° of pure abduction to 90° forward elevation.

Hawkins-Kennedy test with the arm in forward elevation (a, b) and with the arm in abduction (c)

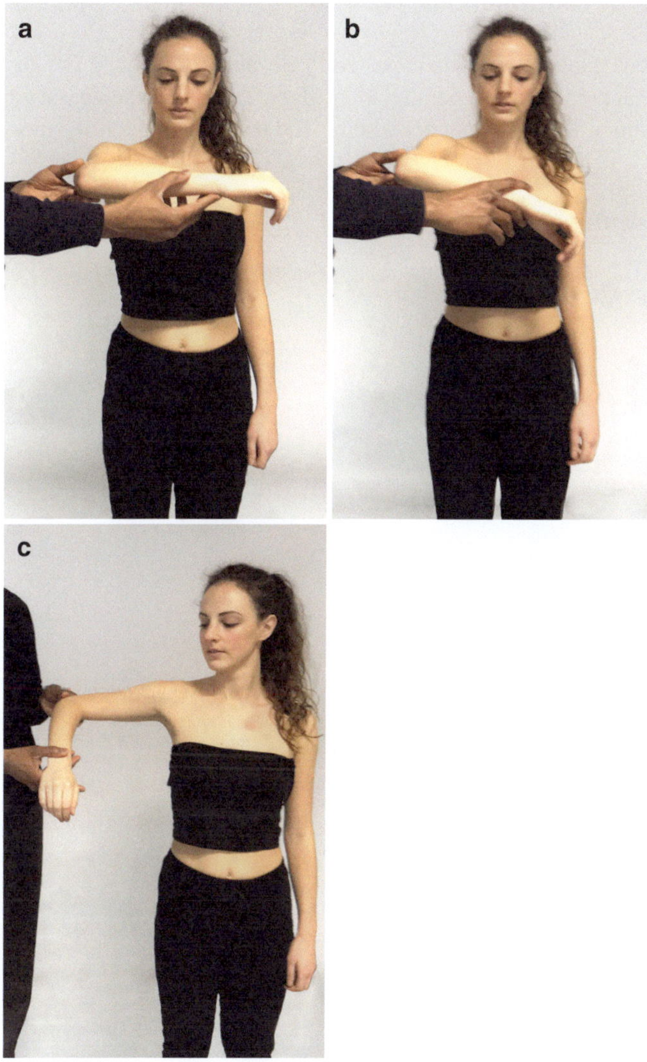

5.7.2 ACJt Pain Provoking Tests

5.7.2.1 Cross-Body Adduction Test [23]

With a patient standing, the arm is passively elevated forwards to 90° and internally rotated so that the forearm is parallel to the floor. The arm is then passively adducted by the examiner across the patient's body. The test is positive if it causes pain over the ACJt.

Cross adduction test

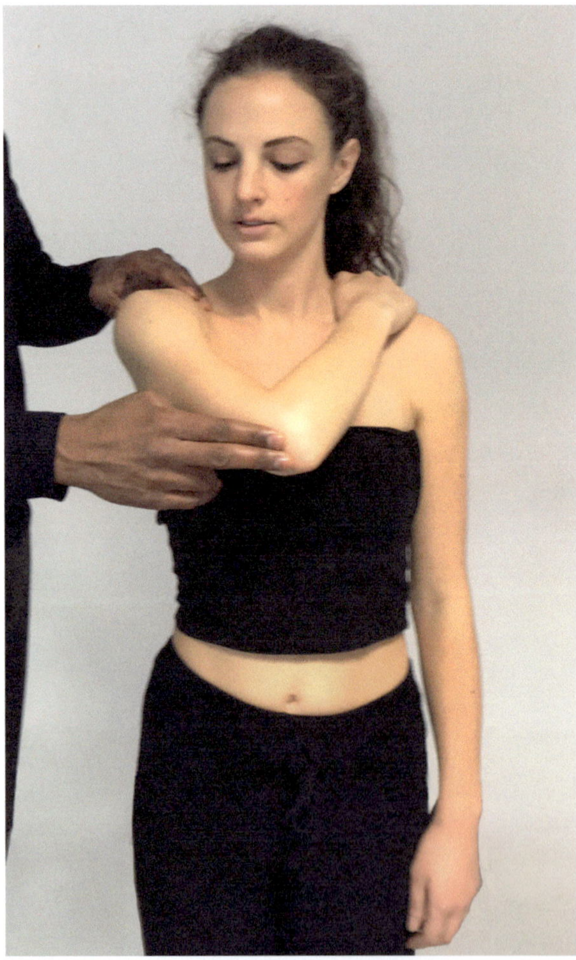

5.7.2.2 **Paxinos Sign** [24]

The patient is sitting with the affected arm by the side. The examiner places one hand over the shoulder with the thumb on the posterolateral part of the acromion. The examiner's opposite index finger is placed over the superior mid-part of the clavicle. The examiner applies pressure to the acromion in an antero-superior direction and to the clavicle in an inferior direction. The test is positive if it causes or aggravates pain in the ACJt.

5.7.3 Labrum Tear Pain Provoking Tests

5.7.3.1 **O'Brien's Test for Superior Labrum Anterior Posterior (SLAP) Tear** [25]

With the patient standing, the arm is elevated forwards to 90° and placed at 10–15° of adduction and full internal rotation (thumb pointing down). The patient is asked to hold the arm in that position and resist a downward force applied by the examiner over the distal forearm. This is repeated with the arm in the same position but in full external rotation (palm facing upwards). The test is positive if the first manoeuvre causes or aggravates pain which improves with the latter manoeuvre. The location of experienced pain may guide towards its origin:

- Pain felt deeply in the glenohumeral joint is suggestive of labrum tear
- Pain felt over the ACJt is suggestive of ACJt arthropathy

O'Brien's test

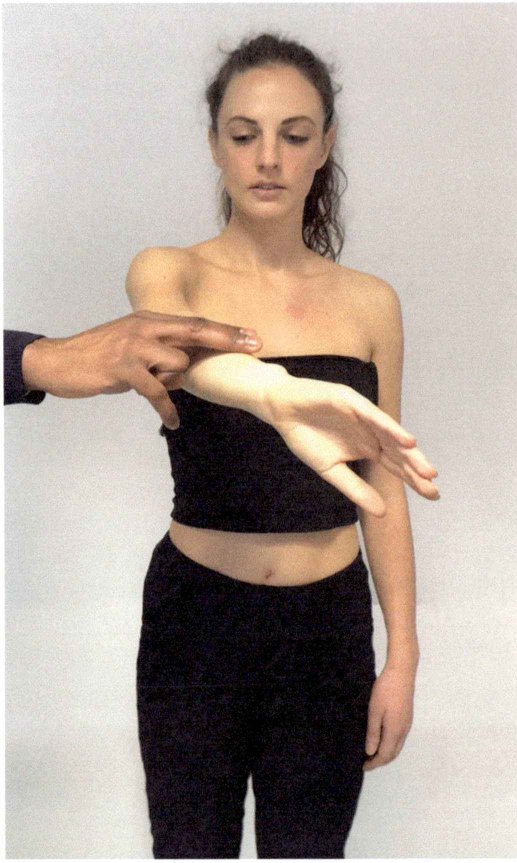

5.7.3.2 Jerk Test for Posterior Labrum Tear [26]

This aims to displace the humeral head posteriorly. The patient is sitting. The examiner stabilises the scapula with one hand. With the other hand, the examiner abducts the patient's arm to 90° and internally rotates it to 90°. A posterior directed axial force is then applied whilst bringing the arm into adduction. The test is suggestive of the presence of a posterior labrum lesion if this manoeuvrer causes a sharp glenohumeral pain.

5.7.3.3 Kim's Test for Posterior-Inferior Labrum Tear [27]

- The patient is sitting against the back of a chair. The arm is placed in 90° of abduction and internal rotation with the elbow flexed to 90°. The examiner holds the patient's elbow and proximal arm and flexes the arm forwards by 45° whilst applying an axial posterior and inferior force on the proximal arm. The arm is then taken into adduction. The test is positive if this causes posterior shoulder pain with or without a posterior clunk of the humeral head. Essentially Kim's test is a variation of the Jerk test that assesses the posterior-inferior part of the labrum (rather than the posterior labrum) due to the application of an inferior force. During the test the humeral head is also compressed onto the glenoid

5.7.4 Long Head of Biceps Tendon Pain Provoking Tests

5.7.4.1 **Speed's Test** [28]

The arm is elevated forwards to 90° with the elbow fully extended and the forearm supinated (palm facing upwards). The examiner applies a downward force to the forearm which the patient is asked to resist. The test is positive if the patient experiences pain in the bicipital groove area.

Speed's test

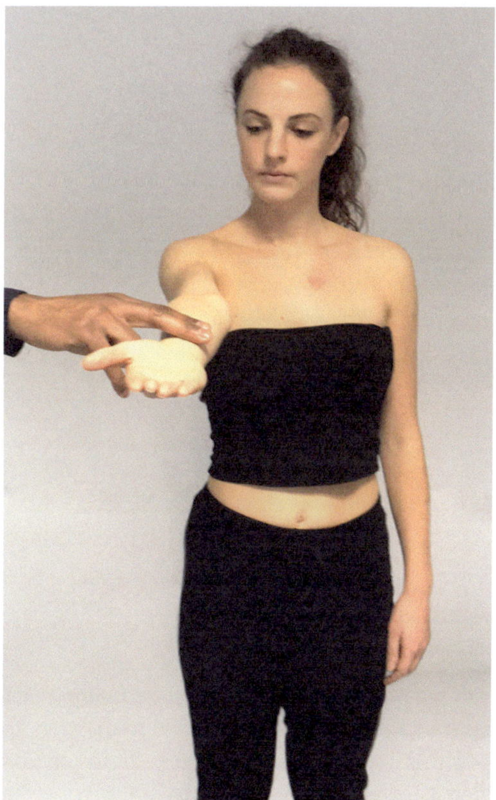

5.7.4.2 Yergason's Test [29]

With the arm by the side and the elbow flexed 90°, the patient is asked to maintain the elbow in full supination against a pronating force applied by the examiner. The test is positive if the patient experiences pain in the bicipital groove area.

Yergason's test

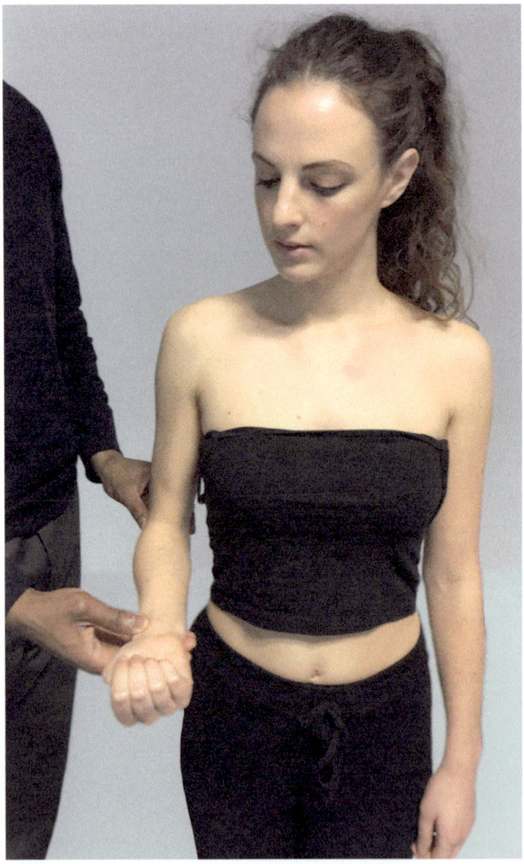

5.8 Laxity Assessment

Hyper-laxity refers to the presence of excessive joint laxity (excessive joint translation or motion). This may be described with regard to the glenohumeral joint of the shoulder as excessive translation of the humeral head in relation to the glenoid. It may also be described as generalised hyper-laxity if it involves multiple joints. The following tests may be used in the assessment of laxity.

5.8.1 *Assessment of Shoulder Laxity*

5.8.1.1 Load and Shift Test [30]

With one hand the examiner supports the patient's arm at about 20° abduction, 20° forward elevation and neutral rotation. With the other hand, the examiner grasps the humeral head between their thumb and index and applies stress in an anterior and then posterior direction to determine the maximum amount of humeral translation that can be achieved in relation to the glenoid and glenoid rim. For a posterior stress, the examiner pushes the humeral head backwards. For anterior stress the examiner pushes the humeral head forwards.

Load and shift test for glenohumeral laxity

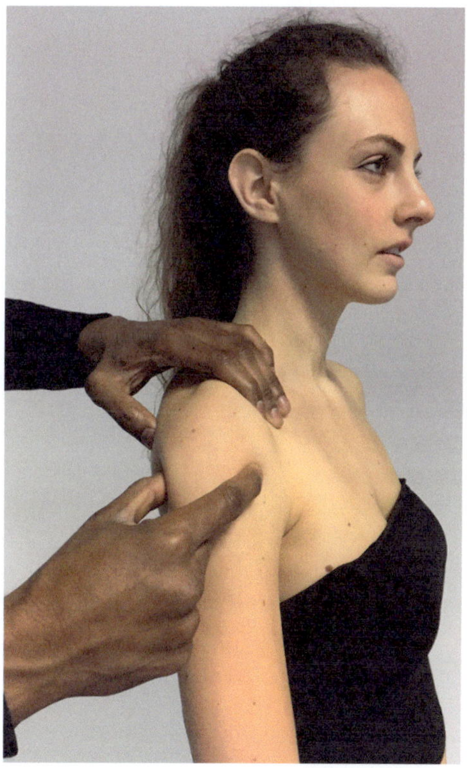

Translation may also be assessed with the arm in 90° of abduction and external rotation (at this position tension of the intact ligaments is expected to limit the amount of achievable anterior translation).

Humeral head translation may be described as:

- Moves forwards but does not sublux
- Subluxes but does not dislocate

- Dislocates but reduces upon removal of the distracting force
- Dislocates but does not reduce upon removal of the distracting force

5.8.1.2 Excessive or Increased External Rotation of the Arm [17, 31]

Excessive or increased passive external rotation of the arm, as compared to the opposite side, with the elbow flexed 90° and pressed to the patient's trunk, is suggestive of anterior laxity or a ruptured subscapularis tendon.

5.8.1.3 Gagey's Sign [32]

With the scapula stabilised by the examiner's forearm, the examiner takes the patient's arm into abduction with the elbow flexed to 90° and the forearm horizontal. Abduction of the glenohumeral joint that is greater than 105° or greater by more than 20° compared to the opposite side is suggestive of inferior glenohumeral laxity.

5.8.1.4 Inferior Sulcus Sign [33, 34]

With the arm by the side in neutral position and the elbow flexed 90°, a longitudinal downwards pull is applied by the examiner on the arm. The shoulder is observed for the development of a sulcus on its lateral aspect between the acromion and humeral head. An inferior humeral head displacement greater than 1 cm from the acromion is suggestive of inferior laxity. Repeating this manoeuvre with the arm placed in 30° of external rotation evaluates any deficiency of the rotator interval or the superior glenohumeral ligament. The inferior sulcus sign may be graded as:

Mild – <1 cm translation
Moderate – 1–2 cm translation
Severe – >2 cm translation

5.8.2 Assessment of Generalised Joint Hyper-laxity

5.8.2.1 Beighton Score [35, 36]

The subject is examined for the presence of the following:

1. Passive dorsiflexion of the little finger beyond 90°
2. Passive thumb opposition to the flexor aspect of the forearm
3. Active elbow hyperextension beyond 10° – patient asked to push elbows as straight as possible
4. Active knee hyperextension beyond 10 – patient asked to push knees as straight as possible
5. Forward flexion of the trunk – patient asked to bend and touch the palms of the hands flat on the floor whilst keeping the knees straight

(a) Little finger hyperextension at the metacarpophalangeal joint

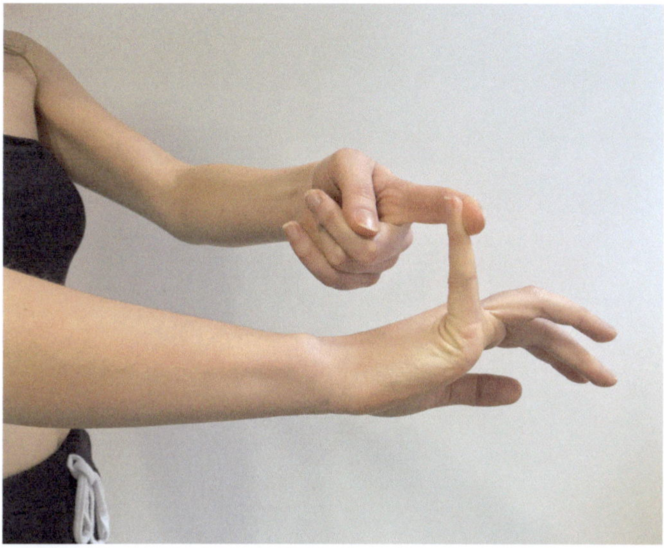

(b) Thumb touching forearm

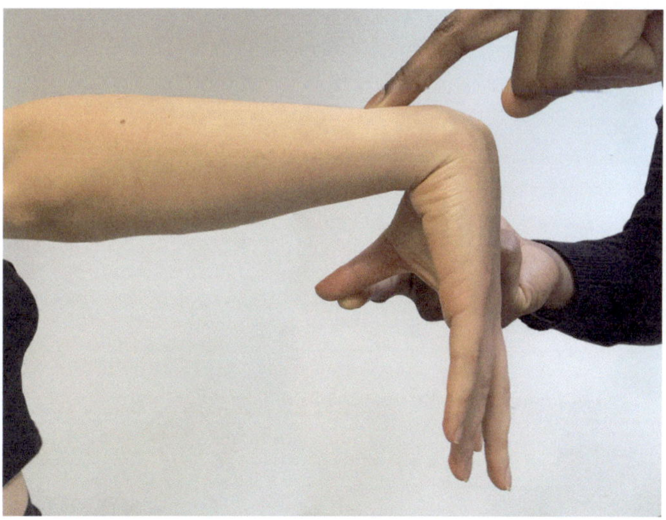

(c) Elbow hyperextension

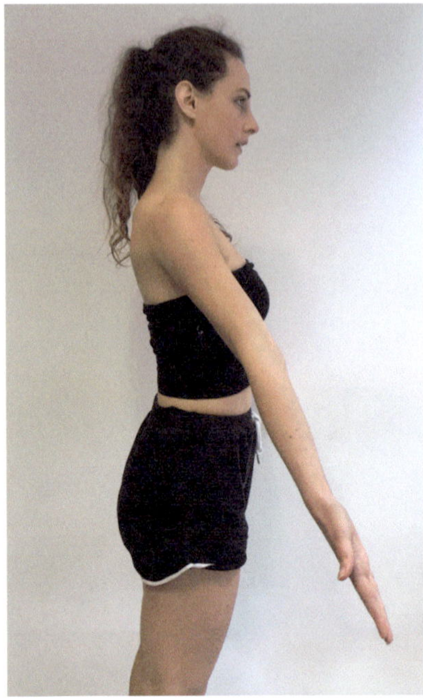

(d) Knee hyperextension

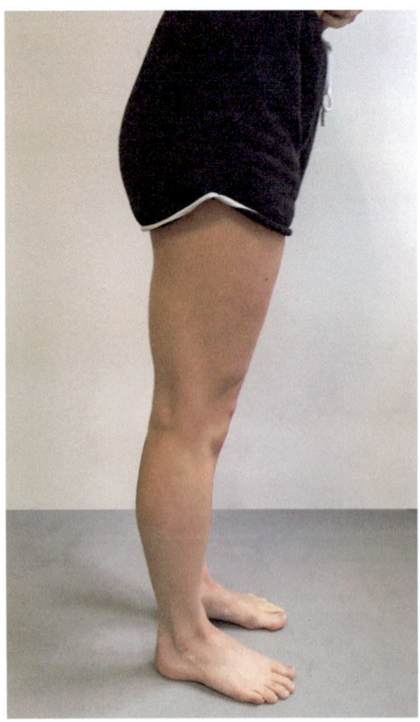

(e) Ability to put palms flat on floor with knees straight

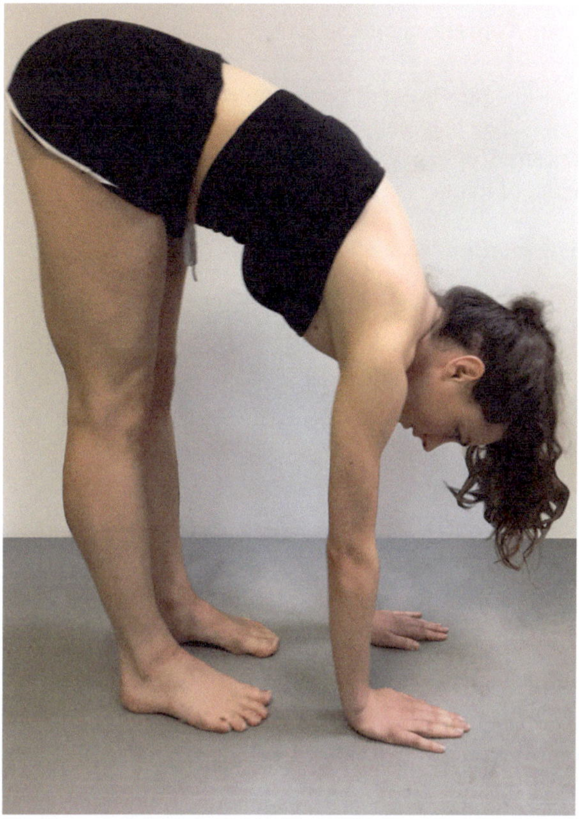

The presence of each of the first four components scores one point for the left and right side, and the presence of the fifth component scores one point, giving a maximum potential score of nine. A score greater than six in adults is suggestive of hyper-laxity.

5.9 Shoulder Instability Tests

Instability refers to joint translation that regardless of its degree cannot be controlled and causes clinical symptoms. Special tests for glenohumeral instability aim to determine if there is symptomatic anterior, posterior or inferior instability. In addition, they try to determine potential contributors to such instability such as abnormal muscle patterning or hyper-laxity.

5.9.1 Tests for Anterior Glenohumeral Instability

5.9.1.1 Anterior Apprehension Test [37, 38]

With the patient standing, sitting or lying supine, the arm is passively placed in 90° of abduction and is then externally rotated as far as possible. The test is positive if this manoeuvre causes or aggravates shoulder discomfort or apprehension that the arm may move out of joint.

Anterior instability apprehension test

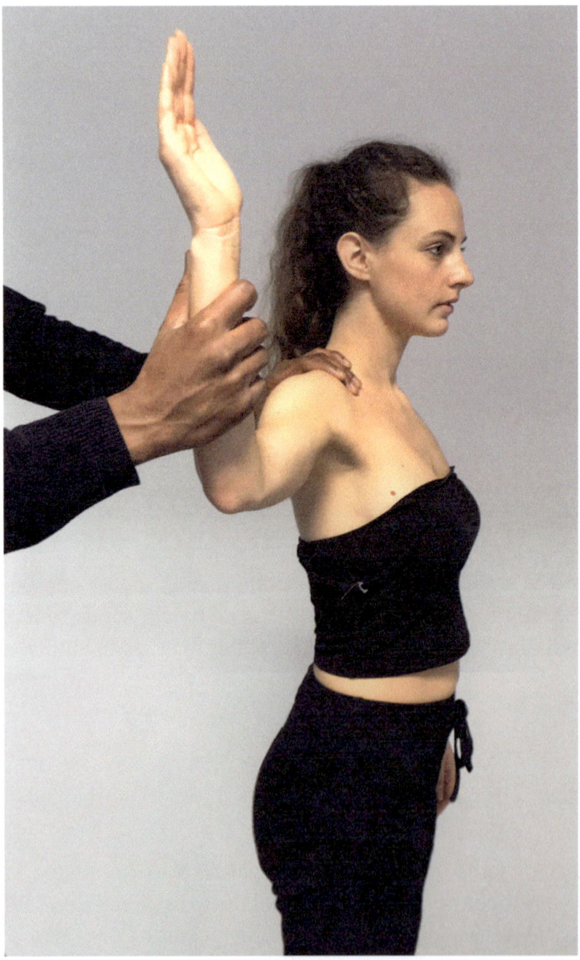

5.9.1.2 Anterior Relocation/Release Test [38, 39]

With the patient standing, sitting or lying supine, the arm is passively placed in 90° of abduction and is then externally rotated. Discomfort or apprehension experienced by the patient in this position is improved by the application of a posterior force on the humeral head by the examiner's hand (relocation). However, subsequent sudden release of this posterior force aggravates the patient's symptoms.

Anterior instability relocation test

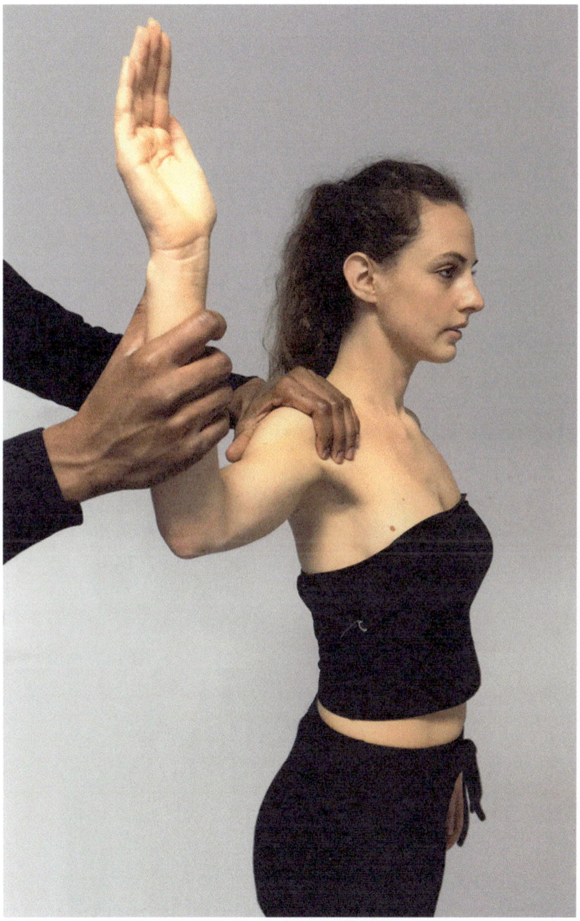

5.9.2 *Tests for Posterior Glenohumeral Instability*

5.9.2.1 **Posterior Apprehension Test** [40]

The patient is standing, sitting or lying supine. The examiner elevates forwards the patient's arm to 90° and internally rotates the arm whilst using the other hand to stabilise the scapula. The patient exhibits apprehension or symptoms of instability. If the above does not elicit apprehension or symptoms of instability, the manoeuvre may be repeated with the additional application of arm adduction.

5.9.2.2 **Jerk Test for Posterior Instability** [27]

This aims to displace the humeral head posteriorly. The patient is sitting. The examiner stabilises the scapula with one hand. With the other hand, the examiner abducts the arm to 90° and internally rotates the arm to 90° and then applies posterior axial loading and adduction to the arm. The test is positive if this manoeuvrer causes a palpable clunk or click of the humeral head. The arm is then passively brought back into abduction and neutral (or external) rotation which may cause a palpable clunk as the shoulder relocates. Often, the clunk of the relocation is more easily felt than the initial clunk of the dislocation.

5.9.2.3 **Posterior Kim's Test for Posterior-Inferior Instability** [26]

The patient is sitting against the back of a chair. The arm is placed in 90° of abduction and internal rotation with the elbow flexed at 90°. The examiner holds the patient's elbow and proximal arm and flexes the arm forwards by 45° whilst applying a posterior and inferior force on the proximal arm. The arm is then taken into adduction. The test is positive for posterior-inferior instability if it causes a posterior clunk of the humeral head. Essentially Kim's test is a variation of the Jerk test that assesses the posterior-inferior part of the labrum (rather than the posterior labrum) due to the application of an inferior force.

5.9.2.4 **Posterior Instability Test**

The patient is standing or sitting. The patients arm is passively placed in 90° forward elevation, internal rotation and adduction. The arm is then brought into abduction and external rotation. The humeral head may be felt or heard dislocating posteriorly during the first part of the manoeuvre or relocating during the second part of the manoeuvre.

Posterior instability test

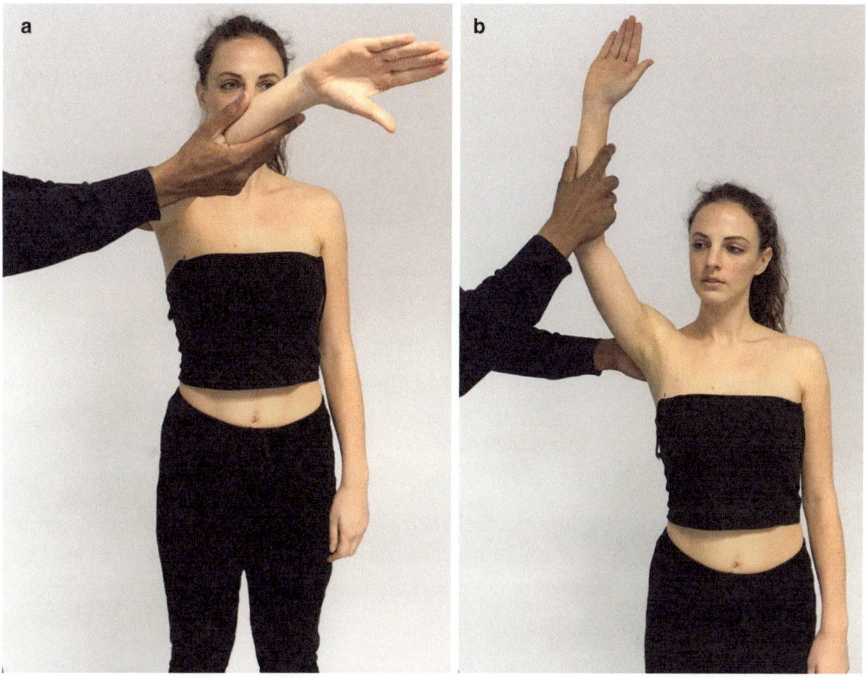

5.9.3 Tests for Inferior Glenohumeral Instability

5.9.3.1 Inferior Sulcus Test [41]

With the arm by the side in neutral position and the elbow flexed to 90°, a longitudinal downwards pull is applied by the examiner on the arm. The shoulder is observed for the development of a sulcus on its lateral aspect between the acromion and humeral head. An inferior humeral head displacement greater than 1 cm from the acromion is suggestive of inferior laxity. It indicates inferior instability if it causes pain, apprehension or symptoms of instability.

5.9.4 *Testing for Abnormal Motion-Driven Glenohumeral Instability* [42, 43]

The patient is asked to perform active arm motion (forward elevation, abduction), whilst the trunk, chest, cervical and thoracic spine are observed for:

- Abnormal movement such as trunk, neck or thoracic side flexion, lumbar extension
- Scapular dysrhythmia – winging, downward scapular rotation
- Abnormal arm motion – internal rotation, elbow extension

The patient is asked to repeat the arm motion, whilst the examiner attempts to correct any aberrant motion such as by:

- Opposing neck or thoracic motion
- Pushing the medial border of the scapula against the chest wall to reduce winging
- Pushing the scapula into upward rotation
- Getting the patient to actively shrug the shoulders to rotate the scapula upwards

If the above manoeuvres improve the arm motion, then this may suggest that correction of any aberrant spinal or scapular movements may improve glenohumeral instability; this can then be incorporated into a physiotherapy regime the patient is prescribed.

5.9.5 *Testing for Abnormal Muscle Patterning*

The patient is asked to move the arm (forward elevation, adduction, abduction and external rotation):

- The examiner observes and palpates the pectoralis major and latissimus dorsi for overactivity – suggestive of muscle patterning
- Whilst attempting forward elevation, the patient also pushes against the examiner's hand applying an external rotation force to compensate for any deficiency in the external rotation activity of infraspinatus – an improvement in forward arm motion is suggestive of infraspinatus underactivity

5.9.5.1 **Hand Squeeze Test** [44]

The hand squeeze test tests for muscle patterning instability. Squeezing the examiner's hand distracts the patient's attention from the affected shoulder, diminishing or abolishing any abnormal muscle activation. The patient elevates the examined arm in pronation, and the shoulder is observed for any posterior humeral head displacement. The patient is then asked to squeeze as hard as possible the examiner's opposite hand with the opposite hand, whilst the affected arm is elevated as previously. The test is regarded positive, if during squeezing with the contralateral hand and elevation of the involved arm, no posterior shoulder dislocation occurs and is suggestive of muscle patterning being a major contributor to the instability. The test is negative if posterior dislocation occurs despite the "hand squeeze".

5.9.6 *Cervical Spine Tests*

5.9.6.1 **Spurling's Test for Cervical Radiculopathy** [45, 46]

The patient is seated. The examiner flexes the patient's cervical spine towards the affected side whilst applying axial compression. The test is positive if it reproduces or worsens the patient's radiculopathy symptoms (pain, paraesthesia radiating down the upper limb).

The test may also be performed by utilising:

- Cervical spine ipsilateral lateral bending, extension and axial compression
- Cervical spine ipsilateral lateral bending, ipsilateral rotation and axial compression

Spurling's test of the cervical spine with no cervical spine rotation (a), with ipsilateral rotation (b)

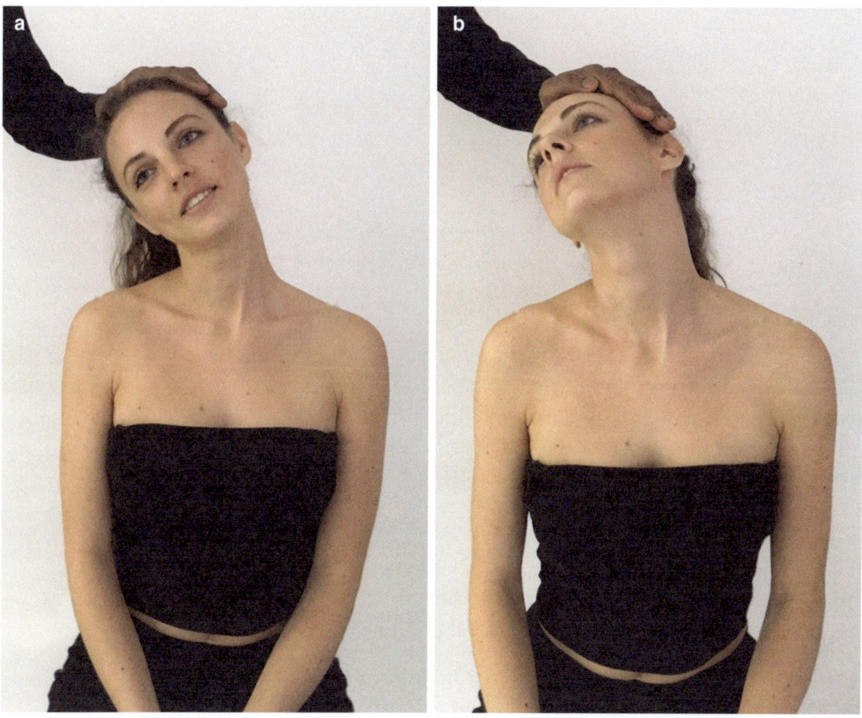

5.9.7 *Thoracic Outlet Syndrome Tests*

Several tests have been described for assessing the presence of thoracic outlet syndrome. It should be emphasised that these have a low specificity and may be positive in a high proportion of normal individuals or in individuals with a nerve lesion occurring at a site other than the thoracic outlet. However, when such tests reproduce the patient's clinical symptoms, they should raise the possibility that symptoms may be of TOS origin.

5.9.7.1 Roos' Test [47]

The patient sits looking forwards and places the arms in 90° of abduction and full external rotation with the elbows flexed 90°. The patient opens and closes the hands in this position for 3 min. The test is positive if it causes pain and paraesthesia, heaviness or hand discolouration or reproduces the patient's clinical symptoms. It tests all three sides of potential thoracic outlet entrapment.

Roos' test

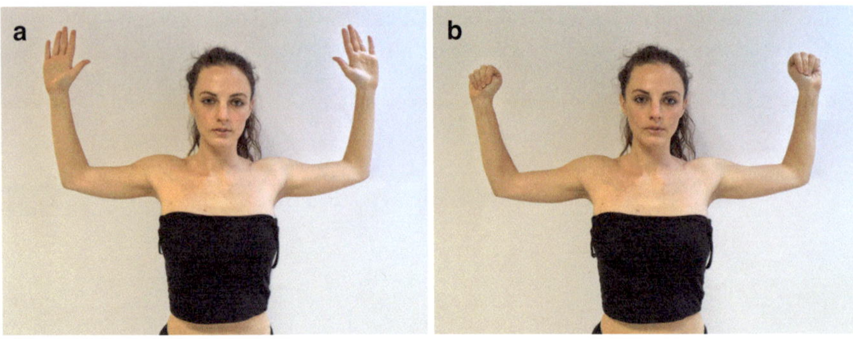

5.9.7.2 Supra-Clavicular Pressure [48]

The patient sits with the arms by the side. The examiner presses in the supraclavicular fossa over the lowest part of the anterior scalene muscle for 30 s. The test is positive if it causes pain and paraesthesia down the arm or if it reproduces the patient's clinical symptoms.

5.9.7.3 Adson's Test [49]

It assesses inter-scalene entrapment. The patient sits with the arms straight resting on their knees. The examiner palpates the radial pulse. The patient is asked to:

1. Take a deep breath in and hold that breath for as long as comfortably possible
2. Elevate the chin (extend the cervical spine)
3. Turn head to the affected side (rotate the cervical spine)

The test is positive if there is a reduction in the strength of the radial pulse or loss of the pulse or reproduction of the patient's symptoms, pain/paraesthesia.

5.9.7.4 Wright's Test [50]

Testing the sub-pectoralis minor space – the patient sits with the arms by the side. The examiner palpates the radial pulse. The patient places the arm in 90° of abduction and full external rotation with the elbow flexed 90°.

Testing the costo-clavicular space – the arm is placed in maximum abduction with the elbow straight, again testing for a reduction in the strength of the radial pulse or loss of the pulse or reproduction of the patient's symptoms.

The test is positive if there is reduction in the strength of the radial pulse or loss of the pulse or reproduction of the patient's symptoms.

5.9.7.5 Costo-Clavicular Test [51]

The patient stands with arms by the side. The radial pulse is palpated. The patient pulls the shoulders back and down whilst pushing the chest outwards (adopting a military posture position). The radial pulse is palpated again looking for a reduction in the strength of the radial pulse or loss of the pulse or reproduction of the patient's symptoms.

5.9.7.6 Upper Limb Tension Test [52]

The patient is sitting or standing and sequentially:

1. Puts arms in 90° abduction, with the elbows straight and palms facing down
2. Dorsiflexes the wrists
3. Bends the neck to touch the ear to the opposite shoulder

After each of the above stages, the patient reports any pain or paraesthesia radiating down the arm which would indicate a positive test. Each of the three steps stretches further the nerve roots of the brachial plexus. A positive test indicates compression of the nerve roots of the brachial plexus (at any side – cervical spine, thoracic outlet).

5.9.8 Core Balance Tests

Several tests may be used to screen for core weakness or inbalance and include the following [53].

5.9.8.1 Single Leg Stance

The patient is asked to stand on one leg at a time. Inability to achieve or maintain this position in a balanced way is suggestive of core weakness or inbalance. The use of the patient's arms to maintain the stance, flexion or twisting of the weight bearing leg may also indicate core weakness.

5.9.8.2 Single Leg Squat

The patient is asked to stand on one leg and do a quarter to half squat. Inability to achieve or maintain this position in a balanced way is suggestive of core weakness or inbalance. The use of the patient's arms to maintain the stance, flexion or twisting of the weight bearing leg may also indicate core weakness.

5.9.8.3 Tri-planar Core Assessment

Sagittal Plane Assessment

The patient is asked to stand about 8 cm from a wall, facing away from the wall. The patient is asked to lean backwards with legs straight until the back of the head touches the wall. This is then repeated whilst standing on one leg at a time.

Frontal Plane Assessment

The patient stands with their side about 8 cm from the wall. The patient is asked to stand on the leg close to the wall and lean towards the wall, with the leg straight, until the side of the shoulder touches the wall. This is then repeated on the other side.

Transverse Plane Assessment

The patient is asked to stand about 8 cm from a wall, facing away from the wall. The patient is asked to stand on one leg and alternately lean, with the leg straight, so as to touch the back of each shoulder on the wall. The same is then repeated by standing on the other leg.

Inability to perform the above tasks in a balanced way is suggestive of core weakness or inbalance.

Learning Pearls

- A difference in the range of passive (and active) glenohumeral motion may not necessarily reflect loss of movement on the side with less motion. It is possible for the side with greater motion to be abnormal such as:
  - Increased external rotation with the arm in abduction seen in chronic stretching of the anterior capsule in overhead throwing activities
  - Rupture of structures that act as static constrains to motion – increased external rotation in subscapularis tears (an intact subscapularis provides a constraint to external rotation)

References

1. Solomon L, Warwick D, Nayagam S. Apley's system of Orthopaedics and fractures. 9th ed. Boca Raton: CRC Press; 2010.
2. Solomon L, Apley A. Physical examination in Orthopaedics. Milton Park: Taylor & Francis; 1997.
3. Hughes PC, Taylor NF, Green RA. Most clinical tests cannot accurately diagnose rotator cuff pathology: a systematic review. Aust J Physiother. 2008;54(3):159–70.

4. Hughes PC, Green RA, Taylor NF. Isolation of infraspinatus in clinical test positions. J Sci Med Sport. 2014;17(3):256–60.
5. Hegedus EJ, Goode A, Campbell S, Morin A, Tamaddoni M, Moorman CT 3rd, Cook C. Physical examination tests of the shoulder: a systematic review with meta-analysis of individual tests. Br J Sports Med. 2008;42(2):80–92.
6. Jain NB, Luz J, Higgins LD, Dong Y, Warner JJ, Matzkin E, Katz JN. The diagnostic accuracy of special tests for rotator cuff tear: the ROW cohort study. Am J Phys Med Rehabil. 2017;96(3):176–18.
7. Sandrey MA. Special physical examination tests for superior labrum anterior-posterior shoulder tears: an examination of clinical usefulness. J Athl Train. 2013;48(6):856–8.
8. Park HB, Yokota A, Gill HS, El Rassi G, McFarland EG. Diagnostic accuracy of clinical tests for the different degrees of subacromial impingement syndrome. J Bone Joint Surg Am. 2005;87(7):1446–55.
9. Jia X, Ji JH, Pannirselvam V, Petersen SA, McFarland EG. Does a positive neer impingement sign reflect rotator cuff contact with the acromion? Clin Orthop Relat Res. 2011;469(3):813–8.
10. Medical Research Council. Aids to the investigation of the peripheral nervous system. Memorandum No. 45. Her Majesty's Stationary Office. London. 1981. Accessed at https://www.mrc.ac.uk/documents/pdf/aids-to-the-examination-of-the-peripheral-nervous-system-mrc-memorandum-no-45-superseding-war-memorandum-no-7/.
11. Hertel R, Ballmer FT, Lombert SM, Gerber C. Lag signs in the diagnosis of rotator cuff rupture. J Shoulder Elb Surg. 1996;5(4):307–13.
12. Jobe FW, Moynes DR. Delineation of diagnostic criteria and a rehabilitation program for rotator cuff injuries. Am J Sports Med. 1982;10(6):336–9.
13. Walch G, Boulahia A, Calderone S, Robinson AH. The 'dropping' and 'hornblower's' signs in evaluation of rotator-cuff tears. J Bone Joint Surg Br. 1998;80(4):624–8.
14. Arthuis M. Obstetrical paralysis of the brachial plexus. I. Diagnosis. Clinical study of the initial period. Rev Chir Orthop Reparatrice Appar Mot. 1972;58(Suppl 1):124–6.
15. Scheibel M, Magosch P, Pritsch M, Lichtenberg S, Habermeyer P. The belly-off sign: a new clinical diagnostic sign for subscapularis lesions. Arthroscopy. 2005;21(10):1229–35.
16. Gerber C, Hersche O, Farron A. Isolated rupture of the subscapularis tendon. J Bone Joint Surg Am. 1996;78(7):1015–23.
17. Gerber C, Krushell RJ. Isolated rupture of the tendon of the subscapularis muscle. Clinical features in 16 cases. J Bone Joint Surg Br. 1991;73(3):389–94.
18. Smith J, Padgett DJ, Kaufman KR, Harrington SP, An KN, Irby SE. Rhomboid muscle electromyography activity during 3 different manual muscle tests. Arch Phys Med Rehabil. 2004;85(6):987–92.
19. Ekstrom RA, Donatelli RA, Soderberg GL. Surface electromyographic analysis of exercises for the trapezius and serratus anterior muscles. J Orthop Sports Phys Ther. 2003;33(5):247–58.
20. Kessel L, Watson M. The painful arc syndrome. Clinical classification as a guide to management. J Bone Joint Surg Br. 1977;59(2):166–72.
21. Neer CS 2nd. Impingement lesions. Clin Orthop Relat Res. 1983;173:70–7.
22. Hawkins RJ, Kennedy JC. Impingement syndrome in athletes. Am J Sports Med. 1980;8(3):151–8.
23. Chronopoulos E, Kim TK, Park HB, Ashenbrenner D, McFarland EG. Diagnostic value of physical tests for isolated chronic acromioclavicular lesions. Am J Sports Med. 2004;32(3):655–61.
24. Walton J, Mahajan S, Paxinos A, Marshall J, Bryant C, Shnier R, Quinn R, Murrell GA. Diagnostic values of tests for acromioclavicular joint pain. J Bone Joint Surg Am. 2004;86-A(4):807–12.
25. O'Brien SJ, Pagnani MJ, Fealy S, McGlynn SR, Wilson JB. The active compression test: a new and effective test for diagnosing labral tears and acromioclavicular joint abnormality. Am J Sports Med. 1998;26(5):610–3.
26. Kim SH, Park JC, Park JS, Oh I. Painful jerk test: a predictor of success in nonoperative treatment of posteroinferior instability of the shoulder. Am J Sports Med. 2004;32(8):1849–55.
27. Kim SH, Park JS, Jeong WK, Shin SK. The Kim test: a novel test for posteroinferior labral lesion of the shoulder--a comparison to the jerk test. J Bone Joint Surg Am. 1966;48(8):1496–502.
28. McLaughlin HL. On the frozen shoulder. Bull Hosp Joint Dis. 1951;12(2):383–93.

29. Yergason RM. Supination sign. J Bone Joint Surg Am. 1931;13(1):160.
30. Hawkins RJ, Schutte JP, Janda DH, Huckell GH. Translation of the glenohumeral joint with the patient under anesthesia. J Shoulder Elb Surg. 1996;5(4):286–92.
31. Mihata T, Lee Y, McGarry MH, Abe M, Lee TQ. Excessive humeral external rotation results in increased shoulder laxity. Am J Sports Med. 2004;32(5):1278–85.
32. Gagey OJ, Gagey N. The hyperabduction test. J Bone Joint Surg Br. 2001;83(1):69–74.
33. Neer CS 2nd, Foster CR. Inferior capsular shift for involuntary inferior and multidirectional instability of the shoulder. A preliminary report. J Bone Joint Surg Am. 1980;62(6):897–908.
34. Silliman JF, Hawkins RJ. Classification and physical diagnosis of instability of the shoulder. Clin Orthop Relat Res. 1993;291:7–19.
35. Beighton P, Horan F. Orthopaedic aspects of the Ehlers-Danlos syndrome. J Bone Jt Surg. 1969;51B:444.
36. Beighton P, Solomon L, Soskolne CL. Articular mobility in an African population. Ann Rheum Dis. 1973;32(5):413–8.
37. Silliman JF, Hawkins RJ. Current concepts and recent advances in the athlete's shoulder. Clin Sports Med. 1991;10(4):693–705.
38. Lo IK, Nonweiler B, Woolfrey M, Litchfield R, Kirkley A. An evaluation of the apprehension, relocation, and surprise tests for anterior shoulder instability. Am J Sports Med. 2004;32(2):301–7.
39. Jobe FW, Kvitne RS, Giangarra CE. Shoulder pain in the overhand or throwing athlete. The relationship of anterior instability and rotator cuff impingement. Orthop Rev. 1989;18(9):963–75.
40. O'Driscoll SW. A reliable and simple test for posterior instability of the shoulder. J Bone Joint Sutg. 1991;73B(Suppl 1):50.
41. McFarland EG, Kim TK, Park HB, Neira CA, Gutierrez MI. The effect of variation in definition on the diagnosis of multidirectional instability of the shoulder. J Bone Joint Surg Am. 2003;85:2138–44.
42. Barrett C. The clinical physiotherapy assessment of non-traumatic shoulder instability. Shoulder Elbow. 2015;7(1):60–71.
43. Watson LA, Pizzari T, Balster S. Thoracic outlet syndrome part 2: conservative management of thoracic outlet. Man Ther. 2010;15:305–14.
44. Van Tongel A, Atoun E, Narvani A, Sforza G, Levy O. The 'hand squeeze' test for posterior 'muscle patterning instability' of the shoulder. Acta Orthop Belg. 2013;79(1):31–5.
45. Spurling RS, Scoville WB. Lateral rupture of the cervical intervertebral discs: a common cause of shoulder and arm pain. Surg Gynecol Obstet. 1944;78:350–8.
46. Anekstein Y, Blecher R, Smorgick Y, Mirovsky Y. What is the best way to apply the Spurling test for cervical radiculopathy? Clin Orthop Relat Res. 2012;470(9):2566–72.
47. Roos DB. Congenital anomalies associated with thoracic outlet syndrome. Anatomy, symptoms, diagnosis, and treatment. Am J Surg. 1976;132(6):771–8.
48. Roos DB. New concepts of thoracic outlet syndrome that explain etiology, symptoms, diagnosis, and treatment. J Vasc Surg. 1979;13:313–21.
49. Adson AW. Surgical treatment for symptoms produced by cervical ribs and the scalenus anticus muscle. Surg Gynecol Obstet. 1947;85(6):687–700.
50. Wright IS. The neurovascular syndrome produced by hyperabduction of the arms. Am Heart J. 1945;29:1–19.
51. Sanders M, Monsour JW, Gerber WF, Adams WR, Thompson N. Scalenectomy versus first rib resection for treatment of thoracic outlet syndrome. Surgery. 1979;85:109–21.
52. Sanders RJ, Hammond SL, Rao NM. Diagnosis of thoracic outlet syndrome. J Vasc Surg. 2007;46(3):601–4.
53. Kibler WB, Press J, Sciascia A. The role of core stability in athletic function. Sports Med. 2006;36(3):189–98.

Chapter 6
Investigations for Shoulder Disorders

Once a clinical impression is made as to the likely source of the patient's symptoms, the aim is to investigate these further, to confirm or dispute the working and alternative diagnoses. Radiological and neurophysiological examinations form the core of investigations for the symptomatic shoulder.

The chapter gives an overview of the potential radiological and neurophysiological tests that are available in the diagnosis of shoulder conditions, helping to guide the reader as to what information they may provide and hence when they could be of use. The value of diagnostic local anaesthetic injections is also discussed.

6.1 Radiological Investigations

Several radiological investigations are available to the shoulder clinician. Their choice is influenced by the question to be answered, working diagnosis, specific structures to assess, radiological resources and radiological expertise availability. Some of the radiological investigations that may be utilised in assessing the shoulder and the clinical situations where they would be preferable are discussed next. Nevertheless, discussion between clinicians and local radiologists may help guide as to the best radiological modality available to answer a specific question.

© Springer Nature Switzerland AG 2019
C. Panayiotou Charalambous, *The Shoulder Made Easy*,
https://doi.org/10.1007/978-3-319-98908-2_6

6.1.1 Plain Radiographs

Preferable for the assessment of bony, calcium-containing and other radio-opaque structures and hence utilised in the imaging of:

- Arthritis
- Fractures
- Abnormal joint displacement (joint instability, superior migration of the humeral head)
- Soft tissue calcification

Several shoulder views have been described [1, 2], but three commonly used are:

1. Anterior-posterior view with the arm in about 30° of external rotation
    (a) Equivalent to looking at the shoulder from the front
    (b) Assesses the glenohumeral joint and acromioclavicular joint (ACJt) and adjacent bony structures
    (c) Localises calcification and other radio-opaque structures in a superior-inferior and medial-lateral direction

Positioning for anterior-posterior view of the shoulder– radiograph

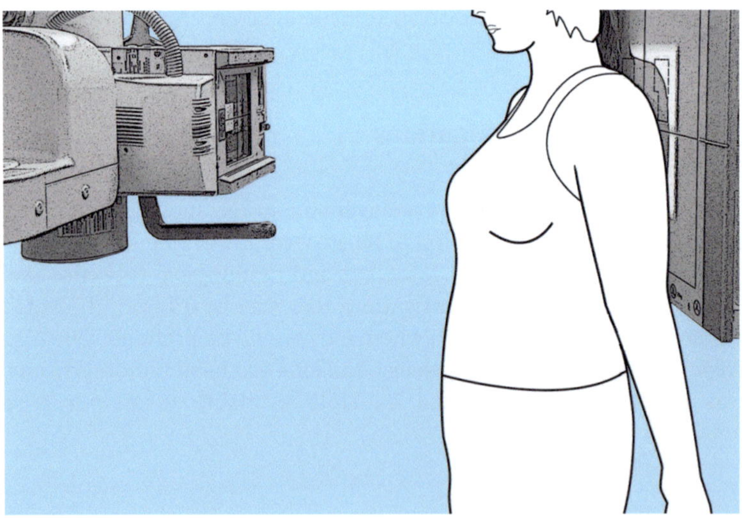

Anterior-posterior radiograph showing the glenohumeral (red arrow) and ACJt (green arrow)

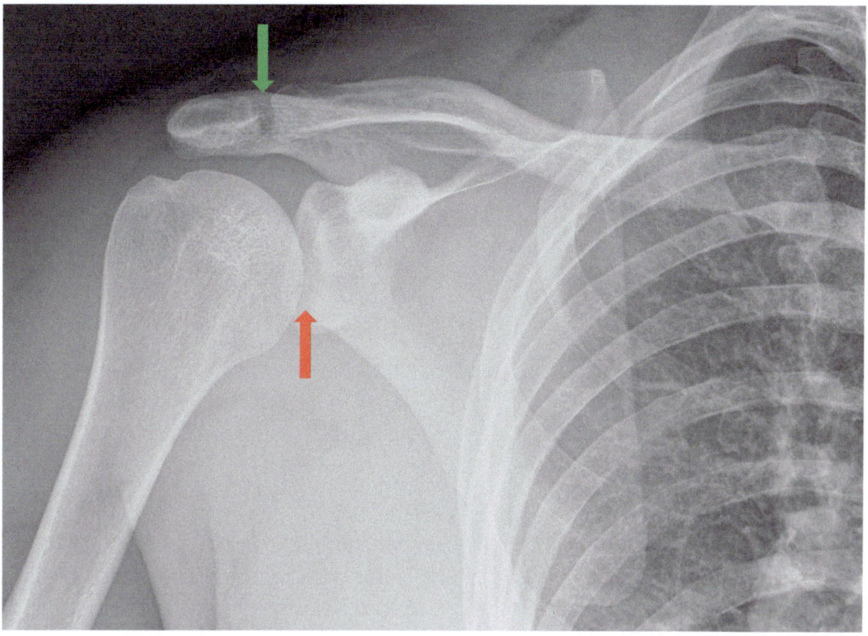

Anterior-posterior radiograph demonstrating the proximal humerus (blue), clavicle (orange), scapula(red), acromion (purple), coracoid (green) and glenoid (yellow)

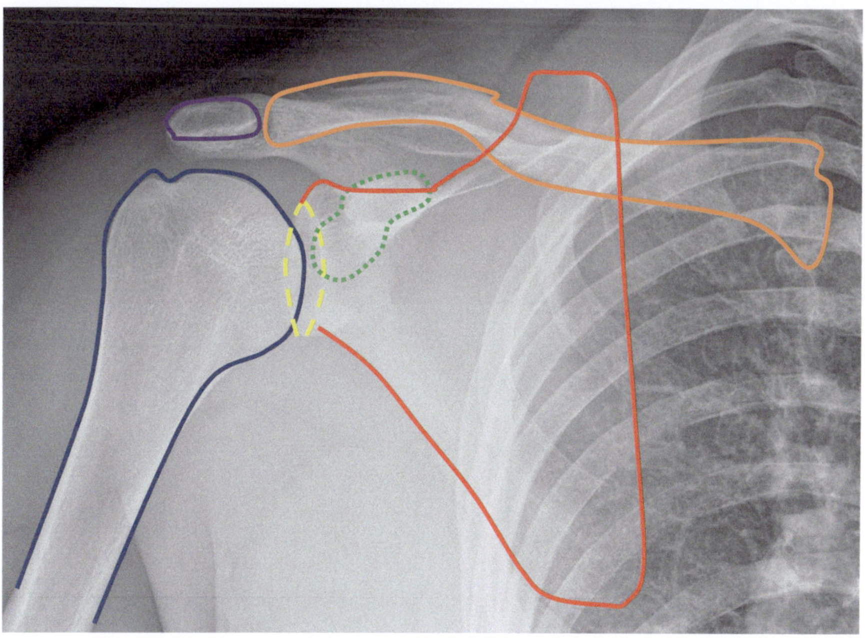

Anterior-posterior radiograph demonstrating the coracoid process (blue outline)

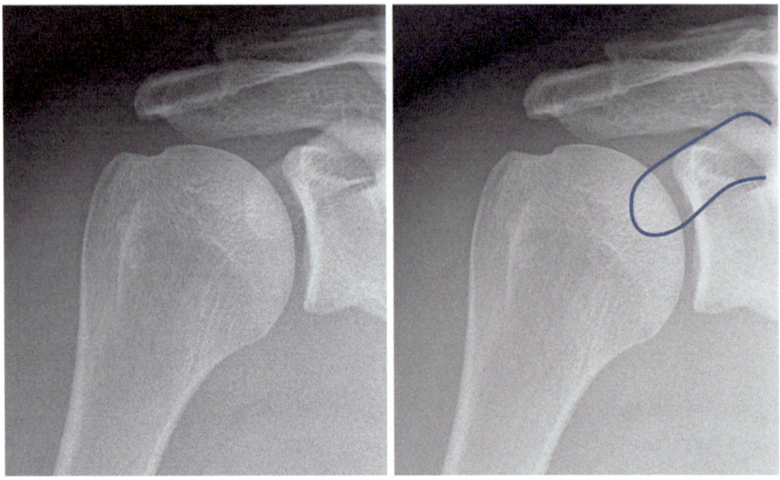

2. Scapular Y view
   (a) Equivalent to looking at the shoulder whilst facing directly at the flat surface of the glenoid. In this view, a "Y" is formed (by the spine of the scapula posteriorly, the coracoid anteriorly and the body of the scapula inferiorly) with the glenoid residing at the centre of this "Y"
   (b) Assesses fractures of the structures forming the three limbs of the "Y" and fractures of the proximal humeral shaft
   (c) Assesses the relation of the humeral head to the glenoid (but the axillary view is preferable for this)
   (d) Localises calcification and other radio-opaque structures in an anterior-posterior and superior-inferior direction

Positioning for scapular view of the shoulder – radiograph

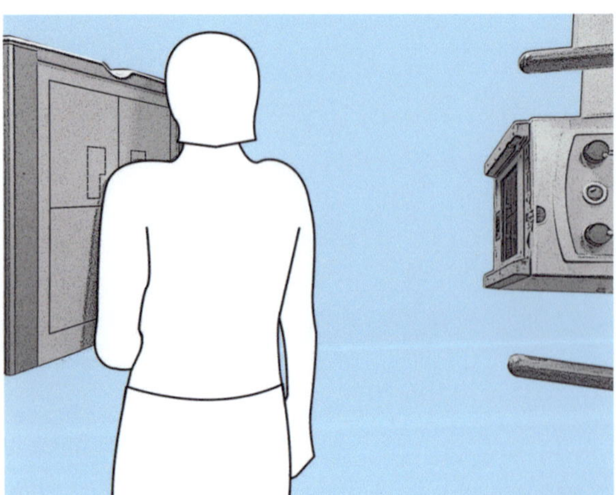

Y scapular view. With the glenohumeral joint intact, the humeral head (blue) is overlying the glenoid (yellow), which is thus difficult to identify. Even if the margins of the glenoid cannot be clearly defined, the glenoid lies in the centre of the Y (green) formed by the coracoid process, spine of the scapula and vertebral body, and these three bony landmarks are usually easy to identify (a). With the humeral head dislocated anteriorly, the outline of the glenoid becomes more evident (b)

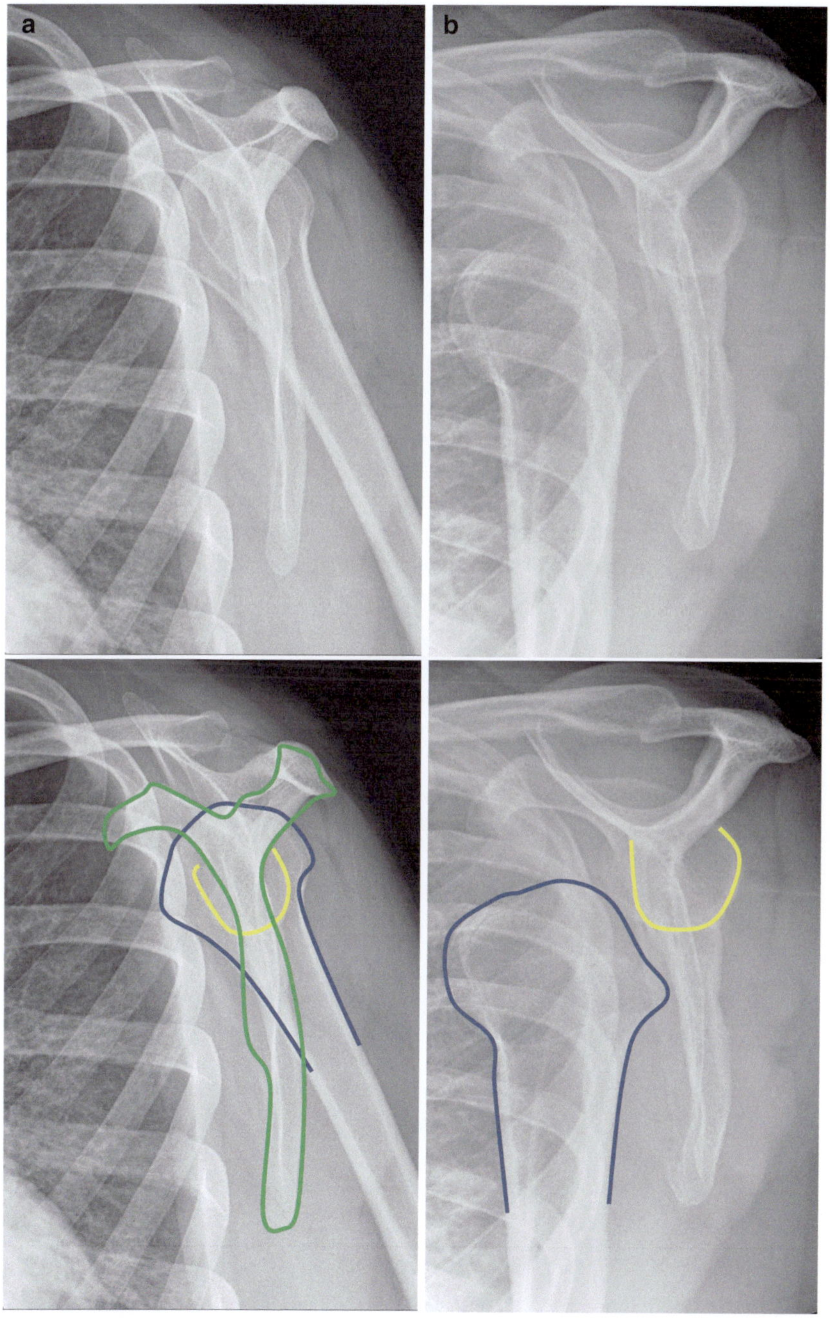

Anterior-posterior radiograph showing a large calcific deposit (yellow arrow) located in the superior cuff. Scapular Y radiograph helps identify the location of the deposit in an antero-posterior direction (red arrow), which can aid surgical excision

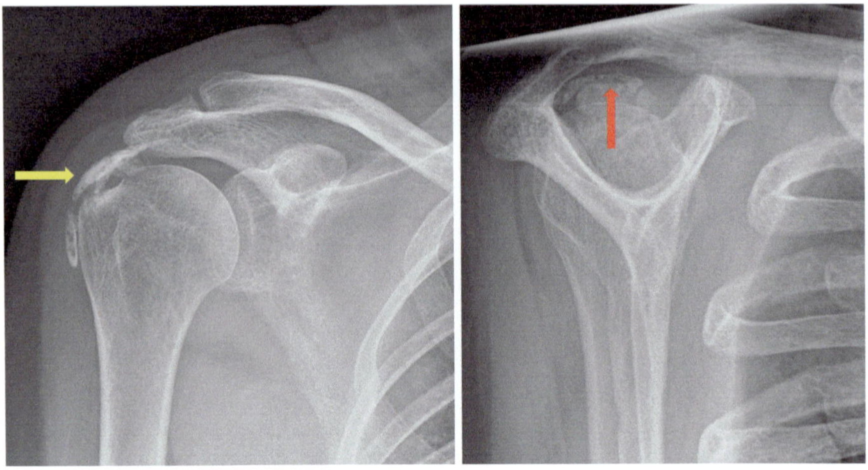

3. Axillary view
   (a) Equivalent to looking at the shoulder from the top down
   (b) Assesses the position of the humeral head in relation to the glenoid in an anterior-posterior direction; hence it is the best view to evaluate subluxation/dislocation of the glenohumeral joint
   (c) Demonstrates the relation of the clavicle to the acromion at the level of the ACJt, in an anterior-posterior direction
   (d) Localises calcification and other radio-opaque structures in an anterior-posterior direction

Positioning for – axillary view of the shoulder – radiograph

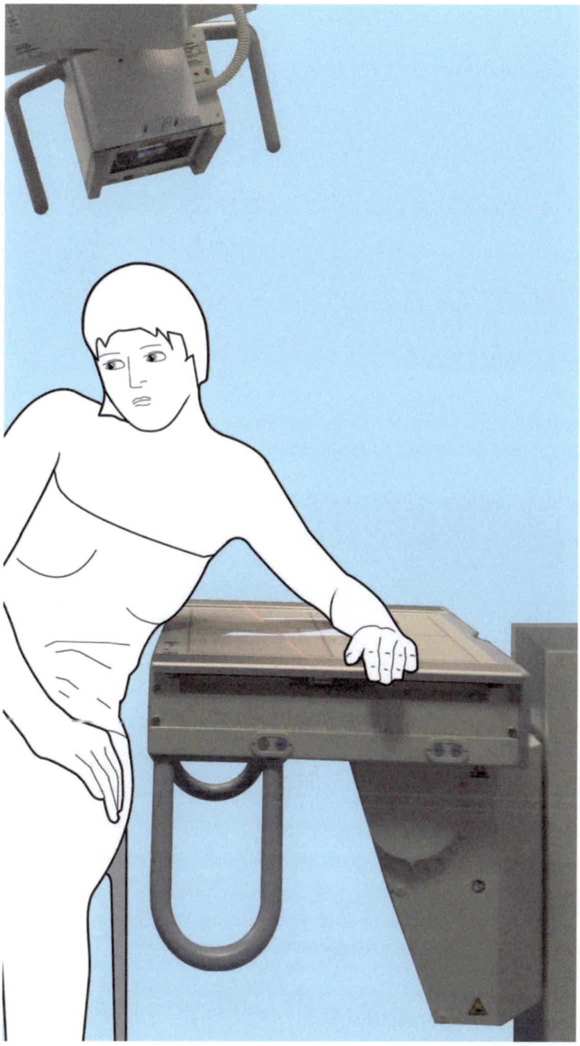

Radiograph – axillary view of the shoulder

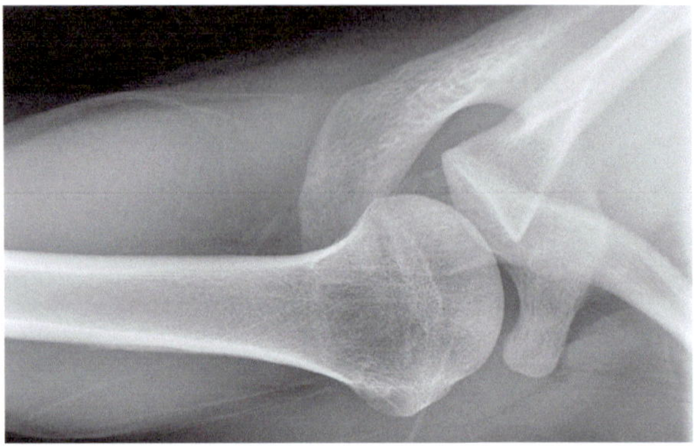

Radiograph – axillary view of the shoulder, outlining the relation between the lateral end of the clavicle (orange) and acromion (purple) at the ACJt

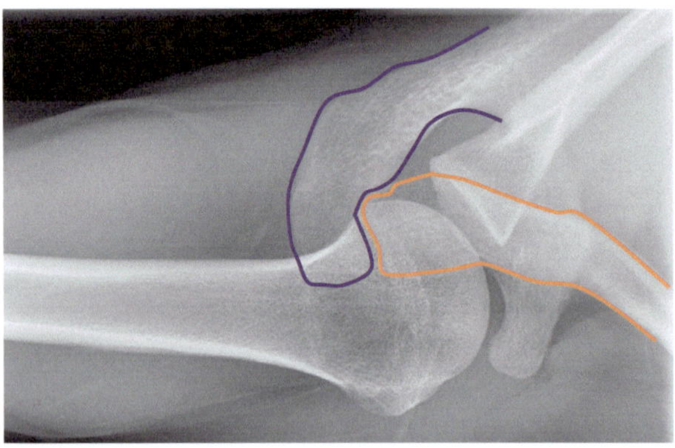

Radiograph – axillary view of the shoulder, outlining the relation between the proximal humerus and humeral head (blue) with glenoid (yellow)

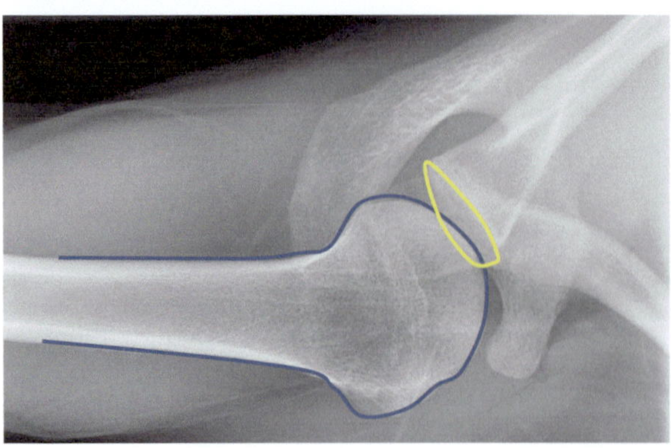

Radiograph – axillary view of the shoulder, outlining the coracoid process (green)

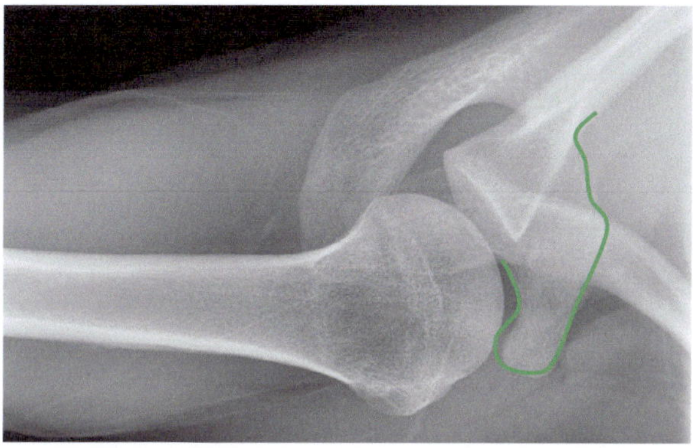

"Light bulb" appearance of the humeral head suggestive of posterior shoulder dislocation (a). An axillary view can accurately determine if this is truly the case or the appearance is due to excessive internal rotation of the humerus (such as in muscle imbalance following a cerebrovascular event (b), or due to placement of the arm in a sling in front of the patient's body)

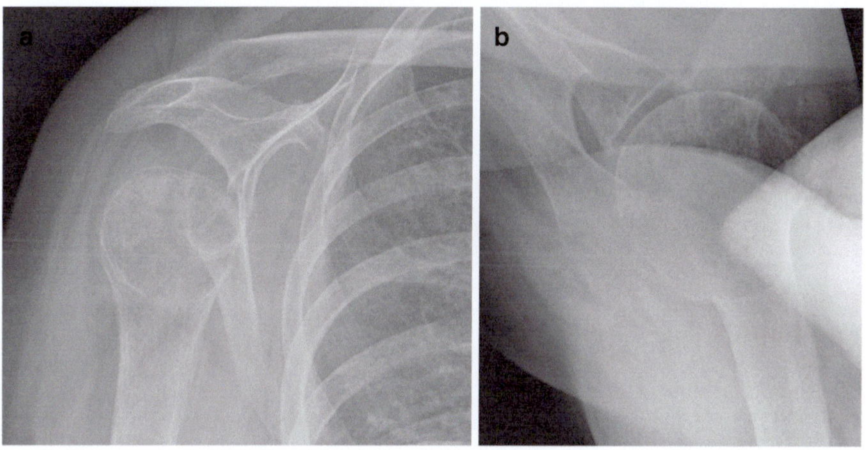

Two views are also described for the sterno-clavicular joint and the ACJt. These are described below:

1. Sterno-clavicular joint view (serendipity view)
    - Used for evaluating the sterno-clavicular joint
    - It is an anterior-posterior view, performed by tilting the X-ray beam 40° towards the direction of the patient's head (cephalad), with the patient supine

- With the sterno-clavicular joint in situ, the clavicle will be in line with the manubrium of the sternum, but this relation is altered in joint dislocation:
  - In anterior dislocation, the medial end of the clavicle lies superior to the manubrium
  - In posterior dislocation, the medial end of the clavicle lies inferior to the sternum

2. ACJt view [3]
   - Used for evaluating the ACJt
   - It is an anterior-posterior view, performed by tilting the X-ray beam 10–15° towards the direction of the patient's head (cephalad)

Positioning for ACJt view – anterior-posterior with cephalad angulation – radiograph

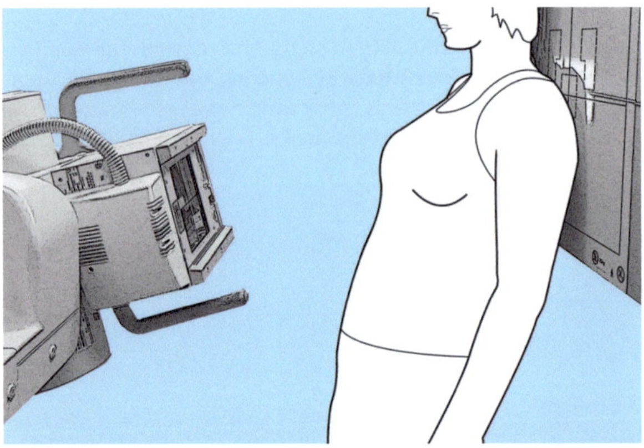

6.1.2 Ultrasound [4–6]

Uses ultrasound waves to assess soft tissues around the shoulder.

- Assesses the superficial soft tissue envelope – skin, subcutaneous tissue, tendons and muscles
- Assesses the presence of glenohumeral, ACJt or sterno-clavicular joint effusion
- Distinguishes between solid and cystic soft tissue swellings. It may also determine if such swellings are vascularised; increased vascularity is indicative of an active inflammatory lesion, infective changes or neoplastic lesions
- Guides injections into the shoulder or fluid aspiration – particularly useful in injecting the bicipital groove to avoid injection into the long head of the biceps tendon substance

During an ultrasound examination, the arm may be actively or passively moved to help stretch the shoulder tendons and hence evaluate their continuity. The arm may also be moved to assess any abnormal displacement of the tendons – such as dynamic dislocation and relocation of the long head of the biceps tendon from the bicipital groove.

Ultrasound is relatively easy and quick to perform, but its accuracy is operator dependent. Some surgeons perform ultrasound as part of their routine clinic evaluation of the shoulder.

6.1.3 Magnetic Resonance Imaging (MRI) [7–9]

The patient is placed in a scanner which applies a magnetic field to create a picture of the structures of the body. Coils placed around the shoulder allow an additional local application of a magnetic field and hence higher quality imaging.

Images are formed with the examined structures constructed using shades of white, grey and black. These can be altered to give multiple versions (sequences) of a particular image to help assess the presented structures. Some commonly utilised MRI sequences are:

- T1-weighted sequence – fluid appears black, muscle grey, fat white
  - Evaluates anatomy – structure
- T2-weighted sequence – fluid appears white, muscle grey, fat white
  - Evaluates pathology – inflammation, infection which show increased fluid levels
- STIR sequence – fat is dark; fluid is bright
  - Evaluates oedema of soft tissue and bones

Images can be obtained in multiple planes, with three commonly used:

- Coronal – equivalent to looking at the shoulder from the front
- Sagittal – equivalent to looking at the shoulder facing directly the flat surface of the glenoid
- Axial – equivalent to looking at the shoulder from the top down

MRI is preferable for the detailed and accurate assessment of:

- Superficial soft tissues of the shoulder – skin, subcutaneous tissue, tendons (continuity, inflammation, degeneration) and muscles (atrophy, fat infiltration)
- Deep soft tissues of the shoulder – labrum, glenohumeral ligaments

- Bone consistency (marrow) – bone oedema, avascular necrosis, infection, inflammation and neoplasia
- Articular cartilage – early degenerative or other chondral changes not evident on plain radiographs

6.1.3.1 Contrast-Enhanced MRI

MRI performed following the intravenous administration of a contrast (dye) fluid, such as gadolinium. This may accumulate in pathological areas which have leaky blood vessels making them look bright.

Preferable for evaluating the presence of:

- Infection
- Inflammation
- Neoplasms

6.1.3.2 MRI Arthrography

MRI performed following the injection of a contrast (dye) fluid into the glenohumeral joint [3, 4]:

- The use of contrast may increase the accuracy of assessing glenohumeral lesions such as labrum tears – the labrum may be detached from the glenoid but still be apposed on the bone giving a false impression that it is intact. The injected contrast inflates the joint and can elevate the detached labrum off the bone, demonstrating a gap between the two and hence confirming the detachment
- Leakage of contrast from the glenohumeral joint into surrounding areas may indicate an abnormal communication between the two such as:
  - Contrast leaking between the labrum and glenoid into the adjacent tissues may indicate labrum detachment
  - Contrast leaking from the glenohumeral space into the subacromial space (normally separated by the rotator cuff tendon) indicates rotator cuff tear

Shoulder arthrogram – contrast (yellow arrow) is injected into the glenohumeral joint via needle (blue arrow)

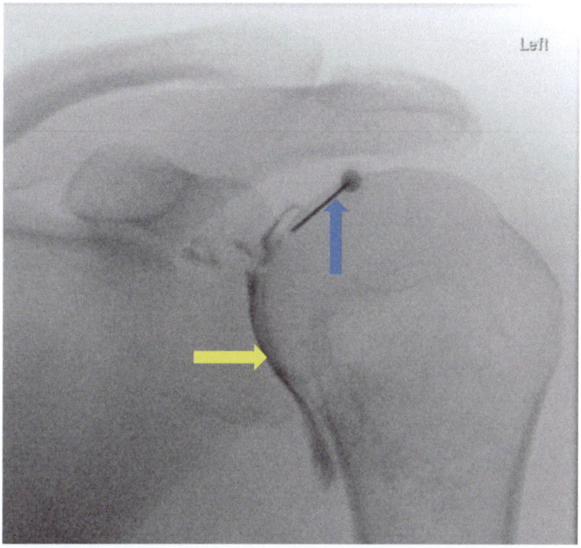

Normal MRI arthrogram. Contrast injected into the glenohumeral joint (red arrow) outlines the limits of that joint, with no escape into the subacromial space, indicating an intact rotator cuff tendon

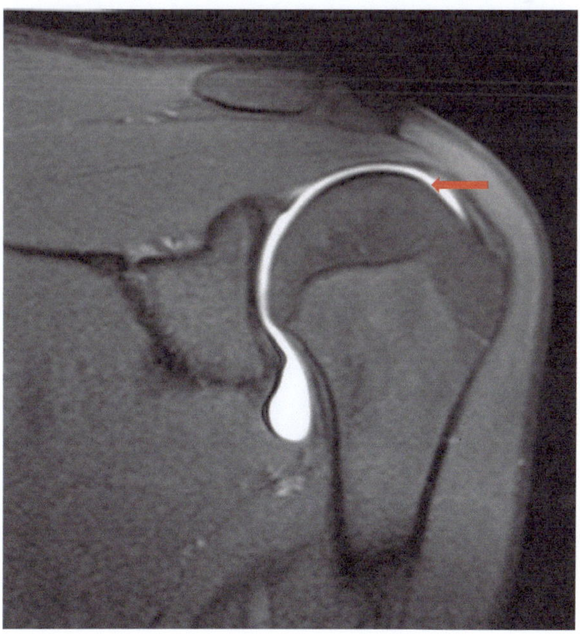

MRI arthrogram, showing an intact superior labrum (yellow arrow) with no contrast escaping between the superior labrum and superior surface of the glenoid

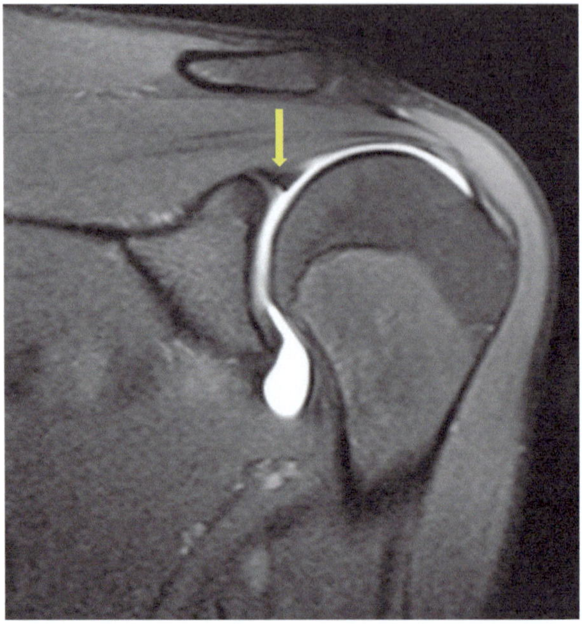

MRI arthrogram, showing an intact anterior (green arrow) and posterior (yellow arrow) labrum, with no contrast escaping between the labrum and glenoid. The red arrow shows an intact subscapularis tendon

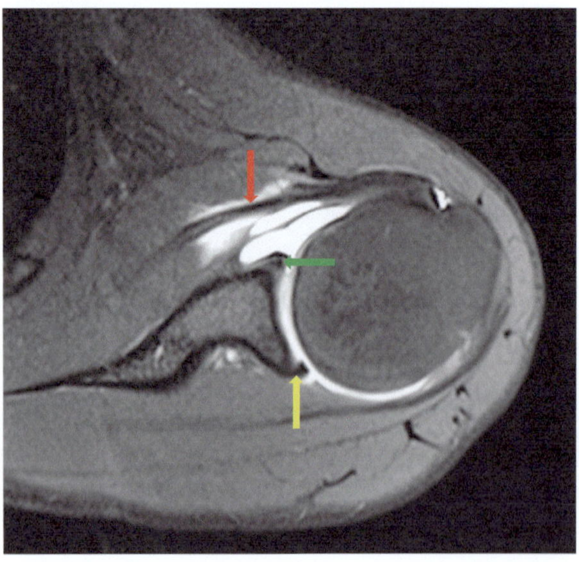

MRI arthrogram, showing the long head of the biceps tendon (green arrow) located in the bicipital groove and surrounded by injected contrast

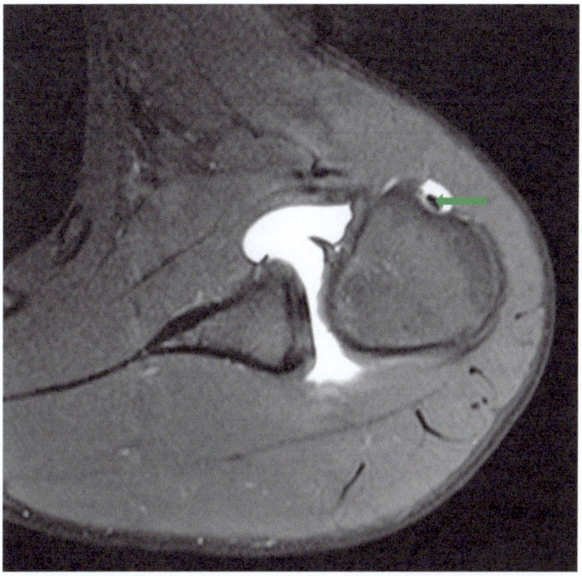

Full-thickness supraspinatus tear (red arrow), allowing escape of contrast injected in the glenohumeral joint (orange arrow) into the subacromial space (green arrow). Following surgical repair and healing of the tear (yellow arrow), such leakage does not occur

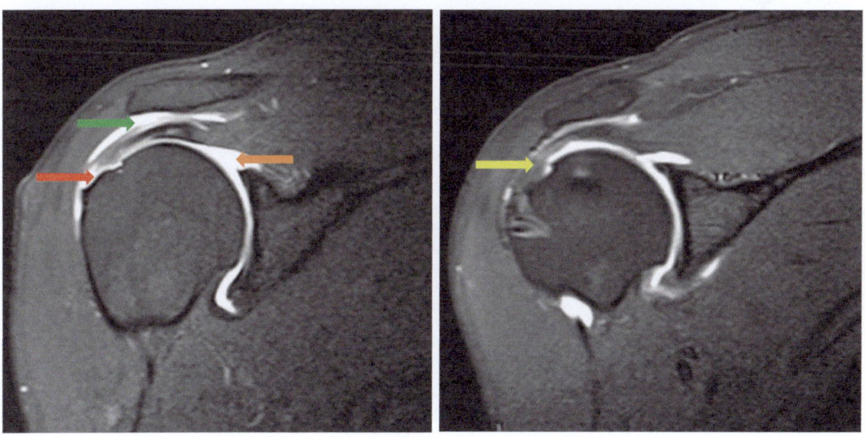

On performing contrast MRI, the shoulder may be placed in:

- Neutral position (with the arm by the side)
- Abduction and external rotation (ABER) – this evaluates the following:
  - Detachments of the anterior-inferior part of the labrum. This shoulder position stretches the inferior glenohumeral ligament pulling the detached labrum away from the glenoid hence allowing easier detection of contrast leakage at labrum tears
  - Partial-thickness articular-side rotator cuff tendon tears. This shoulder position releases tension on the rotator cuff; hence partial tears are not apposed against the humeral head and are thus more easily detected

Positioning for an MRI of the shoulder with the arm by the side

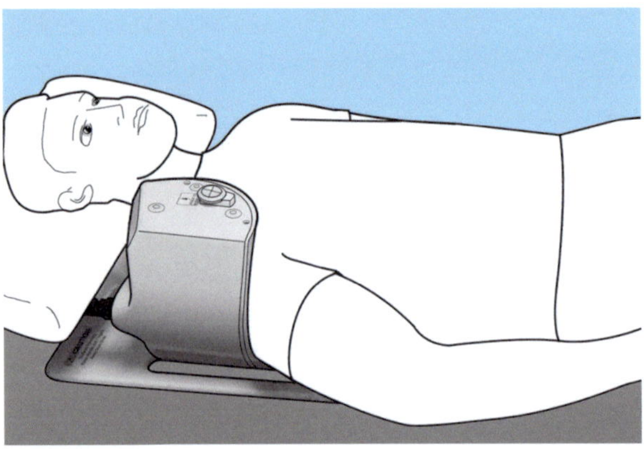

Positioning for an MRI of the shoulder with the arm in abduction and external rotation

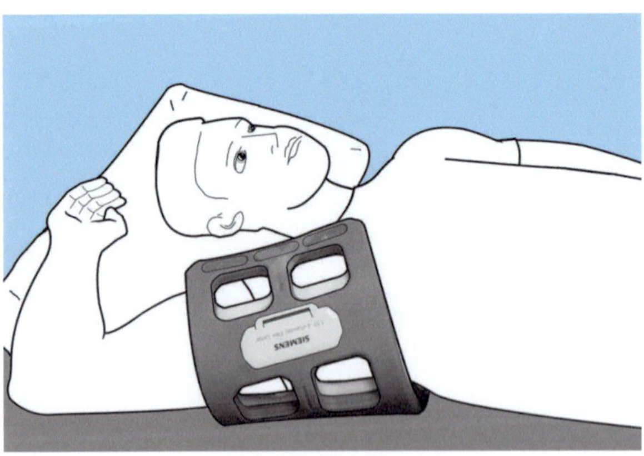

MRI axial section showing the supraspinatus (blue arrow) subscapularis (yellow arrow) and infraspinatus (green arrow) tendons attaching onto the humeral head

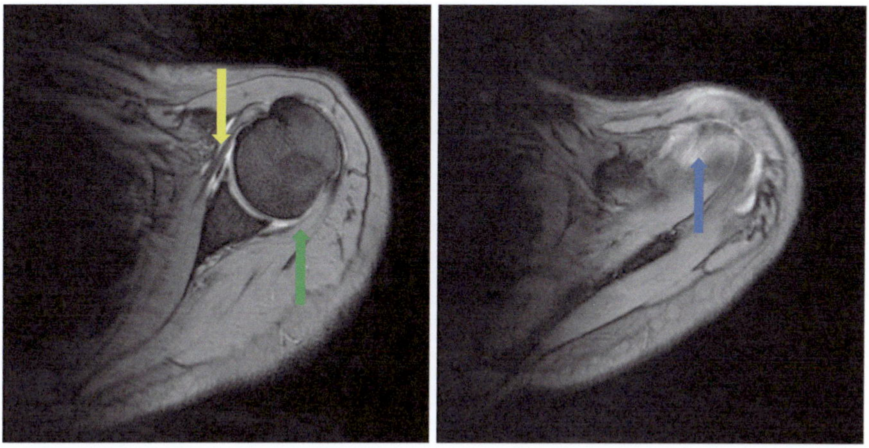

6.1.4 *Computed Tomography* [9]

Mainly assesses the morphology and structure of the bone, although soft tissue evaluation (with or without contrast) is also possible.

- Preferable in the evaluation of bone morphology in planning surgery:
  - Humeral head or glenoid defects in glenohumeral instability surgery
  - Glenoid defects – in shoulder arthroplasty
- Assessment of fractures (confirm presence, determine morphology)
- Evaluation of bone union in fractures

6.1.5 *Bone Scan* [10–11]

- Shoulder bone scan – assesses the perfusion of the shoulder, to determine if there is any increased perfusion (hot spot) consistent with localised increased osteoblastic activity. This may occur in bone regeneration, inflammation or infection
- Whole body bone scan – assesses the whole skeleton for hot spots
  - May help determine if a lesion seen in the shoulder, is isolated to the shoulder or is part of a more generalised problem with similar lesions in other parts of the skeleton. It may thus be used in determine:
    - If an insufficiency fracture is due to localised high chronic loading or associated with similar fractures at other sites suggestive of a metabolic disorder

  - If a neoplastic lesion is isolated to the shoulder (hence likely to be primary) or associated with other skeletal lesions (hence likely to be a metastasis)
  - If shoulder infection is isolated or associated with other foci of infection in the skeleton, suggestive of a source shedding infective emboli

6.1.5.1 Radiolabelled White Cell Bone Scan

White blood cells are obtained from the individual and labelled with radioactive dye. The labelled white cells are then injected into the bloodstream, and their distribution around the shoulder is assessed. An abnormal accumulation of labelled white cells is suggestive of infection or inflammation. Radiolabelled white cell bone scan may help:

- Distinguish between inflammation and infection (with higher white cell accumulation in the latter)
- Distinguish between aseptic and infective loosening of shoulder arthroplasty implants (with higher white cell accumulation in the latter)

6.2 Neurophysiological Investigations for Shoulder Conditions

Neurophysiological investigations of the shoulder and the upper limb may be used in conjunction with clinical findings, to diagnose dysfunction of nerves and muscles which may account for shoulder symptoms. They consist of nerve conduction (NC) studies and electromyography (EMG) [12, 13].

6.2.1 Nerve Conduction Study

This is the examination of conduction along motor and sensory nerves.

Nerve conduction studies may help assess the presence of nerve dysfunction and guide as to its likely cause. In particular they may determine:

- Whether there is involvement of a nerve's myelin or axon fibres
- Whether there is involvement of one or more nerves
- The site of neurological dysfunction (peripheral nerve, plexus, nerve root)
- The pattern of nerve involvement:
  - Long vs. short fibre nerves
  - Large vs. small fibre nerves
  - Focal, multifocal, random nerve involvement

A nerve conduction study involves stimulating and recording over:

1. Two separate points of a peripheral sensory nerve
2. Stimulating a peripheral motor nerve and recording over a muscle

In this way:

1. The time taken for electrical impulses to travel from one point to the other (latency) can be determined, and the speed of electrical transmission (conduction velocity) between the two can be calculated. Slow conduction may indicate a demyelinating neurological disorder or may be due to prolonged transmission at the neuromuscular junction. Focal reduction in conduction velocity may indicate external compression of the nerve at that site
2. The size of electrical activity in the muscle upon nerve stimulation is recorded (compound muscle action potential – CMAP). Similarly, the size of the electrical activity generated in a sensory nerve by its stimulation (sensory nerve action potential – SNAP) is assessed. If the magnitude of such electrical activities is lower than expected, it may suggest that there is loss of axon fibres from the nerve rather than simply loss of myelin. Severe compression of a nerve may with time lead to axon loss

6.2.2 EMG

EMG is the detection of electrical activity from muscles through the percutaneous insertion of fine needle electrodes into muscles. EMG has three main roles:

1. It may help differentiate between a primary muscle disorder and a neurogenic disorder as the cause of muscle weakness or muscle atrophy
2. In dealing with a nerve lesion, it may help determine whether there is involvement of a nerve's myelin sheath or axon fibres, the latter signifying a more severe dysfunction
3. When dealing with a neurogenic disorder, by sampling several muscles, determining the extent and pattern of the muscles affected and taking into account their anatomical innervation, EMG may help localise the lesion and distinguish between:
   (a) Peripheral nerve lesion
   (b) Lesion of the brachial plexus
   (c) Spinal root involvement

EMG recordings mainly aim to assess:

1. The presence of spontaneous electrical activity from the muscle – that is, activity generated in the absence of any voluntary attempt to contract the muscle. The morphology of such spontaneous electrical activity may guide as to the presence of a neurogenic or myopathic disorder:
   (a) Denervated muscle (due to axon loss) may exhibit spontaneous discharges of electrical activity such as fibrillations and fasciculations
   (b) Myotonic discharges are seen in certain myotonias
2. Muscle unit electrical activity
3. The electrical recruitment of muscle fibres upon attempted voluntary contraction

6.3 Diagnostic Shoulder Injections

Local anaesthetic injections may help guide a clinician as to the origin of a patient's pain [14–16]. A local anaesthetic is injected into the area that is considered to be the origin of a patient's pain, and the patient is given time for the local anaesthetic to start working. The patient may be asked to move the arm and see whether the injection has helped the pain.

If the local anaesthetic improves or abolishes the pain, then this indicates that the pain is likely coming from the area that has been injected. If the injection does not reduce the pain, then one needs to consider that the pain may not be coming from that area.

Reduction or elimination of pain by a local anaesthetic injection may also allow one to distinguish between true and apparent (pain-mediated) weakness and between true and apparent (pain-mediated) stiffness. Apparent weakness and apparent stiffness may improve following a reduction in pain (for the duration that the local anaesthetic remains active), whereas true weakness or true stiffness is not helped by pain improvement.

Local anaesthetic injections may be combined with a steroid injection that aims to improve long-term pain. Hence, injections can have both a diagnostic and a therapeutic effect.

Local anaesthetic injections may also help to relax temporarily muscles to determine if that improves a patient's symptoms which may then be attributed to over muscular activity (such as injecting the scalene muscles to help diagnose thoracic outlet syndrome that is secondary to scalene muscle spasm) [17].

Learning Pearls

- An AP radiograph with the arm in a sling in front of the body gives more of a lateral view of the proximal humerus. An AP radiograph with the arm out of sling in about 30° external rotation is preferable
- Different types of radiological investigations may be considered complimentary rather than mutually exclusive, as each may be better at assessing specific components of the musculoskeletal system. Hence, multiple radiological modalities may be necessary as part of the diagnostic workup
- On occasions it may be that "less is more" – a plain radiograph may be preferable to MRI in evaluating advanced arthritis of the glenohumeral joint
- Muscle denervation changes may not become apparent for 2–3 weeks post-nerve injury. Hence, NC studies and EMG studies are better obtained after 3 weeks post-injury or other nerve insults

References

1. Goud A, Segal D, Hedayati P, Pan JJ, Weissman BN. Radiographic evaluation of the shoulder. Eur J Radiol. 2008;68(1):2–15.
2. Tuite MJ, Small KM. Imaging evaluation of nonacute shoulder pain. AJR Am J Roentgenol. 2017;209(3):525–33.
3. Zanca P. Shoulder pain: involvement of the acromioclavicular joint. (analysis of 1,000 cases). Am J Roentgenol Radium Therapy, Nucl Med. 1971;112(3):493–506.
4. Gyftopoulos S, Guja KE, Subhas N, Virk MS, Gold HT. Cost-effectiveness of magnetic resonance imaging versus ultrasound for the detection of symptomatic full-thickness supraspinatus tendon tears. J Shoulder Elb Surg. 2017;26(12):2067–77.
5. Day M, Phil M, McCormack RA, Nayyar S, Jazrawi L. Physician training ultrasound and accuracy of diagnosis in rotator cuff tears. Bull Hosp Jt Dis (2013). 2016;74(3):207–11.
6. Beltran LS, Adler R, Stone T, Surace J, Beltran J, Bencardino JT. MRI and ultrasound imaging of the shoulder using positional maneuvers. AJR Am J Roentgenol. 2015;205(3):W244–54.
7. Gottsegen CJ, Merkle AN, Bencardino JT, Gyftopoulos S. Advanced MRI techniques of the shoulder joint: current applications in clinical practice. AJR Am J Roentgenol. 2017;209(3):544–51.
8. Arirachakaran A, Boonard M, Chaijenkij K, Pituckanotai K, Prommahachai A, Kongtharvonskul J. A systematic review and meta-analysis of diagnostic test of MRA versus MRI for detection superior labrum anterior to posterior lesions type II-VII. Skelet Radiol. 2017;46(2):149–60.
9. Saliken DJ, Bornes TD, Bouliane MJ, Sheps DM, Beaupre LA. Imaging methods for quantifying glenoid and hill-Sachs bone loss in traumatic instability of the shoulder: a scoping review. BMC Musculoskelet Disord. 2015;16:164. https://doi.org/10.1186/s12891-015-0607-1.
10. Love C, Palestro CJ. Nuclear medicine imaging of bone infections. Clin Radiol. 2016;71(7):632–46.
11. Gemmel F, Van den Wyngaert H, Love C, Welling MM, Gemmel P, Palestro CJ. Prosthetic joint infections: radionuclide state-of-the-art imaging. Eur J Nucl Med Mol Imaging. 2012;39(5):892–909.
12. Mohassel P, Chaudhry V. Neurophysiology simplified for imagers. Semin Musculoskelet RadiolS. 2015;19(2):112–20.
13. Mills KR. The basics of electromyography. J Neurol Neurosurg Psychiatry. 2005;76(Suppl 2):ii32–5.
14. McFarland E, Bernard J, Dein E, Johnson A. Diagnostic injections about the shoulder. J Am Acad Orthop Surg. 2017;25(12):799–807.
15. Farshad M, Jundt-Ecker M, Sutter R, Schubert M, Gerber C. Does subacromial injection of a local anesthetic influence strength in healthy shoulders?: a double-blinded, placebo-controlled study. J Bone Joint Surg Am. 2012;94(19):1751–5.
16. Penning LI, De Bie RA, Leffers P, Weijers RE, Walenkamp GH. Empty can and drop arm tests for cuff rupture : improved specificity after sub-acromial injection. Acta Orthop Belg. 2016;82(2):166–73.
17. Bottros MM, AuBuchon JD, McLaughlin LN, Altchek DW, Illig KA, Thompson RW. Exercise-enhanced, ultrasound-guided anterior scalene muscle/Pectoralis minor muscle blocks can facilitate the diagnosis of neurogenic thoracic outlet syndrome in the high-performance overhead athlete. Am J Sports Med. 2017;45(1):189–94.

Chapter 7
Challenges in Managing Shoulder Disorders

Once a diagnosis is reached, using a combination of clinical findings and relevant investigations, the next step is to plan appropriate treatment. The aim of any intervention is to reduce troublesome symptoms and improve function. The clinician has a multitude of options in managing shoulder conditions, and it is a vital skill to decide as to which to employ.

This chapter discusses some of the challenges faced in deciding when and how to intervene when dealing with shoulder complaints. The need to consider the underlying natural history of some conditions and the need to distinguish between findings that may be the source of a patient's symptoms versus incidental asymptomatic findings are also discussed.

This chapter also presents some of the management options in dealing with shoulder conditions with special reference to the intervention ladder.

In managing shoulder conditions, there are several considerations to be made, and these are described next.

7.1 Natural History of Shoulder Disorders

Many shoulder disorders have a natural history of progress which must be taken into account in planning management [1–8]. Hence, when discussing treatment with a patient, one ought to explain that the aim of intervening is to improve current symptoms and speed up recovery rather than change the final outcome:

- It is recognised that adhesive capsulitis is in many cases a self-limiting condition, lasting about 2–3 years following which spontaneous resolution occurs [1, 2]. Intervention aims to improve current symptoms of pain and stiffness, as well as speeding recovery rather than altering the final long-term outcome

In contrast, some conditions may have a natural history of deterioration and worsen with time. Hence, in such circumstances the clinician may discuss the need

© Springer Nature Switzerland AG 2019

C. Panayiotou Charalambous, *The Shoulder Made Easy*,
https://doi.org/10.1007/978-3-319-98908-2_7

to intervene to halt or slow a natural history of further deterioration rather than simply to help with current symptoms:

- There is evidence to suggest that some rotator cuff tears tend to worsen with time, increasing in size and leading to muscular atrophy and fatty infiltration [4–6]. Hence, there may be an argument for intervening early and repairing these rotator cuff tears to halt progression and potentially the worsening of symptoms
- There is evidence to suggest that there is a high risk amongst young active individuals of recurrent dislocation following a first-time glenohumeral dislocation [7, 8]. Hence, there may be an argument for intervening after a first-time dislocation in order to prevent further recurrences which could have a deleterious effect on the shoulder structure and function

7.2 Incidental Findings in the Evaluation of the Shoulder

Certain shoulder radiological or arthroscopic findings may be incidental rather than truly accounting for a patient's symptoms [9–11]. Hence, it is important to correlate such radiological or arthroscopic findings to clinical findings before deciding whether they need addressing. The mere presence of such findings does not necessarily mean they need medical attention. In contrast, intervening in an area that is not the source of the patient's symptoms may itself cause harm and trouble. It is recognised that

- Acromioclavicular joint (ACJt) osteoarthritis
- Degenerative rotator cuff tears
- Degenerative labrum tears

are commonly encountered in the general asymptomatic population and their incidence increases with age. Their presence should thus be correlated with clinical symptoms and signs in considering medical intervention.

7.3 Not All Pathological Shoulder Findings Need Addressing

A symptomatic shoulder may exhibit multiple pathological findings. There is a need to understand which of these contribute to clinical symptoms and which are less relevant. Addressing the major contributors may help one's symptoms, whereas dealing with other findings may confer no additional benefit:

- In glenohumeral arthritis, it is not unusual to find associated labrum tears or degenerative partial tears of the rotator cuff. In the presence of severe arthritis, addressing the arthritis rather than other associated findings may be the main component of intervention

7.4 Clinical Symptoms Originating from Multiple Shoulder Sources

Symptoms may originate from multiple sources, and failure to address all of those may lead to persistent trouble. Such recognition may also help manage patient expectations as part of shared decision-making in discussing clinical intervention:

- Glenohumeral arthritis may be associated with subacromial impingement, ACJt arthritis and long head of the biceps tendinopathy. Simply addressing the loss of glenohumeral cartilage by glenohumeral joint replacement may not relieve the patient's symptoms. Instead, a concurrent subacromial decompression, ACJt excision and biceps tenotomy/tenodesis may be needed along with the replacement arthroplasty [12, 13]
- Pain originating from the subacromial space may co-exist with pain originating from the cervical spine. Hence, shoulder intervention would be expected to improve only part of one's symptoms

Glenohumeral arthritis (red arrow) associated with extensive ACJt arthritis (yellow arrow)

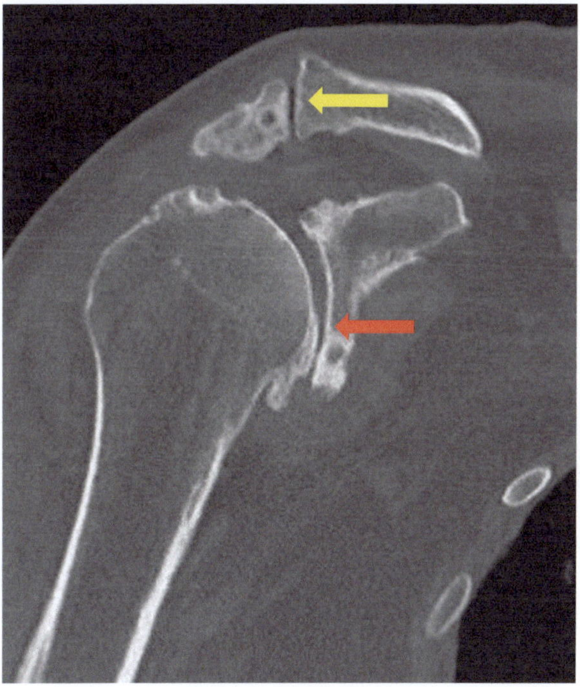

Proximal humerus fracture treated with intramedullary nailing showing non-union. CT scan showing narrowing of the subacromial space (yellow arrow) coexistent with fracture non-union (red arrow). Clinically most symptoms were subacromial in origin

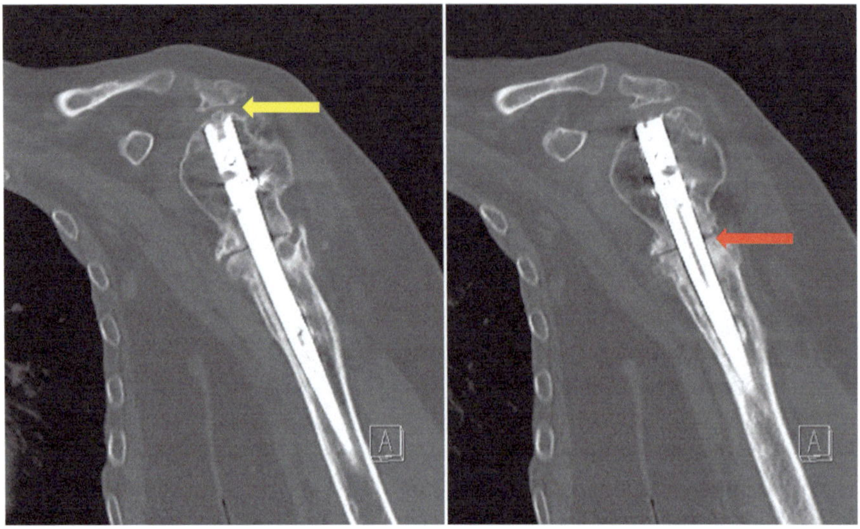

7.5 Systemic/Distant Disorders Causing Shoulder Clinical Symptoms

In dealing with shoulder symptoms, it is essential to enquire about systemic or other multifocal conditions that could involve the shoulder area. Non-shoulder conditions may also be mistaken for shoulder conditions due to referred or similarly presenting symptoms. Hence, broad thinking should be utilised in history taking and clinical examination to help guide appropriate investigations:

- Pain in the shoulder may be referred pain from nearby or distant structures – cervical spine, brachial plexus or diaphragmatic irritation such as in gall bladder disease [14, 15]
- A double crush may exist with part of the pain originating from the shoulder and part of the pain having some other cause. Differentiation and relative quantification of the two may be difficult

Some unusual situations to consider are:

- Constant night pain reported in the shoulder may be due to metastatic cancer rather than the rotator cuff tear that one might expect given the patient's age and symptomatology
- ACJt arthropathy may not be degenerative but secondary to crystal arthropathy involving multiple joints
- A rapid glenohumeral degeneration may not be due to degenerative changes but due to osteomyelitis and septic arthritis, as part of multifocal septic arthritis

7.6 Consider Clinical Symptoms Rather Than Pathology in Shoulder Evaluation

On some occasions the clinical symptoms and signs may not be those expected, given the main underlying pathology or precipitating event. Hence, it is important to obtain a thorough clinical history to clarify the presenting symptoms and carry out a systematic clinical examination to detect the present clinical signs:

- Following glenohumeral joint dislocation, patients often continue with recurrent shoulder instability. However, on occasions a patient may develop substantial glenohumeral stiffness after a shoulder dislocation and relocation, due to a soft tissue inflammatory reaction to the trauma associated with the dislocation. In the latter case, surgical release of contracted tissues rather than repair of detached ligaments may be the preferred surgical intervention
- A patient with a rotator cuff tear may present with pain and limitation of function. Clinical examination may identify the development of associated stiffness. It may be necessary to address the stiffness to regain motion before intervening with regard to the torn rotator cuff or address the stiffness simultaneously with the tear repair [16–18]

7.7 Uncertainty as to How Some Clinical Shoulder Symptoms Are Mediated

In some situations we may not fully understand how the clinical symptoms are mediated and why similar pathologies may cause a wide spectrum of symptom severity amongst patients.

There is evidence that the perception of pain and hence the response to any interventions applied may be influenced by [19–22]:

- Central processing
- Psychological disorders
- Ongoing compensation disputes

This must be taken into account in proposing treatments or in evaluating treatment outcomes.

7.8 Uncertainty as to How Shoulder Interventions Work

In some situations, we may not fully understand how our interventions work [23, 24] and hence why the effects of the same intervention may vary amongst patients:

- In carrying out subacromial decompression surgery, potential ways by which the pain may be relieved include:
  - Resection of the bone to reduce mechanical impingement
  - Bursectomy to remove pain receptors, transmission nerve endings and mediators

  - Washout of the subacromial space reducing the load of inflammatory mediators
  - Debridement of an associated partial rotator cuff tendon tear
  - Central pain processing – placebo effect

  Appreciating such limitations is essential to:

- Plan the relative components of any applied intervention
- Counsel patients with regard to any proposed management

7.9 Lack of Evidence Supporting Shoulder Interventions

When it comes to the treatment conditions, we may have limited high-quality evidence as to the effectiveness of the available interventions and the superiority of one intervention over another [25–27]. Hence:

- It may be preferable to try the least invasive and potentially least harmful interventions first
- It is essential to communicate such uncertainty with patients

7.10 Intervention Management Ladder for Shoulder Disorders

In dealing with shoulder conditions, one may consider the intervention management ladder [28] whereby simple non-invasive interventions are tried prior to proceeding with more complex invasive interventions such as arthroscopic or open shoulder surgery. This management ladder needs to be discussed with the patient, and it is on occasions preferable that one step in the ladder is tried before the next step is attempted. However, some patients may prefer going straight onto the more invasive interventions to avoid time loss and associated functional loss that may occur if the less invasive procedures do not work. Some patients may also have strong views against some interventions (such as injection therapy in needle phobia), and this should also be taken into account in discussing treatment.

Intervention management ladder

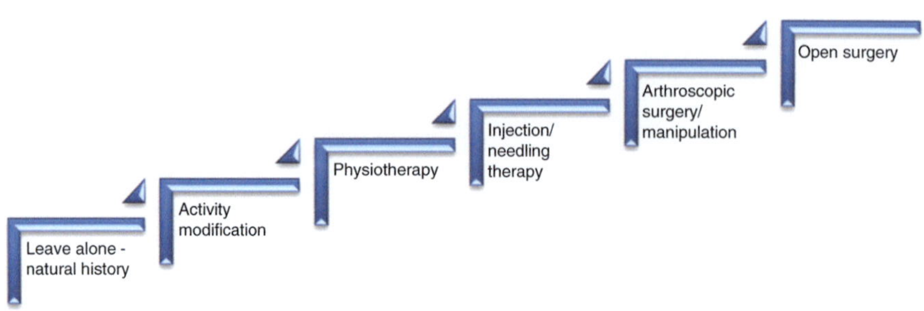

> **Learning Pearls**
> - There is uncertainty in much of what we do
> - One solution does not fit all

References

1. Vastamäki H, Kettunen J, Vastamäki M. The natural history of idiopathic frozen shoulder: a 2- to 27-year follow up study. Clin Orthop Relat Res. 2012;470(4):1133–43.
2. Reeves B. The natural history of the frozen shoulder syndrome. Scand J Rheumatol. 1975;4(4):193–6.
3. Ertan S, Ayhan E, Güven MF, Kesmezacar H, Akgün K, Babacan M. Medium-term natural history of subacromial impingement syndrome. J Shoulder Elb Surg. 2015;24(10):1512–8.
4. Hebert-Davies J, Teefey SA, Steger-May K, Chamberlain AM, Middleton W, Robinson K, Yamaguchi K, Keener JD. Progression of fatty muscle degeneration in Atraumatic rotator cuff tears. J Bone Joint Surg Am. 2017;99(10):832–9.
5. Keener JD, Galatz LM, Teefey SA, Middleton WD, Steger-May K, Stobbs-Cucchi G, Patton R, Yamaguchi K. A prospective evaluation of survivorship of asymptomatic degenerative rotator cuff tears. J Bone Joint Surg Am. 2015;97(2):89–98.
6. Moosmayer S, Tariq R, Stiris M, Smith HJ. The natural history of asymptomatic rotator cuff tears: a three-year follow-up of fifty cases. J Bone Joint Surg Am. 2013;95(14):1249–55.
7. Flint JH, Pickett A, Owens BD, Svoboda SJ, Peck KY, Cameron KL, Biery J, Giuliani J, Rue JP. Recurrent shoulder instability in a young, active, military population and its professional implications. Sports Health. 2018;10(1):54–9.
8. Kardouni JR, McKinnon CJ, Seitz AL. Incidence of shoulder dislocations and the rate of recurrent instability in soldiers. Med Sci Sports Exerc. 2016;48(11):2150–6.
9. Mall NA, Foley E, Chalmers PN, Cole BJ, Romeo AA, Bach BR Jr. Degenerative joint disease of the acromioclavicular joint: a review. Am J Sports Med. 2013;41(11):2684–92.
10. Needell SD, Zlatkin MB, Sher JS, Murphy BJ, Uribe JW. MR imaging of the rotator cuff: peritendinous and bone abnormalities in an asymptomatic population. AJR Am J Roentgenol. 1996;166(4):863–7.
11. Weber SC, Martin DF, Seiler JG 3rd, Harrast JJ. Superior labrum anterior and posterior lesions of the shoulder: incidence rates, complications, and outcomes as reported by American Board of Orthopedic Surgery. Part II candidates. Am J Sports Med. 2012;40(7):1538–43.
12. Tuckman DV, Dines DM. Long head of the biceps pathology as a cause of anterior shoulder pain after shoulder arthroplasty. J Shoulder Elb Surg. 2006;15(4):415–8.
13. Levy O, Copeland SA. Cementless surface replacement arthroplasty of the shoulder. 5- to 10-year results with the Copeland mark-2 prosthesis. J Bone Joint Surg Br. 2001;83(2):213–21.
14. Kandil TS, El Hefnawy E. Shoulder pain following laparoscopic cholecystectomy: factors affecting the incidence and severity. J Laparoendosc Adv Surg Tech A. 2010;20(8):677–82.
15. de Manzoni G, Furlan F, Guglielmi A, Brunelli G, Laterza E, Ricci F, Genna M, Borzellino G, Cordiano C. Acute cholecystitis: ultrasonographic staging and percutaneous cholecystostomy. Eur J Radiol. 1992;15(2):175–9.
16. Cho CH, Jang HK, Bae KC, Lee SW, Lee YK, Shin HK, Hwang I. Clinical outcomes of rotator cuff repair with arthroscopic capsular release and manipulation for rotator cuff tear with stiffness: a matched-pair comparative study between patients with and without stiffness. Arthroscopy. 2015;31(3):482–7.
17. Tauro JC. Stiffness and rotator cuff tears: incidence, arthroscopic findings, and treatment results. Arthroscopy. 2006;22(6):581–6.

18. Chuang TY, Ho WP, Chen CH, Lee CH, Liau JJ, Huang CH. Arthroscopic treatment of rotator cuff tears with shoulder stiffness: a comparison of functional outcomes with and without capsular release. Am J Sports Med. 2012;40(9):2121–7.
19. Ketola S, Lehtinen J, Rousi T, Nissinen M, Huhtala H, Arnala I. Which patients do not recover from shoulder impingement syndrome, either with operative treatment or with nonoperative treatment? Acta Orthop. 2015;86(6):641–6.
20. Wylie JD, Suter T, Potter MQ, Granger EK, Tashjian RZ. Mental health has a stronger association with patient-reported shoulder pain and function than tear size in patients with full-thickness rotator cuff tears. J Bone Joint Surg Am. 2016;98(4):251–6.
21. Dunn WR, Kuhn JE, Sanders R, An Q, Baumgarten KM, Bishop JY, Brophy RH, Carey JL, Holloway GB, Jones GL, Ma CB, Marx RG, McCarty EC, Poddar SK, Smith MV, Spencer EE, Vidal AF, Wolf BR, Wright RW. Symptoms of pain do not correlate with rotator cuff tear severity: a cross-sectional study of 393 patients with a symptomatic atraumatic full-thickness rotator cuff tear. J Bone Joint Surg Am. 2014;96(10):793–800.
22. Kim HM, Caldwell JM, Buza JA, Fink LA, Ahmad CS, Bigliani LU, Levine WN. Factors affecting satisfaction and shoulder function in patients with a recurrent rotator cuff tear. J Bone Joint Surg Am. 2014;96(2):106–12.
23. Neviaser TJ, Neviaser RJ, Neviaser JS, Neviaser JS. The four-in-one arthroplasty for the painful arc syndrome. Clin Orthop Relat Res. 1982;163:107–12.
24. Henkus HE, de Witte PB, Nelissen RGHH, Brand R, van Arkel ERA. Bursectomy compared with acromioplasty in the management of subacromial impingement syndrome: a prospective randomised study. J Bone Joint Surg Br. 2009;91(4):504–10.
25. Ketola S, Lehtinen J, Rousi T, Nissinen M, Huhtala H, Konttinen YT, Arnala I. No evidence of long-term benefits of arthroscopic acromioplasty in the treatment of shoulder impingement syndrome: five-year results of a randomised controlled trial. Bone Joint Res. 2013;2(7):132–9.
26. Ketola S, Lehtinen J, Arnala I, Nissinen M, Westenius H, Sintonen H, Aronen P, Konttinen YT, Malmivaara A, Rousi T. Does arthroscopic acromioplasty provide any additional value in the treatment ofshoulder impingement syndrome?: a two-year randomised controlled trial. J Bone Joint Surg Br. 2009;91(10):1326–34.
27. Beard DJ, Rees JL, Cook JA, Rombach I, Cooper C, Merritt N, Shirkey BA, Donovan JL, Gwilym S, Savulescu J, Moser J, Gray A, Jepson M, Tracey I, Judge A, Wartolowska K, Carr AJ, CSAW Study Group. Arthroscopic subacromial decompression for subacromial shoulder pain (CSAW): a multicentre, pragmatic, parallel group, placebo-controlled, three-group, randomised surgical trial. Lancet. 2018;391(10118):329–38.
28. Charalambous CP. Professionalism in surgery, in career skills for surgeons. Berlin: Springer; 2017. p. 5–46.

Chapter 8
Surgical Interventions for Shoulder Disorders

Surgery lies at the top of the intervention management ladder [1] in dealing with shoulder disorders. This chapter discusses how surgical interventions aim to reduce troublesome symptoms and improve shoulder function, to help guide the clinician patient communication. It also describes the principles of arthroscopic surgery and the various open approaches that may be utilised in shoulder surgery. Some of the common shoulder surgical procedures are presented, along with a description as to what they entail.

8.1 Principles of Surgical Interventions

Surgical interventions may be considered based on what they aim to achieve. This may be to:

- Restore the normal structure of the shoulder as close as possible such as by:
  - Repairing a torn rotator cuff tendon
  - Excising an acromial spur in subacromial impingement
  - Reducing and stabilising an unstable acromioclavicular joint (ACJt)
- Replace a joint to help pain and improve function:
  - Replace the glenohumeral joint in osteoarthritis or rotator cuff arthropathy
- Salvage an unfavourable situation – accept that it is not possible to restore the normal structure of the shoulder but use alternative means to improve one's symptoms:
  - Tuberoplasty in massive rotator cuff tear
  - Tenotomy in long head of the biceps tendon instability and degeneration
  - Muscle transfer in an irreparable rotator cuff tear
  - Fusion in recurrent glenohumeral instability where other modalities have failed or not deemed appropriate

© Springer Nature Switzerland AG 2019

C. Panayiotou Charalambous, *The Shoulder Made Easy*,
https://doi.org/10.1007/978-3-319-98908-2_8

Aims of surgical interventions for shoulder disorders

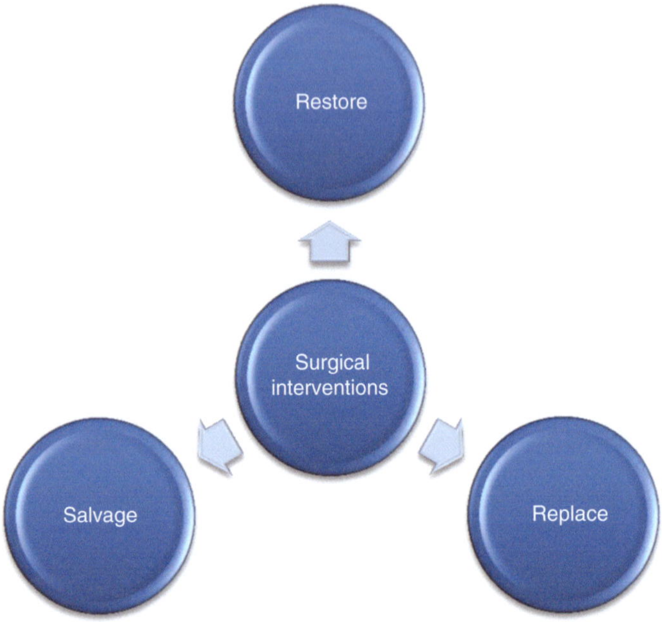

8.2 Arthroscopic and Open Shoulder Surgery

Certain surgical procedures are commonly used in dealing with shoulder conditions, and these are described next.

8.2.1 Arthroscopic Shoulder Surgery

Arthroscopic surgery (Keyhole surgery) utilises portals (small incisions) [2–4] through which:

- A camera is passed to allow visualisation of the glenohumeral joint or subacromial space
- Instruments are passed to carry out a surgical procedure (shaver for shaving and removing the bone, vapour device for dividing or coagulating soft tissue, repair instruments for repairing tears)

During arthroscopic surgery, the shoulder is inflated with fluid (normal saline) to:

- Improve visualisation
- Minimise bleeding

8.2.1.1 Surgical Portals in Arthroscopic Shoulder Surgery

Several portals are available for arthroscopic shoulder surgery, including:

Posterior Portal

Provides access to the:

- Glenohumeral joint
- Subacromial space

Location

- Posterior part of the shoulder about 2 cm inferior and 2 cm medial to the posterior-lateral corner of the acromion (soft spot)

Lateral Portal

Provides access to the subacromial space

Location

- About 1 cm posterior and 4 cm distal to the anterior-lateral corner of the acromion

Anterior Portal

Provides access to the:

- Glenohumeral joint
- Subacromial space
- ACJt

Location

- Anterior part of the shoulder
- Lateral to the coracoid
- Percutaneous needle can help guide exact position under direct arthroscopic visualisation

Superior Portal

Provides access to the:

- Glenohumeral joint
- Subacromial space

Location

- Soft spot between the medial part of the acromion and the posterior part of the lateral end of the clavicle

8.2.2 Open Shoulder Surgery

Open surgery refers to the use of longer incisions to allow access to the internal aspect of the shoulder joint, whereby surgery is performed under direct visualisation. Several approaches are available for open shoulder surgery [5–7], including:

- Anterior – Delto-pectoral approach
  - Access:
    - Subacromial space
    - Glenohumeral joint
  - Incision:
    - From the coracoid process extending distally
    - In line with the delto-pectoral groove
  - Superficial dissection:
    - Retract cephalic vein; incise the delto-pectoral fascia
    - Muscle interval – between deltoid and clavicular head of pectoralis major
  - Deep dissection:
    - Retract conjoined tendon medially
    - If access to the glenohumeral joint is required, this is achieved by subscapularis tendon split or by detachment/division/osteotomy of the subscapularis tendon humeral insertion
- Posterior approach to the shoulder
  - Access:
    - Subacromial space
    - Glenohumeral joint
  - Incision:
    - In line with the spine of the scapula to the posterior part of the acromion
  - Superficial dissection:
    - Muscle plane – between infraspinatus medially and deltoid laterally
  - Deep dissection:
    - Infraspinatus superiorly
    - Teres minor inferiorly
    - If glenohumeral joint access is required, divide the joint capsule

- Lateral – McKenzie approach
  - Access:
    - Subacromial space
    - Proximal humerus
    - Glenohumeral joint
  - Incision:
    - From the tip of the acromion to the lateral aspect of the arm
    - Can be extended to the ACJt allowing access to that joint
  - Superficial dissection:
    - Split deltoid fibres
    - Identify and protect the axillary nerve
  - Deep dissection
    - If access to the glenohumeral joint is required split/detach the rotator cuff tendon

8.3 Patient Positioning for Shoulder Surgery

This aims to:

- Facilitate access to the necessary area
- Minimise intraoperative bleeding

Patient positioning [8–11] includes:

- Beach chair position – patient sat up 60–90°
- On the lateral side – patient lying on the side
- Supine – patient flat

8.4 Minimising Bleeding in Shoulder Surgery

This aims to:

- Minimise any haematological or cardiovascular adverse effects on the patient
- Improve the arthroscopic or open surgical view to facilitate surgery

Certain approaches may be adopted to help minimise intraoperative bleeding [12–19]:

- Joint/space inflation with pressurised fluid
- Beach chair positioning
- Chemical agents – intravenous tranexamic acid, local adrenaline
- Surgical techniques – minimise fluid turbulence, direct pressure

- Anaesthesia induced
  - Hypotension
  - Bradycardia
  - Avoidance of hypercapnia

8.5 Types of Shoulder Surgical Procedures

Several surgical procedures are available in dealing with shoulder conditions, and the following describes what these involve. Most of these (with the exception of realignment osteotomies and arthroplasty procedures) may be performed with arthroscopic or open surgery.

Tendon/ligament repair – if a tendon or ligament is torn through its substance, it may be stitched together by passing sutures through the torn ends. However, in many shoulder conditions, tendon or ligament tears are avulsions from their bony insertions rather than mid-substance tears. Such avulsions may be reattached back to the bone by using:

- Suture anchors – these are screwlike implants (made of metal or non-metallic material) that have sutures attached to them. The anchor is inserted into the bone, and the suture is used to stitch the tendon onto the bone. These may be:
  - Knotted – require the sutures to be tied
  - Knotless – do not require the tying of knots

Bone suture anchors used in reattachment of tendon to the bone

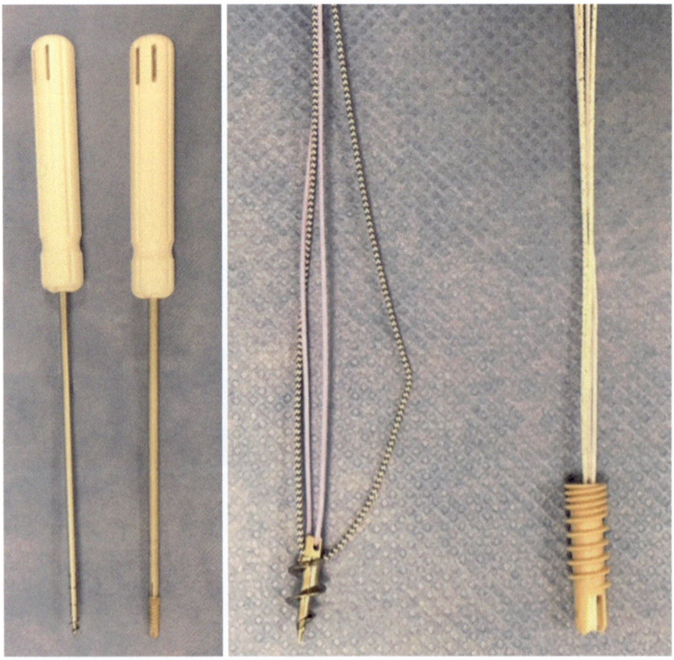

(a) Supraspinatus tendon tear as seen from the subacromial space – arthroscopic view, (b) Metallic suture anchor is inserted through the tendon tear into the humeral head (view from within glenohumeral joint), (c) Suture anchor is buried in the humeral head, with its sutures protruding through the bone, (d) Anchor's sutures as seen from subacromial space, (e) Sutures are passed through the torn tendon, (f) Sutures passed through the tendon are tied (medial row), (g, h) Sutures are then brought over the tendon and stablilised with a lateral knotless anchor (suture bridge technique)

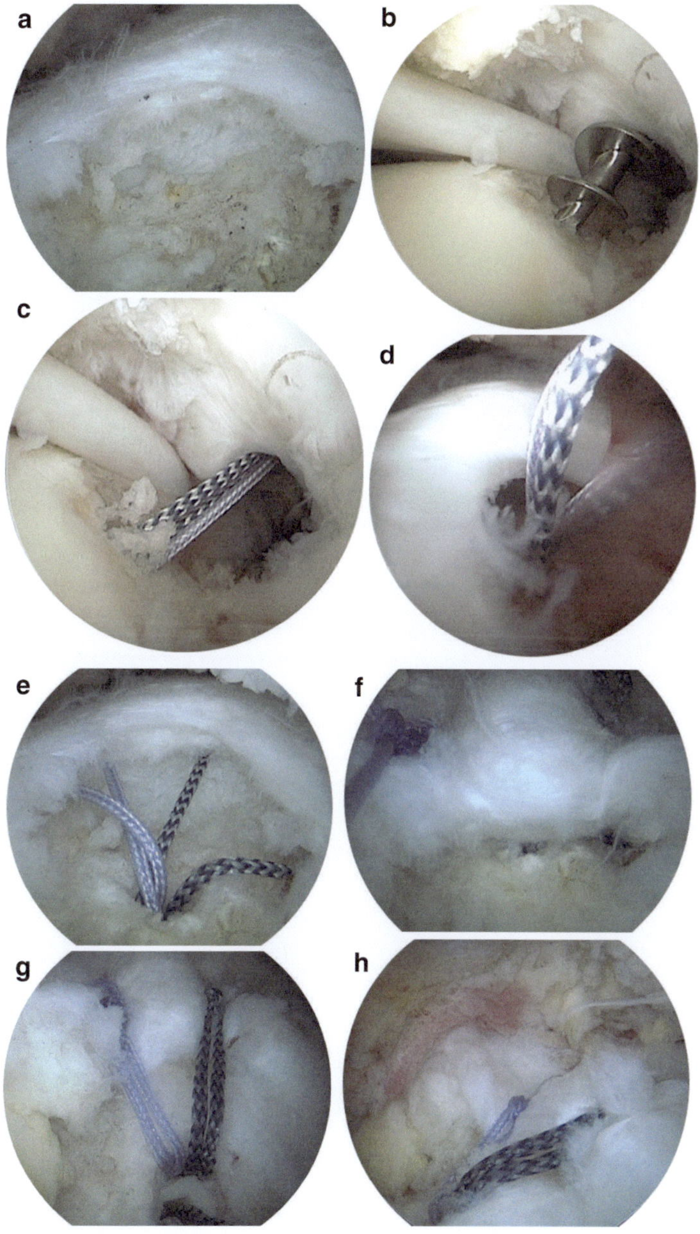

Previous glenohumeral joint antero-inferior labrum repair using metallic anchors (red arrow) which are visible on plain radiograph

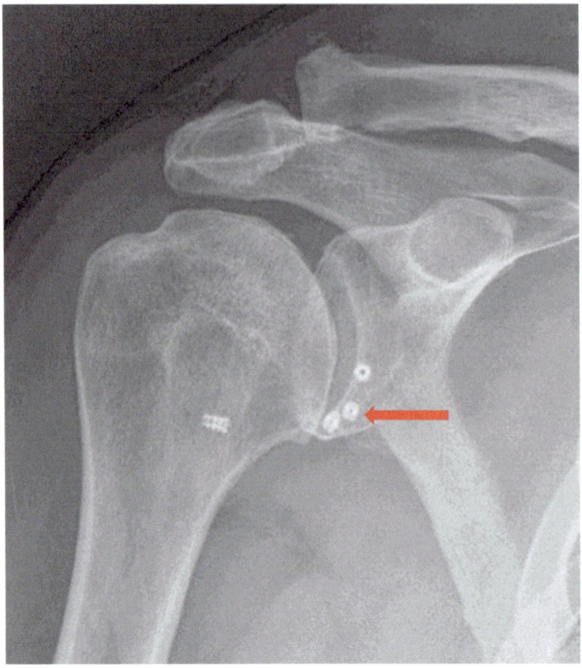

Metallic anchor (yellow arrow) in the humeral head, used to reattach a supraspinatus tendon tear

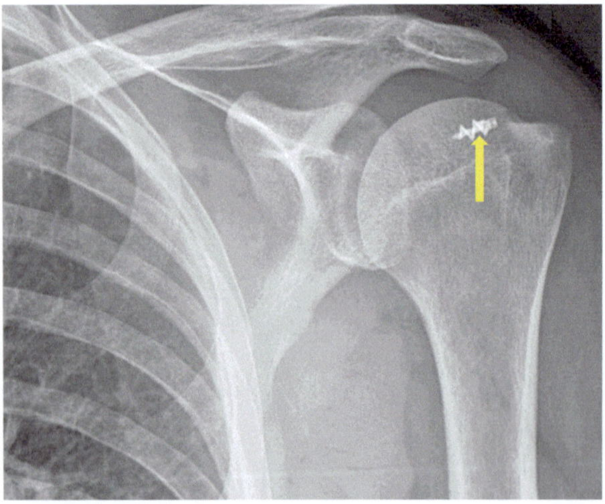

- Bone tunnels – tunnels are drilled through the bone through which sutures are passed which then reattach the tendon or ligament back to the bone

Tendon transfer: this refers to detaching a tendon from its normal insertion, moving it and reattaching it somewhere else. In this way the tendon, and hence the muscle, which has been transferred, may take over the activity of another tendon (muscle) which is torn or dysfunctional. The tendon that is transferred is one the loss of which will not result in further functional loss. For a tendon transfer to be effective, the joint across which it is expected to act has to be mobile; a stiff joint cannot be moved by a transferred tendon no matter how much force is applied.

Tenotomy: the division of a tendon which is then left free (not reattached).

Tenodesis: the reattachment of a tendon at a site away from its normal insertion point. Such a tendon may have ruptured, but it is not feasible to be reattached to its normal site; hence it is reattached back to the bone at a distant site. Alternatively, the tendon may have been surgically divided, or part of the tendon may have been excised to help ease symptoms such as pain.

Bone plasty: the shape of a bone is altered – in the shoulder this may involve smoothening a bone by removing spurs.

Debridement: this may involve:

- Removal of any unstable articular cartilage flaps
- Smoothening of articular cartilage fibrillations
- Excision of unstable tendinous flaps
- Smoothening of tendinous/labrum fraying
- Excision of inflamed/hyperplastic synovium

Osteotomy: this refers to surgical division of a bone. It is part of a realignment procedure whereby the bone is divided, its alignment or orientation is altered and the bone is then fixed in the new position. The bone then heals in this new position. It may be used to:

- Improve joint stability by redirecting a joint surface towards a more stable orientation
- Unload a diseased area by shifting the transmitted forces to a healthy area and hence improve pain

Arthroplasty: this refers to altering the joint in one of several ways:

- Excision arthroplasty – part of the joint is excised – this may stop two arthritic areas rubbing against each other and causing pain such as in ACJt excision
- Fusion arthroplasty – the articular surfaces of a joint are fixed together to stop two arthritic areas rubbing against each other and causing pain
- Replacement arthroplasty – one or both articular surfaces of a joint are replaced
  - Hemi-arthroplasty – only one of the two articulating surfaces is replaced – the humeral head
  - Total shoulder replacement – both articular surfaces are replaced

Several types of shoulder replacement arthroplasty are described [9–11] depending on the characteristics of the components utilised. These include:

- Humeral head resurfacing – the humeral head is reshaped to accommodate a cap which is used to cover the humeral head. The main advantage of this is that it avoids removing the humeral head; hence it is bone preserving. In addition, the native anatomy of the humeral head with regard to its orientation in relation to the humeral shaft and glenoid is maintained
- Stemmed humeral prosthesis – the humeral head is excised and is replaced by a prosthesis that consists of a stem and a head. The stem is inserted into the humeral shaft to which it is stabilised by cement or cementless (press fit) methods
- Anatomic total shoulder replacement – the normal anatomic relation of the humeral head and glenoid is maintained, i.e. a ball replaces the humeral head, and a socket replaces the glenoid
- Reverse total shoulder replacement – the normal anatomic relation of the humeral head and glenoid is reversed – i.e. a ball replaces the glenoid, and a socket replaces the humeral head

References

1. Charalambous CP. Professionalism in surgery. In: Career skills for surgeons. Berlin: Springer; 2017. p. 5–46.
2. Farmer KW, Wright TW. Shoulder arthroscopy: the basics. J Hand Surg Am. 2015;40(4):817–21.
3. Meyer M, Graveleau N, Hardy P, Landreau P. Anatomic risks of shoulder arthroscopy portals: anatomic cadaveric study of 12 portals. Arthroscopy. 2007;23(5):529–36.
4. Snyder SJ, Fasulo GJ. Shoulder arthroscopy: surgical technique. Surg Technol Int. 1993;2:447–53.
5. Chalmers PN, Van Thiel GS, Trenhaile SW. Surgical exposures of the shoulder. J Am Acad Orthop Surg. 2016;24(4):250–8.
6. Hoyen H, Papendrea R. Exposures of the shoulder and upper humerus. Hand Clin. 2014;30(4):391–9.
7. Zlotolow DA, Catalano LW 3rd, Barron OA, Glickel SZ. Surgical exposures of the humerus. J Am Acad Orthop Surg. 2006;14(13):754–65.
8. Mannava S, Jinnah AH, Plate JF, Stone AV, Tuohy CJ, Freehill MT. Basic shoulder arthroscopy: beach chair patient positioning. Arthrosc Tech. 2016;5(4):e731–5.
9. Jinnah AH, Mannava S, Plate JF, Stone AV, Freehill MT. Basic shoulder arthroscopy: lateral decubitus patient positioning. Arthrosc Tech. 2016;5(5):e1069–75.
10. Li X, Eichinger JK, Hartshorn T, Zhou H, Matzkin EG, Warner JP. A comparison of the lateral decubitus and beach-chair positions for shoulder surgery: advantages and complications. J Am Acad Orthop Surg. 2015;23(1):18–28.
11. Peruto CM, Ciccotti MG, Cohen SB. Shoulder arthroscopy positioning: lateral decubitus versus beach chair. Arthroscopy. 2009;25(8):891–6.
12. Hsiao MS, Kusnezov N, Sieg RN, Owens BD, Herzog JP. Use of an irrigation pump system in arthroscopic procedures. Orthopedics. 2016;39(3):e474–8.
13. Yepes H, Al-Hibshi A, Tang M, Morris SF, Stanish WD. Vascular anatomy of the subacromial space: a map of bleeding points for the arthroscopic surgeon. Arthroscopy. 2007;23(9):978–84.
14. Jensen KH, Werther K, Stryger V, Schultz K, Falkenberg B. Arthroscopic shoulder surgery with epinephrine saline irrigation. Arthroscopy. 2001;17(6):578–81.

15. Burkhart SS, Danaceau SM, Athanasiou KA. Turbulence control as a factor in improving visualization during subacromial shoulder arthroscopy. Arthroscopy. 2001;17(2):209–12.
16. Morrison DS, Schaefer RK, Friedman RL. The relationship between subacromial space pressure, blood pressure, and visual clarity during arthroscopic subacromial decompression. Arthroscopy. 1995;11(5):557–60.
17. Levy O, Haddo O, Sforza G, Copeland S, Rath E. "Put your 'extended' finger on the bleeder": the use of direct pressure from the shaver blade to achieve hemostasis. Arthroscopy. 2011;27(6):867–9.
18. Pauzenberger L, Domej MA, Heuberer PR, Hexel M, Grieb A, Laky B, Blasl J, Anderl W. The effect of intravenous tranexamic acid on blood loss and early post-operative pain in total shoulder arthroplasty. Bone Joint J. 2017;99-B(8):1073–9.
19. Lee JH, Min KT, Chun YM, Kim EJ, Choi SH. Effects of beach-chair position and induced hypotension on cerebral oxygen saturation in patients undergoing arthroscopic shoulder surgery. Arthroscopy. 2011;27(7):889–94.

Chapter 9
Shoulder Injection and Needling Therapy

Injection or needling interventions are extensively used in the management of shoulder disorders. This chapter discusses injection therapy, including the types of injectates commonly utilised, their possible underlying mechanisms of action as well as potential associated complications. Techniques commonly used in injecting the shoulder are also presented. In addition, reference is made to dry needling techniques in the management of tendon and muscle disorders as well as the use of barbotage in the treatment of calcific tendinopathy.

9.1 Injection Therapy

Several agents may be injected in the shoulder and these are described below. There is substantial controversy as to the extent of effectiveness of these injectates, and a wide variation is observed in the benefit obtained amongst patients to such injections [1–5]. Patients need to be warned of the possibility that such injections may have no benefit and that even when improvement in symptoms occurs, such improvement may be short-lived. It is not possible to reliably predict at an individual level which patient will benefit the most from shoulder injections.

9.2 Types of Shoulder Injections

Commonly utilised shoulder injections are discussed next.

© Springer Nature Switzerland AG 2019

C. Panayiotou Charalambous, *The Shoulder Made Easy*,
https://doi.org/10.1007/978-3-319-98908-2_9

9.2.1 Steroid Injections

Steroid injections are used for their anti-inflammatory effect to help:

- Improve pain
- Reduce soft tissue inflammation, oedema and joint stiffness

They may be injected into the:

- Subacromial space—for subacromial pain syndrome
- Glenohumeral joint—for adhesive capsulitis, synovitis and arthritis
- ACJt—for arthropathy
- Bicipital groove—for long head of biceps tendinopathy
- Suprascapular notch—to reduce suprascapular nerve symptoms

They are usually administered mixed with a local anaesthetic, which increases the volume of fluid to be injected and hence its distribution area.

There have been concerns with steroid injections in that:

- They may adversely affect supraspinatus tendon cells [6–8] by:
  - Reducing cell proliferation
  - Causing cell degeneration
  - Reducing collagen formation impairing the ability of tendon cells to repair
- They may reduce local immune responses increasing the risk of infection in subsequent arthroplasty procedures [9–11]
- They may be systemically absorbed causing blood sugar elevation in patients with diabetes [12]

9.2.2 Hyaluronic Acid Injections

Hyaluronic acid and its derivatives are available in multiple commercial preparations. Their aim is to supplement the natural hyaluronic acid found in synovial fluid. Depending on the commercial preparation, they may be administered as a single injection or as a course of 3–5 weekly injections.

Hyaluronic acid aims to reduce pain and improve function and may exert its effects by [13–15]:

- Limiting cell death and hence protecting cartilage degeneration
- Reducing inflammation
- Reducing synovial fibrosis
- Reducing synovial new vessel formation

Hyaluronic acid may be injected into the:

- Subacromial space—for subacromial pain syndrome, tendinopathy [16, 17]
- Glenohumeral joint—for degenerative arthritis, adhesive capsulitis [18, 19]

9.2.3 Platelet-Rich Plasma injections

Whole blood is obtained from the patient by venepuncture and is centrifuged. This allows platelets and growth factors (such as TGF-b, PDGF, FGF) which can stimulate tissue healing and regeneration to be separated from the rest of the blood [20–22]. This platelet/growth factor concentrate is then injected at the area of interest such as the:

- Subacromial space—for subacromial pain syndrome, tendinopathy, rotator cuff tears [23, 24]
- Glenohumeral joint—for adhesive capsulitis [25]

9.2.4 Local Anaesthetic Injections

- Local anaesthetic may be administered as a component of other injectates to increase the volume of the administered solution and hence the area into which it can be delivered
- Local anaesthetic injections may be used in isolation as treatment of:
  - Myofascial trigger points [26, 27]
  - Peripheral nerve dysfunction [28]
- Sole local anaesthetic injections may also be used as diagnostic injections [29, 30] to help:
  - Determine if the pain a patient complains originates from the area injected
  - Determine if muscle relaxation improves the patient's symptoms

There have been concerns about the effects of local anaesthetic injections [31, 32] including:

- Cytotoxicity to tenocytes and chondrocytes
- Impairment of the biomechanical properties of tendons
- Induction of tendon cell apoptosis

9.2.5 Normal Saline Injections

Normal saline may be injected into muscular tender spots to help pain originating from such spots. Its effects may be mediated by a mechanical pressure mechanism [33, 34].

9.3 Contra-Indications to Injection Therapy

The following are potential contra-indications to injection therapy:

- Local or systemic infection
- Hypersensitivity to the injectate
- Uncontrolled diabetes
- Acute fracture at the site of injection
- Anticoagulation therapy due to risk of bleeding—current evidence however suggests that routine discontinuation is not necessary as the risk of bleeding is very small [35, 36]

9.4 Potential Complications of Shoulder Injections

Several complications of injection therapy have been described [9, 12, 37, 38]. Some are seen across injectates and some are more injectate specific. These complications must be discussed with the patient prior to injecting the shoulder and include:

- Infection
- Bleeding causing soft tissue haematoma or haemarthrosis
- Neurovascular damage
- Hypersensitivity reactions
- Local pain and tenderness (post-hyaluronic acid injections)
- Subcutaneous fat atrophy, thinning of the skin, loss of pigmentation (steroid injections if adversely injected into subcutaneous tissue)
- Aggravation of pain—post-steroid injections, usually self-limiting
- Menstrual bleeding—heavier, erratic, postmenopausal (post-steroid injections)
- Blood sugar derangement—post-steroid injections

9.5 Shoulder Injection Techniques

Injections into the shoulder area may be administered using radiological imaging guidance such as image intensifier radiography or dynamic ultrasound [39–42]. Such guidance is preferable for injections administered in tight spaces or close to tubular tendons (into which injection is to be avoided) or neurovascular structures. Hence, radiological guidance (to help the accuracy of administration) is preferable for injections into the:

- ACJt—plain radiographs or US
- Bicipital groove—US
- Suprascapular notch—US

ACJt injection with needle (green arrow) inserted under image intensifier control

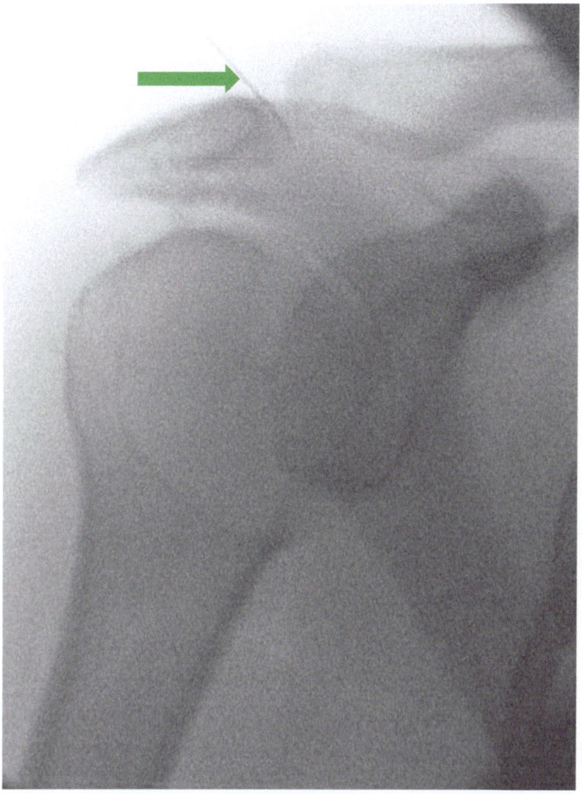

Injections however may be also performed using palpable anatomical landmarks, and the techniques for these are described next.

9.5.1 Glenohumeral Joint Injection

Patient is sitting or standing

- Anterior approach
  - Rotate the proximal humerus internally and externally whilst palpating the anterior part of the shoulder just lateral to the coracoid, feeling for the interval between the humeral head and glenoid
  - Insert the needle into this interval aiming in a posterior and slight medial direction
  - If the needle hits the humeral head, withdraw slightly and direct it more medially

- Posterior approach
  - Identify the soft spot on the posterior part of the shoulder—located about 2 cm inferior and medial to the posterolateral corner of the acromion. This is the entry point
  - Palpate the tip of the coracoid
  - Insert the needle aiming towards the tip of the coracoid

Glenohumeral injection via anterior (a) and posterior (b) approach

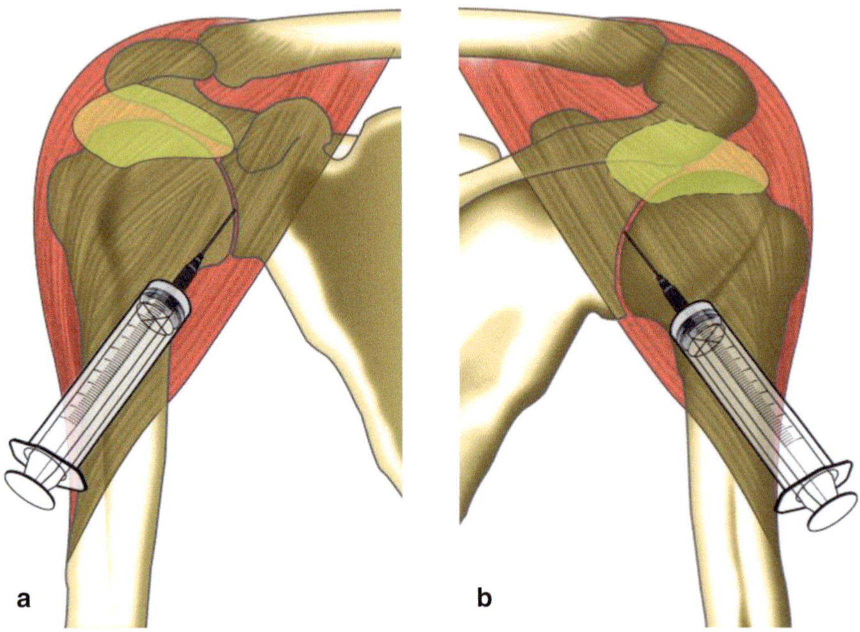

9.5.2 *Subacromial Space Injection*

Patient is sitting or standing with the arm hanging by the side relaxed, so the weight of the arm pulls down the humeral head, increasing the access to the subacromial space.

- Anterior-lateral approach
  - Identify the soft spot inferior to the anterior-lateral part of the acromion—located about 1 cm posterior and inferior to the anterior-lateral corner of the acromion
  - Insert the needle aiming towards the undersurface of the acromion
  - If the needle is directed too horizontally, it will hit the humeral head; if too vertical, it will hit the undersurface of the acromion

- Posterior approach
  - Identify the soft spot on the posterior part of the shoulder—located about 2 cm inferior and medial to the posterolateral corner of the acromion
  - Palpate the posterior border of the acromion
  - Insert the needle aiming towards the undersurface of the acromion directing it towards the anterior-lateral part of the acromion

Subacromial injection via a posterior (a) and lateral (b) approach

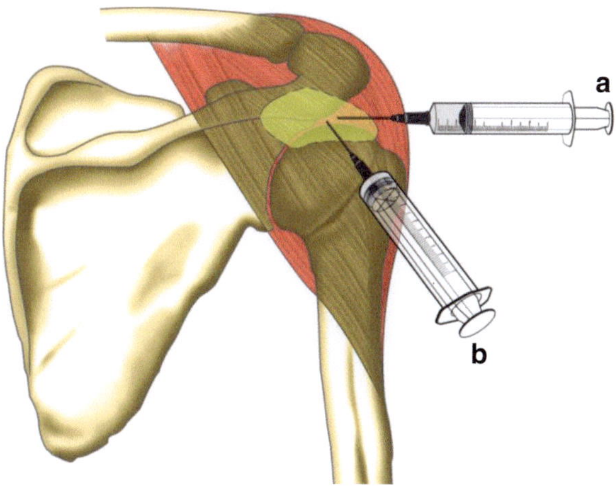

9.5.3 *ACJt Injection*

- Direct superior approach
  - Palpate the lateral end of the clavicle and medial part of the acromion
  - Feel for the depression between the two
  - This is usually located slightly anterior and laterally to the soft spot, located between the medial part of the acromion and posterolateral border of the clavicle
  - Insert the needle aiming inferiorly and slightly medially

ACJt injection—superior approach (a, b)

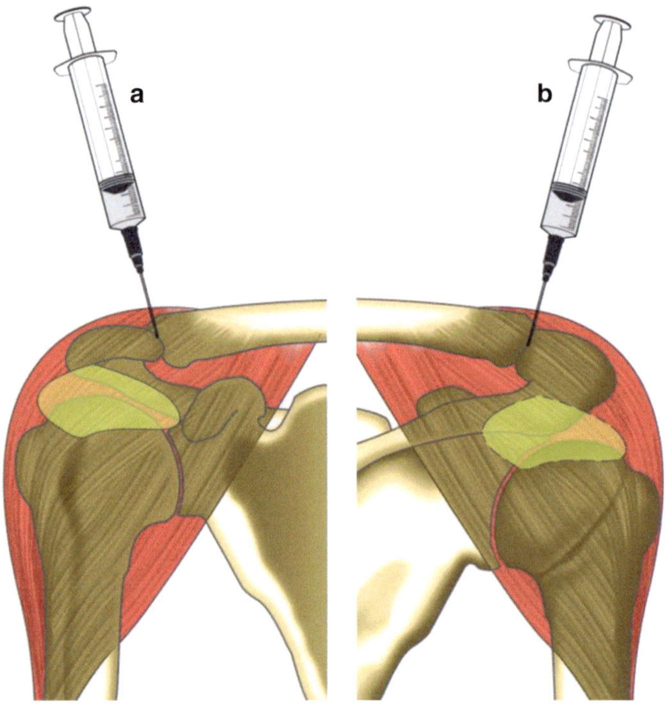

9.5.4 *Bicipital Groove Injection*

- Palpate the anterior part of the shoulder for the bicipital groove
- This can be facilitated by rotating the arm internally and externally
- The bicipital groove is more accessible with the arm in slight internal rotation
- Insert the needle aiming posteriorly
- The needle may go through the biceps tendon and rest on the humeral bone. Withdraw the needle slightly, so it is in the space between the bone and tendon, and inject the solution. There should be minimal resistance during injection; if high resistance is encountered, advance or withdraw the needle further, or reposition, as the needle may be within the tendon substance

9.6 Dry Needling

Dry needling involves the insertion of solid needles (such as acupuncture needles) which aim to create multiple fenestrations in the tissue rather than administer an injectate [43, 44].

This may be in:

- Muscles, in the treatment of muscle tender points
- Tendons
- Ligaments
- Tendon-bone insertion sites

Acupuncture also involves dry needling, but a description of that is beyond the scope of this chapter.

Dry needling may exert its effects by stimulating [34, 45]:

- Local blood flow increasing local oxygen levels
- Activity of fibroblast cells promoting collagen formation, tissue regeneration and healing
- Neural activation of pathways that inhibit pain
- Mechanical pressure effect—activating local reflexes that suppress pain

Technique for dry needling of tendon

- The diseased area of the tendon is identified using dynamic ultrasound
- An acupuncture needle is passed through the skin into the tendon and is used to make multiple fenestrations in the tendon

9.7 Barbotage

Barbotage is a technique used to break down and remove calcific deposits in tendons or ligaments [46].

Technique

- Dynamic ultrasound is used to visualise and localise the calcification
- The calcific deposit is punctured using a percutaneously inserted needle and irrigated with normal saline injected through the needle to break it down
- Once the calcific deposit is broken, the calcium may be aspirated through the same or a second (separately inserted) needle

Learning Pearls

- In assessing a patient who previously had a shoulder injection, it is useful to gather as to which area was injected, as one of several places could have been injected
- Steroid injections may be more preferable in acutely inflamed tissues rather than for chronic noninflammatory pain
- With repetitive administration the effect of steroid injections may diminish—the first injection is considered to be the one most likely to improve one's symptoms
- Steroid injections may exert their effect partly through systemic absorption—on occasions patients report that the injection of one joint helped their pain in other distant joints

References

1. Bouju Y, Bouilleau L, Dubois de Montmarin G, Bacle G, Favard L. Do subacromial ultrasonography findings predict efficacy of intra-bursal injection? Prospective study in 39 patients. Orthop Traumatol Surg Res. 2014;100(8 Suppl):S361–4.
2. Dimitroulas T, Hirsch G, Kitas GD, Klocke R. Clinical outcome of ultrasound-guided steroid injections for chronic shoulder pain. Int J Rheum Dis. 2013;16(4):398–402.
3. Contreras F, Brown HC, Marx RG. Predictors of success of corticosteroid injection for the management of rotator cuff disease. HSS J. 2013;9(1):2–5.
4. Alvarez CM, Litchfield R, Jackowski D, Griffin S, Kirkley A. A prospective, double-blind, randomized clinical trial comparing subacromial injection of betamethasone and xylocaine to xylocaine alone in chronic rotator cuff tendinosis. Am J Sports Med. 2005;33(2):255–62.
5. Gammaitoni AR, Trudeau JJ, Radnovich R, Galer BS, Jensen MP. Predicting response to subacromial injections and lidocaine/tetracaine patch from pretreatment pain quality in patients with shoulder impingement syndrome. Pain Med. 2015;16(7):1333–40.
6. Maman E, Yehuda C, Pritsch T, Morag G, Brosh T, Sharfman Z, Dolkart O. Detrimental effect of repeated and single subacromial corticosteroid injections on the intact and injured rotator cuff: a biomechanical and imaging study in rats. Am J Sports Med. 2016;44(1):177–82.
7. Dean BJ, Franklin SL, Murphy RJ, Javaid MK, Carr AJ. Glucocorticoids induce specific ion-channel-mediated toxicity in human rotator cuff tendon: a mechanism underpinning the ultimately deleterious effect of steroid injection in tendinopathy? Br J Sports Med. 2014;48(22):1620–6.
8. Poulsen RC, Watts AC, Murphy RJ, Snelling SJ, Carr AJ, Hulley PA. Glucocorticoids induce senescence in primary human tenocytes by inhibition of sirtuin 1 and activation of the p53/p21 pathway: in vivo and in vitro evidence. Ann Rheum Dis. 2014;73(7):1405–13.
9. Charalambous CP, Prodromidis AD, Kwaees TA. Do intra-articular steroid injections increase infection rates in subsequent arthroplasty? A systematic review and meta-analysis of comparative studies. J Arthroplast. 2014;29(11):2175–80.
10. Werner BC, Cancienne JM, Browne JA. The timing of total hip arthroplasty after intraarticular hip injection affects postoperative infection risk. J Arthroplast. 2016;31(4):820–3.
11. Chambers AW, Lacy KW, Liow MHL, Manalo JPM, Freiberg AA, Kwon YM. Multiple hip intra-articular steroid injections increase risk of periprosthetic joint infection compared with single injections. J Arthroplast. 2017;32(6):1980–3.
12. Choudhry MN, Malik RA, Charalambous CP. Blood glucose levels following intra-articular steroid injections in patients with diabetes: a systematic review. JBJS Rev. 2016;4(3):372–4. https://doi.org/10.2106/JBJS.RVW.O.00029. pii: 01874474-201603000-00002.
13. Gallorini M, Berardi AC, Berardocco M, Gissi C, Maffulli N, Cataldi A, Oliva F. Hyaluronic acid increases tendon derived cell viability and proliferation in vitro: comparative study of two different hyaluronic acid preparations by molecular weight. Muscles Ligaments Tendons J. 2017;7(2):208–14.
14. Russo F, D'Este M, Vadalà G, Cattani C, Papalia R, Alini M, Denaro V. Platelet rich plasma and hyaluronic acid blend for the treatment of osteoarthritis: rheological and biological evaluation. PLoS One. 2016;11(6):e0157048. https://doi.org/10.1371/journal.pone.0157048. eCollection 2016.
15. Ghosh P, Guidolin D. Potential mechanism of action of intra-articular hyaluronan therapy in osteoarthritis: are the effects molecular weight dependent? Semin Arthritis Rheum. 2002;32(1):10–37.
16. Merolla G, Bianchi P, Porcellini G. Ultrasound-guided subacromial injections of sodium hyaluronate for the management of rotator cuff tendinopathy: a prospective comparative study with rehabilitation therapy. Musculoskelet Surg. 2013;97(Suppl 1):49–56.
17. Penning LI, de Bie RA, Walenkamp GH. The effectiveness of injections of hyaluronic acid or corticosteroid in patients with subacromial impingement: a three-arm randomised controlled trial. J Bone Joint Surg Br. 2012;94(9):1246–52.

18. Lee LC, Lieu FK, Lee HL, Tung TH. Effectiveness of hyaluronic acid administration in treating adhesive capsulitis of the shoulder: a systematic review of randomized controlled trials. Biomed Res Int. 2015;2015:314120. https://doi.org/10.1155/2015/314120.
19. Di Giacomo G, de Gasperis N. Hyaluronic acid intra-articular injections in patients affected by moderate to severe glenohumeral osteoarthritis: a prospective randomized study. Joints. 2017;5(3):138–42.
20. Wu PI, Diaz R, Borg-Stein J. Platelet-rich plasma. Phys Med Rehabil Clin N Am. 2016;27(4):825–53.
21. Mlynarek RA, Kuhn AW, Bedi A. Platelet-rich plasma (PRP) in orthopedic sports medicine. Am J Orthop (Belle Mead NJ). 2016;45(5):290–326.
22. Zhu Y, Yuan M, Meng HY, Wang AY, Guo QY, Wang Y, Peng J. Basic science and clinical application of platelet-rich plasma for cartilage defects and osteoarthritis: a review. Osteoarthr Cartil. 2013;21(11):1627–37.
23. Kesikburun S, Tan AK, Yilmaz B, Yaşar E, Yazicioğlu K. Platelet-rich plasma injections in the treatment of chronic rotator cuff tendinopathy: a randomized controlled trial with 1-year follow-up. Am J Sports Med. 2013;41(11):2609–16.
24. Shams A, El-Sayed M, Gamal O, Ewes W. Subacromial injection of autologous platelet-rich plasma versus corticosteroid for the treatment of symptomatic partial rotator cuff tears. Eur J Orthop Surg Traumatol. 2016;26(8):837–42.
25. Aslani H, Nourbakhsh ST, Zafarani Z, Ahmadi-Bani M, Ananloo ME, Beigy M, Salehi S. Platelet-rich plasma for frozen shoulder: a case report. Arch Bone Jt Surg. 2016;4(1):90–3.
26. Kim DH, Yoon DM, Yoon KB. The effects of myofascial trigger point injections on nocturnal calf cramps. J Am Board Fam Med. 2015;28(1):21–7.
27. Peloso P, Gross A, Haines T, Trinh K, Goldsmith CH, Burnie S, Cervical Overview Group. Medicinal and injection therapies for mechanical neck disorders. Cochrane Database Syst Rev. 2007;3:CD000319.
28. Taskaynatan MA, Yilmaz B, Ozgul A, Yazicioglu K, Kalyon TA. Suprascapular nerve block versus steroid injection for non-specific shoulder pain. Tohoku J Exp Med. 2005;205(1):19–25.
29. McFarland E, Bernard J, Dein E, Johnson A. Diagnostic Injections about the shoulder. J Am Acad Orthop Surg. 2017;25(12):799–807.
30. Bottros MM, AuBuchon JD, McLaughlin LN, Altchek DW, Illig KA, Thompson RW. Exercise-enhanced, ultrasound-guided anterior scalene muscle/pectoralis minor muscle blocks can facilitate the diagnosis of neurogenic thoracic outlet syndrome in the high-performance overhead athlete. Am J Sports Med. 2017;45(1):189–94.
31. Honda H, Gotoh M, Kanazawa T, Nakamura H, Ohta K, Nakamura K, Shiba N. Effects of lidocaine on torn rotator cuff tendons. J Orthop Res. 2016;34(9):1620–7.
32. Kreuz PC, Steinwachs M, Angele P. Single-dose local anesthetics exhibit a type-, dose-, and time-dependent chondrotoxic effect on chondrocytes and cartilage: a systematic review of the current literature. Knee Surg Sports Traumatol Arthrosc. 2018;26(3):819–30.
33. Frost FA, Jessen B, Siggaard-Andersen J. A control, double-blind comparison of mepivacaine injection versus saline injection for myofascial pain. Lancet. 1980;1(8167):499–500.
34. Baldry P. Management of myofascial trigger point pain. Acupunct Med. 2002;20(1):2–10.
35. Yui JC, Preskill C, Greenlund LS. Arthrocentesis and joint injection in patients receiving direct oral anticoagulants. Mayo Clin Proc. 2017;92(8):1223–6.
36. Ahmed I, Gertner E. Safety of arthrocentesis and joint injection in patients receiving anticoagulation at therapeutic levels. Am J Med. 2012;125(3):265–9.
37. Fawi HMT, Hossain M, Matthews TJW. The incidence of flare reaction and short-term outcome following steroid injection in the shoulder. Shoulder Elbow. 2017;9(3):188–94.
38. Charalambous CP, Tryfonidis M, Sadiq S, Hirst P, Paul A. Septic arthritis following intra-articular steroid injection of the knee--a survey of current practice regarding antiseptic technique used during intra-articular steroid injection of the knee. Clin Rheumatol. 2003;22(6):386–90.
39. Messina C, Banfi G, Orlandi D, Lacelli F, Serafini G, Mauri G, Secchi F, Silvestri E, Sconfienza LM. Ultrasound-guided interventional procedures around the shoulder. Br J Radiol. 2016;89(1057):20150372. https://doi.org/10.1259/bjr.20150372.

40. Javed S, Sadozai Z, Javed A, Din A, Schmitgen G. Should all acromioclavicular joint injections be performed under image guidance? J Orthop Surg (Hong Kong). 2017;25(3). 2309499017731633.
41. Hashiuchi T, Sakurai G, Morimoto M, Komei T, Takakura Y, Tanaka Y. Accuracy of the biceps tendon sheath injection: ultrasound-guided or unguided injection? A randomized controlled trial. J Shoulder Elb Surg. 2011;20(7):1069–73.
42. Sabeti-Aschraf M, Lemmerhofer B, Lang S, Schmidt M, Funovics PT, Ziai P, Frenzel S, Kolb A, Graf A, Schueller-Weidekamm C. Ultrasound guidance improves the accuracy of the acromioclavicular joint infiltration: a prospective randomized study. Knee Surg Sports Traumatol Arthrosc. 2011;19(2):292–5.
43. Settergren R. Treatment of supraspinatus tendinopathy with ultrasound guided dry needling. J Chiropr Med. 2013;12(1):26–9.
44. Dunning J, Butts R, Mourad F, Young I, Flannagan S, Perreault T. Dry needling: a literature review with implications for clinical practice guidelines. Phys Ther Rev. 2014;19(4):252–65.
45. Nagraba Ł, Tuchalska J, Mitek T, Stolarczyk A, Deszczyński J. Dry needling as a method of tendinopathy treatment. Ortop Traumatol Rehabil. 2013;15(2):109–16.
46. Gatt DL, Charalambous CP. Ultrasound-guided barbotage for calcific tendonitis of the shoulder: a systematic review including 908 patients. Arthroscopy. 2014;30(9):1166–72.

Chapter 10
Shoulder Physiotherapy: A Surgeon's Perspective

Physiotherapy has an important role to play in reducing troublesome symptoms and improving function in shoulder disorders. Physiotherapy may be the sole modality in the management of shoulder conditions or may compliment surgery, either in optimising a patient for surgery or in enhancing the postsurgical recovery.

This chapter aims to describe some of the principles of shoulder physiotherapy. It is not aimed to be an in-depth analysis of physiotherapy techniques but a basic explanation of terms and principles as perceived by an orthopaedic surgeon. The principles described here may help guide the surgeon in requesting specific physiotherapy for a particular condition and the physiotherapist to appreciate the surgeon's aims and concerns when asking for such therapy. Clear understanding between team members and regular sharing of information is essential in such multidisciplinary care.

Initially some of the physiotherapy nomenclature is presented along with physiotherapy techniques that may be employed in the management of shoulder disorders. The approaches that may be utilised in improving glenohumeral stability, reducing joint stiffness and rehabilitating the shoulder following an injury or surgical repair are then presented. The role of early versus late mobilisation and the role of early loading of the injured or surgically repaired site are also discussed.

10.1 Physiotherapy Nomenclature

Some of the common terms used in physiotherapy [1–5] are presented here. Physiotherapy interventions may be described as:

- Passive—interventions applied to a patient
- Active—activities a patient performs

© Springer Nature Switzerland AG 2019

C. Panayiotou Charalambous, *The Shoulder Made Easy*,
https://doi.org/10.1007/978-3-319-98908-2_10

Limb mobilisation may be described as:

- Passive—movement achieved by the patient using the opposite limb or by the therapist
- Active assisted—movement achieved through action of the limb itself assisted by the opposite limb or by the therapist
- Active—movement achieved solely through action of the limb in consideration

Mobilisation/strengthening exercises may be described as:

- Open kinetic chain active exercises—the distal part of the limb is free (for the upper limb, the hand is free, as in throwing)
- Closed kinetic chain exercises—the distal part of the limb is supported (for the upper limb, the hand is supported, as in rowing)

Muscles contract in order to:

- Maintain a particular position/posture—such as standing still
- Bring about motion—such as arm elevation
- Oppose/decelerate a motion—such as allowing controlled descend of the arm from full elevation, preventing the fall of the elevated arm due to the effect of gravity

Several types of muscle contraction are described:

- Concentric contraction—a type of contraction where the muscle shortens whilst generating a force overcoming an applied resistance—in abducting the arm, the supraspinatus muscle shortens
- Eccentric contraction—a contraction which occurs whilst the muscle lengthens. Essentially the muscle is trying to oppose an applied force, but the applied force is greater than the tension generated by the muscle. This occurs when the abducted arm with a heavy weight in the hand is lowered towards the floor in a controlled fashion. The supraspinatus tenses to oppose the force of the arm weight and the weight held in the hand to allow a slow controlled descend of the arm
- Isometric contraction—an increase in muscle tension without a change in the muscle length. Such contractions are used to maintain posture. Shoulder isometric contractions may involve trying to initiate a movement against firm resistance (such as against a wall)
- Isotonic contraction—contraction where the tension remains constant and leads to either muscle shortening or lengthening. It can either be concentric or eccentric

Eccentric supraspinatus strengthening—right arm is pulled by opposite arm into abduction. Supraspinatus then opposes the slow lowering of the right arm against the effect of gravity

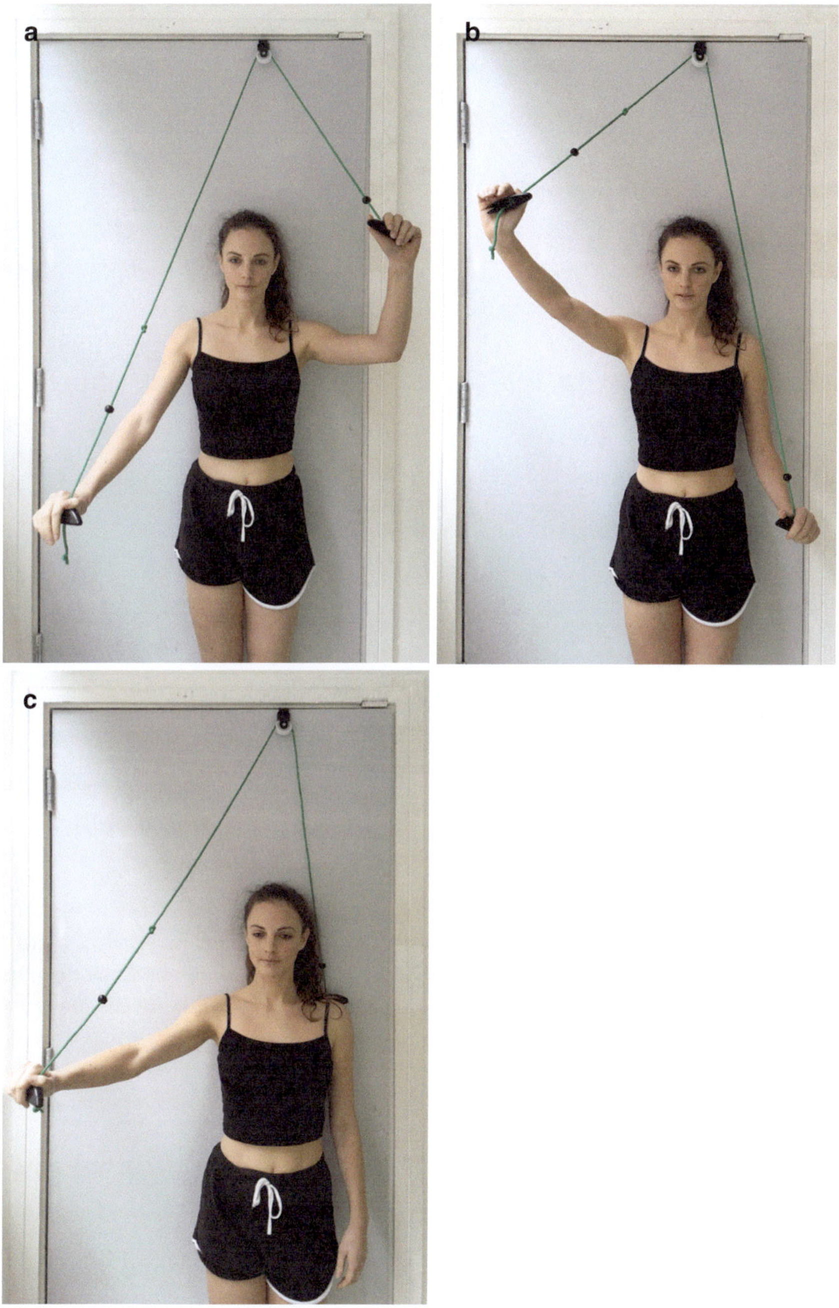

Hence, muscle contractions may help preserve muscle bulk even when limb or joint motion is limited (such as in joint stiffness or when protecting a surgical repair).

Eccentric contractions have been shown to be effective in improving pain and function in tendinopathies through beneficial changes in tendon structure.

Muscles may be described as:

- Agonists—work in synergy
- Antagonists—work in opposition

10.2 Physiotherapy Techniques

Several techniques may be employed in physiotherapy, and some of these are described below.

10.2.1 Local Treatment to Improve Pain

Physiotherapy may reduce pain in multiple ways and some of these are described next.

1. Local passive treatment

According to the gate control theory of pain, activation of nerve endings that transmit touch can lead to inhibition of the transmission of pain signals in the dorsal horn of the spinal cord and hence a reduction in the perception of pain [6, 7]. This may explain why rubbing an area that hurts can improve pain. This is also the basis of several modalities used to improve local pain [8–11] including:

- Transcutaneous electrical nerve stimulation (TENS)
- Heat therapy—this can be applied in the form of a moist heat pack, ultrasound or diathermy. Megapulse is pulsed shortwave diathermy that can heat the deep tissue and increase collagen extensibility. An increase in temperature can lead to an increase in the local vascular response
- Acupuncture—the exact mechanism of the effect of acupuncture is uncertain, but it may involve the release of encephalin and endorphins as well regulate prostaglandin synthesis, all of which can affect pain perception
- Application of localised mechanical pressure or electrical pulsing may have a similar effect

Two-way interaction between physiotherapy modalities and shoulder pain. Pain may limit the ability to strengthen or stretch the shoulder. Similarly, an attempt to strengthen or stretch may further aggravate pain

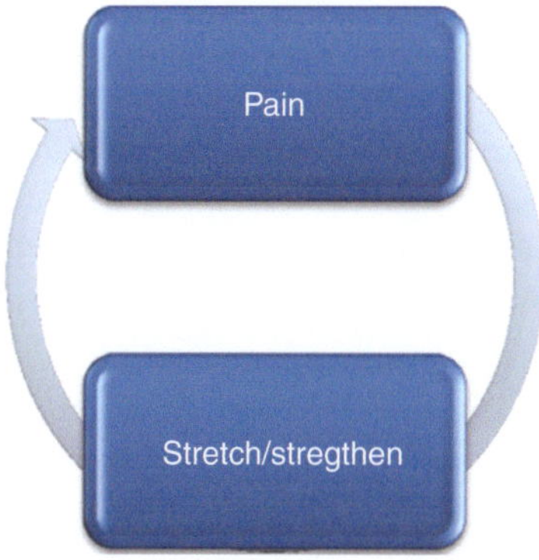

2. Improvement in shoulder biomechanics—this aims to reduce abnormal mechanics which may cause pain by establishing balanced joint control and motion, maintaining joint stability or reducing mechanical impingement. This may be achieved by:
   (a) Posture control
   (b) Proprioception training
   (c) Strengthening/rebalancing muscles
3. Stretching of muscle tender spots

10.2.2 Muscle Strengthening

Muscle strengthening aims to increase:

- Maximum load that can be achieved
- Endurance

In dealing with muscles the aims are to:

1. Awake and recruit inactive muscles
2. Strengthen alternative muscles to compensate for a lost muscle

For example, in massive rotator cuff tendon tears, one may compensate for what has been lost by strengthening the adjacent muscles (such as deltoid) that can have the same function [12–14]. This is analogous to a parachutist whose main parachute fails. The release of a reserve parachute can stop the free fall and allow safe landing—the supraspinatus keeps the arm high up in the air, but when it fails, the deltoid can strengthen and take over. The ability to activate and recruit such muscles may vary from individual to individual; nevertheless patients who in the initial period have substantial arm weakness (pseudo-paralysed arm) and are unable to exert any arm elevation following a supraspinatus tear may achieve normal or near-normal motion with activation and strengthening of the deltoid.

Compensating for a lost muscle (like supraspinatus) by recruiting and strengthening another muscle (like deltoid) is equivalent to releasing a reserve parachute when the primary one fails

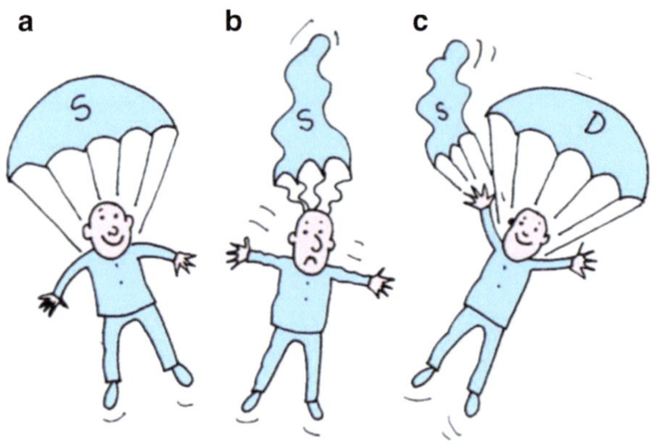

Muscle strengthening may involve:

- Electrical stimulation to recruit inactive muscles
- Isometric/isotonic exercises
- Concentric/eccentric strengthening
- Gradual increase in the:
  - Amount of loading
  - Repetition (cycles) of loading
  - Frequency of loading

Anterior deltoid strengthening—(a) Lying flat assisted, (b) Lying flat—active, (c) Sitting—assisted, (d) Sitting—active, (e) Standing—assisted, (f) Standing—Active

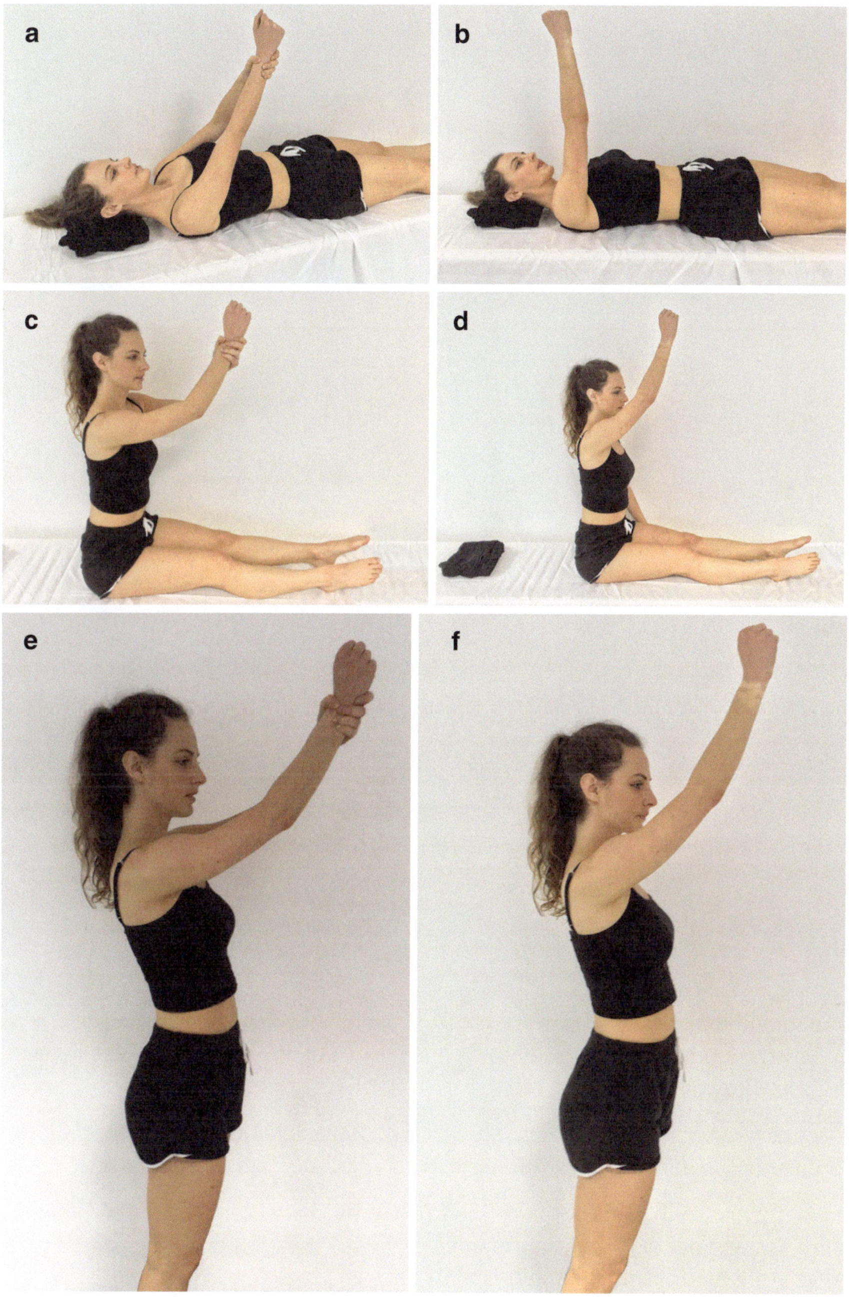

Arm strengthening using resistance band—(a) abduction, (b) external rotation (c) internal rotation

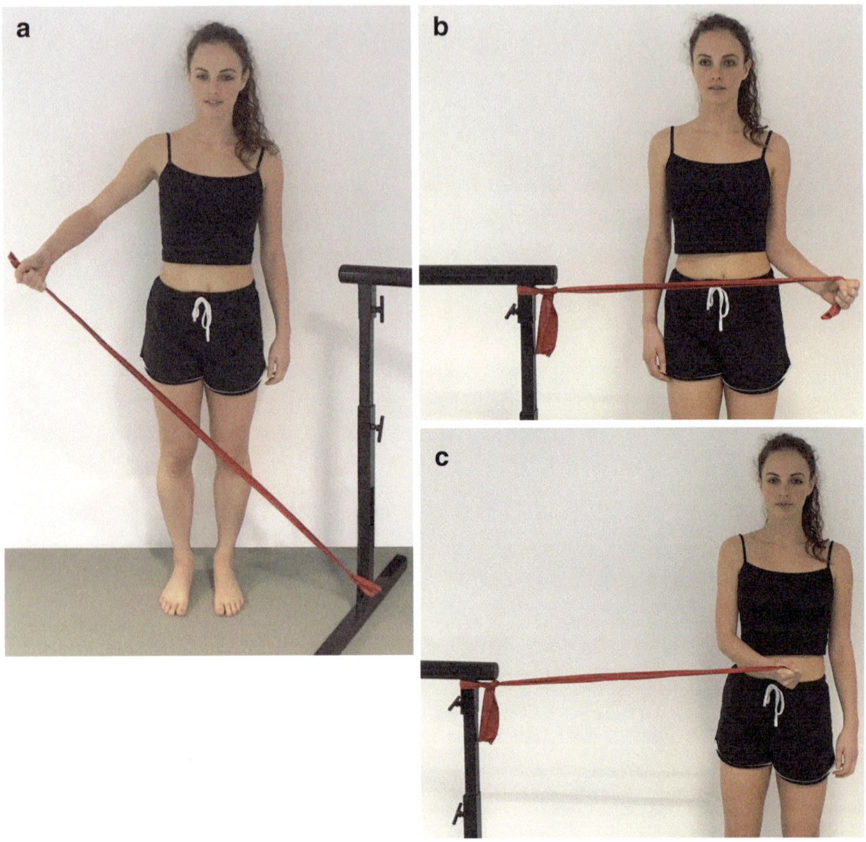

10.2.3 *Joint Mobilisation*

Joint mobilisation may be achieved by:

Passive motion—performed by the therapist or by the patient (such as by using the opposite limb). This aims to:

- Limit the forces transmitted through the affected joint, and, hence, limit any disturbance to healing (soft tissue or bony) that such forces may have

Active assisted motion—performed partly by the patient using the protected body part and partly by assistance provided by the therapist or by the patient (such as by using the opposite limb). This aims to:

- Limit but still allow some forces transmitted through the affected joint, and, hence, limit any disturbance to healing (soft tissue or bony) that such forces may have

Active motion—unaided mobilisation performed by the patient

10.2.4 Core Strengthening and Balancing

The area around the lumbar spine is known as the core [15–19]. It includes the:

- Abdominal muscles anteriorly
- Paraspinals and gluteue posteriorly
- Diaphragm superiorly
- Pelvic floor and hip girdle muscles inferiorly

The core provides the basis upon which muscles of the upper and lower extremities rely to function in a coordinated way. Adequate core strength, endurance and core stability are necessary to provide a stable platform upon which the scapula and upper limb can operate.

A strong core may also eliminate any aberrant activity of muscles connecting the trunk to the humerus, such as the latissimus dorsi.

Core strengthening and balancing improves the strength of the core muscles and facilitates coordination of their activity. This may be the first step in rehabilitation of the upper limb.

10.2.5 Soft Tissue Stretching

This refers to application of a force to elongate the soft tissues. Such force may be applied by:

- The therapist—passive manipulation
- The patient—manipulating own limb using the opposite limb or trunk

Stretching acts on muscles, ligaments and other soft tissues.

- Initial stretching increases the resting length of muscles (sarcomere and connective tissue)
- When a muscle is stretched, its tone initially increases followed by relaxation; further stretching elongates the ligaments

Hence, in stretching exercises a stretching force is applied for about 30 s to allow initial muscle relaxation and subsequent elongation of static soft tissue structures (ligaments) [20, 21].

10.2.6 Proprioception Training

Proprioception [22–26] is the ability to:

- Sense the position of the body, joint or body segment in space (joint position sense/limb position sense)
- Sense any joint or body segment movement (kinaesthesia)
- Process the above sensory inputs to modulate motor output and hence achieve muscle control

Proprioception is the process that allows one to touch their finger to their nose with their eyes closed or, in extreme examples, allows an acrobat to walk blindfolded on a tightrope. The brain develops the ability to process the sensory input in a subconscious way, and this allows voluntary activity to concentrate on other specific actions. Proprioception is believed to play a role in the ability of muscles to coordinate their contraction to maintain joint stability and allows body segments to maintain balance. Proprioception reduces the risk of injury by allowing the body to react in a fast and subconscious way to any sudden changes in the environment which have an effect on the position or movement of the body or body components.

Proprioception allows one to subconsciously control joint position and motion to perform complex and not so complex balancing acts

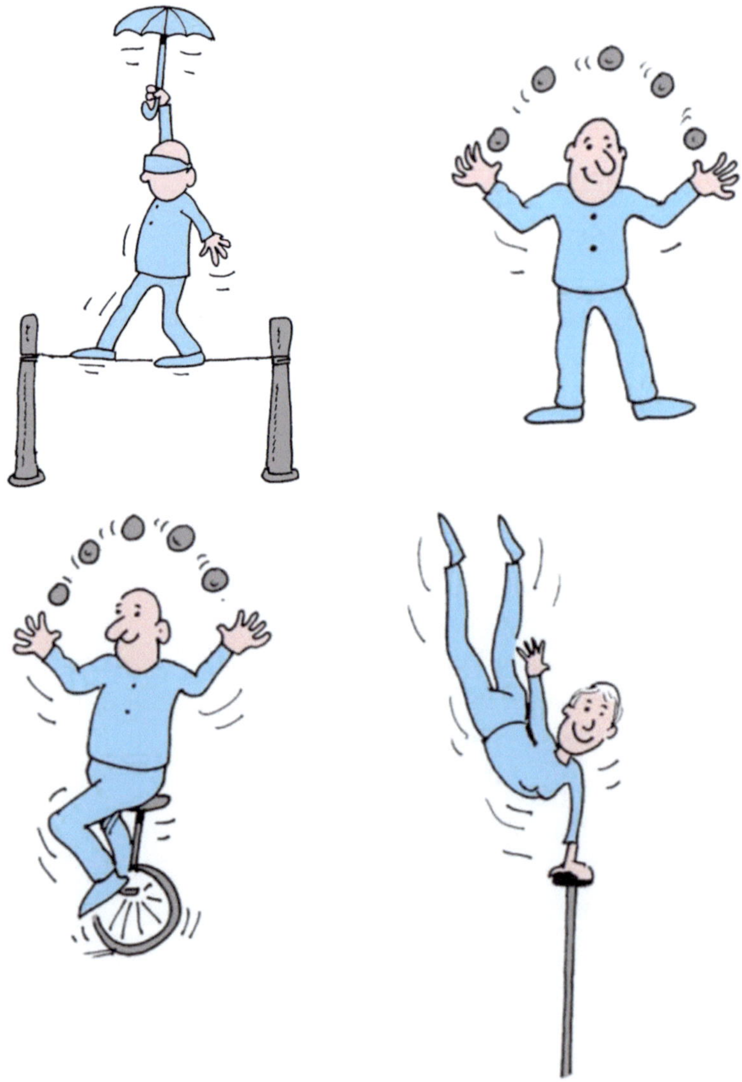

Sensory input originates from receptors found in muscle (muscle spindle) and tendons as well as joint capsules (Golgi body). From these, sensory fibres pass to the dorsal nerve roots and enter the dorsal horn of the spinal cord where they synapse with ascending neurons transmitting impulses to the brain (medulla, thalamus, somatosensory cortex).

Sensory pathways for proprioception—from mechanoreceptors to the central nervous system

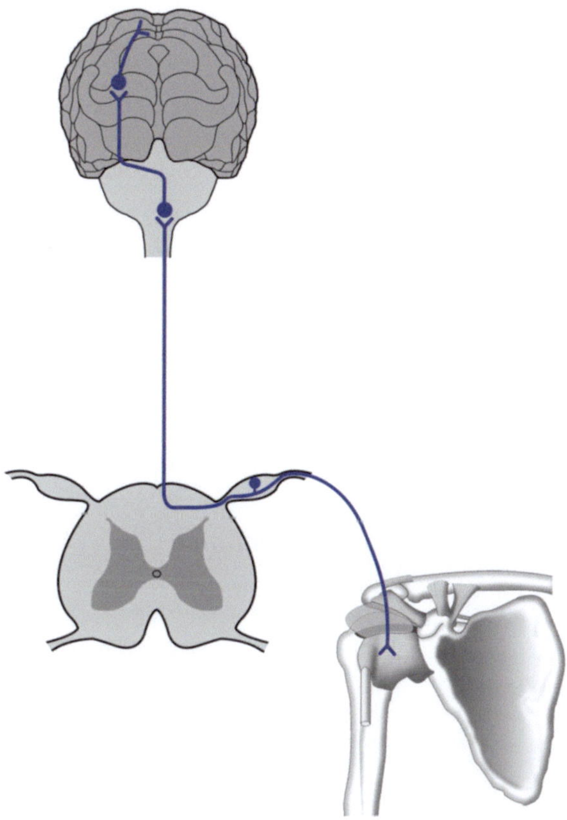

Proprioception relies on adequate sensory input and may be compromised in ligament injuries which result in loss of their bony anchorage [27, 28]. Proprioception may also be impaired in patients who suffer from joint hypermobility [29].

In training for proprioception, three levels may be considered [30, 31]:

1. Static balance activities
2. Dynamic balance activities
3. Coordination and activity training

Proprioceptive exercise for the shoulder may be tailored based on whether the patient aims to achieve open or closed kinetic chain activities. Proprioceptive training exercises [30, 31] include:

- Mirroring movement of the upper extremity—patient tries to match movement of one arm with the other
- Duplicating the position of the upper extremity—one arm is placed in a certain position, and the patient tries to put the opposite arm in same position
- Closed chain mobilisation exercises—patient presses on a trampoline ball rather than a rigid surface
- Balancing on a bouncing ball, wobble board and trampoline

Proprioception may also be enhanced by the application of a sleeve or splint around the shoulder or arm that increases the cutaneous sensory input to the central nervous system.

10.2.7 Biofeedback

The patient is given feedback with regard to muscle contraction to facilitate muscle activation or to inhibit aberrant muscle activity—feedback may be provided by various means such as electronically on a screen [32, 33].

10.2.8 Symptom Modification Techniques

Shoulder symptom modification techniques involve the application of a series of manual interventions to patients with shoulder pain to assess whether these reduce their symptoms [34].

These interventions are applied whilst the patient performs the arm movement that most closely causes their symptoms. The ability of these procedures to improve symptoms is thus assessed. The exact reason why such procedures may reduce symptoms is not known. Nevertheless, if a particular procedure does improve clinical symptoms, then it suggests that a rehabilitation programme could be helpful and exercises that may achieve the same effect as the applied procedure can be utilised as part of that rehabilitation programme.

Shoulder symptom modification procedures may help reduce pain, improve movement or both and include:

1. Humeral head facilitation—aims to influence the position of the humeral head in relation to the glenoid
2. Scapular movement facilitation—aims to change the position of the scapula
3. Spine posture correction—aims to improve the position of the spine

Such facilitation may be achieved by:

- Manual pressure exerted by the examiner
- Taping—to hold a structure (such as the humeral head or scapula) in place
- Recruitment of certain muscle groups such as the external rotators of the humeral head. Glenohumeral external rotation increases the posterior rotator cuff activity, and this can reduce any abnormal scapular motion and thus improve pain

If these facilitation procedures improve the patient's symptoms, they can form the basis for further physiotherapy exercises.

10.3 Physiotherapy for Improving Shoulder Stability

This may be achieved by several ways depending on the possible deficits including:

- Muscle strengthening to improve dynamic stabilisers
- Muscle rebalancing
- Scapular motion coordination
- Core strengthening/balancing
- Proprioceptive training

Glenohumeral joint stability may be improved by coordinating the activities of the rotator cuff, scapular and core muscles

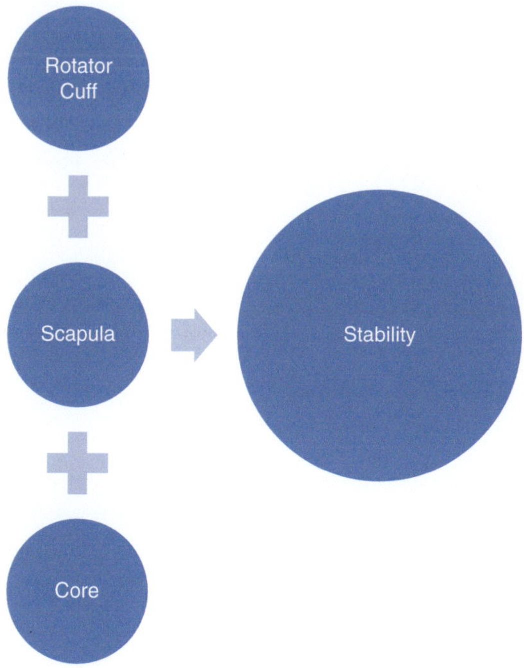

10.4 Physiotherapy to Reduce Joint Stiffness

In trying to improve mobility of a stiff joint, the aims are to:

- Elongate contracted structures
- Relax tense muscles

The following therapy principles may be utilised:

- The direction of stiffness is determined
- Specific exercises are applied for each direction in which there is stiffness
- A stretching force is applied in the direction of necessary soft tissue elongation
- Stretching is applied by the patient or by the therapist
- Pain must be adequately controlled to minimise opposition to the stretching force
- Muscles may be relaxed by:
  - Local massage
  - Chemical means: botulinum toxin injection

Passive stretching exercises of the right shoulder using the opposite arm: (a) external rotation (b) internal rotation

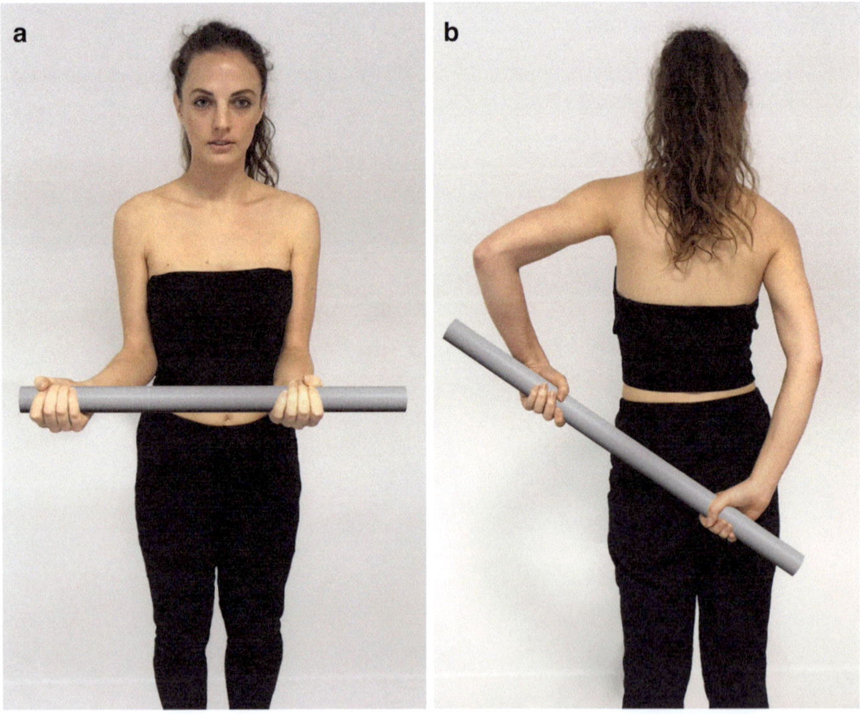

10.5 Rehabilitation of the Shoulder Following a Soft Tissue or Bony Injury

This involves several stages:

1. Rest, control pain and reduce inflammation
2. Protect the site of healing (by limiting motion and loading) by utilising one of various levels of mobilisation:
    (a) Immobilisation
    (b) Passive mobilisation
    (c) Active assisted
    (d) Active
3. Regain motion:
    (a) Active mobilisation
    (b) Passive manipulation
    (c) Stretch soft tissues
4. Strengthen
5. Rehabilitate to improve function, guided to specific functional demands

Steps in rehabilitating the shoulder following a soft tissue or bony injury

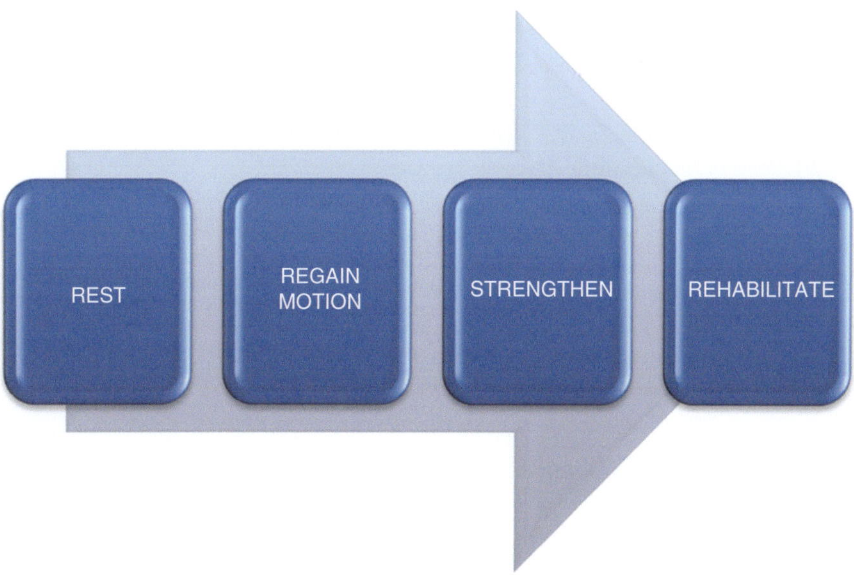

Throughout all stages an attempt is made to maintain muscle bulk and proprioception. Any exercises applied should avoid substantially aggravating the pain which can lead to guarding, apprehension and inhibition of movement and have a counterproductive effect on recovery. The aim of therapy is to avoid or break this vicious cycle. Hence, initially gentle exercises are prescribed which are gradually increased guided by pain.

The protection period lasts for as long as it is necessary for the injured site to heal, which for bone to bone is about 6–12 weeks and tendon to bone or ligament to bone about 8–12 weeks [35, 36].

This protection period is followed by mobilisation to regain active motion, eliminate stiffness and strengthen the arm. These stages are followed by rehabilitation which aims to return the arm and patient to a desirable and achievable functional level. In this phase, goal-orientated tasks and specific functional patterns of activity are introduced which resemble the activities that the individual may face in real life. Finally, the patient is exposed to real-life training.

10.6 Rehabilitation Postsurgical Soft Tissue or Bony Repair

The approach to rehabilitation may similarly be described in five stages following surgical repair:

1. Control pain and reduce inflammation
2. Protect the repair (limiting motion and loading), utilising various levels of mobilisation:
   (a) Immobilisation
   (b) Passive mobilisation
   (c) Active assisted
   (d) Active
3. Regain motion
   (a) Active mobilisation
   (b) Passive manipulation
   (c) Stretch soft tissues
4. Strengthen
5. Rehabilitate to improve function, guided to specific functional demands

Steps in rehabilitating the shoulder following a soft tissue or bony repair

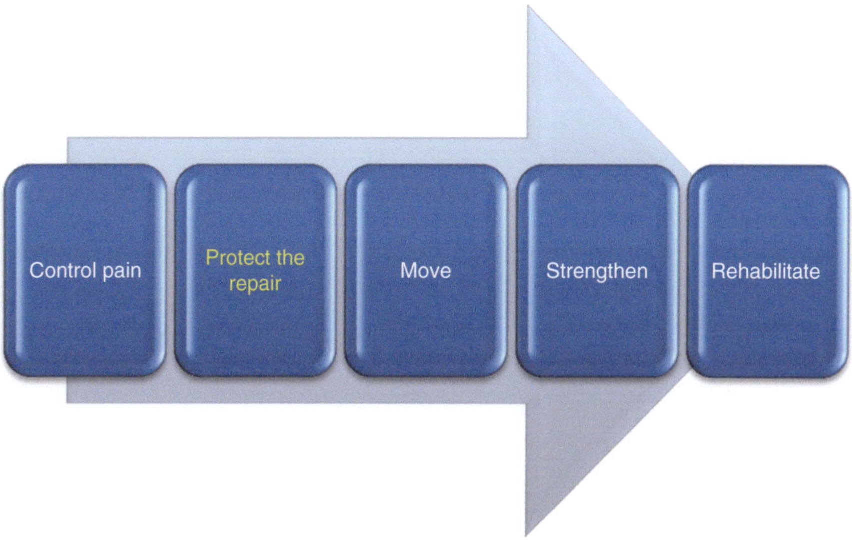

10.7 Early vs. Delayed Mobilisation and Loading

Following a soft tissue or bony injury where natural repair is taking place and following a soft tissue or bony surgical repair, the amount of mobilisation and loading of the area under consideration may need to be limited until sufficient healing has occurred.

This is because there may be a concern that excessive mobilisation or overloading may lead to:

- Gap formation between the apposed tissues at the injured and repair site
- Dysfunction or failure of the repair

It has been shown that in rotator cuff tears [37–43]:

- Delayed mobilisation may confer better strength than early mobilisation
- Low levels of loading may confer better strength than complete unloading
- Tendon cells (fibroblasts) are capable of mechanotransduction—this means that they respond to the application of force by altering their biological activity in terms of collagen, extracellular matrix and growth factor synthesis. In this way mechanical loading can alter the tissue biology
- Forces directed in the line of action of a tendon may facilitate collagen fibre alignment and maturation

There is often a push for early mobilisation in order to avoid or minimise stiffness due to:

- Contracture of soft tissues
- Intra-articular or periarticular adhesion formation

However, there is substantial evidence that although early mobilisation compared to delayed mobilisation may confer less stiffness at early follow-up post-injury or post-surgery, at longer follow-up (1 year or longer), the amount of stiffness and functional outcomes may not differ between such groups [37, 44, 45].

The above suggest that:

- It may not be necessary to have a period of absolute immobilisation or unloading
- Early mobilisation may be:
  - Applied using passive or active assisted exercises
  - Allowed in a range that does not unduly stress and compromise the injured or repair site. For surgical repairs this range of motion may be determined intra-operatively and communicated to the therapist
- Early loading may be applied using:
  - Isometric exercises
- Mobilisation and loading may be guided by:
  - The possibility of impairing a natural or surgical repair site
  - The strength of the surgical repair and the need to protect such a repair rather than by an arbitrary push to mobilise early

Learning Pearls

- Communication between the surgeon and therapist is essential to ensure there is clarity as to what therapy aims to achieve and the extent or pace at which such therapy is applied
- Pain control is essential in allowing patients to perform physiotherapy, and this should form an integral part of therapy

References

1. Uhl TL, Muir TA, Lawson L. Electromyographical assessment of passive, active assistive, and active shoulder rehabilitation exercises. PM R. 2010;2(2):132–41.
2. Active assisted shoulder exercises—Oxford University Hospitals. Accessed at http://www.ouh.nhs.uk/patient-guide/leaflets/files/10874Pshoulder.pdf on 19/3/18
3. Dillman CJ, Murray TA, Hintermeister RA. Biomechanical differences of open and closed chain exercises with respect to the shoulder. J Sport Rehabil. 1994;3:228–38.

4. Gowitzke BA, Milner M. Scientific bases of human movement. Baltimore, MD: Williams and Wilkins; 1988.
5. Padulo J, Laffaye G, Chamari K, Concu A. Concentric and eccentric: muscle contraction or exercise? Sports Health. 2013;5(4):306. https://doi.org/10.1177/1941738113491386.
6. Melzack R, Wall PD. Pain mechanisms: a new theory. Science. 1965;150(3699):971–9.
7. Katz J, Rosenbloom BN. The golden anniversary of Melzack and Wall's gate control theory of pain: celebrating 50 years of pain research and management. Pain Res Manag. 2015;20(6):285–6.
8. Sluka KA, Walsh D. Transcutaneous electrical nerve stimulation: basic science mechanisms and clinical effectiveness. J Pain. 2003;4(3):109–21.
9. Rawe IM. The case for over-the-counter shortwave therapy: safe and effective devices for pain management. Pain Manag. 2014;4(1):37–43.
10. Goats GC. Pulsed electromagnetic (short-wave) energy therapy. Br J Sports Med. 1989;23(4):213–6.
11. Ondrejkovicova A, Petrovics G, Svitkova K, Bajtekova B, Bangha O. Why acupuncture in pain treatment? Neuro Endocrinol Lett. 2016;37(3):163–8.
12. Christensen BH, Andersen KS, Rasmussen S, Andreasen EL, Nielsen LM, Jensen SL. Enhanced function and quality of life following 5 months of exercise therapy for patients with irreparable rotator cuff tears—an intervention study. BMC Musculoskelet Disord. 2016;17:252. https://doi.org/10.1186/s12891-016-1116-6.
13. Levy O, Mullett H, Roberts S, Copeland S. The role of anterior deltoid reeducation in patients with massive irreparable degenerative rotator cuff tears. J Shoulder Elb Surg. 2008;17(6):863–70.
14. Collin PG, Gain S, Nguyen Huu F, Lädermann A. Is rehabilitation effective in massive rotator cuff tears? Orthop Traumatol Surg Res. 2015;101(4 Suppl):S203–5.
15. Huxel Bliven KC, Anderson BE. Core stability training for injury prevention. Sports Health. 2013;5(6):514–22.
16. Willson JD, Dougherty CP, Ireland ML, Davis IM. Core stability and its relationship to lower extremity function and injury. J Am Acad Orthop Surg. 2005;13(5):316–25.
17. Kibler WB, Press J, Sciascia A. The role of core stability in athletic function. Sports Med. 2006;36(3):189–98.
18. Rosemeyer JR, Hayes BT, Switzler CL, Hicks-Little CA. Effects of core-musculature fatigue on maximal shoulder strength. J Sport Rehabil. 2015;24(4):384–90.
19. Radwan A, Francis J, Green A, Kahl E, Maciurzynski D, Quartulli A, Schultheiss J, Strang R, Weiss B. Is there a relation between shoulder dysfunction and core instability? Int J Sports Phys Ther. 2014;9(1):8–13.
20. Magnusson SP. Passive properties of human skeletal muscle during stretch maneuvers. A review. Scand J Med Sci Sports. 1998;8(2):65–77.
21. Bandy WD, Irion JM. The effect of time on static stretch on the flexibility of the hamstring muscles. Phys Ther. 1994;74(9):845–50.
22. Myers JB, Lephart SM. Sensorimotor deficits contributing to glenohumeral instability. Clin Orthop Relat Res. 2002;400:98–104.
23. Warner JJ, Lephart S, Fu FH. Role of proprioception in pathoetiology of shoulder instability. Clin Orthop Relat Res. 1996;**330**:35–9.
24. Jerosch J, Prymka M. Proprioception and joint stability. Knee Surg Sports Traumatol Arthrosc. 1996;4(3):171–9.
25. Nyland JA, Caborn DN, Johnson DL. The human glenohumeral joint. A proprioceptive and stability alliance. Knee Surg Sports Traumatol Arthrosc. 1998;6(1):50–61.
26. Galloway MT, Lalley AL, Shearn JT. The role of mechanical loading in tendon development, maintenance, injury, and repair. J Bone Joint Surg Am. 2013;95(17):1620–8.
27. Jerosch J, Steinbeck J, Clahsen H, Schmitz-Nahrath M, Grosse-Hackmann A. Function of the glenohumeral ligaments in active stabilisation of the shoulder joint. Knee Surg Sports Traumatol Arthrosc. 1993;1(3-4):152–8.

28. Lephart SM, Warner JJ, Borsa PA, Fu FH. Proprioception of the shoulder joint in healthy, unstable, and surgically repaired shoulders. J Shoulder Elb Surg. 1994;3(6):371–80.
29. Smith TO, Jerman E, Easton V, Bacon H, Armon K, Poland F, Macgregor AJ. Do people with benign joint hypermobility syndrome (BJHS) have reduced joint proprioception? A systematic review and meta-analysis. Rheumatol Int. 2013;33(11):2709–16.
30. Partin NB, Stone JA, Ryan EJ, Lueken JS, Timm KE. Upper extremity proprioceptive training. J Athl Train. 1994;29(1):15–8.
31. Borsa PA, Lephart SM, Kocher MS, Lephart SP. Functional assessment and rehabilitation of shoulder proprioception for glenohumeral instability. J Sport Rehabil. 1994;3:84–104.
32. Lim OB, Kim JA, Song SJ, Cynn HS, Yi CH. Effect of selective muscle training using visual EMG biofeedback on infraspinatus and posterior deltoid. J Hum Kinet. 2014;44:83–90.
33. Huang HY, Lin JJ, Guo YL, Wang WT, Chen YJ. EMG biofeedback effectiveness to alter muscle activity pattern and scapular kinematics in subjects with and without shoulder impingement. J Electromyogr Kinesiol. 2013;23(1):267–74.
34. Lewis JS. Rotator cuff tendinopathy/subacromial impingement syndrome: is it time for a new method of assessment? Br J Sports Med. 2009;43(4):259–64.
35. Rodeo SA, Arnoczky SP, Torzilli PA, Hidaka C, Warren RF. Tendon-healing in a bone tunnel. A biomechanical and histological study in the dog. J Bone Joint Surg Am. 1993;75(12):1795–803.
36. St Pierre P, Olson EJ, Elliott JJ, O'Hair KC, McKinney LA, Ryan J. Tendon-healing to cortical bone compared with healing to a cancellous trough. A biomechanical and histological evaluation in goats. J Bone Joint Surg Am. 1995;77(12):1858–66.
37. Lee BG, Cho NS, Rhee YG. Effect of two rehabilitation protocols on range of motion and healing rates after arthroscopic rotator cuff repair: aggressive versus limited early passive exercises. Arthroscopy. 2012;28(1):34–42.
38. Eliasson P, Andersson T, Aspenberg P. Achilles tendon healing in rats is improved by intermittent mechanical loading during the inflammatory phase. J Orthop Res. 2012;30(2):274–9.
39. Eliasson P, Andersson T, Aspenberg P. Rat Achilles tendon healing: mechanical loading and gene expression. J Appl Physiol (1985). 2009;107(2):399–407.
40. Andersson T, Eliasson P, Aspenberg P. Tissue memory in healing tendons: short loading episodes stimulate healing. J Appl Physiol (1985). 2009;107(2):417–21.
41. Hettrich CM, Gasinu S, Beamer BS, Stasiak M, Fox A, Birmingham P, Ying O, Deng XH, Rodeo SA. The effect of mechanical load on tendon-to-bone healing in a rat model. Am J Sports Med. 2014;42(5):1233–41.
42. Killian ML, Cavinatto L, Galatz LM, Thomopoulos S. The role of mechanobiology in tendon healing. J Shoulder Elb Surg. 2012;21(2):228–37.
43. Galatz LM, Charlton N, Das R, Kim HM, Havlioglu N, Thomopoulos S. Complete removal of load is detrimental to rotator cuff healing. J Shoulder Elb Surg. 2009;18(5):669–75.
44. Kim YS, Chung SW, Kim JY, Ok JH, Park I, Oh JH. Is early passive motion exercise necessary after arthroscopic rotator cuff repair? Am J Sports Med. 2012;40(4):815–21.
45. Cuff DJ, Pupello DR. Prospective randomized study of arthroscopic rotator cuff repair using an early versus delayed postoperative physical therapy protocol. J Shoulder Elb Surg. 2012;21(11):1450–5. https://doi.org/10.1016/j.jse.2012.01.025. Epub 2012 May 2.

Chapter 11
Shoulder Pain

Pain may be considered the commonest symptom patients present with. Pain may be an isolated complaint or, quite often, be associated with other symptoms such as weakness, paraesthesia, stiffness or instability.

This chapter discusses some of the potential sources of shoulder pain and gives guidance as to the principles used in identifying the origin of pain. These include, amongst others, pain's nature, location, onset and clinical examination findings. Furthermore, this chapter describes the principles of investigating and managing the painful shoulder.

11.1 Sources of Shoulder Pain

Several sources of shoulder pain are recognised [1–19]. These are described according to the anatomical structure or area giving rise to pain. These sources of pain are presented below.

Potential sources of shoulder pain

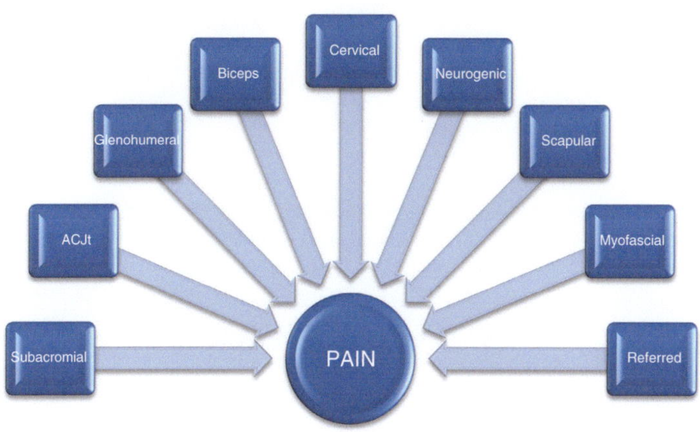

© Springer Nature Switzerland AG 2019

C. Panayiotou Charalambous, *The Shoulder Made Easy*,
https://doi.org/10.1007/978-3-319-98908-2_11

11.1.1 Subacromial Pain Syndrome

This is used to describe pain originating from disorders involving the subacromial space. It is typically felt over the deltoid muscle but can radiate distally towards the elbow and forearm. Pain is usually diffuse rather than localised. The pain over deltoid may be so intense to the extent that patients may find it difficult to accept that the pain felt over the mid-arm area is actually originating from the shoulder. Pain is typically worse on activities involving forward elevation, abduction or internal rotation of the arm such as reaching for a cupboard, combing hair, reaching the back pocket of trousers and reaching the bottom for personal hygiene. Causes of subacromial pain syndrome include:

- Subacromial bursitis
- Rotator cuff tendinopathy
- Calcific tendinopathy
- Rotator cuff tears

Subacromial pain is diffusely felt over deltoid

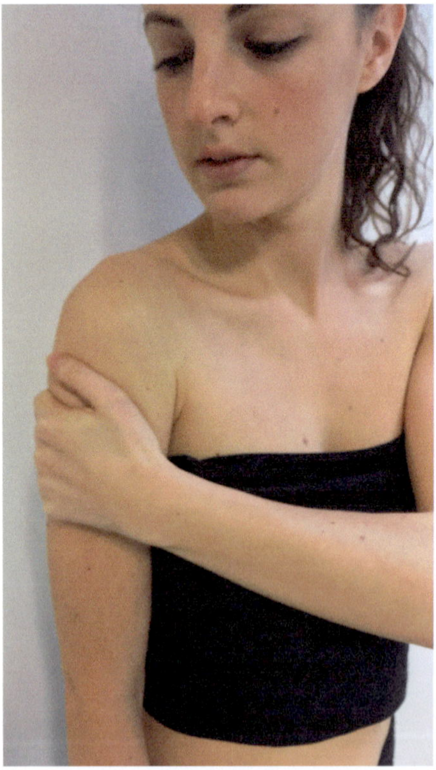

11.1.2 Acromio-Clavicular Joint (ACJt) Pain

This is pain felt on the top of the shoulder, directly over the ACJt. It tends to be well localised with the patient being able to point with a finger to the painful area. ACJt pain may be aggravated by overhead activities such as reaching upper shelves or carrying weights above head level. Causes of ACJt pain include:

- Arthritis
- Post-traumatic sprain
- Instability
- Weightlifter's arm—lateral end of clavicle osteolysis
- Fibrocartilage disc disruption

ACJt pain is very well localised—patient can point to painful area with finger

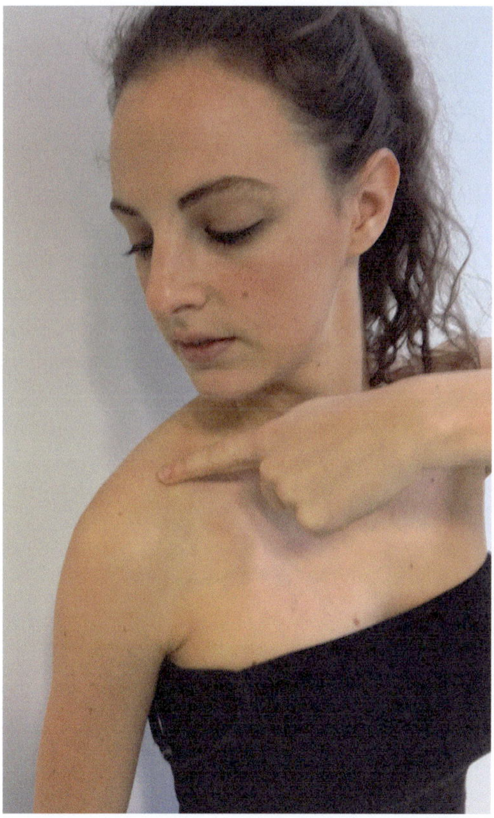

11.1.3 Glenohumeral Joint Pain

This is deep-seated pain, felt within the shoulder joint. Pain originating from the rotator interval may be felt at the front of the shoulder. Pain due to degenerative or inflammatory causes may be constant and dull in nature, aggravated by arm movements at low body level. Pain due to labrum injuries may be worsened by forward elevation and rotation of the arm and be accompanied by clicking or clucking of the shoulder. Similarly, pain due to glenohumeral instability may be vague, dull or burning, constant or intermittent, associated with episodes of subluxation or dislocation of the joint. Causes of glenohumeral joint pain include:

- Arthritis
- Avascular necrosis of the humeral head
- Adhesive capsulitis
- Labrum tears
- Instability

11.1.4 Long Head of the Biceps Tendon Pain Syndrome

This is pain felt in the anterior aspect of the shoulder, in the bicipital groove, radiating to the front of the arm, in line with the biceps muscle. It may be dull, burning or cramp-like pain. It may be worsened by activation of the biceps muscle (during forearm rotation such as when using a screwdriver) or stretching of the biceps muscle.

It may be classified according to the underlying biceps pathology causing pain:

- Intra-articular
  - Superior labrum anterior posterior (SLAP) tear
  - Subluxation/dislocation of the long head of the biceps from the bicipital groove
  - Biceps tendinopathy
- Extra-articular
  - Constriction synovitis in the bicipital groove
  - Tendon subluxation/dislocation
  - Biceps tendinopathy

11.1.5 Cervical Origin Pain

Cervical spine pain may have two sources of origin occurring together or in isolation:

1. Mechanical pain—this is pain originating from the bones, articulations, discs or ligamentous structures of the cervical spine. Such pain is usually felt in line with

the cervical spine and referred to the paraspinal and peri-scapular muscles such as trapezius. Causes of mechanical cervical spine pain include degeneration, arthritis or any other congenital or acquired disturbance of spinal anatomy and function

2. Neurogenic pain—this is pain experienced due to cervical nerve root compression or irritation and may be felt anywhere in the area of innervation of that nerve root. Such pain tends to be burning or sharp, associated with paraesthesia, and may radiate down the arm, forearm or hand, in the area of distribution of the nerve root involved (dermatome). Causes of neurogenic cervical spine pain include—spinal foraminal stenosis, disc prolapse, cervical spine degeneration or any other lesion that compresses or irritates the cervical nerve roots (infection, neoplasia)

Pain felt over the top of the shoulder area is likely of muscular or cervical spine origin rather than of shoulder origin

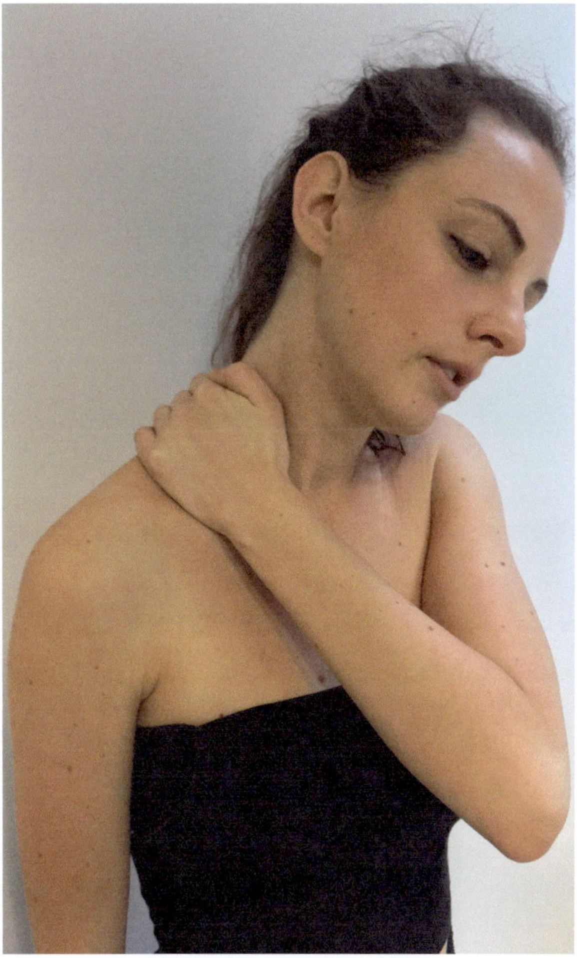

Plain radiograph (lateral view) of the cervical spine showing extensive arthritic changes (red arrow). MRI shows associated cord compression (red arrow)

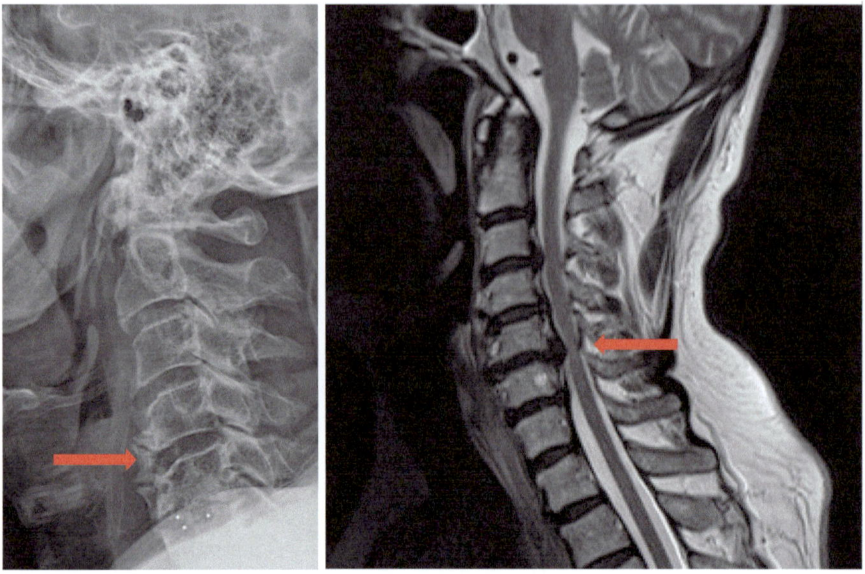

11.1.6 Thoracic Outlet or Peripheral Nerve: Neurogenic

Dysfunction of the nerves innervating the shoulder region may cause pain. Such pain is often dull and non-specific, felt in the area of cutaneous sensory innervation or deep distribution of that nerve. Some of the nerves which must be considered are:

- Suprascapular nerve
- Axillary
- Long-thoracic
- Dorsal scapular

Dysfunction of these nerves may occur at the level of the brachial plexus, as in neurogenic thoracic outlet syndrome or more peripherally.

11.1.7 Scapular Pain

This is pain felt over or near the scapula region. Causes include:

- Snapping scapula
- Scapula dyskinesia

Pain felt over the scapular area may also originate from the thoracic spine.

11.1.8 Pain Referred from a Distal Site

This is pain felt over the shoulder but originates from a distant site:

- Abdominal origin
  - Intra-abdominal pathology—cholecystitis
  - Post-laparoscopic surgery

11.1.9 Myofascial Pain

This is pain that originates from local shoulder, scapular or paraspinal muscles. This is usually felt in the muscle affected and is worsened by movement, muscle stretching or certain body postures. Causes include:

- Muscle spasm—due to overcompensating for dysfunction of other muscles, abnormal shoulder or scapular function or position
- Muscle contracture

Myofascial pain may affect:

- A large part of the muscle
- Isolated trigger points

11.2 Identifying the Origin of Shoulder Pain

Clinical history and examination are used to determine the origin of pain and hence guide appropriate investigations and management. The following characteristics of pain may help point towards a likely diagnosis.

11.2.1 Pain Location

The area where pain is felt may point as to its possible origin, and certain patterns are recognised. However, the shoulder region is densely innervated, with overlap in the nerves innervating certain structures and hence overlap in the area whereby pain from these structures is experienced. In line with this, Gerber et al. attempted to characterise the pattern of pain caused by selective irritation of the ACJt and of the subacromial space. They injected hypertonic saline solution into the ACJt and into the subacromial space of healthy volunteers. Irritation of the ACJt produced pain directly over the joint but also pain in the anterior-lateral part of the neck, in the trapezius-supraspinatus region and in the anterior-lateral part of deltoid. Irritation of the subacromial space produced pain in the region of the lateral acromion, the deltoid muscle and occasionally the forearm and fingers.

In addition, determining the area or structure of pain origin is not the full answer, as various pathologies involving on area or a structure may present with pain and must thus be considered in the differential diagnosis.

Nevertheless, the following suggests how the location of pain may guide to its origin:

The location where shoulder pain is felt may guide as to its area or disorder of origin

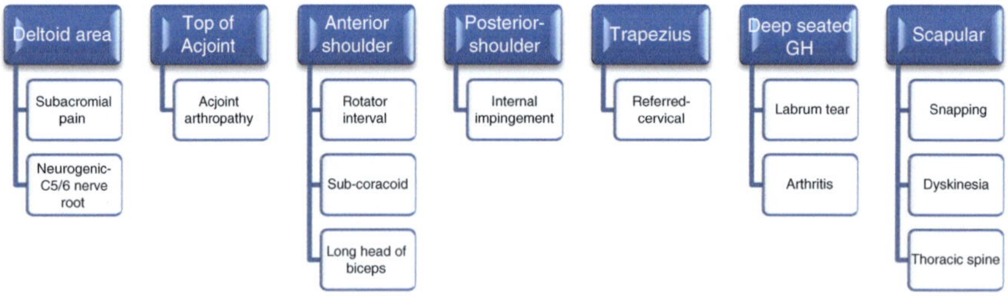

Area of experienced pain varies according to its site of origin

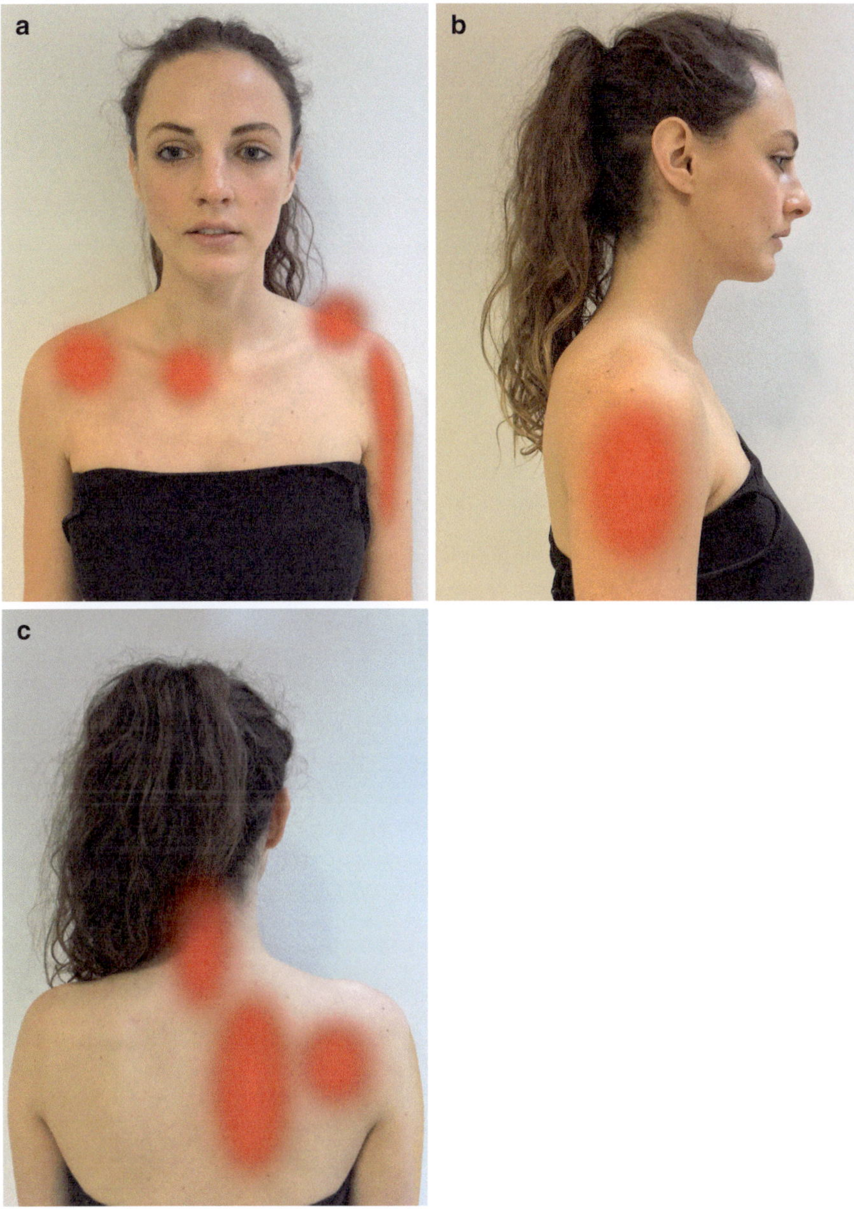

11.2.2 Pain Onset

The onset of pain may also point to a particular area of origin and possible diagnosis. Certain conditions in the shoulder are associated with sudden onset severe pain with no precipitating factor and include:

1. Adhesive capsulitis
2. Calcific tendinopathy
3. Parsonage turner syndrome
4. Infection—septic arthritis, osteomyelitis

11.2.3 Patient's Age

The patient's age may point towards a likely cause for the pain, with some painful conditions being more common in certain age groups. This may apply to both pain of subacromial origin as well as pain of glenohumeral joint origin.

The patient's age may guide as to the potential cause of subacromial pain syndrome

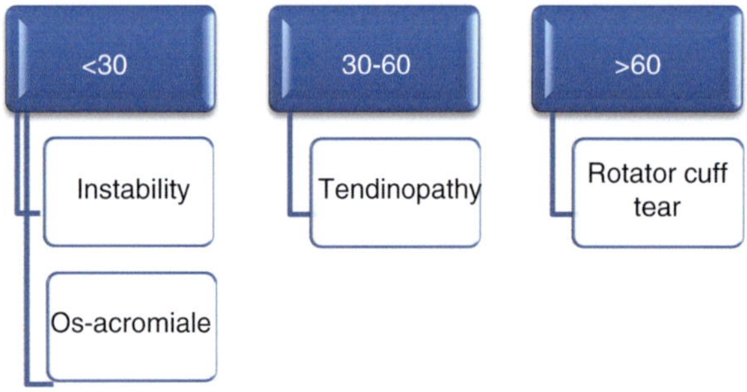

The patient's age may guide as to the potential cause of glenohumeral pain

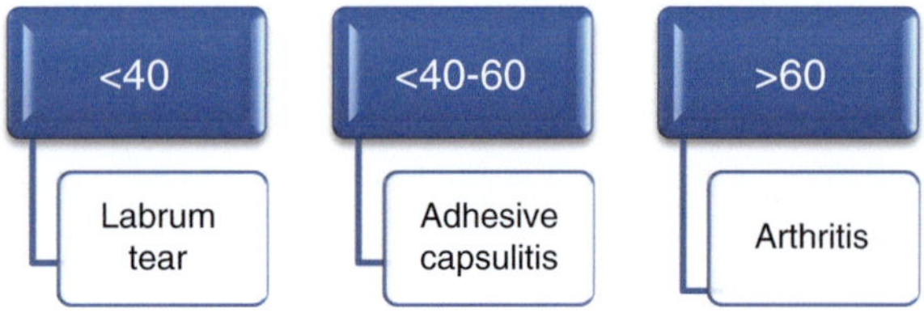

11.2.4 Symptoms Associated with Shoulder Pain

Pain is often accompanied by other shoulder symptoms, the presence of which may help determine the underlying shoulder disorder.

The presence of other clinical symptoms in addition to pain, may guide as to the cause of shoulder pain

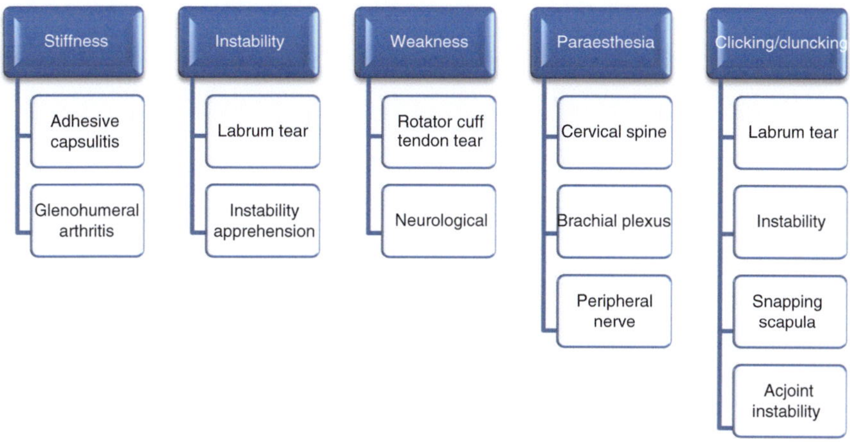

11.2.5 Palpable Shoulder Tenderness

During clinical examination the shoulder is palpated for tenderness. The area of tenderness may guide to the source of pain.

Potential sources of shoulder pain as guided by the area of palpable tenderness

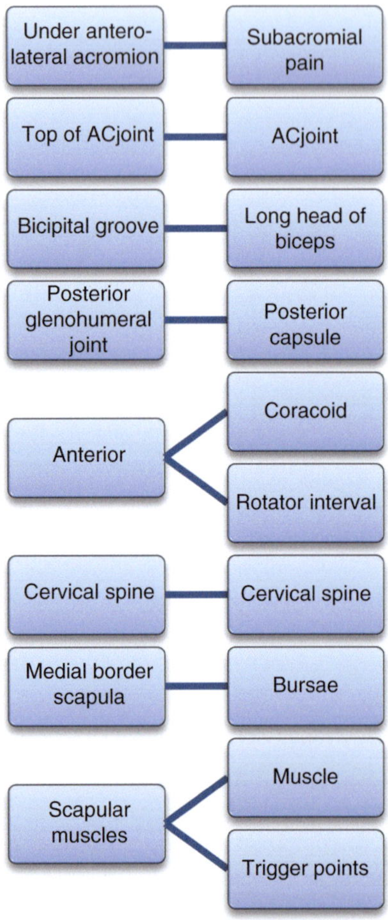

11.2.6 Shoulder Pain Provoking Clinical Tests

Certain clinical special tests, when positive, may point towards a particular origin of pain.

Potential sources of shoulder pain as guided by positive pain provoking clinical tests

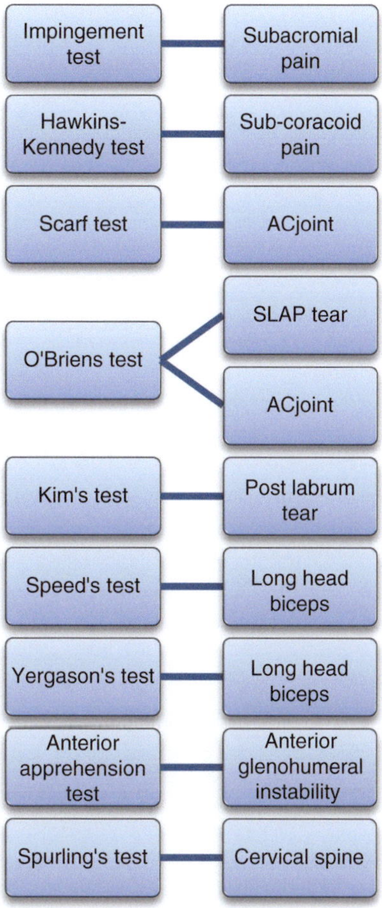

11.3 Investigations for Shoulder Pain

Investigations for the painful shoulder are directed towards confirming the working diagnosis and excluding alternative diagnoses. These include:

- Diagnostic local anaesthetic injections
- Radiological
  - Plain radiographs
  - MRI/CT Scan
  - Bone scan
- Neurophysiological
  - Nerve conduction studies
  - Electromyography
- Arthroscopic evaluation

MRI showing cervical spine disc protrusion with spinal indentation (red arrows)

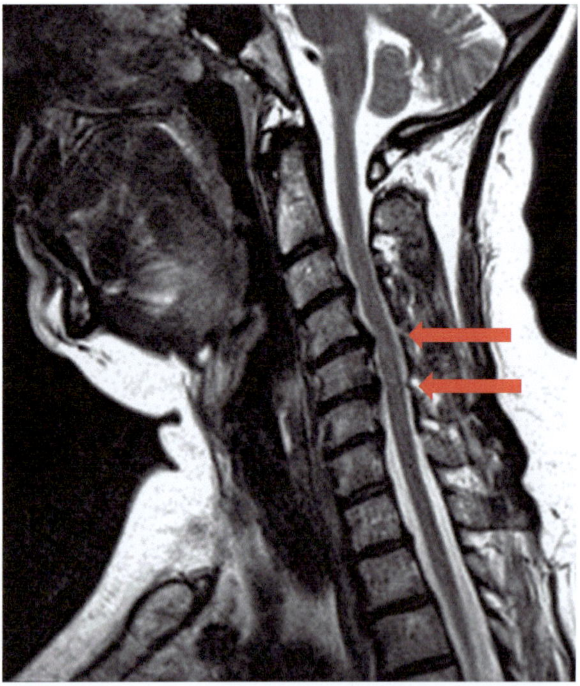

Bone scan showing a hot spot in the spine of the scapula. MRI suggested this was an osteoid osteoma

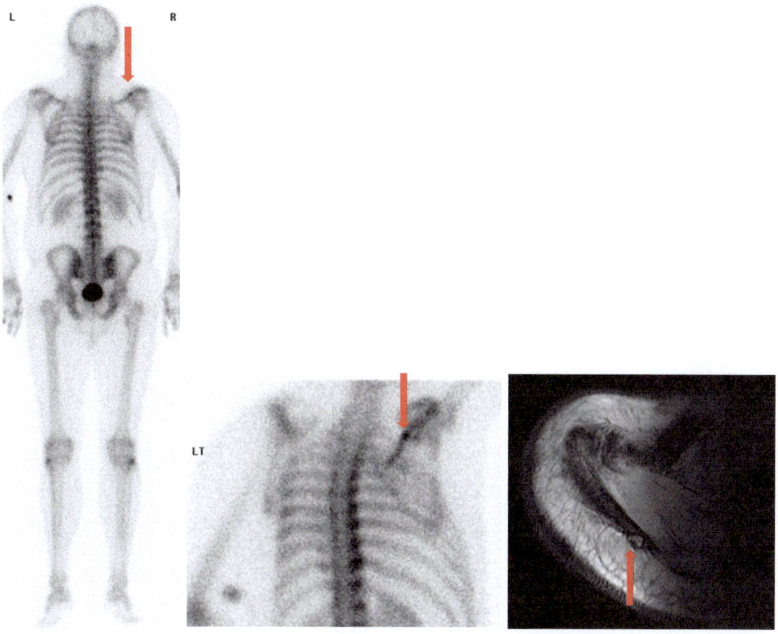

Painful shoulder showing benign cystic lesion in the proximal humerus

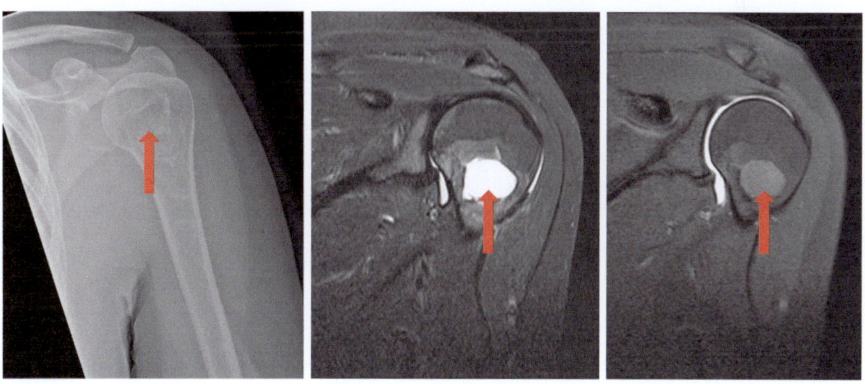

Diagnostic local anaesthetic injections involve injecting local anaesthetic into the area that is considered to be the source of pain. An improvement in pain whilst the local anaesthetic works suggests that the area injected is the origin of pain. Such injections may be administered in the:

- Subacromial space
- Glenohumeral joint
- ACJt
- Bicipital groove
- Suprascapular notch
- Scalene or pectoralis minor muscle in the diagnosis of thoracic outlet syndrome
- Muscle trigger points

11.4 Management of Shoulder Pain

Management of shoulder pain involves:

- Symptomatic control of pain
- Tackling the underlying condition causing the pain

The exact management may be influenced by the working diagnosis, but the management ladder may guide as to the approach utilised, although on occasions initial steps may be bypassed.

Management ladder for shoulder pain

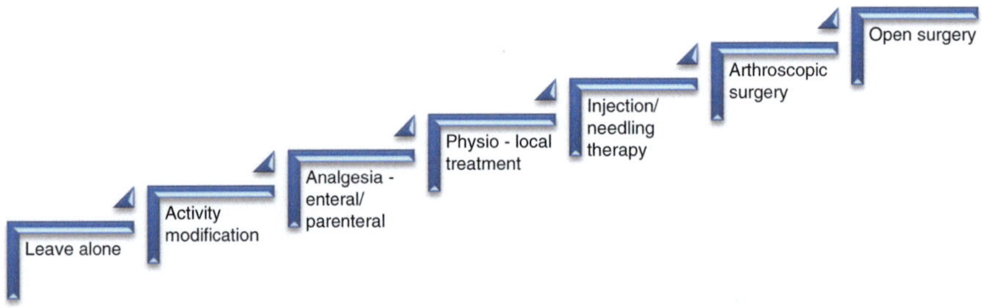

Surgical procedures for the painful shoulder may involve:

- Soft tissue procedures
  - Repair
  - Excision
  - Release
  - Reconstruction
  - Transfer
  - Decompression

- Bony procedures
  - Excision
  - Reconstruction
  - Decompression
- Arthroplasty procedures
  - Realignment
  - Excision
  - Replacement
  - Interposition
  - Fusion

Surgical interventions for pain are directed towards the underlying cause. It must be considered that in some instances we may not be exactly sure as to the origin of the pain or the part of a surgical intervention that actually helps to improve the pain.

If one looks at arthroscopic surgery for subacromial space pain syndrome due to rotator cuff tendon tendinopathy, the following may be performed as part of the procedure:

- Washout of glenohumeral joint and subacromial space
- Debridement of any associated glenohumeral or subacromial synovitis
- Excision of the subacromial bursa
- Debridement of any rotator surface cuff tendon fibrillations
- Release of the coraco-acromial ligament
- Acromioplasty
- Excision of inferior ACJt osteophytes

Extensive subacromial space synovitis associated with a supraspinatus tendon tear

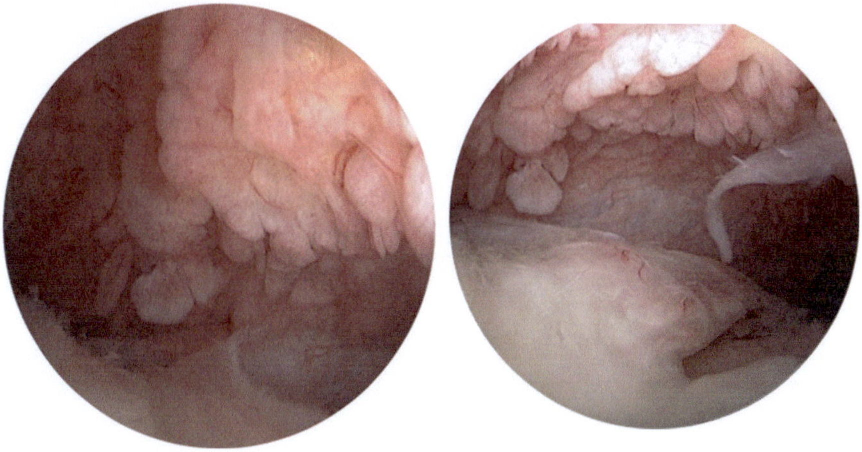

There is controversy as to which of the above components of the procedure, or if any at all, are important in alleviating pain; a recent multicentre randomised trial in the United Kingdom compared arthroscopic subacromial decompression with sham surgery (arthroscopic evaluation) in the management of subacromial pain syndrome. It was shown that arthroscopic subacromial acromioplasty offered no substantial benefit over sole arthroscopic evaluation (looking inside the shoulder), suggesting that the benefit of surgery may be at least partly mediated by a placebo effect [20].

Learning Pearls

- Various pathological conditions may cause similar clinical symptoms and give similar clinical examination signs—subacromial impingement, subacromial bursitis, rotator cuff tendinopathy, rotator cuff calcific tendinopathy and small rotator cuff tear may present with a similar clinical history and similar clinical examination findings

  Hence, it may be very difficult or impossible to distinguish between various potential pathologies that cause pain originating from an area solely based on clinical grounds. Radiological and other investigations are thus often needed to determine the exact diagnosis

References

1. Murphy RJ, Carr AJ. Shoulder pain. BMJ Clin Evid. 2010;2010:1107.
2. Kandil TS, El Hefnawy E. Shoulder pain following laparoscopic cholecystectomy: factors affecting the incidence and severity. J Laparoendosc Adv Surg Tech A. 2010;20(8):677–82.
3. Gray M, Wallace A, Aldridge S. Assessment of shoulder pain for non-specialists. BMJ. 2016;355:i5783.
4. Burbank KM, Stevenson JH, Czarnecki GR, Dorfman J. Chronic shoulder pain: part I. Evaluation and diagnosis. Am Fam Physician. 2008;77(4):453–60.
5. Kennedy DJ, Mattie R, Nguyen Q, Hamilton S, Conrad B. Glenohumeral joint pain referral patterns: a descriptive study. Pain Med. 2015;16(8):1603–9.
6. Diercks R, Bron C, Dorrestijn O, Meskers C, Naber R, de Ruiter T, Willems J, Winters J, van der Woude HJ, Dutch Orthopaedic Association. Guideline for diagnosis and treatment of subacromial pain syndrome: a multidisciplinary review by the Dutch Orthopaedic Association. Acta Orthop. 2014;85(3):314–22.
7. Sergienko S, Kalichman L. Myofascial origin of shoulder pain: a literature review. J Bodyw Mov Ther. 2015;19(1):91–101.
8. van der Bruggen W, Arens AI, van der Drift MA, de Geus-Oei LF, Gotthardt M, Oyen WJ. Referred shoulder pain in a patient with small cell lung cancer. Adrenal gland metastases. Neth J Med. 2013;71(4):203–6.
9. Argyriou AA, Solomou E, Papadimitriou K, Kraniotis P, Peroukides S, Karanasios P, Kalofonos HP. Large cell neuroendocrine carcinoma of the lung metastatic to the shoulder joint, causing suprascapular nerve palsy. J Pain Symptom Manag. 2011;42(6):e1–3.

10. Butt MA. Shoulder pain: unusual presentation of transitional cell cancer of bladder. ANZ J Surg. 2008;78(9):822. https://doi.org/10.1111/j.1445-2197.2008.04663.x.
11. Moghadam FM, Bahremand GH, Vejdani A. Shoulder pain as the first sign of a hepatic fibrolamellar carcinoma in a young man. J Gastrointestin Liver Dis. 2008;17(2):234–6.
12. Saha E, Dziadzio M, Irving K, Chambers A, Higgens C. Unusual cause of painful shoulder in an elderly woman with rheumatoid arthritis. Clin Rheumatol. 2007;26(9):1549–51.
13. Smith CC, Bevelaqua AC. Challenging pain syndromes: Parsonage-Turner syndrome. Phys Med Rehabil Clin N Am. 2014;25(2):265–77.
14. Hill LJ, Jelsing EJ, Terry MJ, Strommen JA. Evaluation, treatment, and outcomes of suprascapular neuropathy: a 5-year review. PM R. 2014;6(9):774–80.
15. DB P, Berg JH, Thal R. Neck and shoulder pain: differentiating cervical spine pathology from shoulder pathology. J Surg Orthop Adv. 2009;18(4):170–4.
16. Gaskill T, Millett PJ. Snapping scapula syndrome: diagnosis and management. J Am Acad Orthop Surg. 2013;21(4):214–24.
17. Raynor MB, Kuhn JE. Utility of features of the patient's history in the diagnosis of atraumatic shoulder pain: a systematic review. J Shoulder Elb Surg. 2016;25(4):688–94.
18. Raney EB, Thankam FG, Dilisio MF, Agrawal DK. Pain and the pathogenesis of biceps tendinopathy. Am J Transl Res. 2017;9(6):2668–83.
19. Khazzam M, George MS, Churchill RS, Kuhn JE. Disorders of the long head of biceps tendon. J Shoulder Elb Surg. 2012;21(1):136–45.
20. Beard DJ, Rees JL, Cook JA, Rombach I, Cooper C, Merritt N, Shirkey BA, Donovan JL, Gwilym S, Savulescu J, Moser J, Gray A, Jepson M, Tracey I, Judge A, Wartolowska K, Carr AJ, CSAW Study Group. Arthroscopic subacromial decompression for subacromial shoulder pain (CSAW): a multicentre, pragmatic, parallel group, placebo-controlled, three-group, randomised surgical trial. Lancet. 2018;391(10118):329–38.

Chapter 12
Shoulder Weakness

Shoulder weakness can be defined as loss of strength or power of shoulder motion due to inability to create an adequate force. This may be painless or associated with pain. This chapter discusses the concepts of true and apparent weakness and discusses the causes of shoulder weakness, its investigation and management.

12.1 True Versus Apparent Shoulder Weakness

In dealing with shoulder weakness, it is essential to distinguish between true and apparent weakness.

Apparent weakness may be due to:

- Pain
- Instability

Apparent weakness may be due to the patient being reluctant to move the arm or exert a strong force across the arm as that would cause pain; the patient may refer to this reduction of joint motion as weakness. Apparent weakness may also be seen in underlying glenohumeral instability whereby the patient avoids a particular arm movement because that may lead to humeral head subluxation or dislocation. Patients with glenohumeral instability may complain of weakness manifested as inability or difficulty to move the shoulder in a particular direction, difficulty or inability to carry a weight, early fatigue (inability to hold the arm in a particular position or carry a weight for a necessary duration of time). Hence, it is essential to establish whether one is dealing with true weakness where there is loss of active motion due to inability to create sufficient force strength across a joint.

When examining for weakness, it is essential to minimise pain. Pain may be improved by asking the patient to take simple analgesia (sufficient to control pain) and then waiting until that works before assessing strength. Alternatively, an injection of local anaesthetic into the painful area (such as the subacromial space or glenohumeral joint) may temporarily reduce pain, allowing the examiner to assess strength [1–3].

© Springer Nature Switzerland AG 2019

C. Panayiotou Charalambous, *The Shoulder Made Easy*,
https://doi.org/10.1007/978-3-319-98908-2_12

12.2 Causes of Shoulder Weakness

In evaluating the cause of weakness, one must consider the normal control of motor activities. Control of motion begins in the primary motor cortex of the brain's frontal lobe. Like other parts of the body, the shoulder is represented in the primary motor cortex. Upper motor neurons in the primary motor cortex give rise to nerve fibres. These fibres descend through the brain stem where most of them cross to the opposite side of the body and form the cortical spinal tract that descends through the spine. These nerve fibres terminate at the appropriate spinal level whereby they synapse and pass messages to lower motor neurons, cell bodies of which are located in the grey matter of the spinal cord in the ventral horn. Ventral horn lower motor neurons then transmit nerve signals through the ventral roots and from there through peripheral roots to muscles. Transmission occurs from the nerve to the muscle at the neuromuscular junction, leading to muscle fibre activation and contraction. Activation and contraction allows a muscle to act via its tendon (and through its tendon insertion) onto the bone to apply a force and influence movement. In addition to the above pathway, there are neurons which originate in the brain stem (basal ganglia) and which influence other aspects of motion such as coordination [4, 5]. Hence, it can be seen that shoulder weakness can be the result of a deficit occurring anywhere in a pathway that starts in the brain and finishes at the tendon bone junction, as described below.

Motor pathways from brain to shoulder muscles

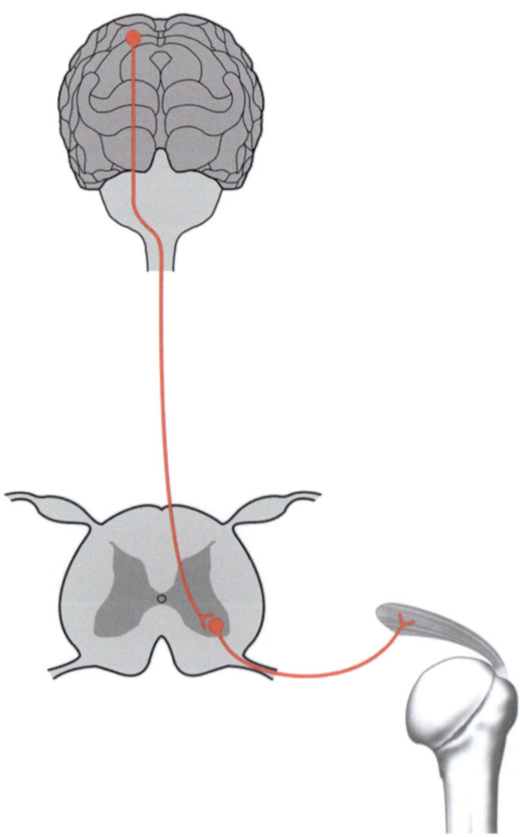

- Neurological causes of weakness
  - Upper neurone lesion

    Brain
    Spinal cord
  - Lower motor neurone lesion

    Spinal cord
    Peripheral nerve
  - Neuromuscular junction
- Muscular causes of weakness
  - Myopathies
  - Muscular ruptures
- Tendinous causes of weakness
  - Tear
  - Bony avulsion

Causes of shoulder weakness

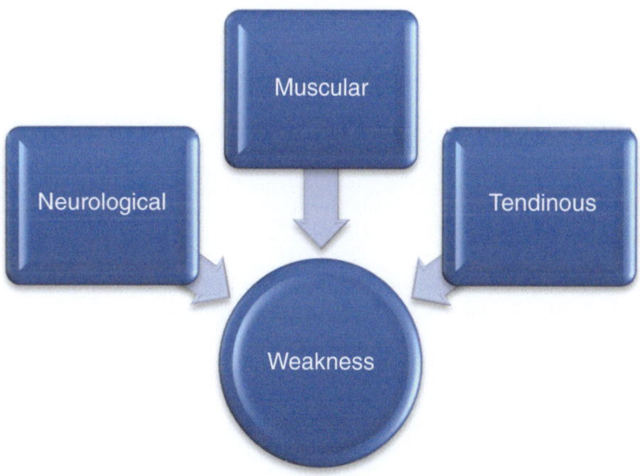

12.3 Identifying the Cause of Shoulder Weakness

In trying to determine the cause of shoulder weakness, some of the factors to consider in the clinical history and clinical examination are:

- Painful or painless weakness?
- Involves one or multiple muscles?
- Isolated shoulder or multiple joint weakness?
- Unilateral or bilateral weakness?
- Gradual or sudden onset?

- Onset related to precipitating factor such as trauma?
- Fluctuating, constant or deteriorating loss of strength?
- Associated sensory symptoms?
- Family history of neuromuscular conditions?
- History of exposure to muscle or nerve toxic conditions?
- History of muscle or nerve toxic medications?
- Muscles involved innervated by one common nerve or multiple nerves?
- Does the weakness follow a peripheral nerve pattern, spinal root or central nervous system (spinal cord or brain) pattern?
- Lower or upper motor neurone symptoms and signs?
- Loss of muscle bulk-wasting?
- Associated rigidity or lack of coordination?

Nerve and muscle activity may be affected by various conditions that are sought of in the clinical history and include:

- Inflammatory disorders (e.g. rheumatological disorders)
- Endocrine disorders (e.g. thyroid dysfunction)
- Metabolic conditions (e.g. diabetes mellitus)
- Neoplasia (e.g. paraneoplastic syndromes, direct infiltration)
- Infection
- Alcohol
- Medicines

- *Painful weakness* may be due to:
  - Inflammation—as that seen with tendon tears
  - Mechanical factors
    - Superior migration of the humeral head which abuts the acromion, as seen in massive rotator cuff tears
  - Nerve dysfunction—nerve irritation, compression, intrinsic neuritis
- *Upper motor neuron lesions* may lead to:
  - Minimal muscle atrophy (although some atrophy may develop because of disuse)
  - Absence of fasciculations
  - Increased spasticity
  - Exaggerated reflexes [6, 7]
- *Lower motor neuron lesions* may lead to:
  - Decreased muscle tone
  - Decreased reflexes
  - Muscle atrophy
  - Fasciculations [6, 7]
- *Associated sensory symptoms* may point to a neurological rather than an intrinsic muscular cause

- *Fluctuating strength* may be associated with:
  - Myopathy such as myasthenia gravis
  - Central disorders such as transient ischaemic attacks which come on suddenly and last for a short time
- *Onset of weakness*
  - Sudden traumatic—may suggest structural failure such as tendon tear
  - Sudden non-traumatic—may suggest a neurological cause such as neuritis or central nerve system dysfunction
  - Gradual onset—may suggest degenerative tendon tear or neuromuscular cause
- *Distribution of weakness*
  - Neuromuscular conditions (neuropathies, myopathies) tend to affect multiple joints or body parts rather than one muscle or joint
  - Myopathies tend to be proximal and bilateral
- *Tone and coordination*
  - Rigidity or lack of coordination such as that seen in Parkinson's disease may manifest as weakness because of difficulty in performing motor activities
- *Family history*
  - Some neuropathies or myopathies are hereditary and family history should be sought

Frequently encountered causes of shoulder weakness include:

- Apparent weakness related to shoulder pain
- True weakness related to:
  - Rotator cuff tendon tear
  - Cervical spondylosis causing nerve root impingement
  - Suprascapular nerve palsy
  - Axillary nerve palsy

But one has to keep in mind the potential alternatives.

12.3.1 Investigations for Shoulder Weakness

Investigations of the weak shoulder aim to confirm the presence of true weakness and its likely cause and exclude any possible alternative diagnoses. These include:

- Radiological
  - Plain radiographs
  - MRI/CT scan

- Neurophysiological
  - Nerve conduction studies
  - Electromyography
- Diagnostic local anaesthetic injections
- Arthroscopic evaluation

12.4 Management of Shoulder Weakness

Management of weakness involves:

- Addressing the structures involved in the neuromuscular control of motion that may be deficient
- Addressing the underlying condition that may have let to changes in the properties of these structures (such as the underlying infection, inflammatory arthritis, poorly controlled diabetes)
- Addressing the structures the discontinuity of which may account for the mechanical loss of motion (such as a torn tendon)
- Strengthening alternative muscles to take over and compensate for what is lost [8–10]

In tackling the deficient structures, the management ladder is followed although on occasion initial steps may be bypassed.

Management ladder for shoulder weakness

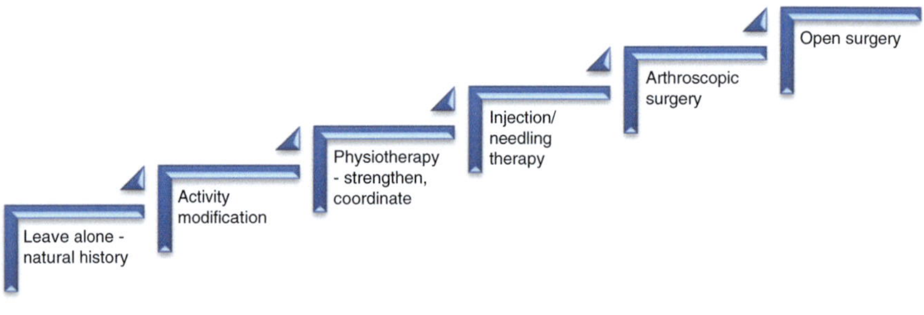

Learning Pearls

The presence of weakness may be objective based on clinical examination, but also subjective based on how the patient perceives their arm strength compared to their usual strength; the examiner may not be able to elicit the weakness that the patient experiences

References

1. Charalambous CP. Investigations for shoulder disorders. In: Charalambous CP, editor. The shoulder made easy. Springer; 2019. pp. 123–43.
2. McFarland E, Bernard J, Dein E, Johnson A. Diagnostic injections about the shoulder. J Am Acad Orthop Surg. 2017;25(12):799–807.
3. Farshad M, Jundt-Ecker M, Sutter R, Schubert M, Gerber C. Does subacromial injection of a local anesthetic influence strength in healthy shoulders?: A double-blinded, placebo-controlled study. J Bone Joint Surg Am. 2012;94(19):1751–5.
4. Martini FH, Nath JL, Bartholomew EF, editors. Fundamentals of anatomy & physiology. San Francisco: Benjamin-Cummings Publishing Company; 2011.
5. Rea P, editor. Essential clinical anatomy of the nervous system. New York: Elsevier Inc; 2015.
6. Reeves AG, editor. Disorders of the nervous system: a primer. 3rd ed: Imperial Company Printers; 1995.
7. Garg N, Park SB, Vucic S, Yiannikas C, Spies J, Howells J, Huynh W, Matamala JM, Krishnan AV, Pollard JD, Cornblath DR, Reilly MM, Kiernan MC. Differentiating lower motor neuron syndromes. J Neurol Neurosurg Psychiatry. 2017;88(6):474–83.
8. Christensen BH, Andersen KS, Rasmussen S, Andreasen EL, Nielsen LM, Jensen SL. Enhanced function and quality of life following 5 months of exercise therapy for patients with irreparable rotator cuff tears - an intervention study. BMC Musculoskelet Disord. 2016;17:252. https://doi.org/10.1186/s12891-016-1116-6.
9. Levy O, Mullett H, Roberts S, Copeland S. The role of anterior deltoid reeducation in patients with massive irreparable degenerative rotator cuff tears. J Shoulder Elb Surg. 2008;17(6):863–70.
10. Collin PG, Gain S, Nguyen Huu F, Lädermann A. Is rehabilitation effective in massive rotator cuff tears? Orthop Traumatol Surg Res. 2015;101(4 Suppl):S203–5.

Chapter 13
Shoulder Stiffness

Stiffness is a condition whereby there is loss of passive joint motion. This may be painless or associated with pain. This chapter discusses the concepts of true and apparent stiffness and discusses the causes of shoulder stiffness, its investigation and management.

13.1 True Versus Apparent Shoulder Stiffness

In dealing with shoulder stiffness it is essential to distinguish between true and apparent stiffness.

Apparent limitation of motion may be due to:

- Pain
- Weakness

Patients may be reluctant to move their arm as that would cause pain and may refer to this reduction of joint motion as "stiffness". Similarly, they may be unable to move the arm due to weakness but describe this loss of motion as "stiffness". Hence, it is essential to determine whether one is dealing with true stiffness, where there is loss of passive motion.

© Springer Nature Switzerland AG 2019

C. Panayiotou Charalambous, *The Shoulder Made Easy*,
https://doi.org/10.1007/978-3-319-98908-2_13

13.2 Passive vs. Active Shoulder Motion

In describing active and passive movements of the shoulder, one may consider the analogy to driving of a car. Car motion requires the driver pressing the gas pedal and creating an electric signal, electrical circuits communicating this to the engine, fuel burning and creating energy and the generated force being transmitted to the wheels. Car motion also requires a good set of wheels and tyres and a smooth surface on which to move along.

If the gas pedal were to be broken and the signal could not be initiated, or if the electric circuits fell apart, or if the fuel ran out, then the car would not actively move. Nevertheless, the driver could still get out and pull the car along happily, as long as there was no mechanical obstruction and the tyres as well as the road surface were smooth (analogous to passive motion).

Similarly, active shoulder motion requires an effective neuromuscular system, from brain stimulation to muscle contraction and force transmission via tendons to bones. It also requires smooth articular surfaces that can easily move relative to each other and soft tissue envelopes (ligaments, muscles, tendons) that have some slack, allowing motion to occur before they become taut. If this neuromuscular and musculotendinous system is disrupted, then active motion may not be feasible with the patient not being able to move their arm. Nevertheless, the examiner will still be able to hold and move the patient's arm (passive motion).

However, in the case of the car, if the tyres were clamped or if the wheels fell in deep road potholes, no matter how hard the driver presses on the gas and no matter how much force the engine creates the car is unlikely to move (loss of active motion). Similarly, no matter how hard one pulls on the rope, the car is also unlikely to move along (loss of passive motion).

A car that runs out of petrol can still be pulled passively along. If, however, its wheels are clamped or if they fall in deep road potholes, the car can move neither actively nor passively. Likewise, loss of passive motion of the shoulder signifies a mechanical block

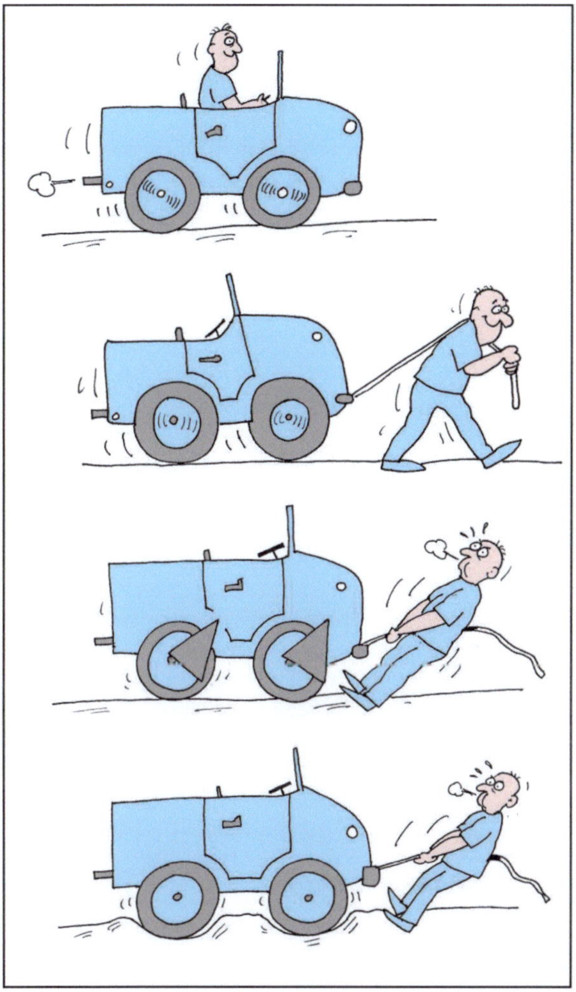

Along similar lines, if the soft tissue envelopes of the glenohumeral joint (capsule, ligaments, tendons, muscles) contract and shorten, swell and thicken and lose their slack, or if the articulating surfaces are worn, irregular, with bumps or projecting osteophytes, no matter how hard the muscles contract, or how much effort the patient makes, the arm is unlikely to move (loss of active motion). This loss of motion will be observed even when the examiner holds the patient's arm and tries to move it (loss of passive motion).

In examining for loss of passive motion, one must ensure that there is no compensatory misleading motion in the nearby joints, such as at the elbow or at the scapulo-thoracic articulation:

- In assessing external rotation of the glenohumeral joint, the elbow is placed and held (by the examiner) by the side of the patient's trunk, and then the arm is taken into external rotation, to avoid the elbow masking the loss of glenohumeral motion
- In assessing forward elevation or abduction of the glenohumeral joint, the scapula must be stabilised to ensure that no compensatory motion occurs at the scapulo-thoracic articulation. The point at which the scapula starts moving will mark the limit of pure glenohumeral joint motion

Stiffness may be described in various ways [1–5] as below.

13.3 Direction of Shoulder Motion Loss

The direction of motion loss may be:

- Global—affecting all directions
- In one or more specific directions

The direction of motion loss may be influenced by the underlying pathology. In adhesive capsulitis, external rotation is usually affected due to thickening and contracture of the anterior capsule, coraco-humeral and glenohumeral ligaments, but loss in other directions may also occur. In missed chronic anterior dislocation, internal rotation may be mostly affected as the humeral head is locked anteriorly out of the glenoid.

13.4 Cause of Shoulder Stiffness

This may be:

- Congenital
- Acquired
    - Idiopathic (adhesive capsulitis)
    - Traumatic (including surgery and seizures)
    - Dislocation, fracture mal-union, adhesions, capsular contracture, metalwork
    - Degenerative
    - Inflammatory
    - Infective—septic arthritis

13.5 Structure Limiting Shoulder Motion

The structure limiting motion may be:

- Soft tissue
  - Capsule
  - Muscle-tendon
  - Ligaments
  - Adhesions

    Intra-articular
    Periarticular
    Extra-articular

- Bony

  Intra-articular
  Periarticular
  Extra-articular

  The structure causing stiffness may guide its management.

Inflamed rotator internal and thickened middle glenohumeral ligament in adhesive capsulitis

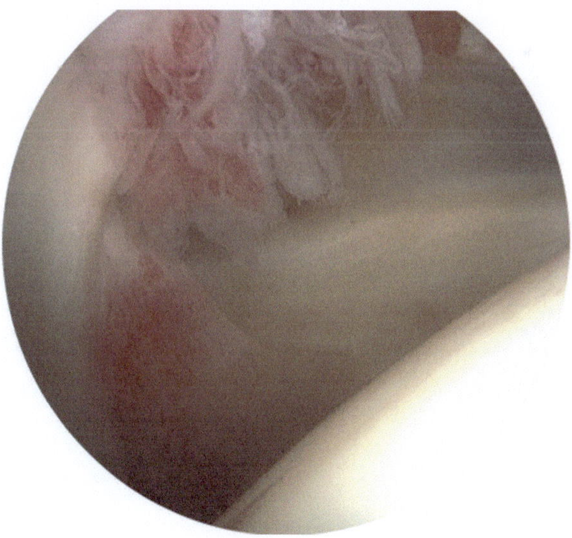

Stiffness may be described according to the structure limiting motion

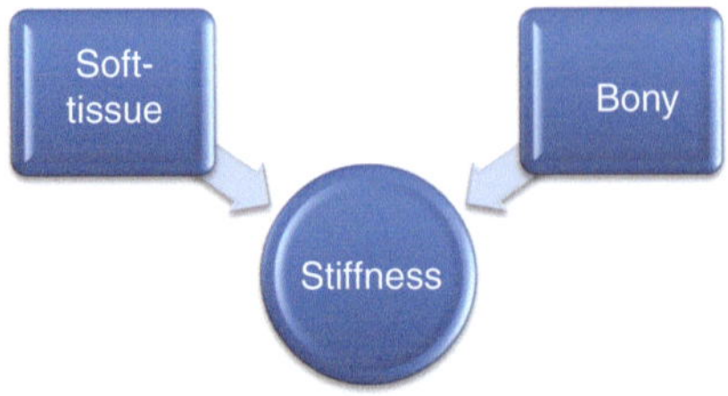

Collapse of the central part of the humeral head. Patient presented with substantial limitation of loss of motion at least partly due to bony mechanical block

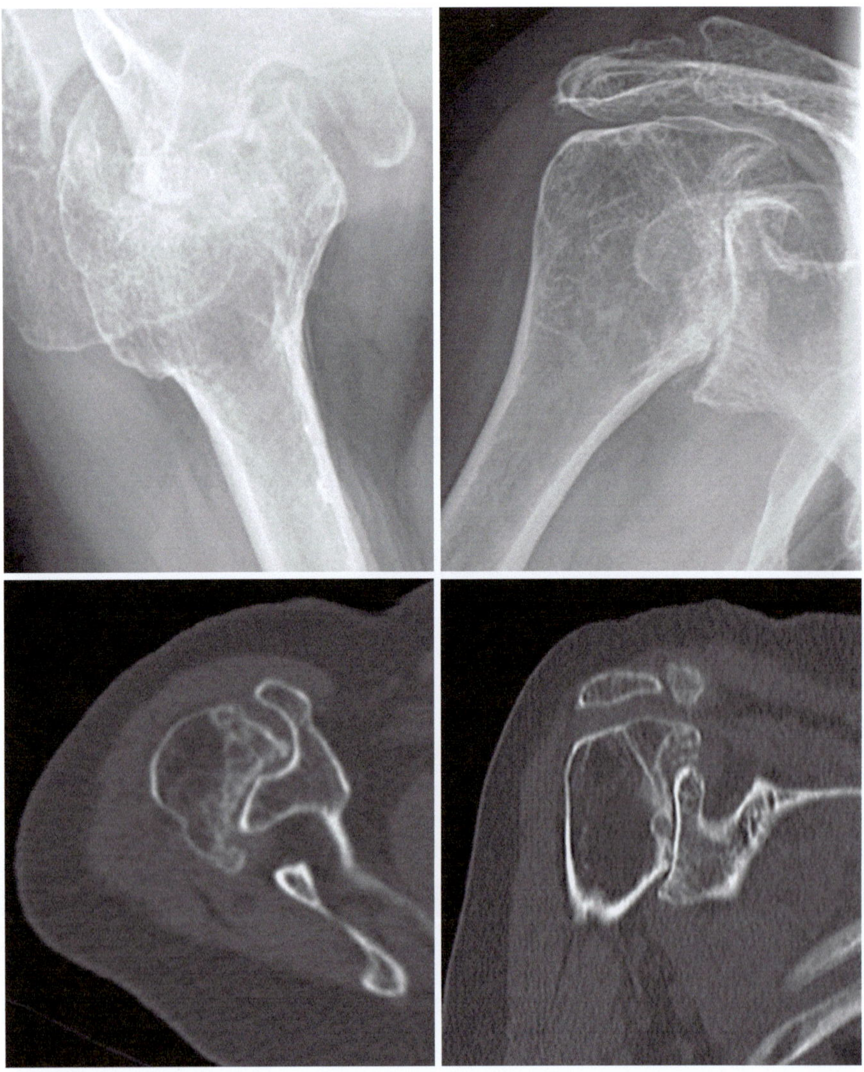

13.6 Differential Diagnoses of Shoulder Stiffness

Some of the most common causes of glenohumeral joint stiffness encountered in clinical practice and which must be considered in the differential diagnosis are:

- Adhesive capsulitis
- Glenohumeral arthritis
  - Degenerative
  - Inflammatory
  - Avascular necrosis of the humeral head
  - Rotator cuff arthropathy
- Post-traumatic stiffness—surgery, missed dislocation, fracture mal-union, adhesions
- Septic arthritis

A thorough clinical history will usually identify the most likely cause. Patient's age may also guide as to the likely diagnosis accounting for the observed stiffness.

The patient's age may guide as to the potential cause of shoulder stiffness

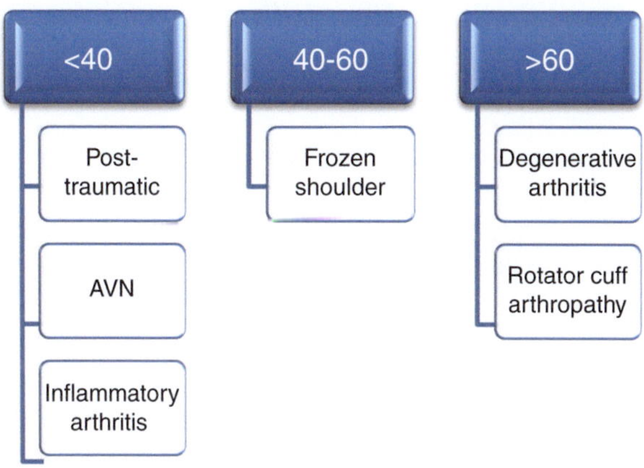

13.7 Investigations for Shoulder Stiffness

Investigations of the stiff shoulder aim to confirm the working diagnosis (as to the presence of true stiffness) and its likely cause, and exclude any possible alternative diagnoses. These include:

- Radiological
  - Plain radiographs
  - MRI/CT scan
  - Bone scan

- Neurophysiological
  - Nerve conduction studies
  - Electromyography
- Haematological
  - Inflammatory markers
  - HgA1c
- Arthroscopic evaluation

When faced with a painful shoulder in which it is difficult to determine if there is true or apparent stiffness, one may attempt to minimise pain and re-examine for movement. Such reduction in pain may be achieved by:

- Adequate oral or parenteral analgesia
- Shoulder local anaesthetic injections
- Examination under regional or general anaesthesia

13.8 Management of Shoulder Stiffness

Management of stiffness [6–9] involves:

- Tackling the structures (soft tissue or bony) that account for the mechanical block to motion
- Tackling the underlying condition that may have let to changes in the properties of these structures (including underlying infection, inflammatory arthritis, poorly controlled diabetes)

In tackling the deranged structures, the management ladder may be followed even though on occasions initial steps may be bypassed.

Management ladder for shoulder stiffness

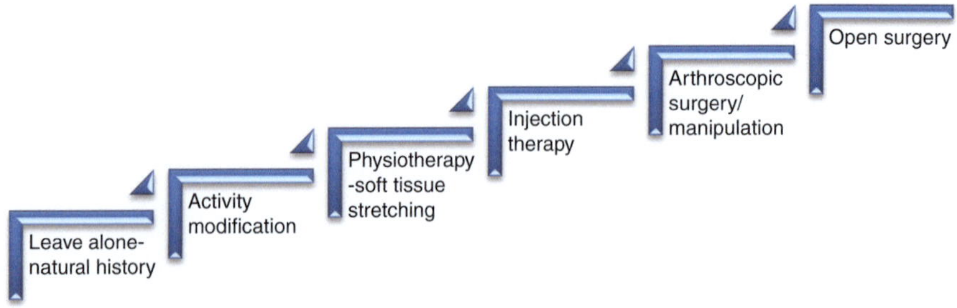

In some cases of stiffness, the underlying process has a natural history of improvement; adhesive capsulitis has been shown to improve in most patients over a period of 2–3 years [6]; hence any intervention aims to speed recovery rather than alter the final outcome. Some patients may not experience much trouble from their stiffness as their day-to-day activities do not require full shoulder movement or may be able to adjust their activities and thus manage to cope with lack of shoulder motion. Hence, there is a good argument in many cases for leaving things alone.

- Non-surgical management
  - Physiotherapy aims to stretch the soft tissue structures contributing to stiffness
  - Steroid injections may reduce glenohumeral joint inflammation helping to improve pain and also reduce any inflammatory-related changes in the soft tissues that contribute to stiffness
- Surgical management

  This is directed towards the structures contributing to loss of motion and may include:

- Soft tissue
  (a) Stretching (manipulation)
  (b) Release (arthroscopic or open division)
  (c) Lengthening (of contracted tendons or muscles)
- Bony
  (a) Reposition (reducing a dislocated joint)
  (b) Realignment (osteotomy)
  (c) Resection (impinging osteophytes)
  (d) Bone replacement (button replacement of osteochondral defects)
  (e) Joint arthroplasty (interposition, partial or total joint replacement)

Learning Pearls

- Patients may function well in performing activities of daily living with ranges of motion well below the maximum range of shoulder motion that is achierable in a healthy joint
- In stretching the painful stiff shoulder (with patient or clinician performed stretching exercises) prior adequate control of pain is required. Failure to adequately control pain may cause patient apprehension or muscle spasm, hindering the ability to perform sufficient stretching of the soft tissue envelop. Pain control may be achieved with oral or parenteral analgesia, with intra-articular steroid injections or with local anaesthetic nerve blocks

References

1. Itoi E, Arce G, Bain GI, Diercks RL, Guttmann D, Imhoff AB, Mazzocca AD, Sugaya H, Yoo YS. Shoulder stiffness: current concepts and concerns. Arthroscopy. 2016;32(7):1402–14.
2. Tauro JC, Paulson M. Shoulder stiffness. Arthroscopy. 2008;24(8):949–55.
3. Franceschi F, Papalia R, Palumbo A, Vasta S, Maffulli N, Denaro V. Management of postoperative shoulder stiffness. Sports Med Arthrosc Rev. 2011;19(4):420–7.
4. Neviaser AS, Neviaser RJ. Adhesive capsulitis of the shoulder. J Am Acad Orthop Surg. 2011;19(9):536–42.
5. Vezeridis PS, Goel DP, Shah AA, Sung SY, Warner JJ. Postarthroscopic arthrofibrosis of the shoulder. Sports Med Arthrosc Rev. 2010;18(3):198–206.
6. Vastamäki H, Kettunen J, Vastamäki M. The natural history of idiopathic frozen shoulder: a 2- to 27-year followup study. Clin Orthop Relat Res. 2012;470(4):1133–43.
7. Goldberg BA, Scarlat MM, Harryman DT 2nd. Management of the stiff shoulder. J Orthop Sci. 1999;4(6):462–71.
8. Elhassan B, Ozbaydar M, Massimini D, Higgins L, Warner JJ. Arthroscopic capsular release for refractory shoulder stiffness: a critical analysis of effectiveness in specific etiologies. J Shoulder Elb Surg. 2010;19(4):580–7.
9. Warner JJ, Greis PE. The treatment of stiffness of the shoulder after repair of the rotator cuff. Instr Course Lect. 1998;47:67–75.

Chapter 14
Shoulder Instability

This is a condition where there is symptomatic translation of one articulating surface in relation to another. The patient may experience pain, discomfort or apprehension, along with a feeling of the joint slipping out of place.

Shoulder instability may involve the glenohumeral, acromio-clavicular (ACJt) or sterno-clavicular joints.

This chapter discusses the principles in diagnosing, describing, classifying, investigating and managing instability around the shoulder. The need to differentiate between instability and laxity is also discussed.

14.1 Describing Shoulder Instability

Shoulder instability may be described in various ways, and some of these are presented below.

14.1.1 According to the Joint Involved

One or more joints may be simultaneously affected by instability.

© Springer Nature Switzerland AG 2019
C. Panayiotou Charalambous, *The Shoulder Made Easy*,
https://doi.org/10.1007/978-3-319-98908-2_14

Instability may involve one or more of the shoulder joints

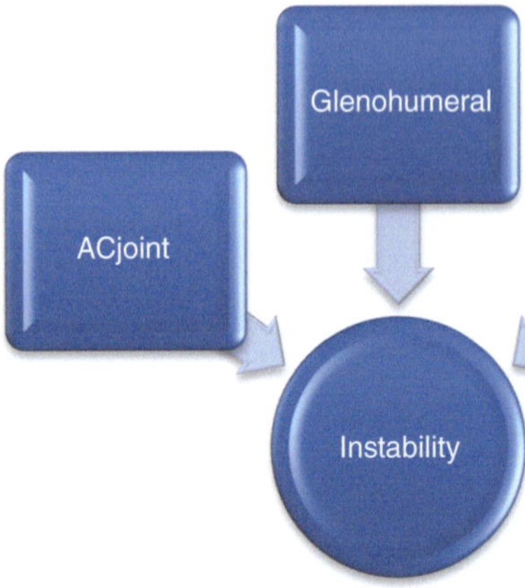

14.1.2 Number of Instability Episodes

- First time instability—refers to the first episode of instability
- Recurrent instability—more than one episode of instability

14.1.3 Degree of Translation

- Subluxation
- Dislocation

One articulating surface may sublux (displace but still remain in partial contact with the opposite articulating surface) or fully dislocate (with loss of all articular contact).

14.1.4 Reducibility

- Spontaneously reducible
- Spontaneously irreducible

Upon dislocation, the articulating surface may either spontaneously relocate or be locked in a dislocated position and need to be reduced medically (by closed or open means).

14.1.5 According to the Direction of Translation of One Articulating Surface to the Other

- Glenohumeral joint—translation of the humeral head in relation to the glenoid:
  - Anterior
  - Posterior
  - Multidirectional—instability occurs in two or more directions (but usually instability in one direction predominates)
- ACJt—translation of the lateral end of the clavicle in relation to the acromion
  - Superior
  - Inferior
  - Anterior
  - Posterior
- Sterno-clavicular joint—translation of the medial end of the clavicle in relation to the sternum
  - Anterior
  - Posterior

The direction of instability can be determined by:

- Clinical history—identifying the provocative position that reproduces instability symptoms
- Clinical examination
  - Visual inspection
  - Palpation
  - Instability provocation tests
- Radiographs or other radiological investigations
  - If there is intermittent instability, there is a need to review any radiological investigations obtained at the time of shoulder dislocation.

14.1.6 According to Its Initiating Event

- Congenital
- Acquired
  - Traumatic—as a result of specific, substantial trauma
  - Atraumatic—occurring with no precipitating substantial trauma
  - Micro-traumatic—as a result of repetitive soft tissue injury (as seen in overhead throwers, football and tennis players, and weight lifters)

14.1.7 According to Presence of Volition

- Voluntary—the patient can dislocate the shoulder at will, by influencing muscular contraction or by placing the shoulder in a particular position
- Involuntary—the patient cannot achieve the above

14.2 Causes of Shoulder Instability [1–8]

Instability may be due to disruption or inefficiency of dynamic or static stabilisers.
Static

- Detached
- Torn
- Stretched

Dynamic

- Weak
- Dis-coordinated
- Lack of stable platform to act upon

Abnormal Muscle Patterning—this describes incoordinated contraction of the muscles acting across the glenohumeral joint. Under normal conditions, such muscles contract in a coordinated way to maintain compression of the humeral head on the glenoid during shoulder motion. However, if one of these muscles contracts more intensely than it should, it may exceed the force of the opposing muscles and pull the humeral head in a particular direction causing subluxation or dislocation. Such imbalance may also occur if the activity of one muscle is less than what it should be [1, 2].

Defective Proprioception—for the muscles to contract in a balanced way, the brain must receive necessary proprioceptive feedback, with regard to the position of the glenohumeral joint, upper limb and overall body in space [3, 4].

Excessive Joint Laxity—the capsule and glenohumeral ligaments contribute to joint stability. However, if these are lax, their contributory stabilising effect diminishes [5–7].

Insufficient Core Control—glenohumeral stability is partially achieved by the coordinated contraction of muscles acting across the joint. Such muscles have attachments to the scapula, the vertebral column and all the way down to the pelvis. Hence, motion of the scapula and core may influence glenohumeral joint stability. The underlying core on which some movement occurs ought to be steady and balanced [8–10]. This may be considered analogous to try to lift a weight whilst standing on a stable rigid platform as compared to a rolling ball.

14.3 Clinical Symptoms of Shoulder Instability

- Feeling of abnormal displacement—this may range from:
  - Feeling "wobbly"
  - "Popping in and out"
  - "Popping out and can't go back" and "coming out to the edge"
  - "Coming out fully"
- Pain, vague and arm heaviness
- Clicking and clunking
- Dead arm syndrome and paraesthesia
- Dislocation where the humeral head comes out of joint. The patient may need to go to the hospital to have a reduction under sedation or general anaesthesia, or in some cases the patient may be able to reduce the shoulder themselves
- Subluxation where the shoulder almost comes out of joint with particular movements but then spontaneously reduces
- Apprehension—fear of placing the arm in a particular position because the shoulder may come out of joint

Symptoms may be aggravated by arm position according to the direction of instability as observed in glenohumeral instability:

- Anterior instability—arm abduction and external rotation—throwing position
- Posterior instability—90° of arm forward flexion, abduction and internal rotation
- Inferior instability—holding weight with arm by the side

14.4 Clinical Signs of Shoulder Instability [11–13]

These aim to assess:

- Apprehension, subluxation, dislocation and relocation of the examined joint
- Direction of instability
- Laxity of the unstable joint
- Generalised joint laxity
- Abnormal muscle patterning
- Scapular dyskinesia
- Core weakness/in-balance

14.5 Investigations for Shoulder Instability

Investigations of the unstable shoulder aim to confirm the presence of instability, determine its likely cause and identify any structural lesions that may be amenable to surgical intervention. These include:

- Radiological
  - Plain radiographs
  - MRI/MRI arthrogram/CT scan
- Neurophysiological
  - Nerve conduction studies
  - Electromyography
- Examination under general anaesthesia—joint translation and laxity are assessed with the patient under general anaesthesia to abolish pain and allow muscle relaxation
- Arthroscopic evaluation

14.6 Management of Shoulder Instability

Management depends on:

- Symptoms—severity and frequency
- Underlying cause
- Direction of instability

Management aims to relocate the joint (if dislocated) and improve joint stability to minimise the risk of further subluxations or dislocations. In doing so, surgery may help to improve associated functional loss, apprehension or pain.

Non-surgical [14–18]

- Activity modification and avoiding unstable arm positions
- Physiotherapy to address deficits in:
  - Core imbalance—core strengthening
  - Scapular dysrhythmia—strengthening of scapular muscles
  - Proprioception—proprioceptive training
  - Abnormal muscle patterning—biofeedback, inhibit overactive and enhance underactive muscles and improve neuromuscular control
  - Rotator cuff weakness—rotator cuff muscle strengthening and balance

It should be noted that non-surgical management does not specifically address any damaged or stretched static joint restraints but aims to improve stability by enhancing the function of dynamic stabilisers (through strengthening, better control and coordination).

Surgical [6, 19–25]

If symptoms do not improve with non-surgical intervention and patient has structural lesions that are amenable to surgery, surgery may be considered. Structural derangements are corrected either directly or indirectly.

- Directly—correct the structural defect itself
- Indirectly—compensate for the structural defect

Surgical interventions for stability may be described according to the structures addressed as:

- Soft tissue procedure
- Bony procedure
- Combined soft tissue/bony procedure

It is important to recognise that:

- Surgery addresses only structural defects; hence, other contributors to instability may still need dealing with
- Correcting structural defects may facilitate the correction of other contributors such as:
  - Proprioception
  - Abnormal muscle patterning

14.7 Special Situations of Shoulder Instability

There are certain considerations that must be made in some specific instability scenarios, and these are described below.

14.7.1 Epilepsy

Patients with epilepsy may have seizures during which they exhibit uncontrolled body movements and uncontrolled strong shoulder muscle contractions. These patients may sustain shoulder dislocations as they injure themselves during the uncontrolled body movements or due to the uncontrolled muscle contractions displacing one part of the joint over the other [26–28]. Anterior and posterior glenohumeral joint dislocations are associated with epileptic fits, but ACJt and sterno-clavicular dislocations may also occur.

In managing a patient with epilepsy and shoulder instability, there is need to control the epilepsy as uncontrolled fits:

- May predispose to further instability
- May lead to failure of any shoulder stabilisation surgery

14.7.2 *First-Time Dislocator*

It is recognised that an initial dislocation of the glenohumeral and sterno-clavicular joints (anterior-traumatic) is associated with an increased risk of subsequent instability, especially in young and high functional demand individuals [29–31]. When faced with a first-time shoulder dislocator of the glenohumeral or sterno-clavicular joint, the consideration is to either:

- Reduce the dislocated joint and also intervene surgically to stabilise the joint to minimise the risk of subsequent dislocations
- Reduce the dislocated joint, observe and rehabilitate and only consider intervening if recurrent dislocations occur

At the moment, there is no high-quality evidence supporting one approach over the other; hence, the second option is favoured by the author as that is the least invasive approach.

14.7.3 *Non-compliant Patients*

Certain patient groups may be less likely to comply with medical guidance following surgical intervention such as soft tissue stabilisation surgery. Such patients may be those with learning difficulties and history of alcohol or substance abuse. Options for this group of patients include:

- Symptomatic treatment avoiding surgical intervention
- Surgical intervention with more robust surgical procedures such as fusion arthroplasty

14.8 Instability vs. Hyper-laxity

Laxity is a physiological condition that is different to instability but may predispose to the development of shoulder instability.

Lax joints are thought to have longer and more stretchable ligaments and other static stabilisers which permit greater translation of the articular surfaces, leading to higher range of motion. Most patients with hyper-laxity do not have instability as they can maintain their joints in situ (such as through dynamic control) despite being able to achieve greater range of motion than the average norm. Hence, they do not have any symptoms of abnormal joint translation [32–34].

Excessive joint translation does not equate to instability. Similarly, it is possible to have shoulder instability without hyper-laxity. Hyper-laxity, however, may increase the risk of shoulder instability.

Some causes of hyper-laxity are described below:

Congenital

- Benign joint hypermobility syndrome (may affect up to 20% of the population, more common in females, Asians and Africans) [35, 36]
- Connective tissue disorders
  - Ehlers-Danlos syndrome
  - Marfan's syndrome
  - Osteogenesis imperfecta

Acquired

- Repetitive micro-trauma causing stretching of the capsule and ligaments—in athletes such as swimmers, gymnasts and pitchers [37, 38]

Generalised joint laxity per se does not require any treatment and is usually asymptomatic.

References

1. Jaggi A, Noorani A, Malone A, Cowan J, Lambert S, Bayley I. Muscle activation patterns in patients with recurrent shoulder instability. Int J Shoulder Surg. 2012;6(4):101–7.
2. Barden JM, Balyk R, Raso VJ, Moreau M, Bagnall K. Atypical shoulder muscle activation in multidirectional instability. Clin Neurophysiol. 2005;116(8):1846–57.
3. Gilman S. Joint position sense and vibration sense: anatomical organisation and assessment. J Neurol Neurosurg Psychiatry. 2002;73(5):473–7.
4. Lephart SM, Warner JJ, Borsa PA, Fu FH. Proprioception of the shoulder joint in healthy, unstable, and surgically repaired shoulders. J Shoulder Elb Surg. 1994;3(6):371–80.
5. Saccomanno MF, Fodale M, Capasso L, Cazzato G, Milano G. Generalized joint laxity and multidirectional instability of the shoulder. Patient Saf Surg. 2015;9:15. https://doi.org/10.1186/s13037-015-0062-9.
6. Sewell MD, Al-Hadithy N, Le Leu A, Lambert SM. Instability of the sternoclavicular joint: current concepts in classification, treatment and outcomes. Bone Joint J. 2013;95-B(6):721–31.
7. Lee HJ, Kim NR, Moon SG, Ko SM, Park JY. Multidirectional instability of the shoulder: rotator interval dimension and capsular laxity evaluation using MR arthrography. Skelet Radiol. 2013;42(2):231–8.
8. Huxel Bliven KC, Anderson BE. Core stability training for injury prevention. Sports Health. 2013;5(6):514–22.
9. Willson JD, Dougherty CP, Ireland ML, Davis IM. Core stability and its relationship to lower extremity function and injury. J Am Acad Orthop Surg. 2005;13(5):316–25.
10. Kibler WB, Press J, Sciascia A. The role of core stability in athletic function. Sports Med. 2006;36(3):189–98.
11. Charalambous CP. Clinical examination of the shoulder. In: Charalambous CP, editor. The shoulder made easy. Springer; 2019. pp. 77–122.
12. Levine WN, Sonnenfeld JJ, Shiu B. Shoulder instability: common problems and solutions. Clin Sports Med. 2018;37(2):161–77.
13. Valencia Mora M, Ibán MÁR, Heredia JD, Gutiérrez-Gómez JC, Diaz RR, Aramberri M, Cobiella C. Physical exam and evaluation of the unstable shoulder. Open Orthop J. 2017;11:946–56.
14. Jaggi A, Lambert S. Rehabilitation for shoulder instability. Br J Sports Med. 2010;44(5):333–40.

15. Warby SA, Ford JJ, Hahne AJ, Watson L, Balster S, Lenssen R, Pizzari T. Comparison of 2 exercise rehabilitation programs for multidirectional instability of the glenohumeral joint: a randomized controlled trial. Am J Sports Med. 2018;46(1):87–97.
16. Watson L, Balster S, Warby SA, Sadi J, Hoy G, Pizzari T. A comprehensive rehabilitation program for posterior instability of the shoulder. J Hand Ther. 2017;30(2):182–92.
17. Burkhead WZJ, Rockwood CAJ. Treatment of instability of the shoulder with an exercise program. J Bone Joint Surg Am. 1992;74(6):890–6.
18. Buss DD, Lynch GP, Meyer CP, Huber SM, Freehill MQ. Nonoperative management for in-season athletes with anterior shoulder instability. Am J Sports Med. 2004;32(6):1430–3.
19. Randelli P, Cucchi D, Butt U. History of shoulder instability surgery. Knee Surg Sports Traumatol Arthrosc. 2016;24(2):305–29.
20. Bankart AS. Recurrent or habitual dislocation of the shoulder-joint. Br Med J. 1923;2(3285):1132–3.
21. Patel RM, Amin NH, Lynch TS, Miniaci A. Management of bone loss in glenohumeral instability. Orthop Clin North Am. 2014;45(4):523–39.
22. Johnson SM, Robinson CM. Shoulder instability in patients with joint hyperlaxity. J Bone Joint Surg Am. 2010;92(6):1545–57.
23. Neer CS 2nd, Foster CR. Inferior capsular shift for involuntary inferior and multi-directional instability of the shoulder. A preliminary report. J Bone Joint Surg Am. 1980;62(6):897–908.
24. Stucken C, Cohen SB. Management of acromioclavicular joint injuries. Orthop Clin North Am. 2015;46(1):57–66.
25. Groh GI, Wirth MA. Management of traumatic sternoclavicular joint injuries. J Am Acad Orthop Surg. 2011;19(1):1–7.
26. Thangarajah T, Lambert SM. Management of recurrent shoulder instability in patients with epilepsy. J Shoulder Elb Surg. 2016;25(8):1376–84.
27. Goudie EB, Murray IR, Robinson CM. Instability of the shoulder following seizures. J Bone Joint Surg (Br). 2012;94(6):721–8.
28. Bühler M, Gerber C. Shoulder instability related to epileptic seizures. J Shoulder Elb Surg. 2002;11(4):339–44.
29. Robinson CM, Howes J, Murdoch H, Will E, Graham C. Functional outcome and risk of recurrent instability after primary traumatic anterior shoulder dislocation in young patients. J Bone Joint Surg Am. 2006;88(11):2326–36.
30. Robinson CM, Seah M, Akhtar MA. The epidemiology, risk of recurrence, and functional outcome after an acute traumatic posterior dislocation of the shoulder. J Bone Joint Surg Am. 2011;93(17):1605–13.
31. Wasserstein DN, Sheth U, Colbenson K, Henry PD, Chahal J, Dwyer T, Kuhn JE. The true recurrence rate and factors predicting recurrent instability after nonsurgical management of traumatic primary anterior shoulder dislocation: a systematic review. Arthroscopy. 2016;32(12):2616–25.
32. Emery RJ, Mullaji AB. Glenohumeral joint instability in normal adolescents. Incidence and significance. J Bone Joint Surg (Br). 1991;73(3):406–8.
33. McFarland EG, Campbell G, McDowell J. Posterior shoulder laxity in asymptomatic athletes. Am J Sports Med. 1996;24(4):468–71.
34. Jia X, Ji JH, Petersen SA, Freehill MT, McFarland EG. An analysis of shoulder laxity in patients undergoing shoulder surgery. J Bone Joint Surg Am. 2009;91(9):2144–50.
35. Hakim A, Grahame R. Joint hypermobility. Best Pract Res Clin Rheumatol. 2003;17(6):989–1004.
36. Jessee EF, Owen DS Jr, Sagar KB. The benign hypermobile joint syndrome. Arthritis Rheum. 1980;23(9):1053–6.
37. Laudner K, Meister K, Noel B, Deter T. Anterior glenohumeral laxity is associated with posterior shoulder tightness among professional baseball pitchers. Am J Sports Med. 2012;40(5):1133–7.
38. Bigliani LU, Codd TP, Connor PM, Levine WN, Littlefield MA, Hershon SJ. Shoulder motion and laxity in the professional baseball player. Am J Sports Med. 1997;25(5):609–13.

Chapter 15
Shoulder Paraesthesia

Paraesthesia refers to altered or reduced sensation. It may involve the shoulder area or may extend to involve part or all of the upper limb. Paraesthesia may be associated with other shoulder symptoms or occur in isolation. This chapter discusses potential sources of paraesthesia as well as principles of diagnosing, investigating and managing paraesthesia involving the shoulder and upper limb.

15.1 Sensory Pathways

In evaluating the cause of paraesthesia, one must consider the normal control of sensation (touch, temperature or pain).

Crude touch, pain and temperature are perceived by tactile, pain and temperature receptors in the skin and soft tissues which stimulate nerves the cell bodies of which are in the dorsal root ganglia of the spinal cord at the corresponding level. These nerve fibres synapse and pass messages to upper neurons the cell bodies of which are located in the dorsal horn of the spinal cord. The fibres of these upper neurons cross to the opposite site and ascend through the spinal cord as the spinothalamic tracts to the thalamus from which further neurons transmit signals to the primary sensory cortex in the frontal lobe of the brain.

© Springer Nature Switzerland AG 2019

C. Panayiotou Charalambous, *The Shoulder Made Easy*,
https://doi.org/10.1007/978-3-319-98908-2_15

Sensory pathways for pain and crude touch

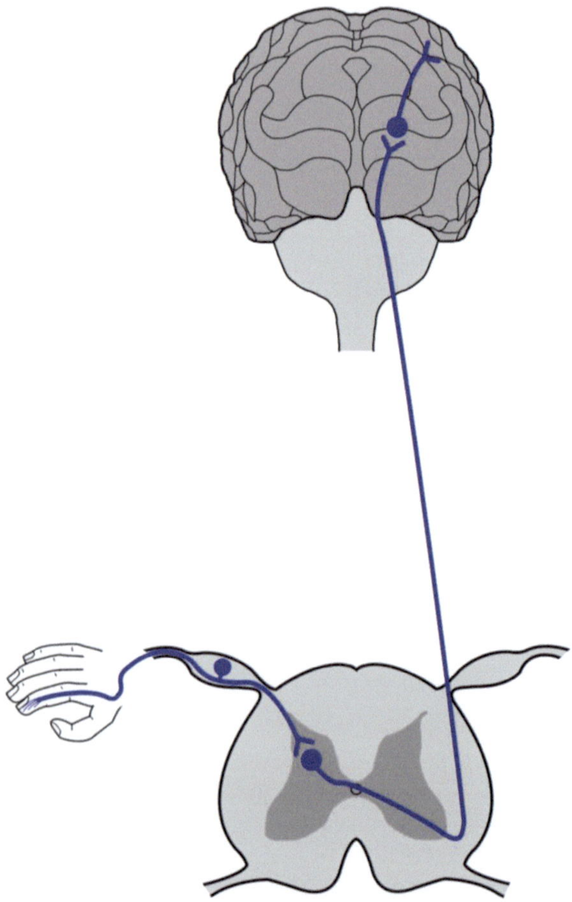

Specific touch is perceived by tactile receptors in the skin and soft tissues which stimulate nerves the cell bodies of which are in the dorsal root ganglia of the spinal cord at the corresponding level. These nerve fibres ascend through the posterior columns of the cord to the medulla where they synapse with neurons that cross to the opposite site and pass to the thalamus where they further synapse with neurons that pass to the primary sensory cortex in the frontal lobe of the brain [1–3].

Sensory pathways for specific touch

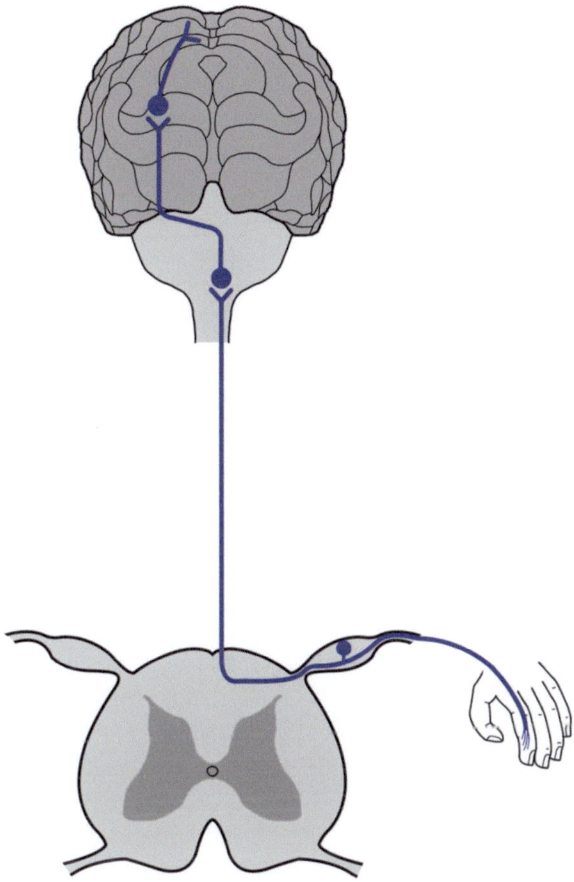

Like other parts of the body, the shoulder and upper limb are represented in the primary sensory cortex.

15.2 Sites of Neurological Dysfunction

As demonstrated by the pathways described above, paraesthesia can be the result of a deficit occurring anywhere between the soft tissue receptors and the brain. These include:

- Peripheral nerve
- Brachial plexus
- Cervical spine nerve roots
- Spinal cord
- Brain

15.3 Causes of Neurological Dysfunction

Nerve fibre activity may be impaired due to [4–6]:

- Ischaemia
- Demyelination—leading to a reduction in conduction velocity
- Axonal degeneration—loss of nerve fibres—leading to a reduction/inability to transmit electrical signals

  Nerve fibre activity may be affected by:

- Extrinsic lesions that affect the perfusion, metabolism or structure of the nerve such as:
  - Compression
  - Traction
  - Discontinuity—nerve laceration
- Intrinsic lesions—that affect the perfusion, metabolism and, hence, structure or function of the nerve:
  - Inflammatory conditions (e.g. rheumatological)
  - Endocrine disorders (e.g. thyroid dysfunction)
  - Metabolic conditions (e.g. diabetes mellitus)
  - Neoplasia—paraneoplastic syndromes
  - Infection
  - Vitamin deficiency
  - Toxins
  - Alcohol
  - Medicines

The above principles may be applied to all the levels of nerves, from the central nervous system to peripheral nerves.

Nerve compression may lead to:

- Perineural oedema
- Demyelination
- Degeneration of distal axons
- Nerve sprout formation
- Regeneration of nerve fibres
- Remyelination

The severity of paraesthesia may be related to the degree and duration of compression and extent of nerve damage:

- Intermittent paraesthesia may be due to intermittent compression that causes intermittent interruption of the neural microcirculation by oedema
- Constant paraesthesia may signify more severe constant compression associated with demyelination; symptoms recover once compression is relieved, but this recovery can take time
- Constant sensory loss may be due to severe compression leading to axon degeneration; symptoms fail to recover fully once compression is relieved

Nerve traction that stretches nerves can have detrimental effects on nerve function similar to compression by:

- Increasing intra-neural pressure
- Impairing nerve blood flow

If nerve gliding is limited, it may lead to local nerve stretching with limb motion. Suddenly applied substantial nerve traction may also lead to nerve discontinuity.

15.4 Conditions Leading to Shoulder Paraesthesia

Some of the common conditions causing shoulder paraesthesia are:

- Shoulder instability—causing dead arm syndrome
- Cervical spondylosis causing nerve root impingement
- Suprascapular nerve palsy
- Axillary nerve palsy
- Parsonage Turner syndrome
- Brachial plexus lesion
- Thoracic outlet syndrome

Other conditions to consider include:

- Syringomyelia
- Cerebrovascular accident
- Multiple sclerosis

15.5 Clinical Symptoms in Shoulder Paraesthesia

Patients may complain of:

- Altered sensation
- Pins and needles
- Reduced sensation
- Tingling
- Numbness
- Dead arm
- Associated shoulder symptoms—pain, instability, weakness, stiffness

15.6 Clinical Examination in Shoulder Paraesthesia [7]

- Assess overall posture
- Shoulder examination looking for evidence of instability
- A full neurological examination is carried out including:
  - Objective assessment of the integrity of sensation—light touch, pain, temperature, joint position sense
  - Mapping of the area of paraesthesia—in some cases, symptoms may not be associated with an objective demonstration of neurological dysfunction
  - Muscle activity:

    Strength
    Wasting

  - Reflexes
  - Tests for cervical spine nerve root dysfunction
  - Tests for thoracic outlet syndrome (Roo's, hyper-abduction, Tinel's)
  - Tests for peripheral nerve lesion (Tinel's, Phalen's)
  - Lower limb strength, coordination, clonus

15.7 Identifying the Cause of Paraesthesia [2, 8]

In trying to determine the cause of paraesthesia, factors to consider are:

- *Painful vs. painless*
  - Associated pain may suggest:

    A lesion stimulating nociceptors and also impairing nerve function
    An extrinsic lesion irritating the nerve
    An intrinsic lesion causing nerve dysfunction—neuritis

- *Distribution*
  - Nerve:

    Single peripheral nerve distribution
    Multiple peripheral nerve distribution
    Dermatomal

  - Unilateral or bilateral?

    If symptoms are bilateral consider a higher lesion (spinal cord, brain) although some peripheral neuropathies such as carpal tunnel syndrome may be bilateral

- *Associated weakness or muscle atrophy*
  - Their presence may signify a substantial disruption of nerve function rather than intermittent nerve fibre ischaemia
  - An upper motor neuron lesion is associated with:

    Minimal atrophy (although some atrophy may develop because of disuse)
    Absent fasciculations
    Increased spasticity
    Exaggerated stretch reflexes

  - A lower motor neuron lesion leads to:

    Decreased muscle tone
    Decreased reflexes
    Atrophy
    Fasciculations

- *Gradual vs. sudden onset*
- *Precipitating factor*
  - None
  - Trauma
  - Surgery
- *Intermittent vs. constant*
- *Family history of neurological conditions*
  - Certain neuropathies are hereditary
- *Aggravating factors*

  Posture
  Overhead activities
  Computer activities

- *Worse at night*
  - Relief of nerve pressure
  - Aggravation of nerve pressure

    Sleeping with arm overhead—causing thoracic outlet obstruction
    Sleeping with wrists flexed—aggravating carpal tunnel compression

15.8 Investigations for Shoulder Paraesthesia

Investigations of paraesthesia aim to confirm the working diagnosis. These include:

- Radiological imaging of the nerve pathways and related bony and soft tissue structures
  - Plain radiographs
  - Ultrasound/MRI/CT scan
- Neurophysiological
  - Nerve conduction studies
  - EMG studies
- Blood tests to exclude systemic causes of nerve dysfunction including
  - Inflammatory markers
  - B12 levels
  - Urea, electrolytes, calcium
  - HgA1c

MRI showing cervical spine disc protrusion with spinal indentation (red arrow)

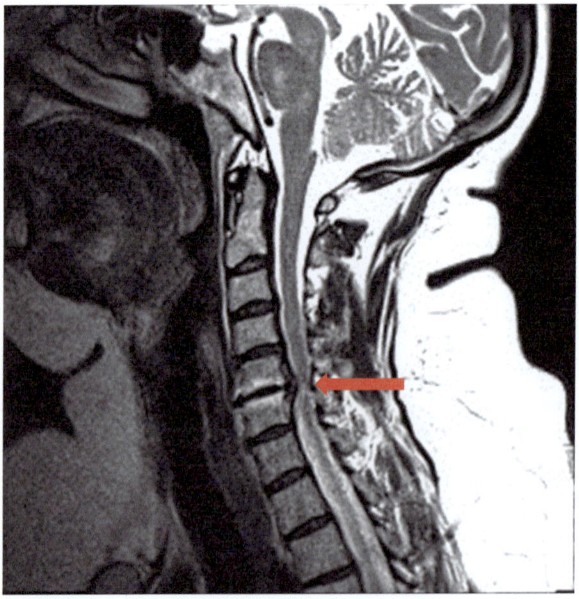

15.9 Management of Shoulder Paraesthesia

Management of paraesthesia [9–16] involves:

- Leave alone
- Symptomatic control of paraesthesia especially if painful:
  - Simple analgesia

    Non-steroidal anti-inflammatories
  - Neuropathic analgesia

    Gabapentin
    Pregabalin
    Low-dose amitriptyline
  - Local massage
  - Acupuncture
  - Sensory re-education:

    Touching objects of different textures
    Identifying different temperatures
    Identifying different pressures
    Determining joint/limb position
- Addressing the underlying condition that may have led to changes in the intrinsic properties of nerves (such as the underlying infection, inflammatory arthritis, vasculitis, poorly controlled diabetes)
- Addressing the extrinsic causes of nerve dysfunction

15.10 Management of Extrinsic Causes of Nerve Dysfunction

In dealing with extrinsic causes of nerve dysfunction, the following management ladder may be considered although on occasions initial steps may be bypassed.

Management ladder for extrinsic causes of nerve dysfunction

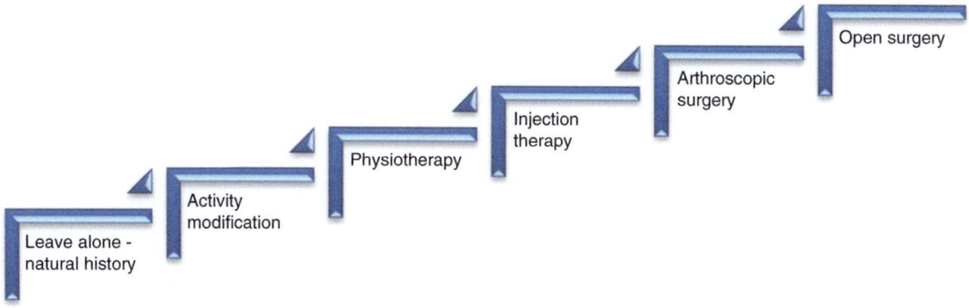

- Leave alone
- Activity modification:
  - Avoid exaggerating factors, positions and repetitive activities
- Physiotherapy:
  - Improve shoulder biomechanics
  - Reduce nerve traction by posture control
  - Improve scapular control
  - Reduce compression:

    Relax tense muscles
    Stretch tense, hypertrophied muscles
    Cervical spine traction
  - Mobilise nerves:

    Stretch
    Local massage
- Injection therapy—reduce compression:
  - Steroid injections to reduce perineural inflammation
  - Local anaesthetic injections to reduce muscle spasm
  - Botulinum toxin injections to reduce muscle spasm
- Arthroscopic surgery:
  - Decompress nerves
  - Improve shoulder biomechanics—such as by improving shoulder stability
- Open surgery:
  - Improve shoulder biomechanics—such as stabilisation surgery
  - Decompress nerves
  - Nerve transfers
  - Nerve grafts

Learning Pearls

- There may be absence of objective findings on clinical neurological examination, despite complaints of paraesthesia. This may be due to intermittent nerve compression or traction (analogous to leg numbness that one may experience when staying in an awkward sitting or kneeling posture for too long or the arm numbness when sleeping on the arm for too long but which quickly resolves once that posture is corrected). Intermittent compression may be positional or posture related or due to some internal pathology such as tight muscles, impinging structures or otherwise. Hence, the absence of objective neurological findings should not cast doubt on the validity of symptoms

References

1. Rea P. Essential clinical anatomy of the nervous system. New York: Elsevier Inc; 2015.
2. Reeves AG, editor. Disorders of the nervous system: a primer. 3rd ed. West Lebanon: Imperial Company Printers; 1995.
3. Gilman S, Newman SW. Manter and Gatz's essentials of clinical neuroanatomy and neurophysiology, vol. 8. Philadelphia: FA Davis; 1992.
4. Mackinnon SE. Pathophysiology of nerve compression. Hand Clin. 2002;18(2):231–41.
5. Burnett MG, Zager EL. Pathophysiology of peripheral nerve injury: a brief review. Neurosurg Focus. 2004;16(5):E1.
6. Rempel D, Dahlin L, Lundborg G. Pathophysiology of nerve compression syndromes: response of peripheral nerves to loading. J Bone Joint Surg Am. 1999;81(11):1600–10.
7. Charalambous CP. Clinical examination of the shoulder. In: Charalambous CP, editor. The shoulder made easy. Springer; 2019. pp. 77–122.
8. McKnight JT, Adcock BB. Paresthesias: a practical diagnostic approach. Am Fam Physician. 1997;56(9):2253–60.
9. Deli G, Bosnyak E, Pusch G, Komoly S, Feher G. Diabetic neuropathies: diagnosis and management. Neuroendocrinology. 2013;98(4):267–80.
10. Moore RA, Derry S, Aldington D, Cole P, Wiffen PJ. Amitriptyline for neuropathic pain in adults. Cochrane Database Syst Rev. 2015;7:CD008242. https://doi.org/10.1002/14651858.CD008242.
11. Yang CP, Hsieh CL, Wang NH, Li TC, Hwang KL, Yu SC, Chang MH. Acupuncture in patients with carpal tunnel syndrome: a randomized controlled trial. Clin J Pain. 2009;25(4):327–33.
12. Oud T, Beelen A, Eijffinger E, Nollet F. Sensory re-education after nerve injury of the upper limb: a systematic review. Clin Rehabil. 2007;21(6):483–94.
13. Childress MA, Becker BA. Nonoperative management of cervical radiculopathy. Am Fam Physician. 2016;93(9):746–54.
14. Peolsson A, Söderlund A, Engquist M, Lind B, Löfgren H, Vavruch L, Holtz A, Winström-Christersson A, Isaksson I, Öberg B. Physical function outcome in cervical radiculopathy patients after physiotherapy alone compared with anterior surgery followed by physiotherapy: a prospective randomized study with a 2-year follow-up. Spine (Phila Pa 1976). 2013;38(4):300–7.
15. Bottros MM, AuBuchon JD, McLaughlin LN, Altchek DW, Illig KA, Thompson RW. Exercise-enhanced, ultrasound-guided anterior scalene muscle/pectoralis minor muscle blocks can facilitate the diagnosis of neurogenic thoracic outlet syndrome in the high-performance overhead athlete. Am J Sports Med. 2017;45(1):189–94.
16. Godoy IR, Donahue DM, Torriani M. Botulinum toxin injections in musculoskeletal disorders. Semin Musculoskelet Radiol. 2016;20(5):441–52.

Chapter 16
Shoulder Noise

Symptoms of crepitus, clicking or clunking are often described around the shoulder, either in isolation or accompanying other complaints such as those of pain or instability. This chapter discusses some of the causes of such symptoms, along with the investigation and management of the underlying causative disorders.

16.1 Clinical Symptoms of Shoulder Noise

- Audible shoulder noise on arm motion
- Soft or loud
- Clicking, clunking, popping, grating, snapping
- May occur in isolation or be associated with other symptoms including:
  - Pain
  - Instability
  - Locking/jamming
  - Reduced arm motion
  - Weakness
  - Shoulder swellings—scapular, acromio-clavicular joint (ACJt)

16.2 Clinical Signs of Shoulder Noise

- Audible shoulder noise (including clicking, clunking, friction, grating, snapping, flipping)
- Palpable crepitus
- Signs consistent with underlying disorder causing noise

© Springer Nature Switzerland AG 2019

C. Panayiotou Charalambous, *The Shoulder Made Easy*,
https://doi.org/10.1007/978-3-319-98908-2_16

16.3 Sources of Abnormal Shoulder Noise

The abnormal shoulder noises may come from several areas, but sometimes it is difficult to determine their exact origin. Similarly, on occasions it may be challenging for the clinician and patient to reach an agreement as to where the abnormal noise is coming from.

Potential sources of shoulder noise

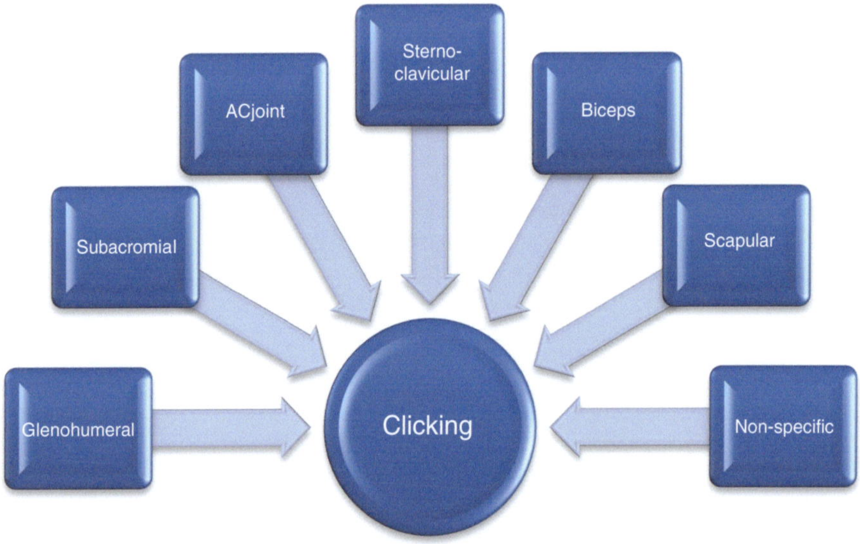

Potential pathologies affecting parts of the shoulder that can give rise to clicking or clucking are shown next. These noises may be physiological or may reflect a mechanical event such as abnormal translation or mechanical contact between two surfaces [1–7].

Spectrum of disorders that may give rise to shoulder noise

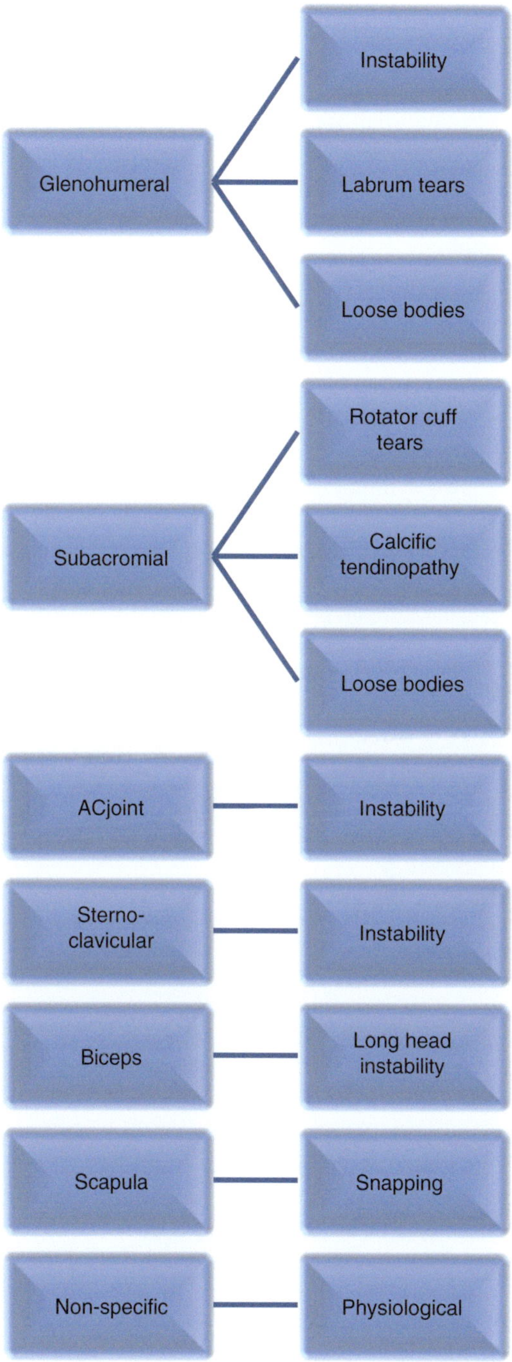

16.4 Investigations for Shoulder Noise

- Radiological
  - Plain radiographs
  - Dynamic ultrasound/MRI/MRI arthrogram/CT scan
- Neurophysiological
  - Nerve conduction studies
  - Electromyography
- Arthroscopic evaluation

16.5 Management of Shoulder Noise

This depends on clinical symptoms. If there are no associated symptoms such as pain or instability, symptoms of clunking or clinking may be left alone with reassurance. If there are associated symptoms or the symptoms of shoulder noise are troublesome, then management is directed at the underlying cause. The management ladder may be followed, although on occasions initial steps may be bypassed.

Management ladder for troublesome shoulder noise

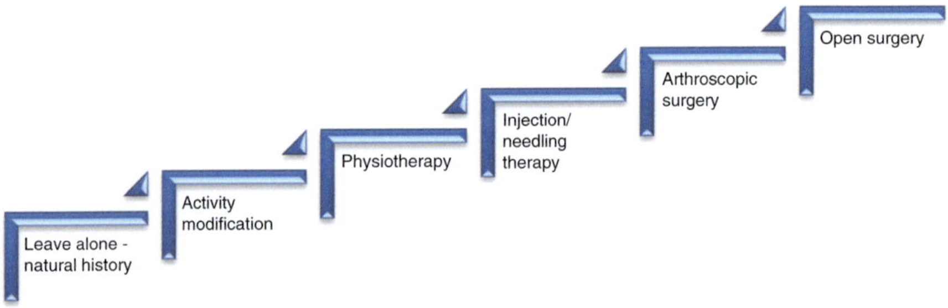

Learning Pearls
- The examiner may not be able to hear the noise the patient describes but may be able to feel it on palpation
- Physiological joint noises are common and all the clinician may need to provide is reassurance

References

1. Liu SH, Henry MH, Nuccion S, Shapiro MS, Dorey F. Diagnosis of glenoid labral tears. A comparison between magnetic resonance imaging and clinical examinations. Am J Sports Med. 1996;24(2):149–54.
2. O'Kane JW, Toresdahl BG. The evidenced-based shoulder evaluation. Curr Sports Med Rep. 2014;13(5):307–13.
3. Jeong JH, Shin SJ. Arthroscopic removal of proud metallic suture anchors after Bankart repair. Arch Orthop Trauma Surg. 2009;129(8):1109–15.
4. Gaskill T, Millett PJ. Snapping scapula syndrome: diagnosis and management. J Am Acad Orthop Surg. 2013;21(4):214–24.
5. Merolla G, Cerciello S, Paladini P, Porcellini G. Snapping scapula syndrome: current concepts review in conservative and surgical treatment. Muscles Ligaments Tendons J. 2013;3(2):80–90.
6. Pierce RO Jr. Internal derangement of the sternoclavicular joint. Clin Orthop Relat Res. 1979;141:247–50.
7. Huylebroek J, van Hedent E, van Overschelde J. Correlation of computed arthrotomography with arthroscopy of the glenohumeral joint. Acta Orthop Belg. 1991;57(Suppl 1):83–8.

Chapter 17
Shoulder Swellings

Patients may present with a visible or palpable swelling around the shoulder. This chapter focuses on how to describe such swellings and on the clinical symptoms and signs to be sought when dealing with these. Principles of investigating and managing shoulder swellings are also discussed.

17.1 Types of Shoulder Swellings

The spectrum of swellings that may be encountered in the shoulder region is very broad [1–16]. Such swellings may be described in several ways including the ones below:

17.1.1 According to Aggressiveness of the Swelling

A swelling that is rapidly and constantly getting bigger is more worrying that one that fluctuates in size or is diminishing in size.

Aggressive swellings may be painless but may also cause constant severe pain if complicated by:

- local infiltration of surrounding tissues, pressure on nearby nerves, or intra-substance bleeding

© Springer Nature Switzerland AG 2019

C. Panayiotou Charalambous, *The Shoulder Made Easy*,
https://doi.org/10.1007/978-3-319-98908-2_17

Benign swellings may cause pain due to pressure effects or may be associated with pain originating from the underlying tissue that gives rise to the swelling as seen in:

- Arthritis of the acromio-clavicular joint (ACJt) associated with an ACJt cyst

Description of neoplastic shoulder swellings according to their aggressiveness

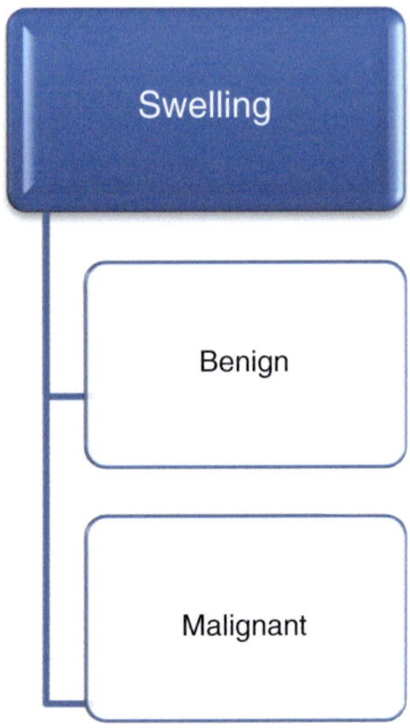

17.1.2 *According to the Anatomical Origin of the Swelling*

Description of shoulder swellings according to their anatomical origin (with examples given)

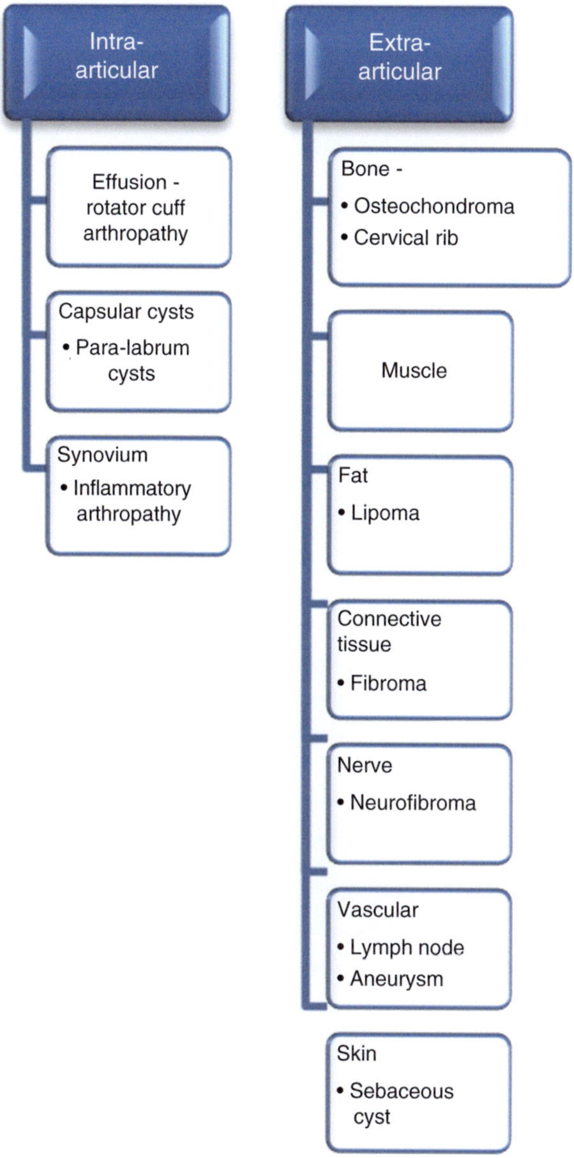

17.1.3 According to Swelling Composition

Description of shoulder swellings according to their composition

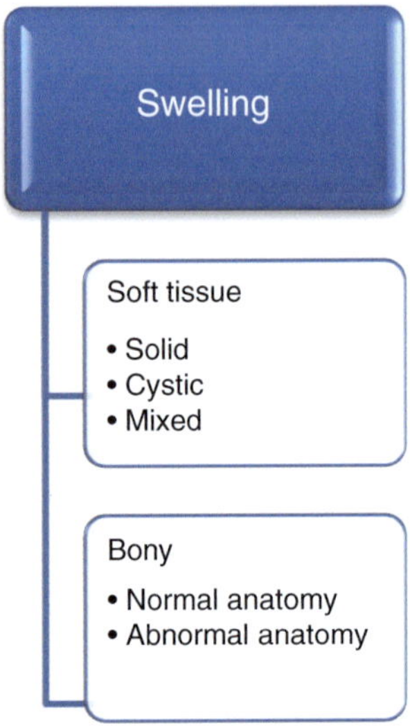

17.1.4 According to the Precipitating Cause of the Swelling

Description of shoulder swellings according to their precipitating cause

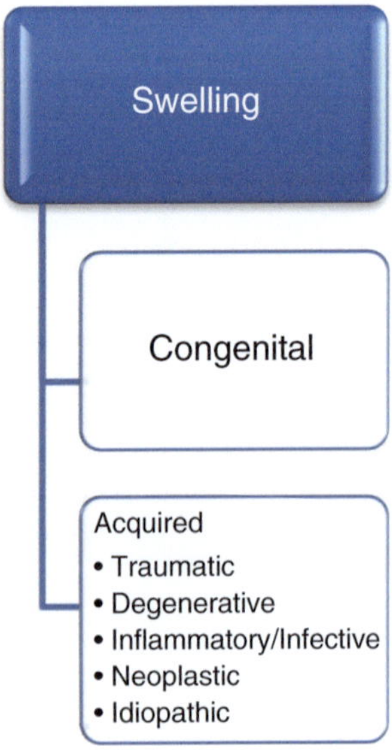

Large diffuse swelling of the shoulder due to rotator cuff arthropathy

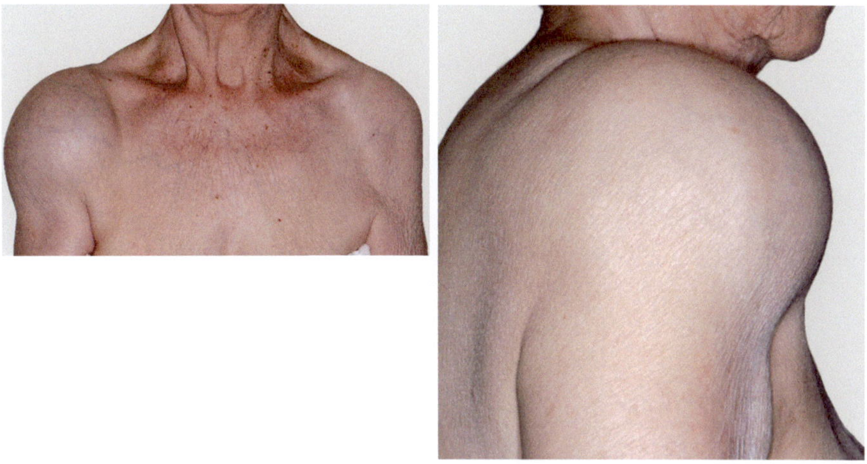

Swelling at the top of the ACJt found to be a lipoma

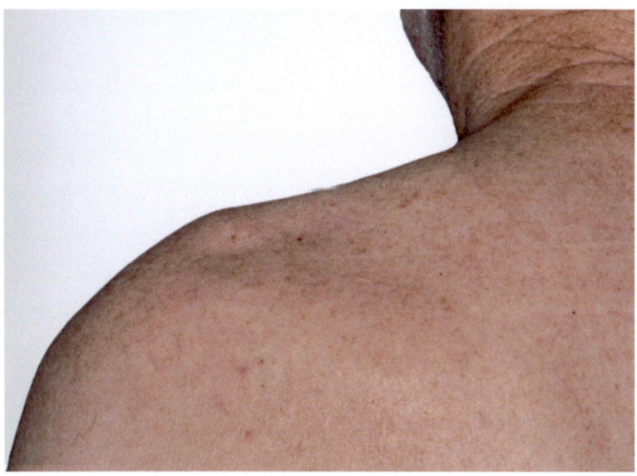

Soft tissue swelling over left scapula, found to be a lipoma

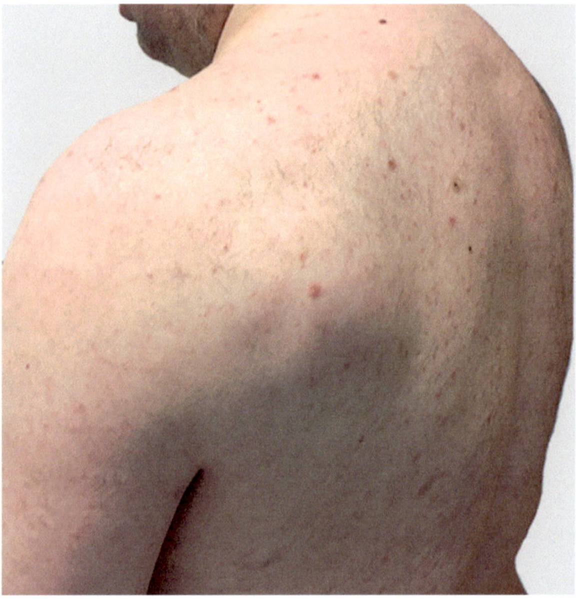

ACJt dislocation with bony lump (lateral end of clavicle) seen at the level of the ACJt

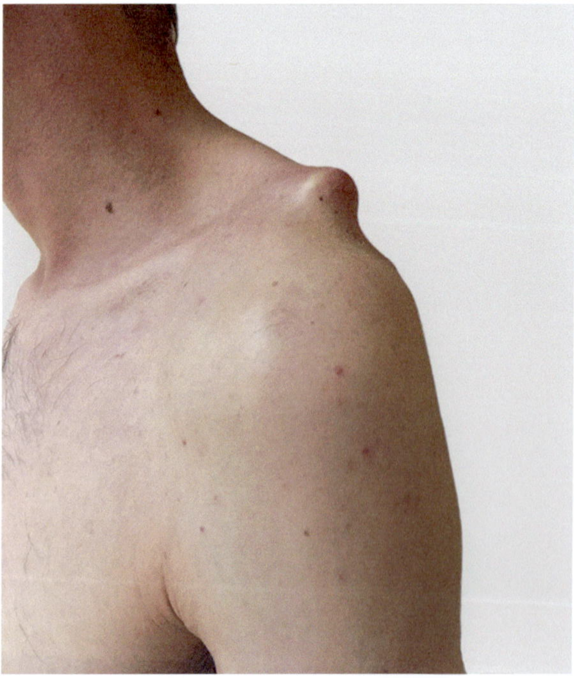

Swelling over ACJt—ACJt cyst

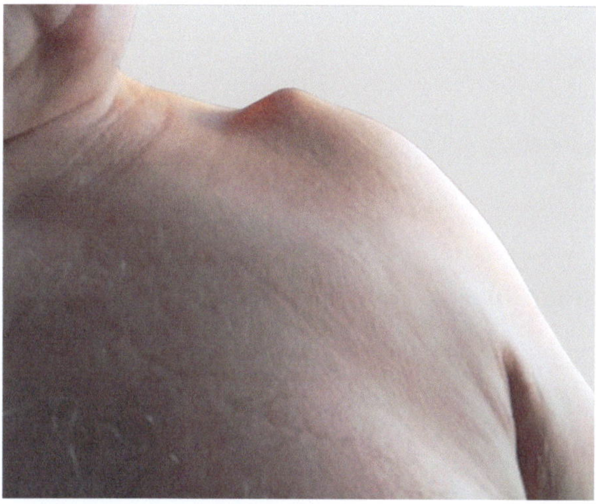

17.2 Clinical Symptoms of Shoulder Swellings

- Complaint of lump, swelling, prominence, deformity, asymmetry between sides, "something out of place", "something sticking out", noticed by patient or brought to the patient's attention by others
- Onset—sudden/gradual, precipitating factor such as trauma, no precipitating event
- Constant size and shape or changing with arm movement or time
- Getting bigger/smaller/fluctuating in size
- Speed of change
- Associated symptoms—pain, paraesthesia, clicking/clucking, instability

17.3 Clinical Examination for Shoulder Swellings

- Location
- Shape
- Size
- Origin—tracing its base—localised to skin, subcutaneous tissue, muscle, bone

- Consistency—firm, soft, fluctuant
- Mobility—freely mobile, tethered to underlying tissues, reduced by muscle contraction
- Specials tests:
  - Pulsatile
  - Transillumination
  - Tinel's sign

17.4 Investigations for Shoulder Swellings

- Radiological
  - Plain radiographs
  - MRI/CT scan
  - Bone scan
- Neurophysiological
  - Nerve conduction studies
  - Electromyography
- Arthroscopic/open evaluation
  - Sample biopsy
  - Excision biopsy

MRI scan showing cystic lesion at the superior aspect of the shoulder close to the ACJt (red arrow) confirmed with Ultrasound (yellow arrow)

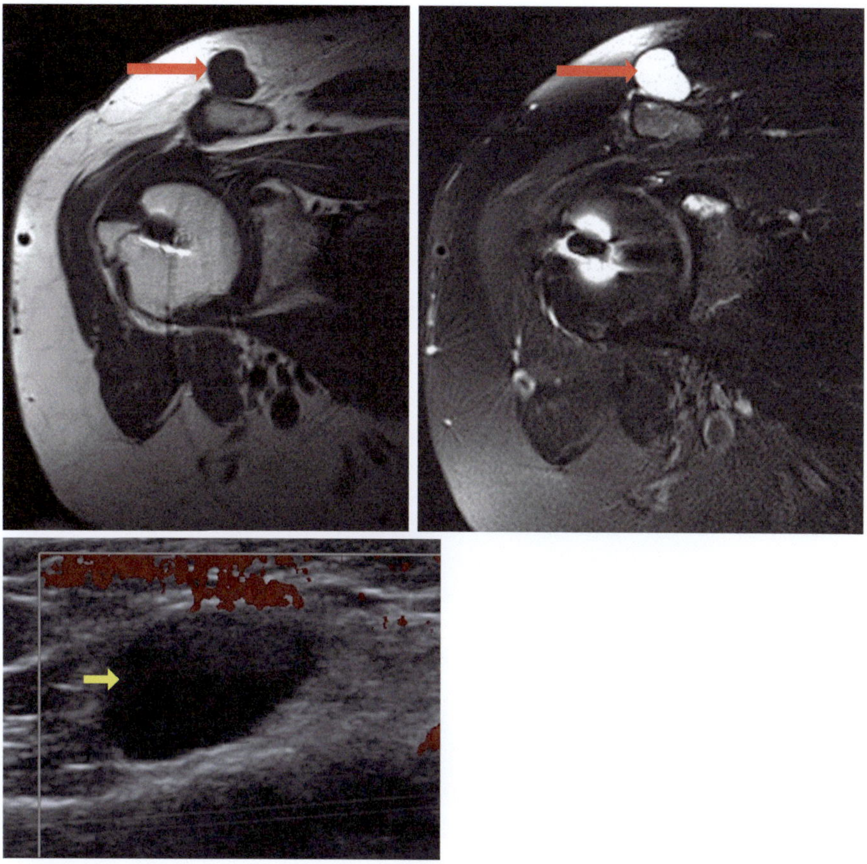

Exostosis (red arrow) arising from the anterior part of the lateral end of the clavicle-palpable as hard swelling on clinical examination

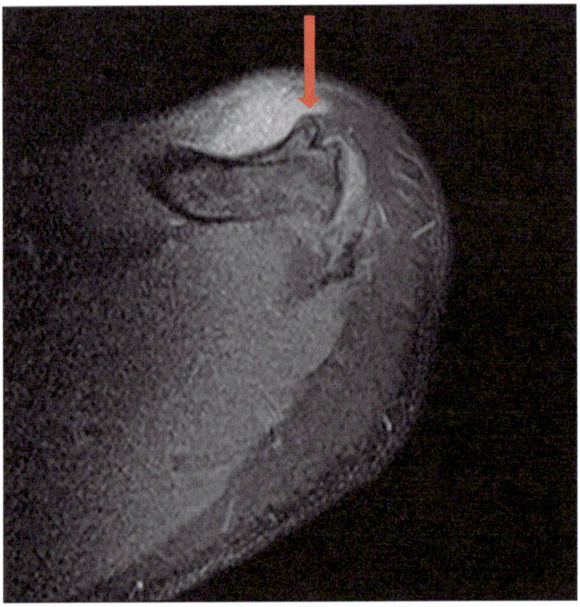

Swelling over ACJt shown to be lipoma on MRI (red arrow)

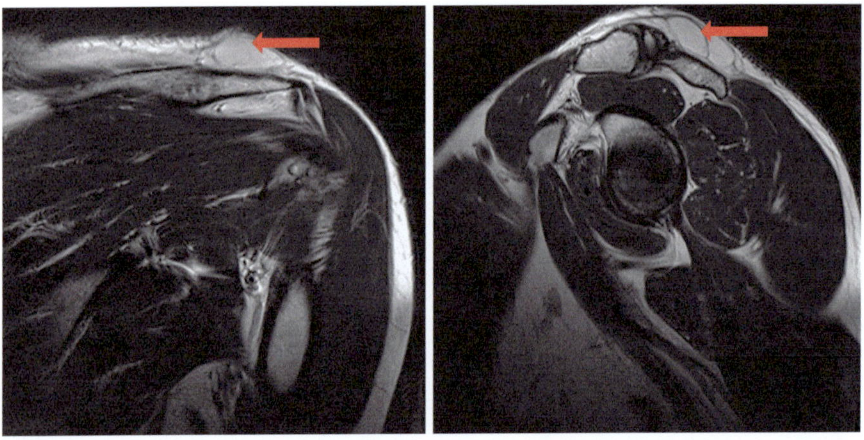

A palpable hard swelling on the anterior aspect of the shoulder, turned out to be an exostosis (red arrows) arising from the proximal humerus

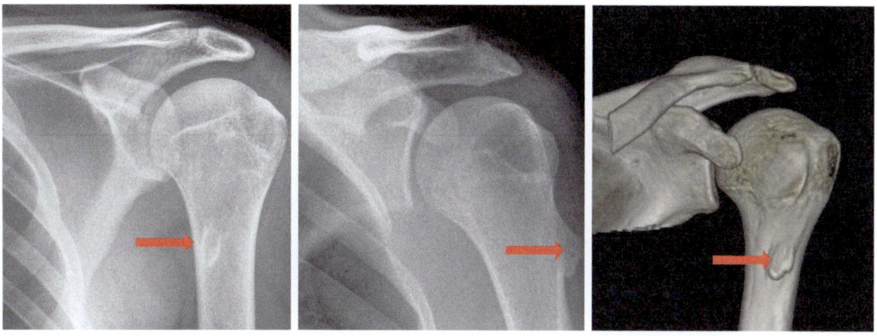

MRI showing lipoma in peri-scapular area

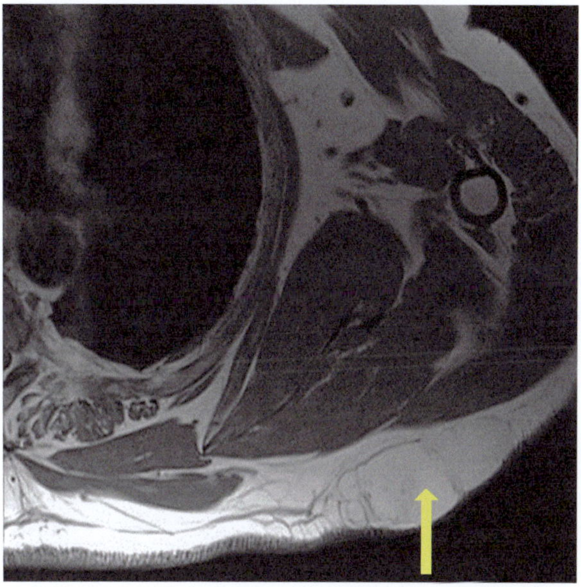

17.5 Management of Shoulder Swellings

This will depend on symptoms, nature and aggressiveness of the swelling. Asymptomatic (non-infective and non-malignant) swellings may be left alone with reassurance. If symptomatic then management may involve:

- Addressing the swelling
- Addressing the underlying condition that may have led to the swelling

The management ladder may be followed, although on occasions initial steps may be bypassed.

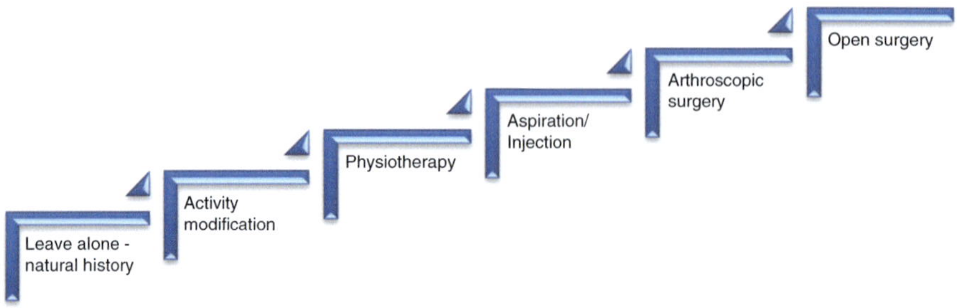

Learning Pearls

- Worrying features of soft tissue swellings include:
  - Recent increase in size
  - Location deep to the subcutaneous fascia
  - Limited mobility relative to deep tissues
  - Size greater than 4 cm
  - Indeterminate nature on imaging

  The nature of such swellings may need verification by biopsy which is better done at a centre that is capable of extensive excision of the swelling if this proved to be malignant. Hence, early referral to a regional soft tissue tumour unit is recommended.

- Lipomas around the shoulder area may have an intramuscular extension, which must be sought for on imaging, as this would complicate an attempted surgical excision

References

1. Westhovens R, Dequeker J. Musculoskeletal manifestations of benign and malignant tumors of bone. Curr Opin Rheumatol. 2003;15(1):70–5.
2. Damron TA, Beauchamp CP, Rougraff BT, Ward WG Sr. Soft-tissue lumps and bumps. Instr Course Lect. 2004;53:625–37.
3. Frassica FJ, McCarthy EF, Bluemke DA. Soft-tissue masses: when and how to biopsy. Instr Course Lect. 2000;49:437–42.
4. Verbeek BM, Kaiser CL, Larque AB, Hornicek FJ, Raskin KA, Schwab JH, Chen YL, Lozano Calderón SA. Synovial sarcoma of the shoulder: A series of 14 cases. J Surg Oncol. 2017;117(4):788–96. https://doi.org/10.1002/jso.24889.
5. Ruigrok D, Soetekouw R, Stockmann HB, van Krimpen K, Chesaru I, Sulzer MA. Soft-tissue mass as a rare presentation of sarcoidosis. Ned Tijdschr Geneeskd. 2014;158(4):A6441.

6. Tantisricharoenkul G, Tan EW, Fayad LM, McCarthy EF, McFarland EG. Malignant soft tissue tumors of the biceps muscle mistaken for proximal biceps tendon rupture. Orthopedics. 2012;35(10):e1548–52.
7. Carbone S, Candela V, Passaretti D, Cinotti G, Della Rocca C, Giannicola G, Gumina S. Subdeltoid lipomas: a consecutive series of 13 cases. Musculoskelet Surg. 2012;96(Suppl 1):S53–6.
8. Park HW, Jo H, Moon SH, Baek S. Painful Intramuscular Lipoma of the Infraspinatus: unusual location and presentation. Orthopedics. 2016;39(2):e370–3.
9. Kapetanakis S, Papathanasiou J, Dermon A, Dimitrakopoulou A, Ververidis A, Chloropoulou P, Kazakos K. Unusual intramuscular lipoma of deltoid muscle. Folia Med (Plovdiv). 2010;52(2):68–71.
10. Dympep B, Khangarot S, Hadke N. An unusual presentation of traumatic pseudoaneurysm of axillary artery mimicking soft tissue tumor. J Surg Case Rep. 2012;2012(10):17.
11. Castelino-Prabhu S, Stoll LM, Li QK. Metastatic retinoblastoma presenting as a left shoulder soft tissue mass: FNA findings and review of the literature. Diagn Cytopathol. 2010;38(6):440–6.
12. Cleeman E, Auerbach JD, Springfield DS. Tumors of the shoulder girdle: a review of 194 cases. J Shoulder Elb Surg. 2005;14(5):460–5.
13. Elbardouni A, Kharmaz M, Salah Berrada M, Mahfoud M, Elyaacoubi M. Well-circumscribed deep-seated lipomas of the upper extremity. A report of 13 cases. Orthop Traumatol Surg Res. 2011;97(2):152–8.
14. Hiller AD, Miller JD, Zeller JL. Acromioclavicular joint cyst formation. Clin Anat. 2010;23(2):145–52.
15. Nowak DD, Covey AS, Grant RT, Bigliani LU. Massive acromioclavicular joint cyst. J Shoulder Elb Surg. 2009;18(5):e12–4.
16. Ersoy H, Pomeranz SJ. Milwaukee shoulder syndrome. J Surg Orthop Adv. 2017;26(1):54–7.

Chapter 18
Rotator Cuff Tendinopathy

This is condition where there is disease of the rotator cuff tendon. It may be considered a spectrum of disorders ranging from acute inflammation to chronic degeneration. Tendinopathy may eventually lead to tendon tear. Tendinopathy may also be associated with calcium deposits within the tendon.

18.1 Rotator Cuff Tendinopathy Pathology

Neer [1] described three stages of rotator cuff tendon disease:

1. Oedema and haemorrhage of the tendon and bursa
2. Tendinitis and fibrosis
3. Partial or full thickness tears

Tendinopathy may involve:

- The tendon substance
- The tendon's bony insertion—enthesis
- Both

Degeneration may involve the tendon's:

- Outer surface (articular or bursal side)
- Internal substance
- Combined (outer surface and internal substance)

An acutely inflamed tendon may appear macroscopically swollen (oedematous) and show increased vascularity. A degenerate tendon may appear macroscopically frayed or delaminated (with separation of its various layers). Tendinopathy involving the internal substance of the tendon may not be identified by examining the outer surface of the tendon, and the tendon may look normal on visual inspection.

© Springer Nature Switzerland AG 2019

C. Panayiotou Charalambous, *The Shoulder Made Easy*,
https://doi.org/10.1007/978-3-319-98908-2_18

Articular side of supraspiantus insertion (a) intact, (b) degenerate

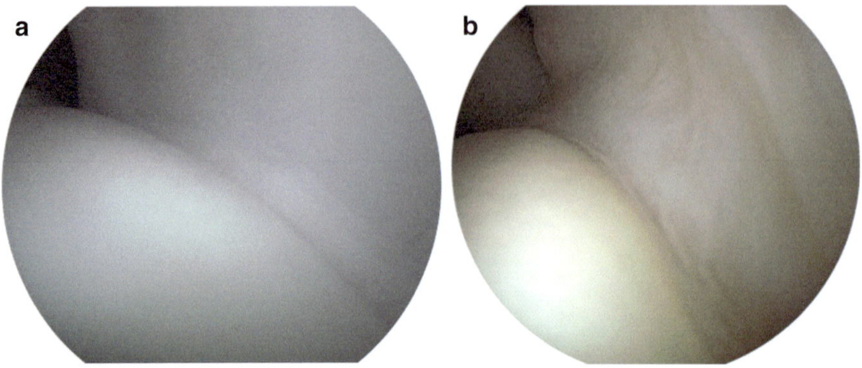

Bussal side of supraspinatus (a) intact, (b) frayed and degenerate

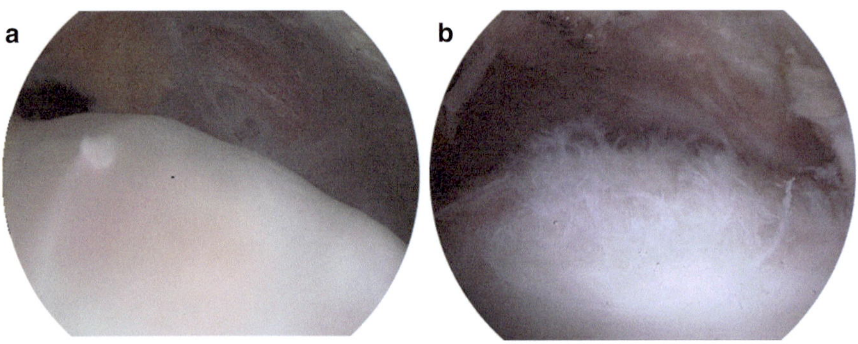

Superior edge of subscapularis (a) intact, (b) frayed and degenerate

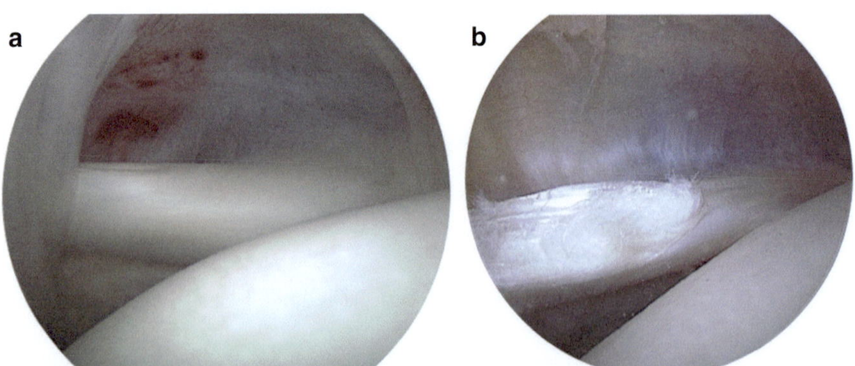

Depending on the stage and the underlying cause, tendinopathy may be associated with [2–4]:

- Inflammatory cells infiltration
- Decreased tendon cell component
- Collagen fibre abnormalities – thinning and disorganisation
- Increased concentrations of matrix metalloproteinase and reduced tissue inhibitors of matrix metalloproteinases leading to increased break down of extra-cellular matrix
- Neovascularisation—new vessel formation
- Neo-innervation—new nerve formation

18.2 Causes of Rotator Cuff Tendinopathy [5–11]

- Extrinsic
  These are external forces acting on the tendon:
  - Impingement —compression and rubbing of the tendon by surrounding structures (subacromial, sub-coracoid, internal impingement)
  - Tensile overload—excessive force application (acute trauma or repetitive use)
- Intrinsic
  These are changes originating within the tendon itself, rather than due to some extrinsic cause:
  - Inflammation
  - Aging
  - Hypo-perfusion
  - Calcium deposition
- Combination of intrinsic and extrinsic causes

18.3 Clinical Symptoms of Rotator Cuff Tendinopathy

- Pain—subacromial pain syndrome, sub-coracoid pain, glenohumeral pain
- Apparent weakness
- Apparent stiffness

18.4 Clinical Signs of Rotator Cuff Tendinopathy [12]

Positive pain provocation tests

- Subacromial impingement test
- Hawkins-Kennedy test
- Pain on loading the rotator cuff tendon—such as when examining for cuff strength

18.5 Investigations for Rotator Cuff Tendinopathy

Plain radiographs

- Calcific deposits in tendon

MRI scan

- High signal areas indicating tendinopathy
- Partial thickness tears—fluid signal with thinning of the tendon or an incomplete gap in the tendon

MRI showing tendinopathy of the supraspinatus tendon, appearing as bright signals within the tendon, but without extending to the tendon surface

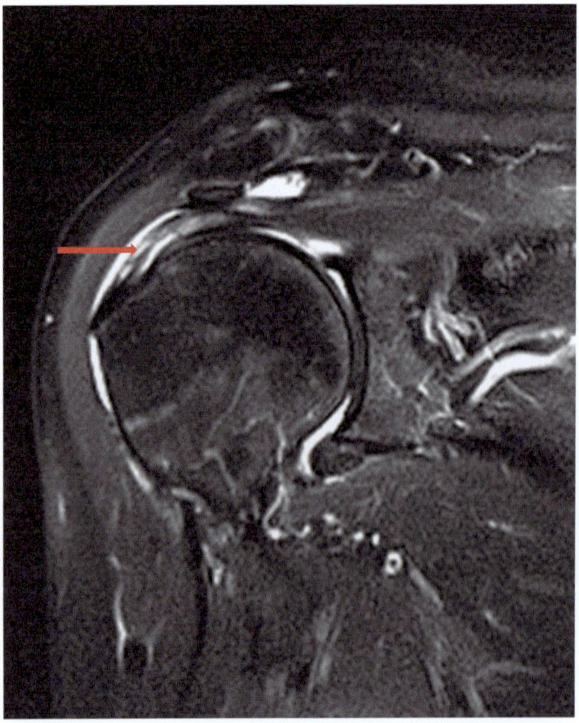

MRI showing supraspinatus tendinopathy with central cystic degeneration but no tear

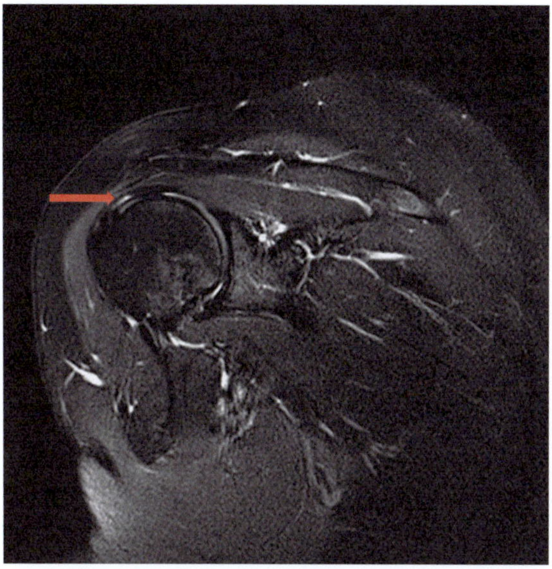

Rotator cuff tendinopathy due to subacromial and sub-coracoid impingement as well as due to internal impingement are described next. Tendinopathy associated with calcium deposits is also described.

References

1. Neer CS 2nd. Impingement lesions. Clin Orthop Relat Res. 1983;173:70–7.
2. Millar NL, Hueber AJ, Reilly JH, Xu Y, Fazzi UG, Murrell GA, McInnes IB. Inflammation is present in early human tendinopathy. Am J Sports Med. 2010;38(10):2085–91.
3. Rees JD, Stride M, Scott A. Tendons--time to revisit inflammation. Br J Sports Med. 2014;48(21):1553–7.
4. DE Giorgi S, Saracino M, Castagna A. Degenerative disease in rotator cuff tears: what are the biochemical and histological changes? Joints. 2014;2(1):26–8.
5. Neviaser A, Andarawis-Puri N, Flatow E. Basic mechanisms of tendon fatigue damage. J Shoulder Elb Surg. 2012;21(2):158–63.
6. Harrison AK, Flatow EL. Subacromial impingement syndrome. J Am Acad Orthop Surg. 2011;19(11):701–8.
7. Seitz AL, PW MC, Finucane S, Boardman ND 3rd, Michener LA. Mechanisms of rotator cuff tendinopathy: intrinsic, extrinsic, or both? Clin Biomech (Bristol Avon). 2011;26(1):1–12.
8. Mehta S, Gimbel JA, Soslowsky LJ. Etiologic and pathogenetic factors for rotator cuff tendinopathy. Clin Sports Med. 2003;22(4):791–812.
9. Notarnicola A, Fischetti F, Gallone D, Moretti L, Pignataro P, Tafuri S, Moretti B. Overload and neovascularization of shoulder tendons in volleyball players. BMC Res Notes. 2012;5(1):397. https://doi.org/10.1186/1756-0500-5-397.
10. Brewer BJ. Aging of the rotator cuff. Am J Sports Med. 1979;7(2):102–10.
11. Neer CS 2nd. Anterior acromioplasty for the chronic impingement syndrome in the shoulder: a preliminary report. J Bone Joint Surg Am. 1972;54(1):41–50.
12. Charalambous CP. Clinical examination of the shoulder. In: Charalambous CP, editor. The shoulder made easy. Basel: Springer; 2019.

Chapter 19
Subacromial Impingement

This is a condition whereby there is an abnormal mechanical contact (compression or rubbing) of the rotator cuff tendon or subacromial bursa as it traverses the subacromial space [1–3]. This may occur at rest or on arm movement (forward elevation, abduction, internal rotation).

The subacromial space is the space between the humeral head and greater tuberosity inferiorly and the acromion and coraco-acromial ligament superiorly. The rotator cuff tendon traverses this space (with the subacromial bursa on its superior surface) and may be trapped between the floor and roof of the subacromial space. Neer described the anterior-inferior acromion as the main area involved in subacromial impingement [3]. In most arm activities, the arm is elevated forwards in relation to the rest of the body. Forward arm elevation places the supraspinatus tendon under the anterior edge of the acromion, coraco-acromial ligament and inferior part of the acromio-clavicular joint(ACJt) [3–5]. Hence, this is the area of the rotator cuff affected most often by mechanical impingement. The long head of the biceps tendon is closely related to the anterior edge of the supraspinatus tendon; hence, it may also be involved in the subacromial impingement. The lateral edge of the acromion may contribute to impingement when the arm is abducted.

In principle, any pathology which reduces the effective distance between the floor and roof of the subacromial space, or increases the contents of the space, may cause impingement. This may be likened to a person finding themselves in a low-ceiling room. In such a room, one can happily sit down (analogous to the arm by the side) and even stand up with their head just escaping the ceiling (analogous to lifting the arm in a non-pathological subacromial space). Nevertheless, if there were a chandelier hanging from the roof (analogous to an acromial spur or a mass lesion of the subacromial space), one would not happily stand up.

Similarly, if the floor of the room is covered with big boxes and one has to stand on these (analogous to a greater tuberosity mal-union or a superior humeral head migration), the situation would be uncomfortable. The dimensions of the room may not change, but the person may become effectively taller by wearing high heels or

© Springer Nature Switzerland AG 2019

C. Panayiotou Charalambous, *The Shoulder Made Easy*,
https://doi.org/10.1007/978-3-319-98908-2_19

standing on tiptoes (analogous to a swollen tendon, scapular dyskinesia, calcific tendinopathy) which again would mean one hitting the head on the roof.

Subacromial impingement is like a person trying to stand in a room without hitting its roof. A chandelier hanging off the roof, big boxes on the floor, or high heels effectively reduce the height of the room available for comfortable standing. One, however, may experience a bad headache even in a high ceiling room

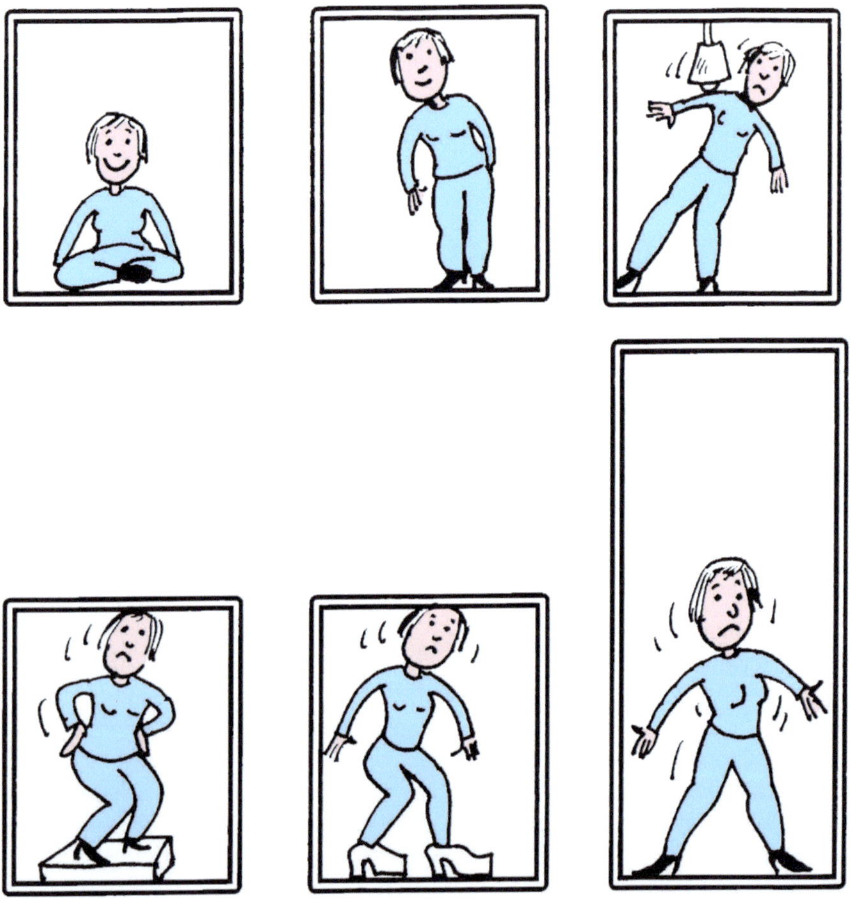

Mechanical subacromial impingement may be due to multiple factors [6–11] including:

- *Scapular dysfunction*—deficient or un-coordinated scapular muscle activity can lead to impingement. The serratus anterior and trapezius stabilise the scapula and cause upward rotation of the scapula during arm elevation, giving the humeral head adequate space to avoid pressing on the acromion

- *Tight posterior capsule*—this may lead to an increase in anterior superior humeral head translation during forward arm elevation, leading to subacromial space narrowing
- *Superior migration of the humeral* head due to rotator cuff dysfunction—weakness or imbalance of these muscles may lead to impingement. Weakness or dysfunction of the infraspinatus and subscapularis can lead to a dysfunctional horizontal muscle force couple, with superior humeral head translation
- *A lateral or anterior down sloping acromion*—this may be more likely to press on the underlying tendon. Bigliani [12] described three types of acromion on radiographs:

1. Flat
2. Curved
3. Hooked

Acromion types- (a) flat, (b) curved, (c) hooked

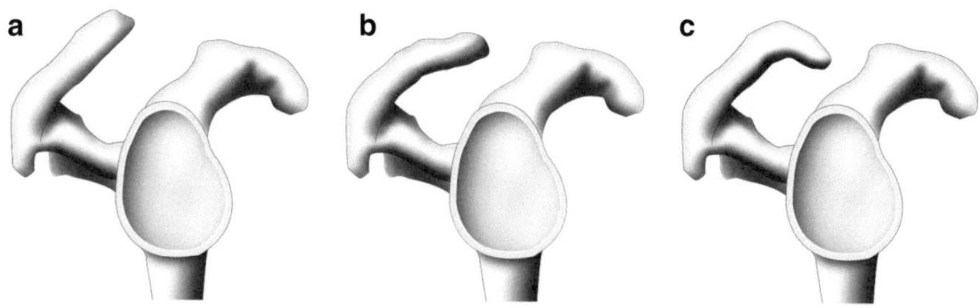

The most common acromion type encountered is I. Type III is the one most commonly associated with rotator cuff tears. Wang et al. [13] reported that with age the shape of the acromion may change from flat to curved or hooked, possibly due to traction forces on the acromion. Acromial fractures and lateral end of the clavicle fractures that mal-unite in a low-lying position may also cause impingement.

- *Acromial spurs*—may be caused by traction of the coraco-acromio ligament and may be located at the lateral, medial or distal end of the acromion
- *Clavicular spurs*—located at the inferior part of the lateral end of the clavicle
- *Hypertrophy of the coraco-acromial ligament*—this ligament may be almost as hard as the bone
- *Mal-united greater tuberosity fracture*—in a more superior position
- *Mass lesion*—bursa fibroma, loose bodies in synovial chondromatosis

Inferior acromial spur (anterior-posterior view (a) and side view (b))

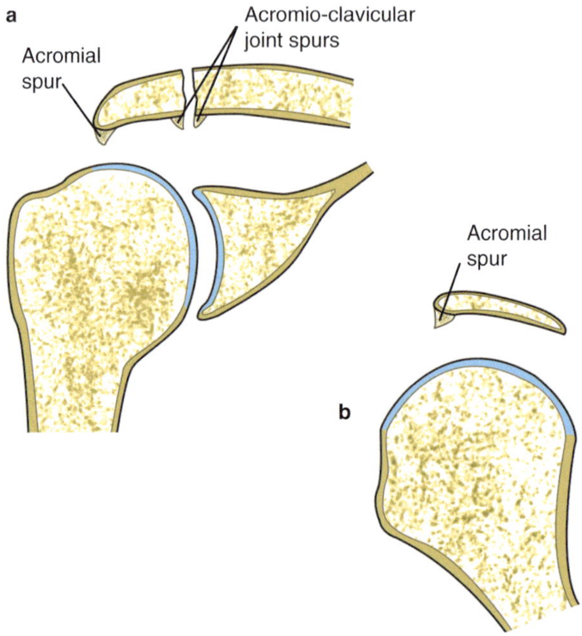

Inferior acromial spur (red arrow)

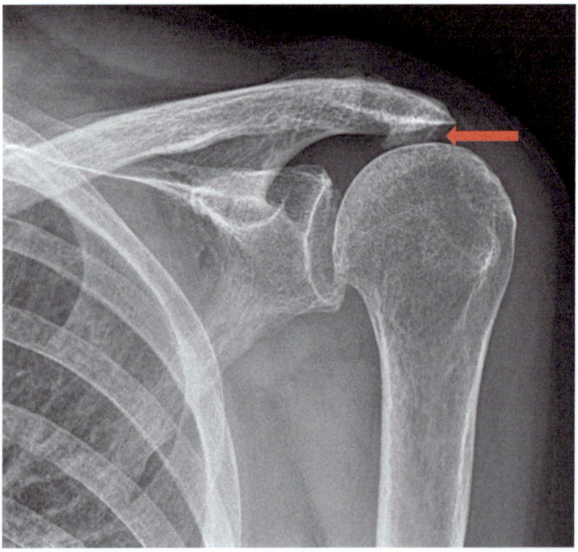

Anteror inferior acromial spur (red arrows)

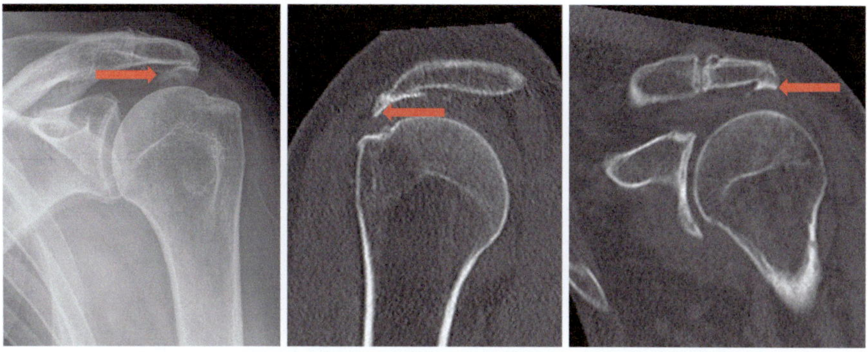

Inferior ACJt spur (red arrows)

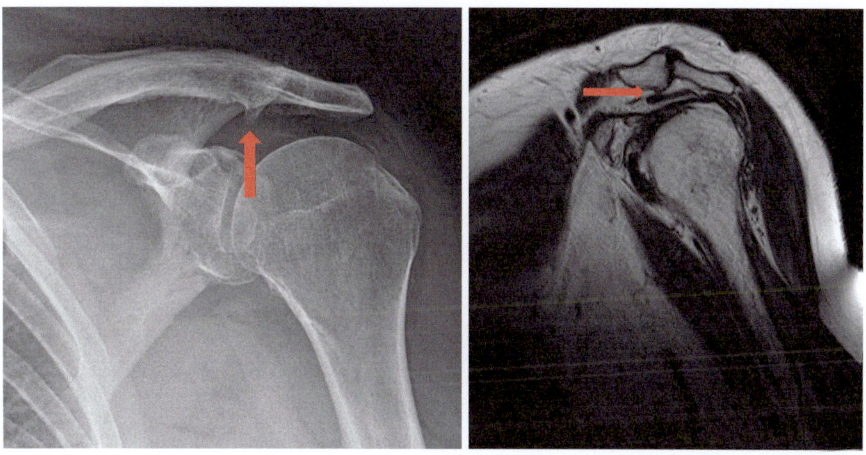

Superior displaced greater tuberosity fracture, which effectively narrows the subacromial space (red arrow) predisposing to mechanical impingement

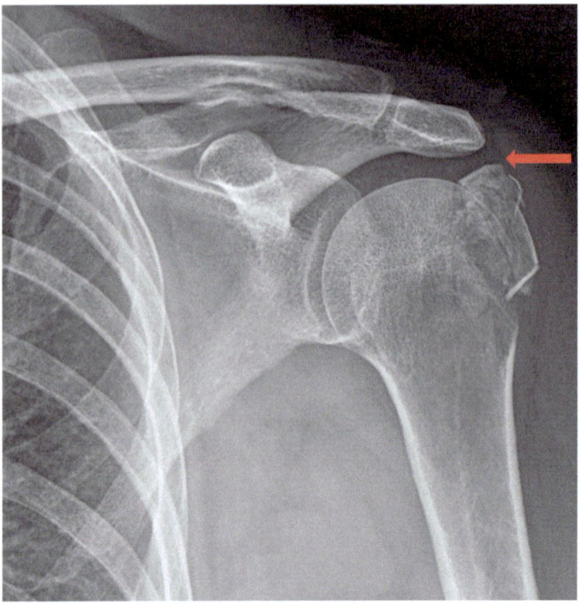

MRI showing sub-chondrtal cyst in the greater tuberosity suggestive of subacromial impinegment (yellow arrow)

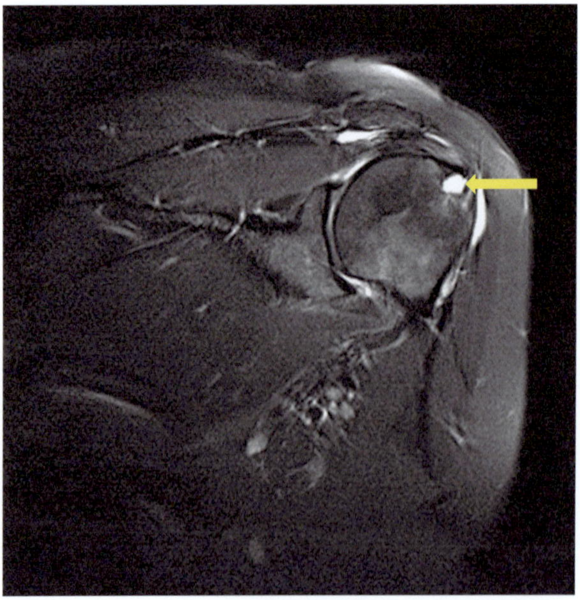

MRI scan showing acromial inferior spur (yellow arrow) causing supraspinatus tendinopathy (red arrow)

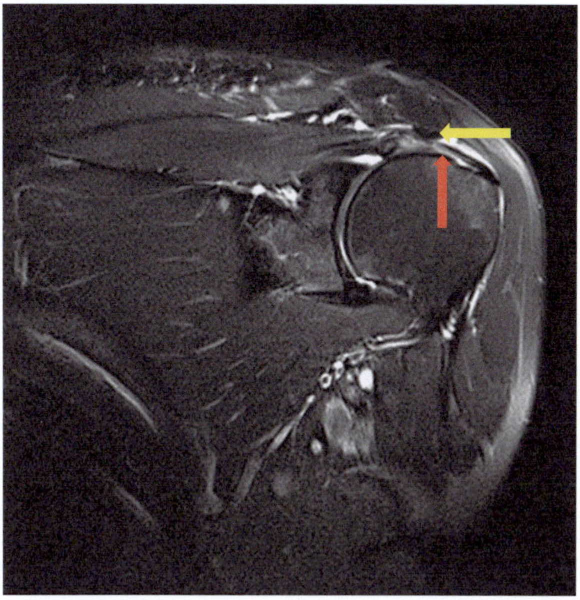

Large anterior-inferior a cromial spur as seen following the release of the coraco-acromial ligament (arthroscopic view)

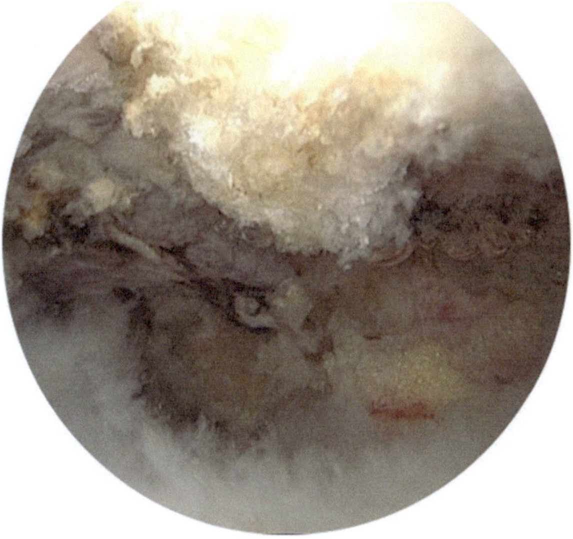

Multiple loose bodies in the sub-acromial space in synovial chondromatosis

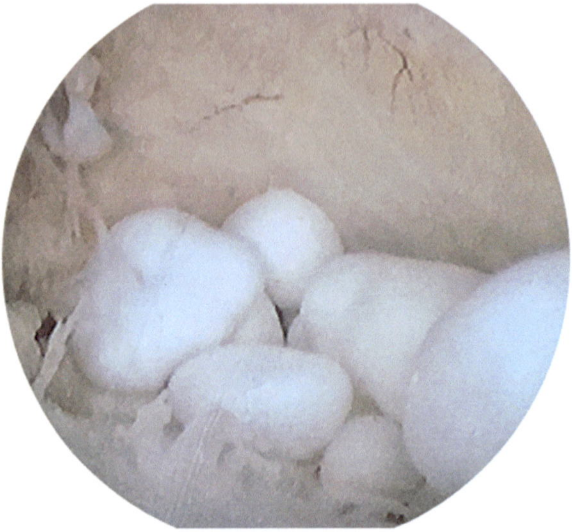

19.1 Clinical Symptoms of Subacromial Impingement

- Pain at the lateral part of the shoulder, over deltoid, aggravated by forward flexion, internal rotation or abduction

19.2 Clinical Signs of Subacromial Impingement

- Subacromial tenderness
- Positive subacromial impingement test

19.3 Investigations for Subacromial Impingement

- Plain radiographs—look for calcific deposits and greater tuberosity cysts
- MRI—look for rotator cuff tendinopathy, tears and subacromial mass lesions
- CT scan—assess acromial morphology (in rare complex cases)

Large inferior acromial spur (red arrow)

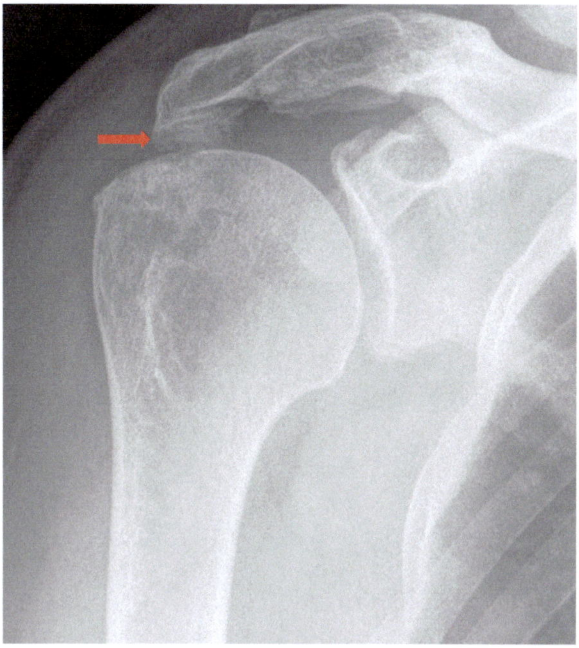

Anterior-inferior acromial spur (red arrow), with corresponding area of cyst formation on the greater tuberosity of the humeral head (yellow arrow) on which impingement occurs

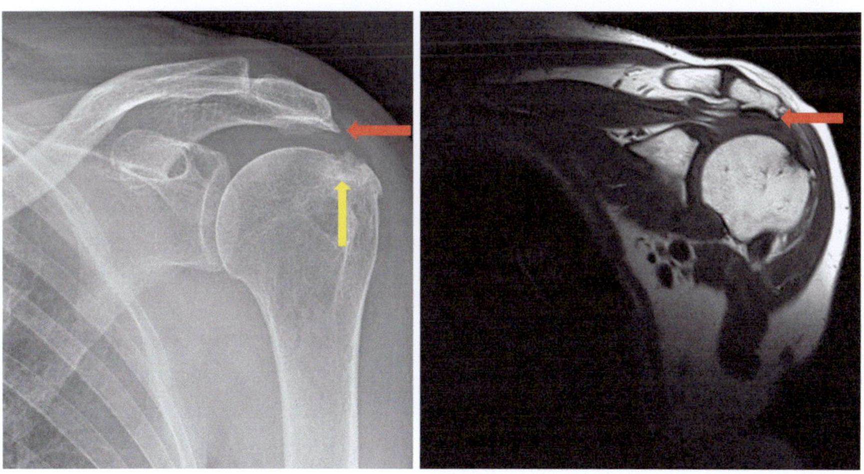

MRI showing subacromial bursitis (red arrow) with intact supraspinatus tendon

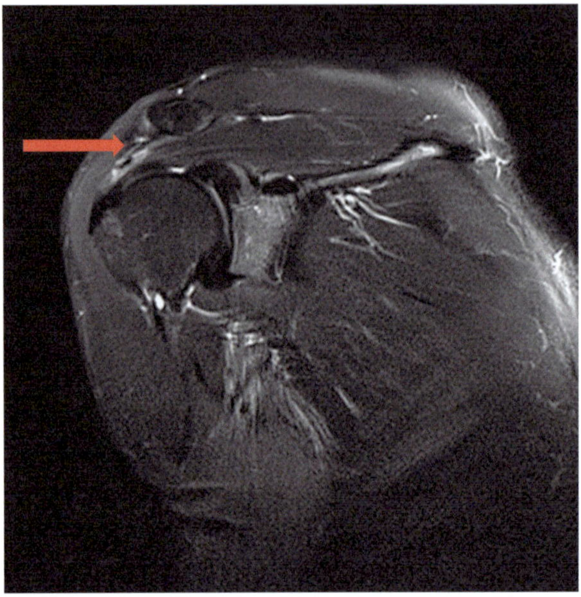

19.4 Management of Subacromial Impingement

This is influenced by the underlying cause of the tendinopathy and may be non-surgical or surgical. The ladder of interventions may be utilised.

Non-surgical Interventions [14–22]

- Rest, activity modification, local passive therapy
- Posture improvement
- Eccentric exercises of the rotator cuff
- Strengthening of scapular and glenohumeral stabilisers
- Posterior shoulder capsule stretching
- Subacromial:
  - Steroid injections
  - Hyaluronate injections
  - PRP injections
- Rotator cuff tendon needling

Surgical Interventions [23–33]

Surgical interventions aim at removing any inflammatory tissue and increasing the space through which the tendon traverses to minimise the risk of external compression during arm elevation. These include:

- Bursectomy +/− acromioplasty—arthroscopic or open. In acromioplasty, the anterior, anterior-inferior and part of the lateral acromion are removed
- Coplaning of the ACJt—involves removing inferior spurs
- Excision of subacromial mass lesions
- Tuberoplasty (with detachment and reattachment of the rotator cuff tendon)
- Osteotomy and reposition of a mal-united greater tuberosity fracture

The effect of treatment for subacromial pain syndrome is highly heterogeneous [34–36]. This may be related to diversity of the pathology of the underlying disease. Hence, it is not possible to predict reliably at an individual level who will benefit from surgical or non-surgical intervention.

Learning Pearls

- Not all subacromial pain may be attributed to mechanical pressure. In the same way of the person standing in a room, not all headache may be attributed to banging the head on the roof as one can be standing in a tall room with ample space but still have a headache due to a migraine attack (analogous to acute bursitis or tendinopathy) or due to tension headache because of cervical spondylosis (analogous to a degenerate tendon) or because they have been thinking too much (analogous to tendon overuse)
- Assessment of the acromial-humeral distance is not a highly reliable process in routine clinical practice, as it can be influenced by various parameters. The acromial-humeral distance is dynamic rather than static varying with arm and scapula position. Although substantial superior migration of the humeral head with abutment of the under surface of the acromion may be easily appreciated, lesser degrees are more difficult to recognise

References

1. Harrison AK, Flatow EL. Subacromial impingement syndrome. J Am Acad Orthop Surg. 2011;19(11):701–8.
2. Mehta S, Gimbel JA, Soslowsky LJ. Etiologic and pathogenetic factors for rotator cuff tendinopathy. Clin Sports Med. 2003;22(4):791–812.
3. Neer CS 2nd. Anterior acromioplasty for the chronic impingement syndrome in the shoulder: a preliminary report. J Bone Joint Surg Am. 1972;54(1):41–50.
4. Mackenzie TA, Herrington L, Horlsey I, Cools A. An evidence-based review of current perceptions with regard to the subacromial space in shoulder impingement syndromes: Is it important and what influences it? Clin Biomech (Bristol, Avon). 2015;30(7):641–8.
5. Bureau NJ, Beauchamp M, Cardinal E, Brassard P. Dynamic sonography evaluation of shoulder impingement syndrome. AJR Am J Roentgenol. 2006;187(1):216–20.

6. Muraki T, Yamamoto N, Zhao KD, Sperling JW, Steinmann SP, Cofield RH, An KN. Effect of posteroinferior capsule tightness on contact pressure and area beneath the coracoacromial arch during pitching motion. Am J Sports Med. 2010;38(3):600–7.
7. Michener LA, McClure PW, Karduna AR. Anatomical and biomechanical mechanisms of subacromial impingement syndrome. Clin Biomech (Bristol, Avon). 2003;18(5):369–79.
8. Kibler WB, Sciascia A, Wilkes T. Scapular dyskinesis and its relation to shoulder injury. J Am Acad Orthop Surg. 2012;20(6):364–72.
9. Page P. Shoulder muscle imbalance and subacromial impingement syndrome in overhead athletes. Int J Sports Phys Ther. 2011;6(1):51–8.
10. Nordenson U, Garofalo R, Conti M, Linger E, Classon J, Karlsson J, Castagna A. Minor or occult shoulder instability: an intra-articular pathology presenting with extra-articular subacromial impingement symptoms. Knee Surg Sports Traumatol Arthrosc. 2011;19(9):1570–5.
11. Struyf F, Nijs J, Baeyens JP, Mottram S, Meeusen R. Scapular positioning and movement in unimpaired shoulders, shoulder impingement syndrome, and glenohumeral instability. Scand J Med Sci Sports. 2011;21(3):352–8.
12. Bigliani LU, Ticker JB, Flatow EL, Soslowsky LJ, Mow VC. The relationship of acromial architecture to rotator cuff disease. Clin Sports Med. 1991;10(4):823–38.
13. Wang JC, Shapiro MS. Changes in acromial morphology with age. J Shoulder Elb Surg. 1997;6(1):55–9.
14. Saito H, Harrold ME, Cavalheri V, McKenna L. Scapular focused interventions to improve shoulder pain and function in adults with subacromial pain: A systematic review and meta-analysis. Physiother Theory Pract. 2018;34(9):1–18.
15. Frizziero A, Vittadini F, Barazzuol M, Gasparre G, Finotti P, Meneghini A, Maffulli N, Masiero S. Extracorporeal shockwaves therapy versus hyaluronic acid injection for the treatment of painful non-calcific rotator cuff tendinopathies: preliminary results. J Sports Med Phys Fitness. 2017;57(9):1162–8.
16. Alizadehkhaiyat O, Roebuck MM, Makki AT, Frostick SP. Postural alterations in patients with subacromial impingement syndrome. Int J Sports Phys Ther. 2017;12(7):1111–20.
17. Tahririan MA, Moezi M, Motififard M, Nemati M, Nemati A. Ultrasound guided platelet-rich plasma injection for the treatment of rotator cuff tendinopathy. Adv Biomed Res. 2016;5:200. https://doi.org/10.4103/2277-9175.190939.
18. Gebremariam L, Hay EM, van der Sande R, Rinkel WD, Koes BW, Huisstede BM. Subacromial impingement syndrome--effectiveness of physiotherapy and manual therapy. Br J Sports Med. 2014;48(16):1202–8.
19. Rha DW, Park GY, Kim YK, Kim MT, Lee SC. Comparison of the therapeutic effects of ultrasound-guided platelet-rich plasma injection and dry needling in rotator cuff disease: a randomized controlled trial. Clin Rehabil. 2013;27(2):113–22.
20. Lewis JS. A specific exercise program for patients with subacromial impingement syndrome can improve function and reduce the need for surgery. J Physiother. 2012;58(2):127. https://doi.org/10.1016/S1836-9553(12)70093-0.
21. Cummins CA, Sasso LM, Nicholson D. Impingement syndrome: temporal outcomes of nonoperative treatment. J Shoulder Elb Surg. 2009;18(2):172–7.
22. Arroll B, Goodyear-Smith F. Corticosteroid injections for painful shoulder: a meta-analysis. Br J Gen Pract. 2005;55(512):224–8.
23. Dong W, Goost H, Lin XB, Burger C, Paul C, Wang ZL, Zhang TY, Jiang ZC, Welle K, Kabir K. Treatments for shoulder impingement syndrome: a PRISMA systematic review and network meta-analysis. Medicine (Baltimore). 2015;94(10):e510. https://doi.org/10.1097/MD.0000000000000510.
24. Kolk A, Thomassen BJW, Hund H, de Witte PB, Henkus HE, Wassenaar WG, van Arkel ERA, Nelissen RGHH. Does acromioplasty result in favorable clinical and radiologic outcomes in the management of chronic subacromial pain syndrome? A double-blinded randomized clinical trial with 9 to 14 years' follow-up. J Shoulder Elb Surg. 2017;26(8):1407–15.
25. Farfaras S, Sernert N, Rostgard Christensen L, Hallström EK, Kartus JT. Subacromial decompression yields a better clinical outcome than therapy alone: a prospective randomized study of

patients with a minimum 10-year follow-up. Am J Sports Med. 2018;46(6):1397–407. https://doi.org/10.1177/0363546518755759.
26. Beard DJ, Rees JL, Cook JA, Rombach I, Cooper C, Merritt N, Shirkey BA, Donovan JL, Gwilym S, Savulescu J, Moser J, Gray A, Jepson M, Tracey I, Judge A, Wartolowska K, Carr AJ, CSAW Study Group. Arthroscopic subacromial decompression for subacromial shoulder pain (CSAW): a multicentre, pragmatic, parallel group, placebo-controlled, three-group, randomised surgical trial. Lancet. 2018;391(10118):329–38.
27. Donigan JA, Wolf BR. Arthroscopic subacromial decompression: acromioplasty versus bursectomy alone--does it really matter? A systematic review. Iowa Orthop J. 2011;31:121–6.
28. Davis AD, Kakar S, Moros C, Kaye EK, Schepsis AA, Voloshin I. Arthroscopic versus open acromioplasty: a meta-analysis. Am J Sports Med. 2010;38(3):613–8.
29. Chen AL, Rokito AS, Zuckerman JD. The role of the acromioclavicular joint in impingement syndrome. Clin Sports Med. 2003;22(2):343–57.
30. Barber FA. Coplaning of the acromioclavicular joint. Arthroscopy. 2001;17(9):913–7.
31. Killen MC, Charalambous CP. Arthroscopic Tuberoplasty for a Malunited Greater Tuberosity Fracture: A Case Report. Ortop Traumatol Rehabil. 2015;17(6):637–40.
32. Calvo E, Merino-Gutierrez I, Lagunes I. Arthroscopic tuberoplasty for subacromial impingement secondary to proximal humeral malunion. Knee Surg Sports Traumatol Arthrosc. 2010;18(7):988–91.
33. Ogawa K, Matsumura N, Yoshida A. Modified osteotomy for symptomatic malunion of the humeral greater tuberosity. J Orthop Trauma. 2014;28(12):e290–5.
34. Kappe T, Knappe K, Elsharkawi M, Reichel H, Cakir B. Predictive value of preoperative clinical examination for subacromial decompression in impingement syndrome. Knee Surg Sports Traumatol Arthrosc. 2015;23(2):443–8.
35. Taheriazam A, Sadatsafavi M, Moayyeri A. Outcome predictors in nonoperative management of newly diagnosed subacromial impingement syndrome: a longitudinal study. MedGenMed. 2005;7(1):63.
36. Mair SD, Viola RW, Gill TJ, Briggs KK, Hawkins RJ. Can the impingement test predict outcome after arthroscopic subacromial decompression? J Shoulder Elb Surg. 2004;13(2):150–3.

Chapter 20
Sub-coracoid Impingement

This is a condition where there is impingement of the anterior part of the rotator cuff (subscapularis) by the coracoid process. The anterior part of the rotator cuff (subscapularis) is caught between the coracoid process and the lesser tuberosity of the humeral head. Sub-coracoid impingement may lead to subscapularis tears [1–5].

20.1 Causes of Sub-coracoid Impingement [6–10]

- Primary
  - Congenital such as an abnormally shaped or positioned (lateralised) coracoid
- Acquired
  - Displaced humeral or scapular fracture mal-union or non-union
  - Subscapularis calcification or ossification
  - Subscapularis hypertrophy
  - Anterior- superior migration of the humeral head (due to cuff insufficiency, glenohumeral instability, scapular dyskinesia, anterior acromioplasty)
  - Ganglion cysts or other mass lesions in the sub-coracoid area

© Springer Nature Switzerland AG 2019

C. Panayiotou Charalambous, *The Shoulder Made Easy*,
https://doi.org/10.1007/978-3-319-98908-2_20

Impingement of the subscapularis tendon by the coracoid tip (sub-coracoid impingement)

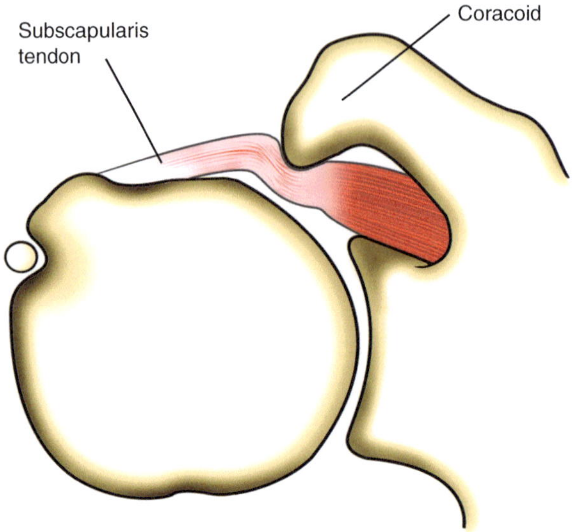

20.2 Clinical Symptoms of Sub-coracoid Impingement

- Pain at the anterior part of the shoulder aggravated by forward flexion, internal rotation and adduction

20.3 Clinical Signs of Sub-coracoid Impingement

- Tender coracoid process
- Positive Hawkins-Kennedy test

20.4 Investigations for Sub-coracoid Impingement

- Plain radiographs—look for subscapularis calcium deposits
- MRI—look for rotator cuff tendinopathy, tears and secondary causes of impingement
- CT scan—assess coracoid morphology

20.5 Management of Sub-coracoid Impingement

- Physiotherapy, steroid injections
- Surgery
  - Primary causes—coracoplasty, open or arthroscopic [11, 12]
  - Acquired causes—addressing the cause with or without coracoplasty

Learning Pearls
- Sub-coracoid impingement may occur in isolation or may coexist with subacromial pathology
- Often sub-coracoid impingement becomes more apparent following sub-acromial decompression and rotator cuff surgery when the patient continues with symptoms that had been attributed to a subacromial origin
- Sub-coracoid impingement is largely a clinical rather than radiological diagnosis [13]

References

1. Osti L, Soldati F, Del Buono A, Massari L. Subcoracoid impingement and subscapularis tendon: is there any truth? Muscles Ligaments Tendons J. 2013;3(2):101–5.
2. Patte D. The subcoracoid impingement. Clin Orthop Relat Res. 1990;254:55–9.
3. Gerber C, Terrier F, Ganz R. The role of the coracoid process in the chronic impingement syndrome. J Bone Joint Surg (Br). 1985;67(5):703–8.
4. Lo IK, Burkhart SS. The etiology and assessment of subscapularis tendon tears: a case for subcoracoid impingement, the roller-wringer effect, and TUFF lesions of the subscapularis. Arthroscopy. 2003;19(10):1142–50.
5. Dugarte AJ, Davis RJ, Lynch TS, Schickendantz MS, Farrow LD. Anatomic Study of Subcoracoid Morphology in 418 Shoulders: Potential Implications for Subcoracoid Impingement. Orthop J Sports Med. 2017;5(10) https://doi.org/10.1177/2325967117731996.
6. Demirhan M, Eralp L, Atalar AC. Synovial chondromatosis of the subcoracoid bursa. Int Orthop. 1999;23(6):358–60.
7. Gumina S, Postacchini F, Orsina L, Cinotti G. The morphometry of the coracoid process - its aetiologic role in subcoracoid impingement syndrome. Int Orthop. 1999;23(4):198–201.
8. Peidro L, Serra A, Suso S. Subcoracoid impingement after ossification of the subscapularis tendon. J Shoulder Elb Surg. 1999;8(2):170–1.
9. Garofalo R, Conti M, Massazza G, Cesari E, Vinci E, Castagna A. Subcoracoid impingement syndrome: a painful shoulder condition related to different pathologic factors. Musculoskelet Surg. 2011;95(Suppl 1):S25–9.
10. Arrigoni P, Brady PC, Burkhart SS. Calcific tendonitis of the subscapularis tendon causing subcoracoid stenosis and coracoid impingement. Arthroscopy. 2006;22(10):1139.e1–3.
11. Kowalsky MS, Bell JE, Ahmad CS. Arthroscopic treatment of subcoracoid impingement caused by lesser tuberosity malunion: a case report and review of the literature. J Shoulder Elb Surg. 2007;16(6):e10–4.
12. Park JY, Lhee SH, Oh KS, Kim NR, Hwang JT. Is arthroscopic coracoplasty necessary in subcoracoid impingement syndrome? Arthroscopy. 2012;28(12):1766–75.
13. Giaroli EL, Major NM, Lemley DE, Lee J. Coracohumeral interval imaging in subcoracoid impingement syndrome on MRI. AJR Am J Roentgenol. 2006;186(1):242–6.

Chapter 21
Shoulder Internal Impingement

Internal impingement of the shoulder is a condition whereby there is excessive contact of the greater tuberosity of the humeral head with the poster-superior part of the glenoid when the arm is placed in abduction and external rotation. This leads to compression of the articular side of the rotator cuff tendons (supraspinatus and infraspinatus) and the labrum between these bony structures [1–3].

This may lead to:

- Articular-side rotator cuff tears
- Posterior-superior labrum lesions

Although some degree of contact between the greater tuberosity and glenoid may occur under normal conditions [4], in internal impingement such contact may be excessive. In contrast to subacromial impingement, in internal impingement the subacromial space is not narrow.

Internal impingement of the rotator cuff tendon and posterior-superior labrum

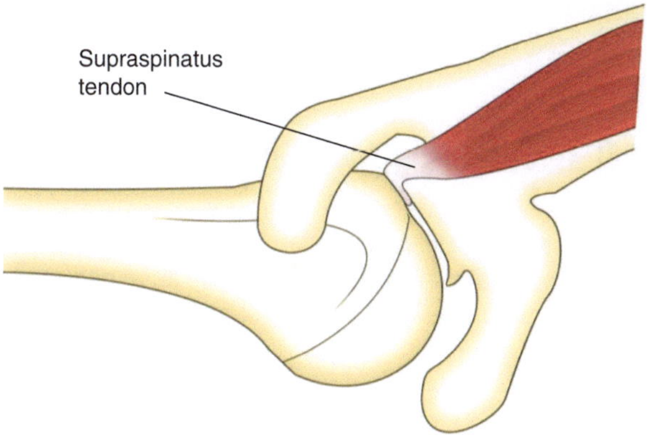

© Springer Nature Switzerland AG 2019
C. Panayiotou Charalambous, *The Shoulder Made Easy*,
https://doi.org/10.1007/978-3-319-98908-2_21

21.1 Glenohumeral Internal Rotation Deficit (GIRD)

Internal impingement has been associated with posterior shoulder tightness and loss of glenohumeral internal rotation. This may be more common in those engaging in throwing activities such as throwing athletes (baseball pitchers).

During throwing, extensive external rotation of the shoulder may cause stretching of the anterior capsule. During the deceleration phase of throwing, the posterior capsule may be injured, sustaining micro-tears which can lead to scarring, capsular hypertrophy and increased capsular stiffness. The resultant deficiency in the integrity of the anterior capsule may lead to anterior micro-instability as well as anterior translation of the humeral head with resultant abutment of the undersurface of the rotator cuff on the posterior glenoid and labrum. The posterior capsular tightness may also lead to reduced internal rotation.

GIRD is defined as lack of internal rotation and excessive external rotation compared to the opposite shoulder. If the total arc of shoulder rotation approximates 180°, a loss of internal rotation and an increase in external rotation are not considered pathological. However, if the loss of internal rotation exceeds the gain of external rotation and there is reduction of the total range of motion (so it less than 180°), then the diagnosis of GIRD may be made. A difference of 20° in internal rotation between the two shoulders is considered significant [5–12].

Loss in internal rotation may also be due to several other causes [7–12] including:

- Alteration to the orientation of the bones (humeral retroversion)
- Muscle stiffness (posterior rotator cuff, teres major) which may be:
  - Short-lived following throwing (due to release of intracellular calcium, fibril contraction and muscle shortening). The extent of loss of internal rotation may be fluctuating due to intermittent transient muscle stiffness and has been shown to decrease up to 15° following a throwing exposure and last for several hours; throwers may notice increased stiffness following pitching with loss of internal rotation which then recovers by the next day
  - Chronic—due to established structural contractures

21.2 Clinical Symptoms of Internal Impingement

- Posterior shoulder pain localised to the joint line
- Associated anterior instability symptoms such as apprehension or a feeling of subluxation with the arm in abduction and external rotation
- Anterior sub-coracoid pain

21.3 Clinical Signs of Internal Impingement

- Posterior glenohumeral joint line tenderness
- Increased external rotation and decreased internal rotation compared to the opposite side

21.4 Investigations for Internal Impingement

- Plain radiographs
  - AP and axillary views to:

    Look for posterior glenoid calcification and spars
- MRI arthrogram
  - Look for labrum/rotator cuff lesions

21.5 Management of Internal Impingement

Non-surgical [13–16]

- Instability is addressed by strengthening the dynamic stabilisers:
  - Rotator cuff strengthening
  - Scapular muscles strengthening
- Posterior shoulder tightness is addressed by:
  - Posterior muscle stretching
  - Posterior capsule stretching

It should be noted that it is important to distinguish between an acceptable change in internal rotation where the total range of motion is preserved and pathological loss of internal rotation where there is loss of total motion. If there is no loss of total motion, then stretching the shoulder to regain internal rotation may lead to increased range of motion and more instability. Furthermore, an increase in external rotation at the expense of internal rotation may offer a functional advantage to the individual (in throwing actions), and any attempt to alter this relation may impair rather than improve one's abilities.

Surgical

- Arthroscopic debridement of rotator cuff tears or labrum lesions [17]
- Glenoidoplasty—removal of any posterior glenoid spurs [18]
- Anterior capsular shift/plication to address anterior instability due to capsular laxity [19]

References

1. Walch G, Liotard JP, Boileau P, Noël E. Postero-superior glenoid impingement. Another impingement of the shoulder. J Radiol. 1993;74(1):47–50.
2. Liu SH, Boynton E. Posterior superior impingement of the rotator cuff on the glenoid rim as a cause of shoulder pain in the overhead athlete. Arthroscopy. 1993;9(6):697–9.

3. Drakos MC, Rudzki JR, Allen AA, Potter HG, Altchek DW. Internal impingement of the shoulder in the overhead athlete. J Bone Joint Surg Am. 2009;91(11):2719–28.
4. Halbrecht JL, Tirman P, Atkin D. Internal impingement of the shoulder: comparison of findings between the throwing and nonthrowing shoulders of college baseball players. Arthroscopy. 1999;15(3):253–8.
5. Rose MB, Noonan T. Glenohumeral internal rotation deficit in throwing athletes: current perspectives. Open Access J Sports Med. 2018;9:69–78.
6. Manske R, Wilk KE, Davies G, Ellenbecker T, Reinold M. Glenohumeral motion deficits: friend or foe? Int J Sports Phys Ther. 2013;8(5):537–53.
7. Kibler WB, Sciascia A, Thomas SJ. Glenohumeral internal rotation deficit: pathogenesis and response to acute throwing. Sports Med Arthrosc Rev. 2012;20(1):34–8.
8. Mihata T, Gates J, McGarry MH, Neo M, Lee TQ. Effect of posterior shoulder tightness on internal impingement in a cadaveric model of throwing. Knee Surg Sports Traumatol Arthrosc. 2015;23(2):548–54.
9. Tehranzadeh AD, Fronek J, Resnick D. Posterior capsular fibrosis in professional baseball pitchers: case series of MR arthrographic findings in six patients with glenohumeral internal rotational deficit. Clin Imaging. 2007;31(5):343–8.
10. Takenaga T, Sugimoto K, Goto H, Nozaki M, Fukuyoshi M, Tsuchiya A, Murase A, Ono T, Otsuka T. Posterior shoulder capsules are thicker and stiffer in the throwing shoulders of healthy college baseball players: a quantitative assessment using shear-wave ultrasound elastography. Am J Sports Med. 2015;43(12):2935–42.
11. Bailey LB, Shanley E, Hawkins R, Beattie PF, Fritz S, Kwartowitz D, Thigpen CA. Mechanisms of shoulder range of motion deficits in asymptomatic baseball players. Am J Sports Med. 2015;43(11):2783–93.
12. Hibberd EE, Oyama S, Myers JB. Increase in humeral retrotorsion accounts for age-related increase in glenohumeral internal rotation deficit in youth and adolescent baseball players. Am J Sports Med. 2014;42(4):851–8.
13. Mine K, Nakayama T, Milanese S, Grimmer K. Effectiveness of stretching on posterior shoulder tightness and glenohumeral internal-rotation deficit: a systematic review of randomized controlled trials. J Sport Rehabil. 2017;26(4):294–305.
14. Tyler TF, Nicholas SJ, Lee SJ, Mullaney M, McHugh MP. Correction of posterior shoulder tightness is associated with symptom resolution in patients with internal impingement. Am J Sports Med. 2010;38(1):114–9.
15. Castagna A, Garofalo R, Cesari E, Markopoulos N, Borroni M, Conti M. Posterior superior internal impingement: an evidence-based review. Br J Sports Med. 2010;44(5):382–8. https://doi.org/10.1136/bjsm.2009.059261.
16. Manske RC, Grant-Nierman M, Lucas B. Shoulder posterior internal impingement in the overhead athlete. Int J Sports Phys Ther. 2013;8(2):194–204.
17. Sonnery-Cottet B, Edwards TB, Noel E, Walch G. Results of arthroscopic treatment of posterosuperior glenoid impingement in tennis players. Am J Sports Med. 2002;30(2):227–32.
18. Lévigne C, Garret J, Grosclaude S, Borel F, Walch G. Surgical technique arthroscopic posterior glenoidplasty for posterosuperior glenoid impingement in throwing athletes. Clin Orthop Relat Res. 2012;470(6):1571–8.
19. Chambers L, Altchek DW. Microinstability and internal impingement in overhead athletes. Clin Sports Med. 2013;32(4):697–707.

Chapter 22
Rotator Cuff Calcific Tendinopathy

This is a condition whereby calcium is deposited in the rotator cuff or other tendons. The calcific deposits consist of calcium carbonated hydroxide [1–5].

22.1 Demographics of Calcific Tendinopathy

- Incidence—about 3%
- More common in females aged 30–50
- May be more common in diabetes and in thyroid disease
- Bilateral—in about 10%
- Rotator cuff tendon involved in decreasing frequency order:
  - Supraspinatus
  - Infraspinatus
  - Subscapularis

22.2 Pathophysiology of Calcific Tendinopathy

Remains unclear. Two theories have been proposed [1, 2]:

1. Passive—Calcium is deposited in degenerate tendon where there is tendon cell necrosis due to ischaemia
2. Active—cell-mediated calcification which is then followed by spontaneous phagocyte resorption. It has been suggested that calcium deposition may reflect a localised attempt of tendons which are weak and have reduced stiffness to increase their stiffness

© Springer Nature Switzerland AG 2019

C. Panayiotou Charalambous, *The Shoulder Made Easy*,
https://doi.org/10.1007/978-3-319-98908-2_22

There may also be an associated crystallisation disorder—phytate is an inhibitor of crystallisation, and its urinary levels have been shown to be reduced in patients with calcific tendinopathy [6, 7].

Three phases have been described:

1. Pre-calcific —Tendon undergoes metaplasia into fibrocartilage
2. Calcific—Calcium forms, is deposited, broken down, and removed by macrophages and phagocytes
3. Post-calcific—Fibroblasts lay down new collagen

The calcium may be in the form of:

- Toothpaste-like fluid
- Sandlike particles
- Small round bodies

The calcium deposits may be:

- Diffuse, infiltrating the tendon substance
- Shelled out lesions

22.3 Clinical Symptoms of Calcific Tendinopathy

- Nonsymptomatic in about 1/3—incidental finding on radiological investigations
- Pain
  - Felt in the subacromial area or in the anterior aspect of the shoulder according to location of calcific deposit
  - May present as:

    Acute-onset pain—sharp pain, may be excruciating, requiring attendance to the accident and emergency department

    Chronic pain—tooth like

Pain may be due to:

- Chemical irritation of the tissue as the body attempts to remove the calcium [8]
- Increase in tendon pressure due to the calcific deposit
- Subacromial/sub-coracoid impingement—caused by bursal thickening or tendon swelling due to the calcium deposit [9]
- Adhesive capsulitis that may accompany calcific tendinopathy [10]

22.4 Clinical Signs of Calcific Tendinopathy

- Tenderness over the affected tendons
- Reduced range of motion:
  - Apparent—due to pain
  - True—due to associated adhesive capsulitis
- Positive impingement test

22.5 Investigations for Calcific Tendinopathy

- Plain radiographs
  - AP and axillary views to:

    Confirm the presence of a calcific deposit
    Determine the location of the calcific deposit in the anterior-posterior and superior-inferior planes
  - Calcific deposits may have a variable appearance:

    Sharply outlined or non-defined border
    Dense or transparent
    Single large deposit or multiple smaller deposits
    Localised or diffuse
- Ultrasound
- MRI scan
  - Look for other pathologies

22.6 Management of Calcific Tendinopathy

Non-surgical

- Observation and analgesia—Most patients improve spontaneously, but some continue to complain of pain with no signs of resorption of the calcific deposits.
- Subacromial space steroid injection
- Extracorporeal shock wave treatment [11, 12]
- Calcific deposit barbotage +/− steroid injection [13]

Calcific deposit (red arrow) involving the superior part of the rotator cuff, appearing as multiple dense bodies on plain radiograph which resolved spontaneously (green arrow)

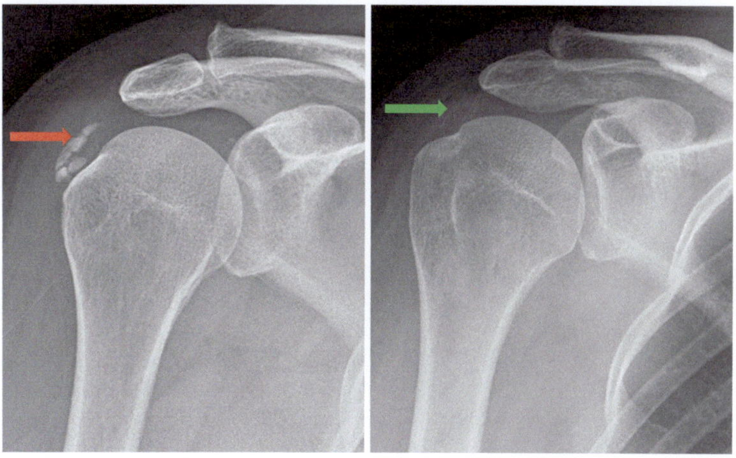

Surgical

- Arthroscopic excision +/− repair of rotator cuff defects created by removing the deposit +/− acromioplasty [14–16]
- Open excision [17]

Calcific deposit identified osthoscopically, its location is confirmed with a needle, and is then scooped out using a curette

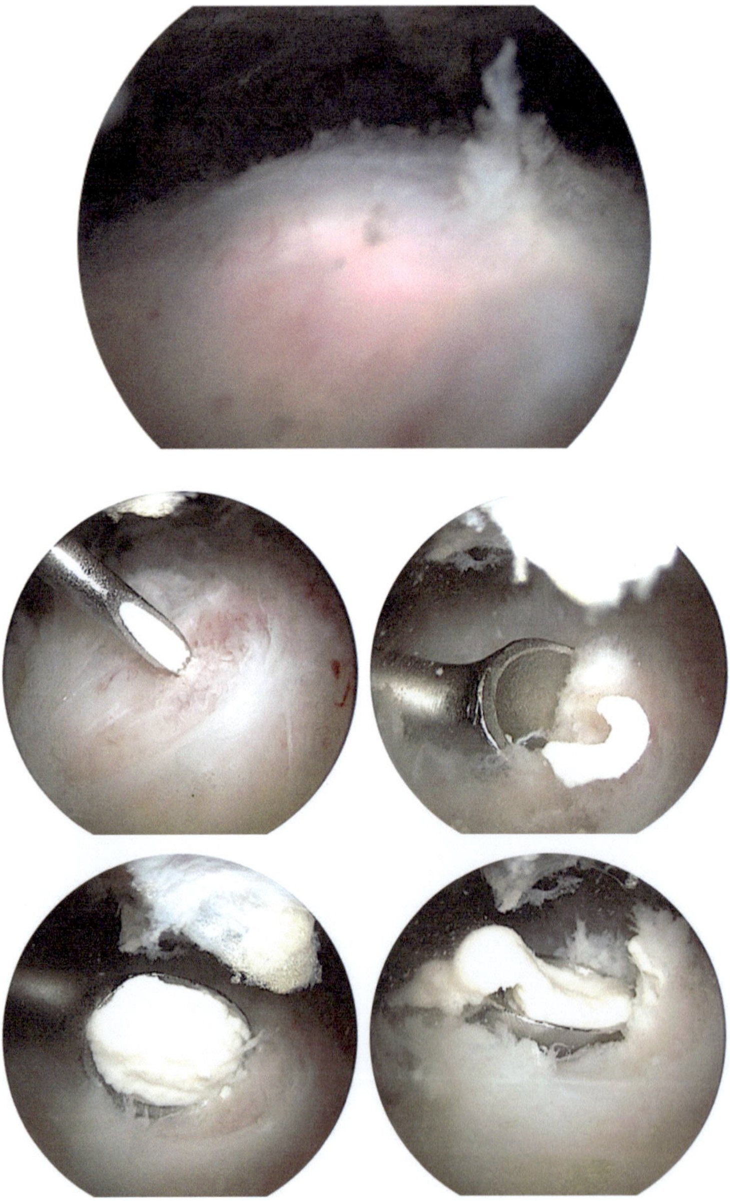

The aim of surgery is to decompress the lesion and remove as much calcium as possible. However, it is understandable that it may not be possible to remove all deposited calcium as that could lead to extensive damage of the tendon [18]. Rarely, the calcium deposit may erode into the greater tuberosity causing osteolysis which is associated with worse prognosis [19]. In those cases, scooping of the bony lesion is also performed at the time of surgery.

Calcific deposit at the distal insertion of the deltoid onto the humerus (red arrow). This helps to remind that tendons other than the rotator cuff may also be affected by calcific tendinopathy

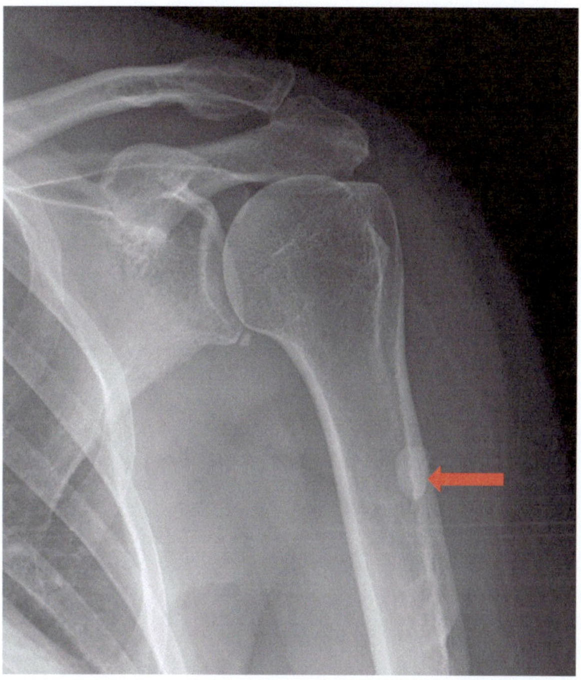

Learning Pearls

- It is important to inform patients that pain can take a substantial time to improve post-surgery

References

1. Oliva F, Via AG, Maffulli N. Physiopathology of intratendinous calcific deposition. BMC Med. 2012;10:95. https://doi.org/10.1186/1741-7015-10.
2. ElShewy MT. Calcific tendinitis of the rotator cuff. World J Orthop. 2016;7(1):55–60.
3. Hurt G, Baker CL Jr. Calcific tendinitis of the shoulder. Orthop Clin North Am. 2003;34(4):567–75.
4. Halverson PB. Crystal deposition disease of the shoulder (including calcific tendonitis and milwaukee shoulder syndrome). Curr Rheumatol Rep. 2003;5(3):244–7.
5. Suzuki K, Potts A, Anakwenze O, Singh A. Calcific tendinitis of the rotator cuff: management options. J Am Acad Orthop Surg. 2014;22(11):707–17.
6. Grases F, Muntaner-Gimbernat L, Vilchez-Mira M, Costa-Bauzá A, Tur F, Prieto RM, Torrens-Mas M, Vega FG. Characterization of deposits in patients with calcific tendinopathy of the supraspinatus. Role of phytate and osteopontin. J Orthop Res. 2015;33(4):475–82.
7. Grases F, Sanchis P, Perello J, Isern B, Prieto RM, Fernandez-Palomeque C, Fiol M, Bonnin O, Torres JJ. Phytate (Myo-inositol hexakisphosphate) inhibits cardiovascular calcifications in rats. Front Biosci. 2006;11(1):136–42.
8. Hackett L, Millar NL, Lam P, Murrell GA. Are the symptoms of calcific tendinitis due to neo-innervation and/or neovascularization? J Bone Joint Surg Am. 2016;98(3):186–92.
9. Arrigoni P, Brady PC, Burkhart SS. Calcific tendonitis of the subscapularis tendon causing subcoracoid stenosis and coracoid impingement. Arthroscopy. 2006;22(10):1139.e1–3.
10. Merolla G, Bhat MG, Paladini P, Porcellini G. Complications of calcific tendinitis of the shoulder: a concise review. J Orthop Traumatol. 2015;16(3):175–83.
11. Louwerens JK, Veltman ES, van Noort A, van den Bekerom MP. The effectiveness of high-energy extracorporeal shockwave therapy versus ultrasound-guided needling versus arthroscopic surgery in the management of chronic calcific rotator cuff tendinopathy: a systematic review. Arthroscopy. 2016;32(1):165–75.
12. Kim YS, Lee HJ, Kim YV, Kong CG. Which method is more effective in treatment of calcific tendinitis in the shoulder? Prospective randomized comparison between ultrasound-guided needling and extracorporeal shock wave therapy. J Shoulder Elb Surg. 2014;23(11):1640–6.
13. Gatt DL, Charalambous CP. Ultrasound-guided barbotage for calcific tendonitis of the shoulder: a systematic review including 908 patients. Arthroscopy. 2014;30(9):1166–72.
14. Balke M, Bielefeld R, Schmidt C, Dedy N, Liem D. Calcifying tendinitis of the shoulder: midterm results after arthroscopic treatment. Am J Sports Med. 2012;40(3):657–61.
15. Yoo JC, Park WH, Koh KH, Kim SM. Arthroscopic treatment of chronic calcific tendinitis with complete removal and rotator cuff tendon repair. Knee Surg Sports Traumatol Arthrosc. 2010;18(12):1694–9.
16. Ranalletta M, Rossi LA, Bongiovanni SL, Tanoira I, Piuzzi N, Maignon G. Arthroscopic removal and rotator cuff repair without acromioplasty for the treatment of symptomatic calcifying tendinitis of the supraspinatus tendon. Orthop J Sports Med. 2015;3(4):2325967115577957. https://doi.org/10.1177/2325967115577957.
17. Rochwerger A, Franceschi JP, Viton JM, Roux H, Mattei JP. Surgical management of calcific tendinitis of the shoulder: an analysis of 26 cases. Clin Rheumatol. 1999;18(4):313–6.
18. Rizzello G, Franceschi F, Longo UG, Ruzzini L, Meloni MC, Spiezia F, Papalia R, Denaro V. Arthroscopic management of calcific tendinopathy of the shoulder--do we need to remove all the deposit? Bull NYU Hosp Jt Dis. 2009;67(4):330–3.
19. Porcellini G, Paladini P, Campi F, Pegreffi F. Osteolytic lesion of greater tuberosity in calcific tendinitis of the shoulder. J Shoulder Elb Surg. 2009;18(2):210–5.

Chapter 23
Rotator Cuff Tears

A condition whereby there is a tear of one or more of the rotator cuff tendons. The rotator cuff consists of subscapularis, supraspinatus, infraspinatus and teres minor [1, 2].

23.1 Causes of Rotator Cuff Tears

- Intrinsic causes
  These refer to changes originating within the tendon rather than due to an extrinsic cause [3–8]. Such changes may be age related and include:
  - Degeneration
  - Hypovascularity—due to the presence of a hypovascular watershed area close to the tendon insertion
  - Decreased cellular component
  - Collagen fibre abnormalities—thinning and disorganisation
  - Increased concentrations of matrix metalloproteinase and reduced tissue inhibitors of matrix metalloproteinases leading to greater breakdown of collagen fibres and weakening of the extracellular matrix
- Extrinsic causes

  These refer to external factors acting on the rotator cuff tendon to cause a tear and include [9–12]:
  - Impingement (subacromial, sub-coracoid, internal impingement)
  - Tensile overload (acute trauma or repetitive use)

© Springer Nature Switzerland AG 2019

C. Panayiotou Charalambous, *The Shoulder Made Easy*,
https://doi.org/10.1007/978-3-319-98908-2_23

  - Subscapularis tears may be traumatic or degenerative. Traumatic tears may be due to forced external rotation or extension of the shoulder with the arm in abduction or as a result of shoulder dislocation. Sub-coracoid impingement may injure the anterior- superior part of the rotator cuff involving the subscapularis tendon
- Combination of intrinsic and extrinsic causes

23.2 Description of Rotator Cuff Tears

Rotator cuff tears may be described in several ways, and these are presented next.

23.2.1 According to the Precipitating Event

1. Acute traumatic—the tendon tears suddenly (due to the application of substantial acute force such as that required to cause a shoulder dislocation)
2. Chronic—the tendon tears gradually over a long time (such as due to chronic repetitive loading or tendon degeneration). Tears occur without the application of substantial force
3. Acute on chronic—a tear exists for a long time, but the subsequent application of a sudden force enlarges the tear. The sudden force required may be much less than that expected to cause a tear in a healthy tendon
4. Iatrogenic—as when removing a calcific deposit

23.2.2 According to the Site of the Tear

- Bony avulsions
- Mid-substance tears
- Muscular-tendinous ruptures

Rotator cuff tears are usually avulsions from the bone rather than divisions of the tendon substance. The term "rotator cuff tendon tear" is hence a misnomer. Rotator cuff tears may also occur at the mid-substance (as in iatrogenic calcium deposit excision) or at the muscular-tendinous junction rather than at the level of the bone tendon interface, but these are unusual. These differ from a classical rotator cuff tear in that the tendon attachment to the humeral head remains intact.

23.2.3 According to the Tendons Torn

1. Subscapularis
2. Supraspinatus
3. Infraspinatus
4. Combined anterior-superior cuff (subscapularis and supraspinatus)
5. Combined posterior-superior cuff (supraspinatus, infraspinatus, teres minor)
6. All tendons

The rotator cuff tendons are flat, sheet tendons rather than tubular. The tendons of the posterior-superior part of the rotator cuff (supraspinatus, infraspinatus, teres minor) merge together before they insert on the humeral head, and it may be difficult to identify exactly where one tendon starts and one tendon finishes [13, 14]. The decision as to which part of the tendon is damaged is to some extent based on the expected anatomical insertion of each part of the rotator cuff tendon on the humeral head.

In more than 90% of cases, rotator cuff disease involves the supraspinatus tendon (in isolation or in combination with other rotator cuff tendons) usually at its distal 1–2 cm from its insertion. Most infraspinatus tendon tears are an extension of a supraspinatus tear. Subscapularis tendon tears may occur as part of a massive rotator cuff tear or in isolation (such as following acute trauma). Teres minor tendon is the least frequently involved.

Superior migration of the humeral head (yellow arrow) due to massive supraspinatus (red arrow) infraspinatus and subscapularis tear, but no associated arthritis. Muscle atrophy and fatty infiltration of the supraspinatus (green arrow) infraspinatus (blue arrow) and subscapularis (orange arrow) is seen

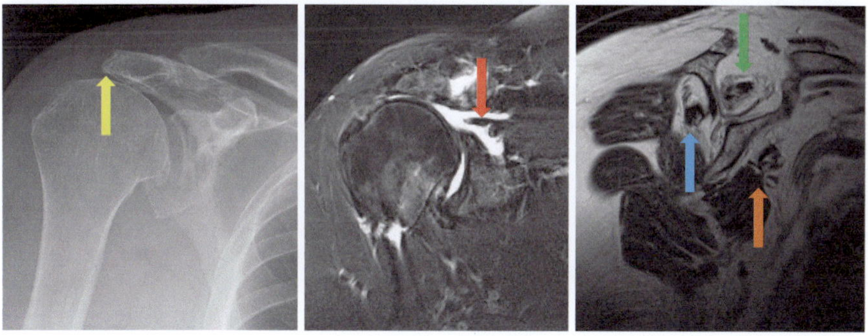

Subscapularis tear (yellow arrow) retracted to the glenoid level with associated medial dislocation of the long head of the biceps tendon (red arrow)

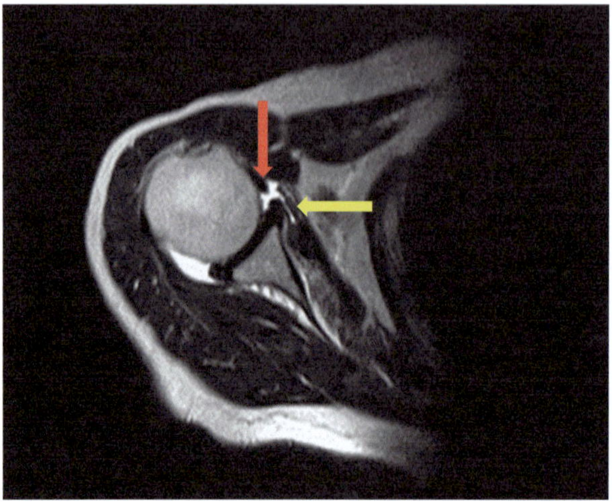

23.2.4 *According to the Length of the Tear*

- Complete (full)
- Incomplete (partial)

The rotator cuff tendons do not attach to a particular point onto the humeral head, but their insertion is several cm long. It is thus possible to have a tear in the tendon which goes all the way across its length or one that involves only part of its length. If the whole of the tendon length is involved, then this is described as a complete (or full) tear. If, however, only part of the rotator cuff tendon length is involved, then it is described as an incomplete length (or partial) tear.

23.2.5 *According to the Tear Thickness* [15]

1. Full thickness
2. Partial thickness

   (a) Articular site
   (b) Bursal site tear
   (c) Intra-substance tear

The rotator cuff tendon does not attach to a particular point on to the humeral head, but its insertion is thick. Hence, it is possible to have a tear in the tendon which goes all the way across the thickness (like a hole) described as a full-thickness tear. Alternatively, it is possible for the undersurface (articular side) or superior surface (bursal side) of the tendon to peel off its attachment from the bone, giving rise to a partial-thickness tear. In this situation, there is no hole in the tendon, and if one were to look into the subacromial space, they would not be able to see through the tendon tear into the glenohumeral joint or vice versa.

Supraspinatus tendon front view: (a) intact tendon, (b) partial thickness articular side tear, (c) partial thickness bursal side tear

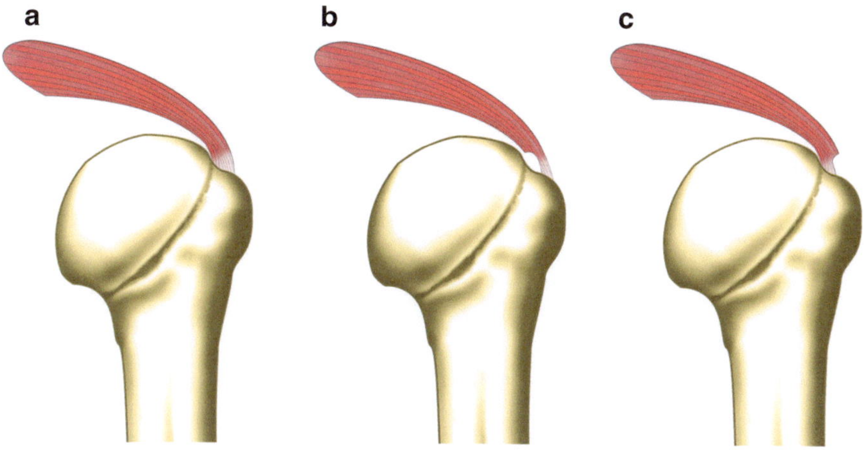

MRI showing partial thickness articular side supraspinatus tear (red arrow)

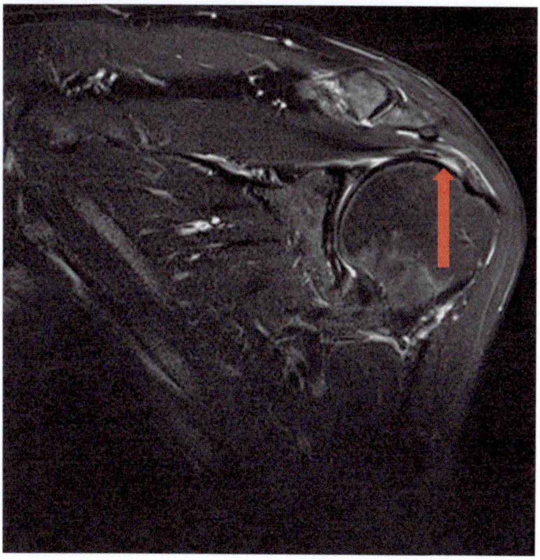

Full thickness supraspinatus tear as seen from glenohumeral joint

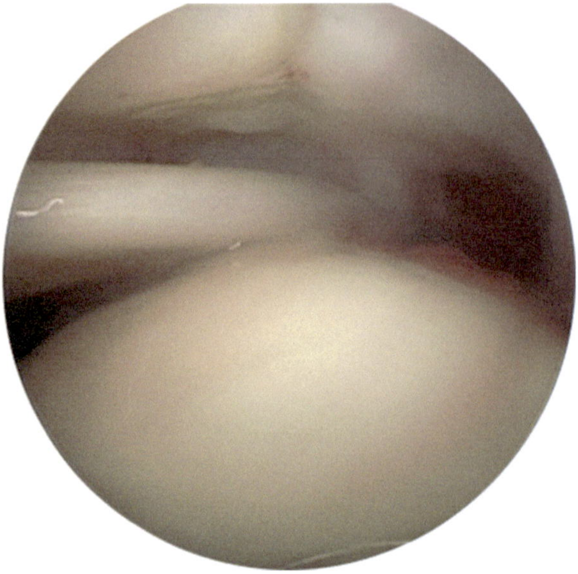

Full thickness supraspinatus tear as seen from subacromial space

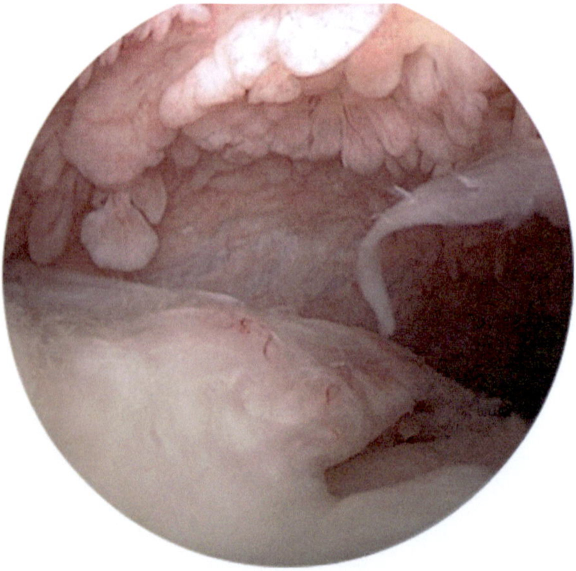

Hence, in describing rotator cuff tears, terminology is important, especially when referring to full or partial. It is important to specify as to whether reference is made to tendon length or thickness.

23.2.6 According to Tear's Shape (Ellman and Gartsman [16])

Tear shape is determined at surgery and may be:

- Crescent
- Triangular
  - L shaped (supraspinatus tears and this tear extends medially through the junction with infraspinatus)
  - Reverse L shaped (supraspinatus tears and this tear extends medially through the rotator cuff interval)
- Trapezoidal (both supraspinatus and infraspinatus tear)
- Massive (three tendon tears)

23.2.7 According to Tear Size (DeOrio and Cofield [17])

Tear size is based on the anterior-posterior length of the tendon detached from the humeral head as assessed at surgery.

1. Small— less than 1 cm
2. Medium—1–3 cm
3. Large—3–5 cm
4. Massive—more than 5 cm

23.2.8 According to the Degree of Retraction (Patte et al. [18])

- Stage 1—Tendon stump remains close to its insertion site
- Stage 2—Retraction to the level of the humeral head
- Stage 3—Retraction to the level of the glenoid

Once a tendon avulses from the bone, it retracts, that is, the edge of the tendon moves away from its insertion site. This is due to:

- Muscle springing away from its insertion
- Muscle contracting
- Muscle shrinking
- Tendon substance lost

Following retraction of the tendon stump, adhesions may form between the retracted tendon and the surrounding structures such as the scapula or the undersurface of the deltoid. Such adhesions may limit a surgeon's ability to pull the tendon back to the bone where it avulsed from upon attempted reattachment surgery. During surgical repair of the torn tendon, division of such adhesions is essential in order to allow the tendon to be mobilised and be pulled back and inserted where it avulsed from. However, despite the release of adhesions, it may still not be possible to return the tendon onto the bone due to changes in the muscle or tendon substance.

Bare humeral head (a) due to massive supraspinatus and infraspinatus tears retracted medial to the glenoid (b)

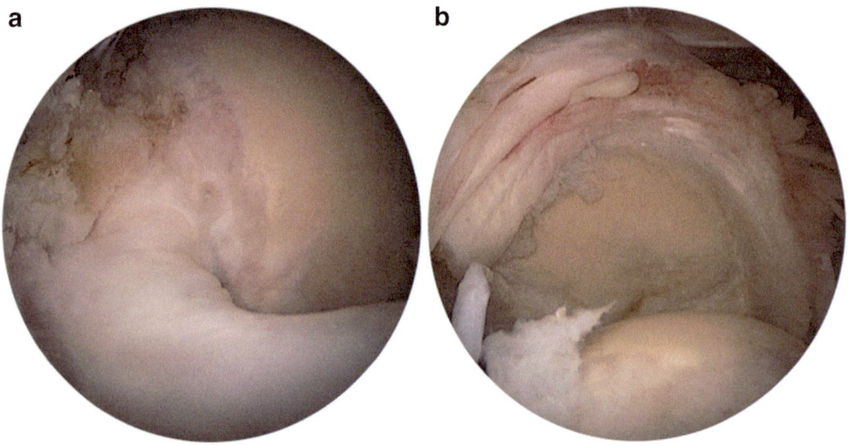

23.2.9 *According to Whether the Tear Can Be Physically Repaired or Not*

1. Repairable
2. Irreparable

   Tendon tears may not be repairable due to several factors including:

- Excessive retraction—cannot re-approximate the tendon to bone
- Poor tendon quality—unable to hold sutures, sutures cutting through the tendon
- Poor bone quality—unable to hold suture anchors or sutures, such as in osteopenic bone (due to old age, immobility or other factors)

Supraspinatus tear (red arrows) but with tendon stump remaining close to its avulsion site

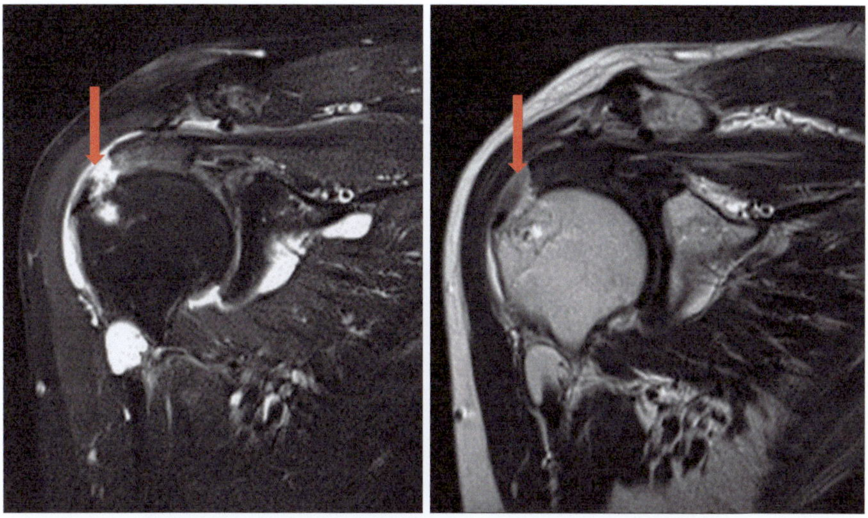

MRI scan showing massive supraspinatus tear with retraction of its stump (red arrow) to the level of the glenoid. No tendon can be seen between the superior part of the humeral head and the glenoid

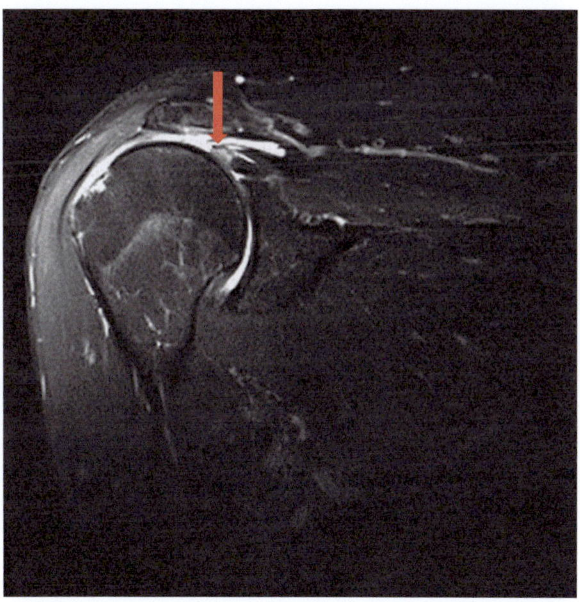

MRI showing re-tear of the supraspinatus tendon (yellow arrow), following a previous repair. The area of high signal in the humeral head (red arrow) is consistent with previous anchor insertion

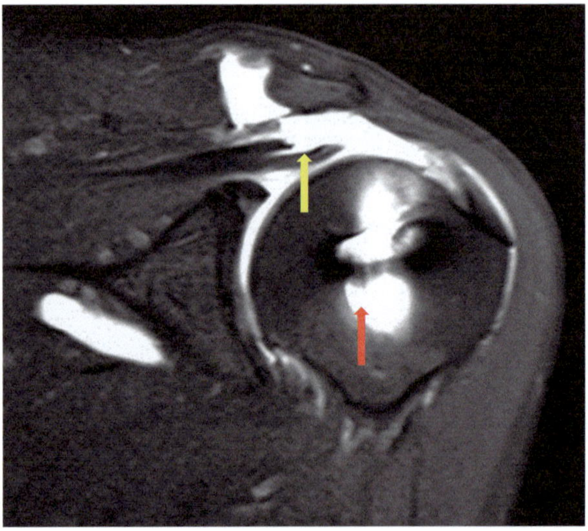

23.2.10 According to the Presence of Associated Muscle Atrophy

The muscle of a torn rotator cuff tendon may atrophy (shrink). Recognising the presence and extent of such atrophy is important as it may be associated with poorer clinical outcomes and may correlate with tear size.

Atrophy of supraspinatus can be assessed quantitatively or qualitatively [19] by:

- Calculating the occupation ratio of the supraspinous fossa by the supraspinatus muscle belly. On the most lateral oblique sagittal image on MRI scan on which the scapular spine is in contact with the rest of the scapula, atrophy is present if the supraspinatus muscle occupies less than half the area of the fossa
- The tangent sign—a line passing from the top of the coracoid process to the top of the spine of the scapula (the tangent) on the most lateral oblique sagittal image on MRI scan on which the scapular spine is in contact with the rest of the scapula; atrophy is present when the superior border of the muscle lies below this line, i.e. it fails to intersect this line (tangent sign positive)

Side view of the scapula demonstrating progression of muscle atrophy in the supraspinatus and infraspinatus muscles

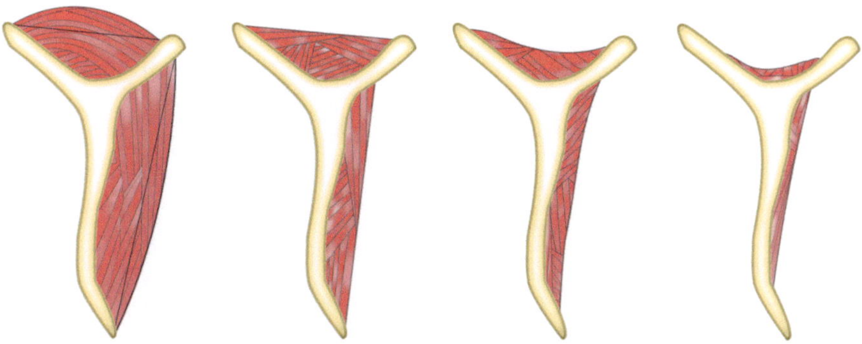

Surgical repair may limit the progression of atrophy but not substantially reverse it [20–22]. Hence, a loss of muscle bulk may limit the success of surgical repair, even when a tendon can be physically reattached to bone.

23.2.11 According to the Presence of Fatty Infiltration

In addition to atrophy, the muscle of a torn rotator cuff tendon may undergo fatty infiltration (replaced by fat).

The severity of fatty infiltration may be staged on CT (as per the original description) or MRI scans using the Goutallier classification [23].

- Stage 0—no fatty deposits
- Stage 1—some fatty straits
- Stage 2—fatty infiltration, but there is still more muscle than fat
- Stage 3—fat equals muscle
- Stage 4—less muscle than fat

MRI showing normal muscle bulk of the supraspinatus (green arrow), infraspinatus (red arrow) and subscapularis (yellow arrow) muscles with no obvious fatty infiltration. Supraspinatus intersects a line (yellow line) passing from the coracoid to the scapular spine

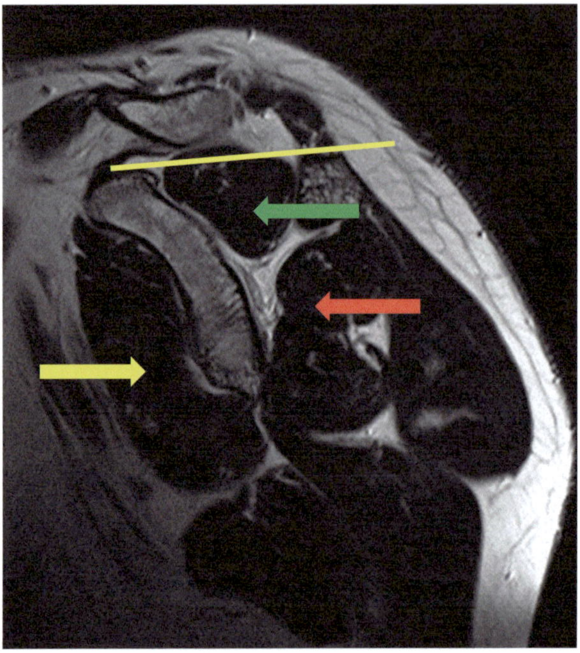

MRI showing atrophy and fatty infiltration of the supraspinatus muscle (red arrow) Supraspinatus lies below a line (yellow line) passing from the coracoid to the scapular spine

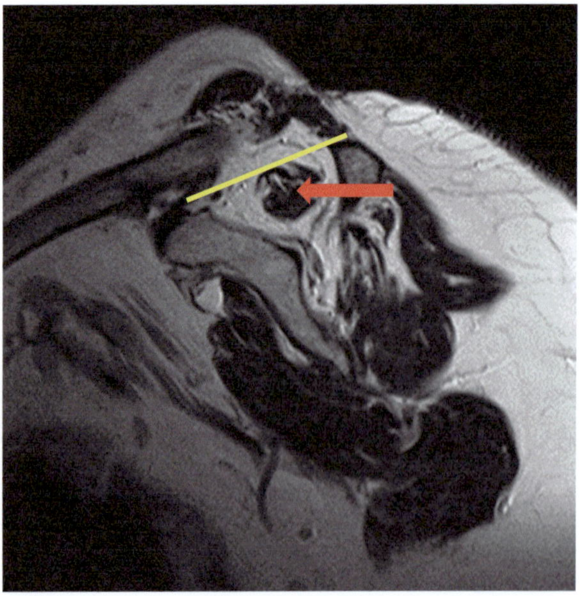

Recognising the presence and extent of such fatty infiltration is important as worse stages of fatty infiltration have been correlated to [24–26]:

- Extent of tear
- Longer duration of tear – moderate supraspinatus fat infiltration seems to appear on average at 3 years after the onset of shoulder symptoms and severe infiltration at an average of 5 years in patients with rotator cuff tears
- Older patient's age

23.3 Prevalence of Rotator Cuff Tears

Rotator cuff tears are common, their prevalence increasing with age. Milgrom et al. [27] reported the prevalence of full- or partial-thickness rotator cuff tears as 5–11% in individuals aged 40–60 but 80% in those older than 70. In their report they noted an increased prevalence after the fifth decade of life.

23.4 Clinical Symptoms of Rotator Cuff Tears [28, 29]

- Pain—at rest or on exertion, night pain
- Weakness of the arm (in one or multiple planes). Patients may complain that they:
  - Cannot elevate the arm
  - Have to throw the arm to get it started during elevation
  - Help the arm with the opposite one, after which arm elevation can be maintained
  - Have inability to reach the mouth with the ipsilateral hand and need to lift the elbow forwards to achieve that
- Stiffness in the presence of degenerative changes
- Difficulty in performing activities of daily life—reaching above head level, reaching back

23.5 Clinical Signs of Rotator Cuff Tears [30]

These will depend on the tendons involved and the severity of tear and include:

- Muscle wasting in supra- and infraspinous fossae
- Tenderness over the subacromial space
- Positive subacromial impingement test
- Positive Hawkins-Kennedy test
- Rotator cuff weakness (reduced active motion, resisted force, lag sign)
- Stiffness—reduced passive motion

23.6 Investigations for Rotator Cuff Tears

- Plain radiograph to look for:
  - Anterior greater tuberosity cysts that may be seen in rotator cuff tears [31]
  - Superior migration of the humeral head
  - Glenohumeral degenerative changes
- Ultrasound scan to assess:
  - Extent of tear
  - Retraction
- MRI scan to assess:
  - Extent of tear
  - Retraction
  - Muscle atrophy
  - Fatty infiltration

MRI arthrogram (especially if done with the arm in abduction and external rotation) is superior to plain MRI and is the investigation of choice in small or partial tears.

23.7 Relation Between Rotator Cuff Tears and Symptoms

It is important to recognise that the presence of rotator cuff tears does not necessarily lead to clinical symptoms. A large proportion of rotator cuff tendon tears are asymptomatic, detected as incidental findings on radiological imaging. It is estimated that only 1 in 15 patients with rotator cuff tears has surgery for symptoms [32].

It has been suggested that only one third of rotator cuff tears cause pain. In addition, Dunn et al. [33] in a cohort study of about 400 patients with non-traumatic full-thickness rotator cuff tears reported that the level of pain was not related to the anatomical features of the tear.

These observations are in line with the fact that:

- Non-surgical treatment of full-thickness tears can be successful in 75% of patients, with pain and function improving despite the tear not healing [34, 35]
- Failure of a rotator cuff tear repair is common, seen in up to 30% of cases. However, some patients who have a failed repair may be pain free with good outcomes that are comparable to those having an intact repair [36, 37]

It is still uncertain as to what causes pain in rotator cuff tears, but a combination of mechanical factors, inflammatory mediators (high levels of inflammatory cytokines have been demonstrated in the subacromial bursa of patients with rotator cuff tears and in the shoulders of animal models of such tears), pain perception and central processing may have a role to play [38–42].

Hinsley et al. [43] used ultrasound to evaluate cuff tendinopathy in a general population cohort. They reported 110 normal tendons, 217 abnormal tendons, 77 partial tears and 124 full-thickness tears. They reported that symptomatic shoulders had a larger median tear size than nonsymptomatic shoulders. When they looked at tear size as a predictor of the presence of pain (trying to decide the point at which full-thickness tears become increasingly likely to be symptomatic), they found the cut-off size to be 2.5 cm; this would be consistent with the difference between single and multi-tendon tears and may signify the point at which altered shoulder biomechanics occur. Nevertheless, they suggested that tear size and type of tear classification systems are not designed to guide treatment and treatment must be individualised.

Curry et al. [44] showed that pain and functional status are not associated with tear size or thickness, fatty infiltration and muscle atrophy. Instead, poor mental health, female sex and increased number of co-morbidities were associated with greater disability scores. Hence, pain and functional disability may have multiple causes and should not be purely related to the characteristics of the tear.

23.8 How Is It Possible to Have a Tendon Tear but No Weakness?

In dealing with rotator cuff tears, a frequent question is how is it possible for a tendon to be torn yet the patient having no symptoms in terms of weakness even when a substantial tear is present.

One may consider an analogy to a person who jumps off a window but holds hanging from a bed sheet. It can be seen that the person can be well supported even when there is a small or a large central tear of the bed sheet or a tear involving the anterior or posterior part of the bed sheet. If the tear progresses and involves the whole of the bed sheet, then there would be no support, and one would fall. However, even if the bed sheet were to be completely ripped apart, one may still be happily supported by alternative means such as a waist harness. Similarly, a tear may be compensated by the remaining intact rotator cuff tendon or by an alternative tendon (such as the deltoid in supraspinatus loss) taking over.

In a tendon with a broad insertion function may persist despite the presence of a partial tear (a, b, c, d). Complete tear (e) may lead to loss of hold, which can be compensated by the action of another muscle (f)

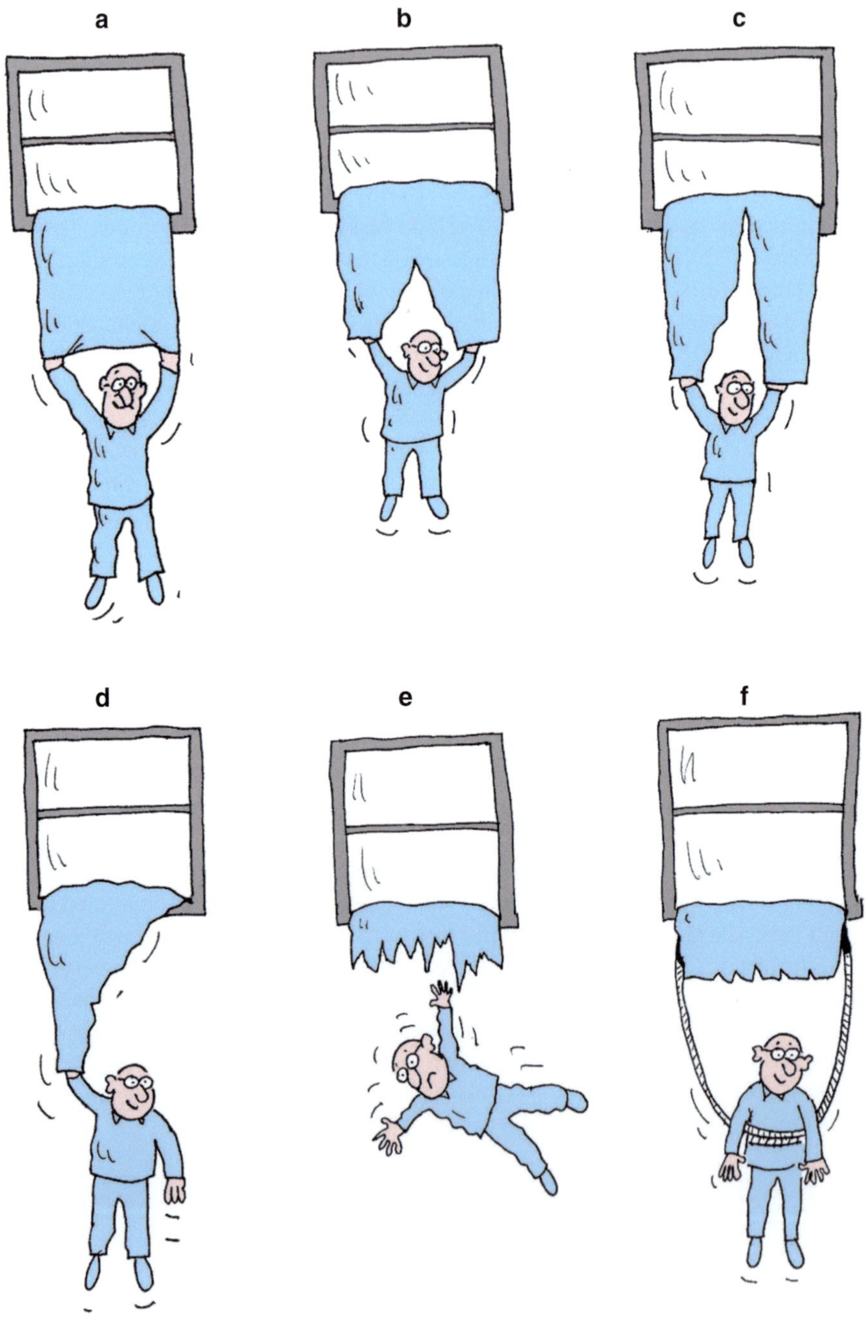

23.9 Considerations in the Treatment of Rotator Cuff Tears

Intervention in rotator cuff tears may aim to:

1. Relieve current troublesome symptoms—reduce pain and improve strength and range of motion and function
2. Limit the deterioration that may occur with time. This is a more controversial indication as it proposes to intervene not for current symptoms but to avoid what may happen in the future

The following are to be considered in contemplating surgical intervention for rotator cuff tears:

- Is the tear likely to worsen (enlarge, retract, muscle detiorate) with time?
- If the tear were to worsen, could the patient's symptoms worsen (an asymptomatic patient becoming symptomatic or a symptomatic patient becoming more severely symptomatic?)
- If the tear were to worsen, would that make surgery more difficult or impossible?
- If the tear were to worsen, would more extensive surgery be necessary?
- If the tear were to worsen, would that impair the clinical outcomes of an applied intervention?

23.9.1 *Tear Progression*

Several stages of rotator cuff tear severity are recognised. In principle, partial-thickness tears may enlarge and propagate into full-thickness tears, with retraction, muscle fatty infiltration and fatty atrophy. Such changes may then lead to degeneration of the glenohumeral joint and cuff tear arthropathy.

Potential progression of rotator cuff tears

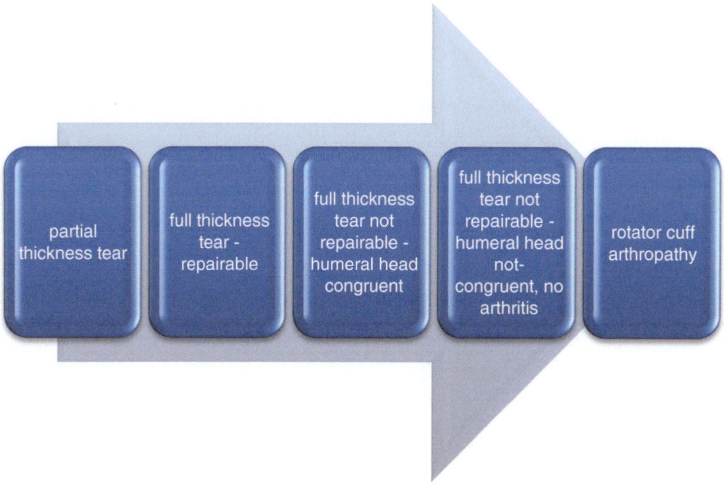

However, there is a controversy as to the temporal relationship and timing of progression between such stages. Similarly, there is a controversy as to the role of surgery in halting such changes.

Denkers et al. [45] studied 37 patients with partial-thickness rotator cuff tears using serial MRI. At a mean of 4.4 years, 76% had no significant progression, 16% had an increase in tear size and 8% progressed to full-thickness tear. Of those with partial tears involving more than 50% of tendon thickness, 55% had tear progression, whereas of those with tears involving less than 50% of tendon thickness, only 14% had tear progression.

Keener et al. [46] evaluated progression of shoulder cuff tears in 224 patients using ultrasound and clinical examination. Tear enlargement was seen in 49% of cases, with a median time to enlargement of 2.8 years. Sixty-one percent of full-thickness tears and 44% of partial-thickness tears enlarged. Tear enlargement was a major risk factor for developing new shoulder pain. The final tear type was related to the risk of new pain development with pain developing in 46% of partial-thickness tears and 50% of full-thickness tears.

Yamaguchi et al. [47] reported that more than half of nonsymptomatic rotator cuff tears become symptomatic within 3 years and a large proportion progresses in size.

Yamanaka et al. [48] reported that about 10% of partial-thickness articular-side tears heal, 10% become smaller, 53% become bigger and 28% become full-thickness tears.

In a study by Connor et al. [49] of 20 elite overhead athletes, the overall prevalence of rotator cuff tears (partial or full thickness) was 40%. Nevertheless, at a 5-year follow-up, none developed shoulder symptoms requiring treatment, nor did they have a reduction in their level of play.

It may thus be concluded that:

- Spontaneous healing of partial tears is rare
- Partial thickness tears do not invariably progress to full-thickness tears
- Rotator cuff tears do not invariably increase in size over time
- In patients with rotator cuff tears, clinical symptoms do not invariably worsen with time
- Symptoms may worsen even if the tear does not change

It may be accepted that some patients with rotator cuff tears will deteriorate with time and become symptomatic, but it seems difficult to reliably predict those at an individual level. The decision to operate for a rotator cuff tear must consider the potential benefits of surgery but also take into account the risk of potential complications of surgery such as infection and stiffness.

Hence, guiding treatment to one's symptoms seems appropriate. If non-surgical treatment fails, then one may consider surgery. An individualised approach, guided by current symptoms, is the author's preferred choice in dealing with such tears. Shared decision-making between clinician and patient has a vital role to play.

23.10 Management of Rotator Cuff Tears

Non-surgical [50–59]

- Analgesia
- Activity modification
- Steroid or hyaluronic injections
- Physiotherapy
  - Local treatment—heat therapy, mega-pulse, ultrasound
  - Addressing scapular dysrhythmia
  - Strengthening—strengthen some of the big muscles of the shoulder (deltoid, pectoralis major and latissimus dorsi) to compensate for the weakness due to a loss of part of the rotator cuff tendon

Non-surgical treatment may help the vast majority of patients with full-thickness, non- traumatic rotator cuff tears. However, patients may experience recurrence of symptoms or intermittent symptoms having good and bad times.

Surgical

Relative indications for surgery:

- Acute traumatic tear
- Failed non-surgical treatment for 3 or more months
- Physiologically young patients
- Physically high-demand patients

Tears occurring following an acute injury may be considered a relative indication for surgery. Decision-making in such cases is challenging as:

- A tear may be present prior to the injury but not causing symptoms—hence a tear identified post-injury may not be a fresh traumatic tear but a chronic, pre-existent degenerative tear

Some patient, tear and injury characteristics which may point towards a chronic pre-existent tear rather than an acute tear are:

- Old patient age—prevalence of degenerative tears increases with age
- Evidence of muscular atrophy or fatty infiltration
- Degenerative tendon changes
- Tendon retraction—however, retraction also may reflect acute springing of the tendon away from its bony origin rather than chronic displacement
- The magnitude of the applied force—could the applied force have caused the tear in a heathy tendon?

Hence, even in post-injury cases, non-surgical management may be initially tried with surgery reserved for resistant cases. However, if there is doubt and especially in situations where there is a substantial arm weakness rather than just pain, early surgical intervention is preferable to fully evaluate the mobility and repairability of the tendon.

23.11 Surgical Options for Rotator Cuff Tears

There are several surgical options [60–100] including:
If tendon tear is repairable:

- Debridement of the torn tendon +/− acromioplasty, without repairing the tear
- Rotator cuff tear repair +/− acromioplasty

If the tendon tear is irreparable:

- Debridement of the torn tendon, but preserving the coraco-acromial ligament
- Tuberoplasty
- Suprascapular nerve ablation
- Superior capsular reconstruction
- Interposition grafts
- Tendon transfers (latissimus dorsi, pectoralis major)
- Subacromial balloon insertion
- Reverse shoulder replacement

23.11.1 Rotator Cuff Tendon Repair

In rotator cuff tendon repair, the aim is to reattach the tendon back to the bone from where it was avulsed. This may be achieved using:

- Suture anchors (screwlike devices which are made either of metallic or non-metallic material and which have sutures attached to them). These anchors are inserted into the bone, and the sutures are used to stitch the tendon down on to the bone
- Sutures passed through bone tunnels—sutures are passed through the tendon. Tunnels are drilled through the humeral head. The sutures are passed through these tunnels and tied over a bone bridge

The number and configuration of sutures, suture anchors and bone tunnels is determined by the size and shape of the tear, as well as tendon and bone quality.

23.11.1.1 Repair of Partial Articular-Side Tendon Tears

A relative indication for repair is symptomatic partial-thickness tendon tears involving more than 50% of the tendon thickness. The thickness of partial tears may be assessed by using the tip of an arthroscopic shoulder shaver. If the tip of a shaver (which is usually about 4.5 mm) can be sunk into the bare area from where the tendon avulsed, then the tear is considered to involve more than 50% of the tendon.

Options for partial-thickness rotator cuff tear repair [101, 102] are:

- Trans-tendon repair—by inserting suture anchors through the intact tendon into the bone (tendon footprint) and using their sutures to repair the tendon
- Conversion of a partial- to full-thickness tear which is then repaired

A potential complication following repair of partial-thickness tears is shoulder stiffness.

23.11.1.2 Repair of Full-Thickness Tendon Tears

Multiple techniques have been described including:

- Single-row repair—one row of suture anchors is used to suture the tendon to the bone. One or more anchors are inserted into the tendon footprint. Their sutures are then passed through the torn tendon edge and are tied securing the tendon edge against the bone
- Double-row repair —two rows of anchors, one medial and one lateral, are used to stitch the tendon to the bone. Their sutures are inserted through the tendon and tied securing the tendon onto the bone (the medial sutures are passed through the medial aspect of the tendon and tied down, and the lateral sutures are passed through the edge of the tendon and tied down). Double-row technique may confer certain advantages including:
  - Increase in the contact area between tendon and bone facilitating healing
  - Biomechanically stronger repair

Supraspinatus tendon full thickness tear (a), repaired with a medial row anchor and knotted sutures (b, c) as well as a suture bridge configuration using a lateral row knotless anchor (d, e)

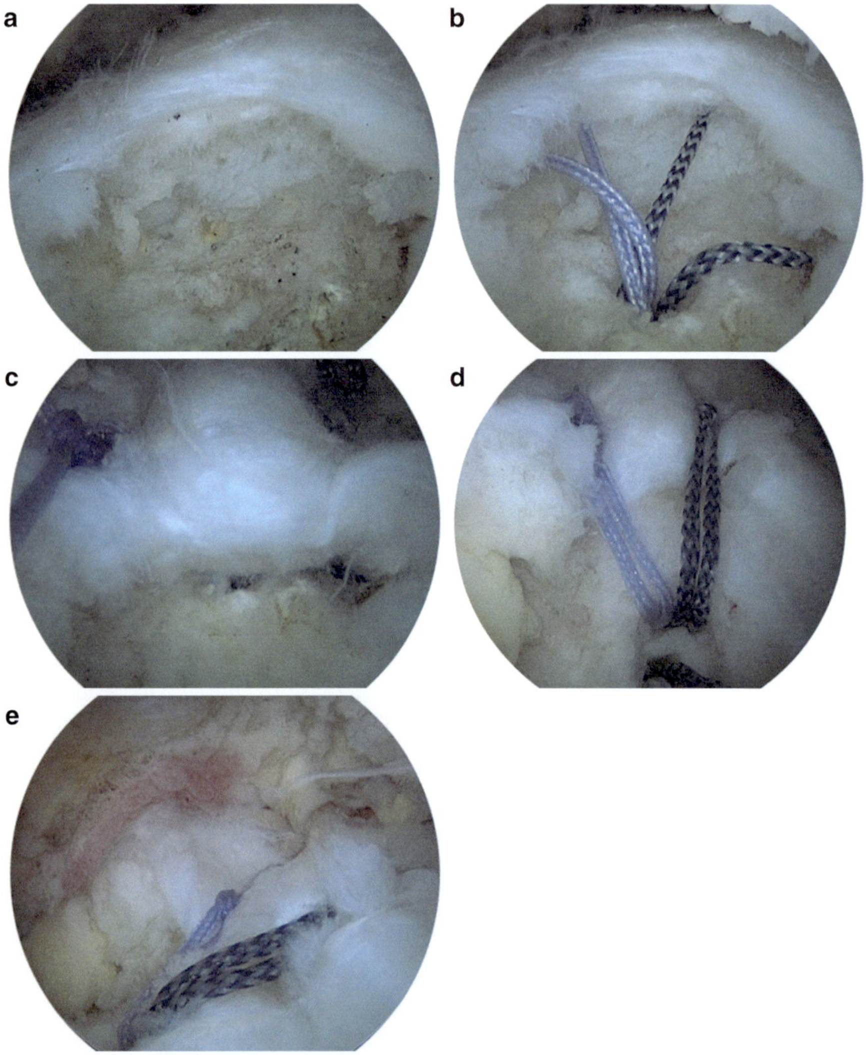

However, clinical studies have failed to consistently show superior clinical outcomes for the double-row technique.

- Suture-bridge repair—a medial row of suture anchors is inserted; the sutures are passed through the tendon and tied but not cut. These sutures are then brought laterally over the tendon and fixed to the lateral part of the humeral head using a knotless anchor. This allows:
  - Compression of the tendon by the sutures throughout the entire tendon footprint hence greater:

Contact pressure between the tendon and bone
Repair strength

Full-thickness rotator cuff tears may be delaminated, that is, the tendon may also be split into superficial and deep layers. Retraction from the bone origin may differ between such layers; the articular-side layer is usually more retracted than the bursal-side layer. Repair techniques may aim to repair both layers combined or repair them in isolation (lamina-specific repair).

It has been shown that in large or massive tears, it is not absolutely essential to reattach the whole of the rotator cuff if that is not technically possible. A tendon repair may not be complete but can still improve function. By partially repairing the rotator cuff, it may be possible to restore the transverse force couple between subscapularis anteriorly and infraspinatus and teres minor posteriorly, hence opposing the superior translation of the humeral head upon deltoid contraction [103].

23.11.2 Tendon Repair Augmentation

There are cases where the free edge of the torn rotator cuff tendon can be approximated to its bony origin to allow a repair, but the tendon substance is very degenerate and of poor quality. This raises concerns that the repair may fail due to the sutures cutting through the tendon. In such circumstances a synthetic ligament can be used to augment the site of the repair. Such a ligament provides a strong scaffold which can hold sutures and hence may increase the chance of a successful repair.

23.11.3 Tendon Bridging

In cases where the tendon is substantially retracted and cannot be re-approximated to its bony origin, an artificial ligament may be used to breach the gap between the tendon edge and the bone. Several types of biological patches have been used made from human skin, swine small intestine, bovine skin, autograft fascia lata and iliotibial ligament.

23.11.4 Tendon Transfer for Rotator Cuff Tears

In cases where the tendon cannot be repaired, another tendon may be used to recreate the function of the torn tendon. The tendon to be utilised is detached from its normal bony insertion, is re-routed and reattached on the bone in such a position as to take over the activity of the lost rotator cuff tendon. The transferred tendon may exert its effects by:

1. Tenodesis effect (equivalent to a passive constrain effect—similar to how ligaments act)
2. Active muscle contraction effect

Tendon transfers may be preferable:

- Where there is marked troublesome weakness, hence need to improve strength
- In younger patients where reverse shoulder arthroplasty is better avoided

Four described tendon transfers for rotator cuff tears are:

1. Latissimus dorsi transfer to the greater tuberosity—latissimus dorsi is detached from its normal insertion is re-routed, and is attached to the greater tuberosity (in the area where normally the supraspinatus tendon inserts) using suture anchors
2. Pectoralis major transfer to the lesser tuberosity to address subscapularis tears (that are associated with or without supraspinatus tears). The superior part of the pectoralis major tendon is often utilised
3. Teres major transfer for supraspinatus/infraspinatus tears
4. Latissimus dorsi transfer for subscapularis tears

Latissimus dorsi tendon transfer for supraspinatus rupture. (a) normal tendon attachment (b) post tendon transfer

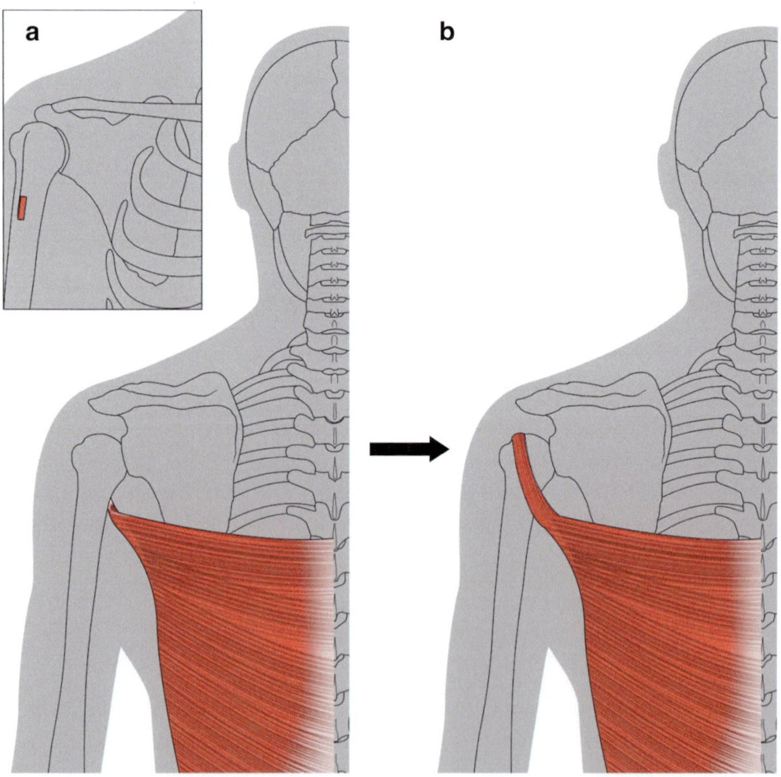

Pectoralis major tendon transfer for subscapularis rupture. (a) normal tendon attachment (b) post tendon transfer

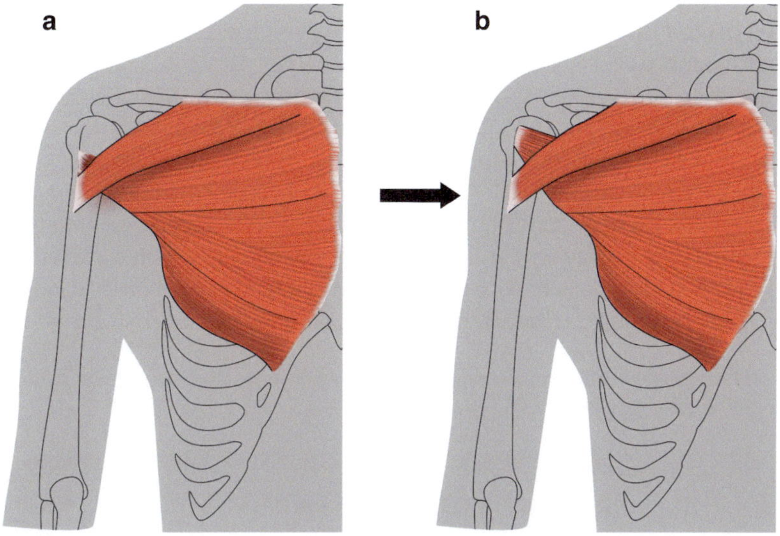

The functional outcome of tendon transfers may vary substantially from patient to patient.

The following are associated with a poor outcome after a transfer:

- Poor deltoid or teres minor function
- Osteoarthritis of the glenohumeral joint
- Glenohumeral joint stiffness

With time the transferred tendon stretches and elongates, and this results in a decreased tenodesis effect. Hence, the beneficial effects of a tendon transfer may deteriorate with time.

23.11.5 Salvage Surgery for Irreparable Rotator Cuff Tears

Of the various surgical options available, some do not aim to repair or replace the torn tendon but to improve pain and strength by alternative means. Some of these are described below. It should be considered that pain may limit the ability of an individual to carry out strengthening exercises of the shoulder and, by improving pain, one may indirectly promote strength.

23.11.5.1 Tuberoplasty

In the presence of a massive rotator cuff tear, upon attempted arm forward elevation or abduction, the humeral head may translate upwards leading to abutment of the greater tuberosity against the inferior surface of the acromion and causing pain. Tuberoplasty involves shaving off the greater tuberosity to increase the distance between the humeral head and the undersurface of the acromion during arm elevation or abduction. This minimises the contact between the two surfaces and may thus improve pain. It is equivalent to performing a subacromial decompression by acromioplasty, but in the case of massive rotator cuff tears, the release of the coraco-acromial ligament (which is the initial part of acromioplasty) is not advisable as it may lead to anterior instability (escape) of the humeral head. Hence, the opposite site (greater tuberosity) is shaved off.

Tuberoplasty-massive supraspinatus and infraspinatus tear leaving a bare greater tuberosity (a) that is athroscopically, excised (b, c)

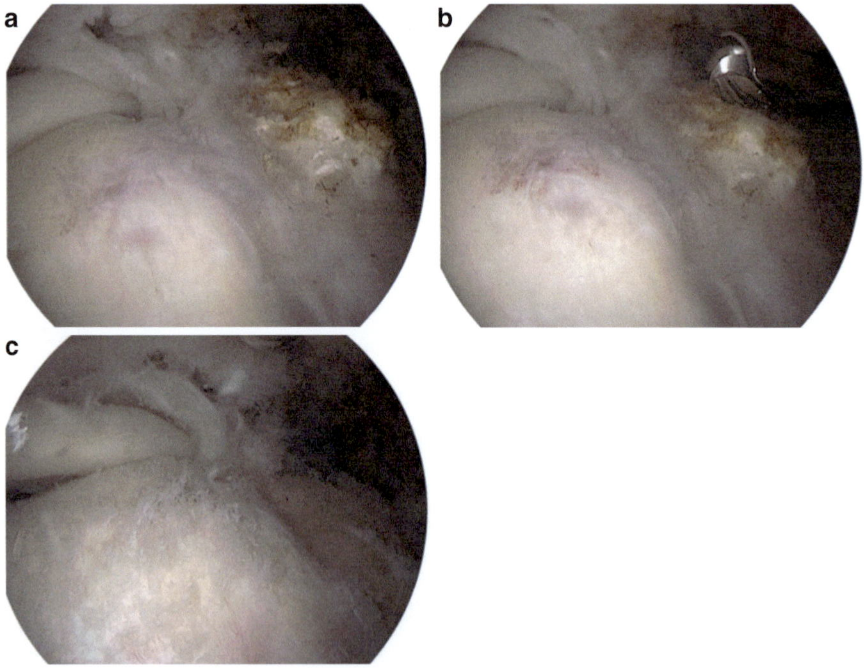

23.11.5.2 Long Head of Biceps Tenotomy/Tenodesis

In rotator cuff tendon tears, the long head of the biceps tendon is often diseased. The long head of the biceps tendon may be degenerative causing pain. It may also be subluxed or dislocated medially out of the bicipital groove. In these cases biceps tenotomy or tenodesis either above or below the bicipital groove or within the groove may be performed [104, 105].

23.11.5.3 Subacromial Spacer [83–85]

This involves the insertion of a bioabsorbable balloon in the subacromial space which is inflated using saline. The balloon pushes the humeral head downwards. The spacer gets reabsorbed, but it may leave behind scar tissue which has a longer-lasting filling effect. Such a spacer may:

- Reduce pain by limiting contact of the humeral head with the acromion
- Improve strength by limiting superior translation of the humeral head and hence improving the glenohumeral biomechanics during arm elevation
- Aid the strengthening of the remaining rotator cuff tendons (anterior and posterior) as well as deltoid, by improving glenohumeral biomechanics

23.11.5.4 Superior Capsular Reconstruction

This involves the reconstruction of the superior capsule of the shoulder. An artificial ligament is sutured to the superior part of the glenoid and to the greater tuberosity of the humeral head to form a passive constraint that limits the superior migration of the humeral head.

23.11.6 Reverse Total Shoulder Arthroplasty

This may help reduce pain and increase strength by improving the biomechanics of the shoulder. Arthroplasty is preferable in rotator cuff tears associated with degenerative changes of the glenohumeral joint; its effects on improving pain tend to be more reliable than its effects on improving range of motion and strength. However, arthroplasty may also be used in the absence of joint degeneration to help address the range of motion and strength.

References

1. Terry GC, Chopp TM. Functional anatomy of the shoulder. J Athl Train. 2000;35(3):248–55.
2. Sinnatamby CS. FRCS last's anatomy: regional and applied. 12th ed. London: Churchill Livingstone Elsevier; 2011.
3. McFarland EG, Maffulli N, Del Buono A, Murrell GA, Garzon-Muvdi J, Petersen SA. Impingement is not impingement: the case for calling it "Rotator Cuff Disease". Muscles Ligaments Tendons J. 2013;3(3):196–200.
4. DE Giorgi S, Saracino M, Castagna A. Degenerative disease in rotator cuff tears: what are the biochemical and histological changes? Joints. 2014;2(1):26–8.
5. Neviaser A, Andarawis-Puri N, Flatow E. Basic mechanisms of tendon fatigue damage. J Shoulder Elb Surg. 2012;21(2):158–63.
6. Seitz AL, McClure PW, Finucane S, Boardman ND 3rd, Michener LA. Mechanisms of rotator cuff tendinopathy: intrinsic, extrinsic, or both? Clin Biomech (Bristol Avon). 2011;26(1):1–12.
7. Via AG, De Cupis M, Spoliti M, Oliva F. Clinical and biological aspects of rotator cuff tears. Muscles Ligaments Tendons J. 2013;3(2):70–9.
8. Maffulli N, Longo UG, Berton A, Loppini M, Denaro V. Biological factors in the pathogenesis of rotator cuff tears. Sports Med Arthrosc Rev. 2011;19(3):194–201.
9. Neer CS 2nd. Impingement lesions. Clin Orthop Relat Res. 1983;173:70–7.
10. Bigliani LU, Ticker JB, Flatow EL, Soslowsky LJ, Mow VC. The relationship of acromial architecture to rotator cuff disease. Clin Sports Med. 1991;10(4):823–38.
11. Lo IK, Burkhart SS. The etiology and assessment of subscapularis tendon tears: a case for subcoracoid impingement, the roller-wringer effect, and TUFF lesions of the subscapularis. Arthroscopy. 2003;19(10):1142–50.
12. Walch G, Liotard JP, Boileau P, Noël E. Postero-superior glenoid impingement. Another impingement of the shoulder. J Radiol. 1993;74(1):47–50.
13. Mochizuki T, Sugaya H, Uomizu M, Maeda K, Matsuki K, Sekiya I, Muneta T, Akita K. Humeral insertion of the supraspinatus and infraspinatus. New anatomical findings regarding the footprint of the rotator cuff. J Bone Joint Surg Am. 2008;90(5):962–9.
14. Gumina S, Borroni M. Classifications of the rotator cuff tears. In: Gumina S, editor. Rotator cuff tear. Cham: Springer; 2017.
15. Ellman H, Gartsman GM. Open repair of full thickness rotator cuff tears. In: Ellman H, Gartsman GM, editors. Arthroscopic shoulder surgery and related procedures. Philadelphia, PA: Lea and Febiger; 1993. p. 181–202.
16. DeOrio JK, Cofield RH. Results of a second attempt at surgical repair of a failed initial rotator cuff repair. J Bone Joint Surg Am. 1984;66:563–7.
17. Patte D. Classification of rotator cuff lesions. Clin Orthop Relat Res. 1990;254:81–6.
18. Zanetti M, Gerber C, Hodler J. Quantitative assessment of the muscles of the rotator cuff with magnetic resonance imaging. Investig Radiol. 1998;33(3):163–70.
19. Gerber C, Fuchs B, Hodler J. The results of repair of massive tears of the rotator cuff. J Bone Joint Surg Am. 2000;82(4):505–15.
20. Gladstone JN, Bishop JY, Lo IK, Flatow EL. Fatty infiltration and atrophy of the rotator cuff do not improve after rotator cuff repair and correlate with poor functional outcome. Am J Sports Med. 2007;35(5):719–28.
21. Chung SW, Kim SH, Tae SK, Yoon JP, Choi JA, Oh JH. Is the supraspinatus muscle atrophy truly irreversible after surgical repair of rotator cuff tears? Clin Orthop Surg. 2013;5(1):55–65.
22. Goutallier D, Postel JM, Bernageau J, Lavau L, Voisin MC. Fatty muscle degeneration in cuff ruptures. Pre- and postoperative evaluation by CT scan. Clin Orthop Relat Res. 1994;304:78–83.
23. Melis B, Wall B, Walch G. Natural history of infraspinatus fatty infiltration in rotator cuff tears. J Shoulder Elb Surg. 2010;19(5):75.

24. Melis B, DeFranco MJ, Chuinard C, Walch G. Natural history of fatty infiltration and atrophy of the supraspinatus muscle in rotatorcuff tears. Clin Orthop Relat Res. 2010;468(6):1498–505.
25. Melis B, Nemoz C, Walch G. Muscle fatty infiltration in rotator cuff tears: descriptive analysis of 1688 cases. Orthop Traumatol Surg Res. 2009;95(5):319–24.
26. Milgrom C, Schaffler M, Gilbert S, van Holsbeeck M. Rotator-cuff changes in asymptomatic adults. The effect of age, hand dominance and gender. J Bone Joint Surg (Br). 1995;77(2):296–8.
27. Minns Lowe CJ, Moser J, Barker K. Living with a symptomatic rotator cuff tear 'bad days, bad nights': a qualitative study. BMC Musculoskelet Disord. 2014;15:228. https://doi.org/10.1186/1471-2474-15-228.
28. Gumina S, Candela V, Passaretti D, Venditto T, Mariani L, Giannicola G. Sleep quality and disturbances in patients with different-sized rotator cuff tear. Musculoskelet Surg. 2016;100(Suppl 1):33–8.
29. Charalambous CP. Clinical examination of the shoulder. In: Charalambous CP, editor. The shoulder made easy. Springer; 2019. pp. 77–122.
30. Suluova F, Kanatli U, Ozturk BY, Esen E, Bolukbasi S. Humeral head cysts: association with rotator cuff tears and age. Eur J Orthop Surg Traumatol. 2014;24(5):733–9.
31. Petri M, Ettinger M, Brand S, Stuebig T, Krettek C, Omar M. Non-operative management of rotator cuff tears. Open Orthop J. 2016;10:349–56.
32. Dunn WR, Kuhn JE, Sanders R, An Q, Baumgarten KM, Bishop JY, Brophy RH, Carey JL, Holloway GB, Jones GL, Ma CB, Marx RG, McCarty EC, Poddar SK, Smith MV, Spencer EE, Vidal AF, Wolf BR, Wright RW. Symptoms of pain do not correlate with rotator cuff tear severity: a cross-sectional study of 393 patients with a symptomatic atraumatic full-thickness rotator cuff tear. J Bone Joint Surg Am. 2014;96(10):793–800.
33. Zoorman RS, More KD, Hollinshead RM, Wiley JP, Brett K, Mohtadi NG, Nelson AA, Lo IK, Bryant D. The rotator cuff quality-of-life index predicts the outcome of nonoperative treatment of patients with a chronic rotator cuff tear. J Bone Joint Surg Am. 2014;96(22):1883–8.
34. Fucentese SF, von Roll AL, Pfirrmann CW, Gerber C, Jost B. Evolution of nonoperatively treated symptomatic isolated full-thickness supraspinatus tears. J Bone Joint Surg Am. 2012;94(9):801–8.
35. Galatz LM, Ball CM, Teefey SA, Middleton WD, Yamaguchi K. The outcome and repair integrity of completely arthroscopically repaired large and massive rotator cuff tears. J Bone Joint Surg Am. 2004;86-A(2):219–24.
36. Russell RD, Knight JR, Mulligan E, Khazzam MS. Structural integrity after rotator cuff repair does not correlate with patient function and pain. J Bone Joint Surg Am. 2014;96(4): 265–71.
37. Sakai H, Fujita K, Sakai Y, Mizuno K. Immunolocalization of cytokines and growth factors in subacromial bursa of rotator cuff tear patients. Kobe J Med Sci. 2001;47(1):25–34.
38. Okamura K, Kobayashi T, Yamamoto A, Shitara H, Osawa T, Ichinose T, Takagishi K. Shoulder pain and intra-articular interleukin-8 levels in patients with rotator cuff tears. Int J Rheum Dis. 2017;20(2):177–81.
39. Yamazaki H, Ochiai N, Kenmoku T, Ohtori S, Sasho T, Miyagi M, Ishikawa T, Kamoda H, Orita S, Sasaki Y, Yamaguchi T, Kijima T, Takahashi K. Assessment of pain-related behavior and pro-inflammatory cytokine levels in the rat rotator cuff tear model. J Orthop Res. 2014;32(2):286–90.
40. Barlow JD, Bishop JY, Dunn WR, Kuhn JE, MOON Shoulder Group. What factors are predictors of emotional health in patients with full-thickness rotator cuff tears? J Shoulder Elb Surg. 2016;25(11):1769–73.
41. Coronado RA, Seitz AL, Pelote E, Archer KR, Jain NB. Are Psychosocial factors associated with patient-reported outcome measures in patients with rotator cuff tears? A systematic review. Clin Orthop Relat Res. 2018;476(4):810–29.

42. Dean BJ, Gwilym SE, Carr AJ. Why does my shoulder hurt? A review of the neuroanatomical and biochemical basis of shoulder pain. Br J Sports Med. 2013;47(17):1095–104.
43. Hinsley H, Nicholls A, Daines M, Wallace G, Arden N, Carr A. Classification of rotator cuff tendinopathy using high definition ultrasound. Muscles Ligaments Tendons J. 2014;4(3):391–7.
44. Curry EJ, Matzkin EE, Dong Y, Higgins LD, Katz JN, Jain NB. Structural characteristics are not associated with pain and function in rotator cuff tears: the row cohort study. Orthop J Sports Med. 2015;3(5):2325967115584596. https://doi.org/10.1177/2325967115584596.
45. Denkers M, Pletsch K, Boorman R, Hollinshead R, Lo IKY. Partial thickness rotator cuff tears: observe or operative. In: Proceedings of the American academy of orthopaedic surgeons annual meeting; February; San Francisco, Calif, USA.
46. Keener JD, Galatz LM, Teefey SA, Middleton WD, Steger-May K, Stobbs-Cucchi G, Patton R, Yamaguchi K. A prospective evaluation of survivorship of asymptomatic degenerative rotator cuff tears. J Bone Joint Surg Am. 2015;97(2):89–98.
47. Yamaguchi K, Tetro AM, Blam O, Evanoff BA, Teefey SA, Middleton WD. Natural history of asymptomatic rotator cuff tears: a longitudinal analysis of asymptomatic tears detected sonographically. J Shoulder Elb Surg. 2001;10(3):199–203.
48. Yamanaka K, Matsumoto T. The joint side tear of the rotator cuff. A followup study by arthrography. Clin Orthop Relat Res. 1994;304:68–73.
49. Connor PM, Banks DM, Tyson AB, Coumas JS, D'Alessandro DF. Magnetic resonance imaging of the asymptomatic shoulder of overhead athletes: a 5-year follow-up study. Am J Sports Med. 2003;31(5):724–7.
50. Levy O, Mullett H, Roberts S, Copeland S. The role of anterior deltoid reeducation in patients with massive irreparable degenerative rotator cuff tears. J Shoulder Elb Surg. 2008;17(6):863–70.
51. Ainsworth R, Lewis JS. Exercise therapy for the conservative management of full thickness tears of the rotator cuff: a systematic review. Br J Sports Med. 2007;41(4):200–10.
52. Gialanella B, Prometti P. Effects of corticosteroids injection in rotator cuff tears. Pain Med. 2011;12(10):1559–65.
53. Bokor DJ, Hawkins RJ, Huckell GH, Angelo RL, Schickendantz MS. Results of nonoperative management of full-thickness tears of the rotator cuff. Clin Orthop Relat Res. 1993;294:103–10.
54. Itoi E, Tabata S. Conservative treatment of rotator cuff tears. Clin Orthop Relat Res. 1992;275:165–73.
55. Itoi E. Rotator cuff tear: physical examination and conservative treatment. J Orthop Sci. 2013;18(2):197–204.
56. Lin JC, Weintraub N, Aragaki DR. Nonsurgical treatment for rotator cuff injury in the elderly. J Am Med Dir Assoc. 2008;9(9):626–32.
57. Boorman RS, More KD, Hollinshead RM, Wiley JP, Mohtadi NG, Lo IKY, Brett KR. What happens to patients when we do not repair their cuff tears? Five-year rotator cuff quality-of-life index outcomes following nonoperative treatment of patients with full-thickness rotator cuff tears. J Shoulder Elb Surg. 2018;27(3):444–8.
58. Kuhn JE, Dunn WR, Sanders R, An Q, Baumgarten KM, Bishop JY, Brophy RH, Carey JL, Holloway BG, Jones GL, Ma CB, Marx RG, McCarty EC, Poddar SK, Smith MV, Spencer EE, Vidal AF, Wolf BR, Wright RW, MOON Shoulder Group. Effectiveness of physical therapy in treating atraumatic full-thickness rotator cuff tears: a multicenter prospective cohort study. J Shoulder Elb Surg. 2013;22(10):1371–9.
59. Kijima H, Minagawa H, Nishi T, Kikuchi K, Shimada Y. Long-term follow-up of cases of rotator cuff tear treated conservatively. J Shoulder Elb Surg. 2012;21(4):491–4.
60. Neumann JA, Zgonis MH, Rickert KD, Bradley KE, Kremen TJ, Boggess BR, Toth AP. Interposition dermal matrix xenografts: a successful alternative to traditional treatment of massive rotator cuff tears. Am J Sports Med. 2017;45(6):1261–8.
61. Steinhaus ME, Makhni EC, Cole BJ, Romeo AA, Verma NN. Outcomes after patch use in rotator cuff repair. Arthroscopy. 2016;32(8):1676–90.

62. Gupta AK, Hug K, Berkoff DJ, Boggess BR, Gavigan M, Malley PC, Toth AP. Dermal tissue allograft for the repair of massive irreparable rotator cuff tears. Am J Sports Med. 2012;40(1):141–7.
63. Audenaert E, Van Nuffel J, Schepens A, Verhelst M, Verdonk R. Reconstruction of massive rotator cuff lesions with a synthetic interposition graft: a prospective study of 41 patients. Knee Surg Sports Traumatol Arthrosc. 2006;14(4):360–4.
64. Modi A, Singh HP, Pandy R, Armstrong A. Management of irreparable rotator cuff tears with the GraftJacket allograft as an interpositional graft. Shoulder Elbow. 2013;5:188–94.
65. Kolk A, Henseler JF, Overes FJ, Nagels J, Nelissen RGHH. Teres major tendon transfer in the treatment of irreparable posterosuperior rotator cuff tears. Bone Joint J. 2018;100-B(3):309–17.
66. Mun SW, Kim JY, Yi SH, Baek CH. Latissimus dorsi transfer for irreparable subscapularis tendon tears. J Shoulder Elb Surg. 2018;27(6):1057–64. pii: S1058-2746(17)30769-3.
67. Gerber C. Latissimus dorsi transfer for the treatment of irreparable tears of the rotator cuff. Clin Orthop Relat Res. 1992;275:152–60.
68. Shin JJ, Saccomanno MF, Cole BJ, Romeo AA, Nicholson GP, Verma NN. Pectoralis major transfer for treatment of irreparable subscapularis tear: a systematic review. Knee Surg Sports Traumatol Arthrosc. 2016;24(6):1951–60.
69. Nelson GN, Namdari S, Galatz L, Keener JD. Pectoralis major tendon transfer for irreparable subscapularis tears. J Shoulder Elb Surg. 2014;23(6):909–18.
70. Gavriilidis I, Kircher J, Magosch P, Lichtenberg S, Habermeyer P. Pectoralis major transfer for the treatment of irreparable anterosuperior rotator cuff tears. Int Orthop. 2010;34(5):689–94.
71. Hawi N, Schmiddem U, Omar M, Stuebig T, Krettek C, Petri M, Meller R. Arthroscopic debridement for irreparable rotator cuff tears. Open Orthop J. 2016;10:324–9.
72. Liem D, Lengers N, Dedy N, Poetzl W, Steinbeck J, Marquardt B. Arthroscopic debridement of massive irreparable rotator cuff tears. Arthroscopy. 2008;24(7):743–8.
73. Park JG, Cho NS, Song JH, Baek JH, Rhee YG. Long-term outcome of tuberoplasty for irreparable massive rotator cuff tears: is tuberoplasty really applicable? J Shoulder Elb Surg. 2016;25(2):224–31.
74. Scheibel M, Lichtenberg S, Habermeyer P. Reversed arthroscopic subacromial decompression for massive rotator cuff tears. J Shoulder Elb Surg. 2004;13(3):272–8.
75. Kenyon P, Mclaughlin-Symon I, Heasley R, Morgan B, Ravenscroft M. Arthroscopic suprascapular neurotomy for the painful irreparable rotator cuff tear. Should Elb. 2015;7(2): 94–9.
76. Nizlan NM, Skirving AP, Campbell PT. Arthroscopic suprascapular neurectomy for the management of severe shoulder pain. J Shoulder Elb Surg. 2009;18(2):245–50.
77. Omid R, Lee B. Tendon transfers for irreparable rotator cuff tears. J Am Acad Orthop Surg. 2013;21(8):492–501.
78. Sethi P, Franco WG. The role of superior capsule reconstruction in rotator cuff tears. Orthop Clin North Am. 2018;49(1):93–101.
79. Pennington WT, Bartz BA, Pauli JM, Walker CE, Schmidt W. Arthroscopic superior capsular reconstruction with acellular dermal allograft for the treatment of massive irreparable rotator cuff tears: short-term clinical outcomes and the radiographic parameter of superior capsular distance. Arthroscopy. 2018;18:30033–1. https://doi.org/10.1016/j.arthro.2018.01.009. pii: S0749-8063.
80. Boutsiadis A, Chen S, Jiang C, Lenoir H, Delsol P, Barth J. Long head of the biceps as a suitable available local tissue autograft for superior capsular reconstruction: "The Chinese Way". Arthrosc Tech. 2017;6(5):e1559–66.
81. Hirahara AM, Andersen WJ, Panero AJ. Superior capsular reconstruction: clinical outcomes after minimum 2-year follow-up. Am J Orthop (Belle Mead NJ). 2017;46(6):266–78.
82. Hirahara AM, Adams CR. Arthroscopic superior capsular reconstruction for treatment of massive irreparable rotator cuff tears. Arthrosc Tech. 2015;4(6):e637–41.
83. Deranlot J, Herisson O, Nourissat G, Zbili D, Werthel JD, Vigan M, Bruchou F. Arthroscopic subacromial spacer implantation in patients with massive irreparable rotator cuff tears: clinical and radiographic results of 39 retrospectives cases. Arthroscopy. 2017;33(9):1639–44.

84. Senekovic V, Poberaj B, Kovacic L, Mikek M, Adar E, Markovitz E, Maman E, Dekel A. The biodegradable spacer as a novel treatment modality for massive rotator cuff tears: a prospective study with 5-year follow-up. Arch Orthop Trauma Surg. 2017;137(1):95–103.
85. Savarese E, Romeo R. New solution for massive, irreparable rotator cuff tears: the subacromial "biodegradable spacer". Arthrosc Tech. 2012;1(1):e69–74.
86. Ernstbrunner L, Suter A, Catanzaro S, Rahm S, Gerber C. Reverse total shoulder arthroplasty for massive, irreparable rotator cuff tears before the age of 60 years: long-term results. J Bone Joint Surg Am. 2017;99(20):1721–9.
87. Sevivas N, Ferreira N, Andrade R, Moreira P, Portugal R, Alves D, Vieira da Silva M, Sousa N, Salgado AJ, Espregueira-Mendes J. Reverse shoulder arthroplasty for irreparable massive rotator cuff tears: a systematic review with meta-analysis and meta-regression. J Shoulder Elb Surg. 2017;26(9):e265–77.
88. Sethi PM, Sheth CD, Pauzenberger L, McCarthy MBR, Cote MP, Soneson E, Miller S, Mazzocca AD. Macroscopic rotator cuff tendinopathy and histopathology do not predict repair outcomes of rotator cuff tears. Am J Sports Med. 2018;46(4):779–85.
89. Vap AR, Mannava S, Katthagen JC, Horan MP, Fritz EM, Pogorzelski J, Millett PJ. Five-year outcomes after arthroscopic repair of partial-thickness supraspinatus tears. Arthroscopy. 2018;34(1):75–81.
90. Katthagen JC, Bucci G, Moatshe G, Tahal DS, Millett PJ. Improved outcomes with arthroscopic repair of partial-thickness rotator cuff tears: a systematic review. Knee Surg Sports Traumatol Arthrosc. 2018;26(1):113–24.
91. Katthagen JC, Vap AR, Tahal DS, Horan MP, Millett PJ. Arthroscopic repair of isolated partial- and full-thickness upper third subscapularis tendon tears: minimum 2-year outcomes after single-anchor repair and biceps tenodesis. Arthroscopy. 2017;33(7):1286–93.
92. Raman J, Walton D, MacDermid JC, Athwal GS. Predictors of outcomes after rotator cuff repair-A meta-analysis. J Hand Ther. 2017;30(3):276–92.
93. Kim DH, Elattrache NS, Tibone JE, Jun BJ, DeLaMora SN, Kvitne RS, Lee TQ. Biomechanical comparison of a single-row versus double-row suture anchor technique for rotator cuff repair. Am J Sports Med. 2006;34(3):407–14.
94. Kim YS, Lee HJ, Jin HK, Kim SE, Lee JW. Conventional En Masse repair versus separate double-layer double-row repair for the treatment of delaminated rotator cuff tears. Am J Sports Med. 2016;44(5):1146–52.
95. DeHaan AM, Axelrad TW, Kaye E, Silvestri L, Puskas B, Foster TE. Does double-row rotator cuff repair improve functional outcome of patients compared with single-row technique? A systematic review. Am J Sports Med. 2012;40(5):1176–85.
96. Abdelshahed M, Mahure SA, Kaplan DJ, Mollon B, Zuckerman JD, Kwon YW, Rokito AS. Arthroscopic rotator cuff repair: double-row transosseous equivalent suture bridge technique. Arthrosc Tech. 2016;5(6):e1297–304.
97. Park MC, ElAttrache NS, Tibone JE, Ahmad CS, Jun BJ, Lee TQ. Part I: footprint contact characteristics for a transosseous-equivalent rotator cuff repair technique compared with a double-row repair technique. J Shoulder Elb Surg. 2007;16(4):461–8.
98. Park MC, Tibone JE, ElAttrache NS, Ahmad CS, Jun BJ, Lee TQ. Part II: biomechanical assessment for a footprint-restoring transosseous-equivalent rotator cuff repair technique compared with a double-row repair technique. J Shoulder Elb Surg. 2007;16(4):469–76.
99. Mochizuki T, Nimura A, Miyamoto T, Koga H, Akita K, Muneta T. Repair of rotator cuff tear with delamination: independent repairs of the infraspinatus and articular capsule. Arthrosc Tech. 2016;5(5):e1129–34.
100. Bayle X, Pham TT, Faruch M, Gobet A, Mansat P, Bonnevialle N. No difference in outcome for open versus arthroscopic rotator cuff repair: a prospective comparative trial. Arch Orthop Trauma Surg. 2017;137(12):1707–12.
101. Sun L, Zhang Q, Ge H, Sun Y, Cheng B. Which is the best repair of articular-sided rotator cuff tears: a meta-analysis. J Orthop Surg Res. 2015;10:84. https://doi.org/10.1186/s13018-015-0224-6.

102. Shin SJ. A comparison of 2 repair techniques for partial-thickness articular-sided rotator cuff tears. Arthroscopy. 2012;28(1):25–33.
103. Nottage WM. Editorial commentary: partial (shoulder rotator) cuff repair: may the force (couple) be with you. Arthroscopy. 2017;33(11):1956–7.
104. Boileau P, Baqué F, Valerio L, Ahrens P, Chuinard C, Trojani C. Isolated arthroscopic biceps tenotomy or tenodesis improves symptoms in patients with massive irreparable rotator cuff tears. J Bone Joint Surg Am. 2007;89(4):747–57.
105. Walch G, Edwards TB, Boulahia A, Nové-Josserand L, Neyton L, Szabo I. Arthroscopic tenotomy of the long head of the biceps in the treatment of rotator cuff tears: clinical and radiographic results of 307 cases. J Shoulder Elb Surg. 2005;14(3):238–46.

Chapter 24
Subacromial Bursitis

This is a condition whereby there is acute or chronic inflammation of the subacromial bursa. It may occur in isolation or in association with rotator cuff tendinopathy or rotator cuff tears. The subacromial bursa may exhibit the spectrum of disorders encountered in other body bursae.

24.1 Causes of Subacromial Bursitis [1–19]

- Extrinsic
  - Acute shoulder or upper limb trauma
  - Chronic micro-trauma to the subacromial space (as in subacromial impingement)
- Intrinsic
  - Inflammation—rheumatoid arthritis, seronegative arthritis, gout
  - Non-traumatic rotator cuff tendinopathy, rotator cuff tears
  - Calcific bursitis/tendinopathy
  - Adhesive capsulitis
  - Reactive (such as to foreign body)
- Combination of intrinsic and extrinsic causes

24.2 Differential Diagnosis of Subacromial Bursitis

The following bursa disorders need to be considered and excluded by consideration of relevant clinical findings and appropriate investigations:

© Springer Nature Switzerland AG 2019

C. Panayiotou Charalambous, *The Shoulder Made Easy*,
https://doi.org/10.1007/978-3-319-98908-2_24

- Infection—bacterial, mycobacterial
- Neoplastic—pigmented villo-nodular synovitis, synovial chondromatosis, synovial sarcomas

24.3 Clinical Symptoms of Subacromial Bursitis

- Subacromial pain syndrome
- Arm weakness
- Arm stiffness
- Shoulder swelling [17, 18]
- Shivers/rigours (if infective)

24.4 Clinical Signs of Subacromial Bursitis [17–19]

- Subacromial tenderness
- Subacromial impingement test
- Apparent or true weakness (latter if associated rotator cuff tear)
- Apparent or true stiffness (latter if associated adhesive capsulitis or other inflammatory process)
- Muscle wasting (if associated rotator cuff tears)
- Fullness of the subacromial space
- Pyrexia (if infective)

24.5 Investigations for Subacromial Bursitis [20–22]

- Plain radiographs—calcific deposits in the subacromial space
- MRI scan:
  - High signal areas in the subacromial bursa
  - Associated tendinopathy and rotator cuff tears
  - "Rice bodies"—granular bodies that may be seen in inflammatory arthritis, infective arthritis (tuberculosis) or reactive arthritis
- Haematological—raised white cell count, ESR, CRP (if infective or associated with underlying inflammatory disorder) and uric acid levels
- Subacromial aspirate:
  - Microscopy for crystals
  - Gram stain and culture to determine if infective
- Subacromial bursa biopsy—open or arthroscopic to determine the cause of inflammation and exclude neoplastic causes

24.6 Management of Subacromial Bursitis

This will be guided by its cause as described below:

24.6.1 Extrinsic: Post-Traumatic, Subacromial Impingement

- Analgesia, anti-inflammatories
- Physiotherapy
- Local treatment to reduce the inflammation
- Address dynamic causes of subacromial impingement (scapular dyskinesis, rotator cuff dysfunction)
- Subacromial steroid injection
- Surgery – Arthroscopic bursectomy +/−acromioplasty +/− repair of associated rotator cuff tears

24.6.2 Intrinsic

- Analgesia, anti-inflammatories
- Physiotherapy
- Subacromial steroid injection
- Disease-modifying drugs (for underlying inflammatory disorder)
- Surgery—arthroscopic bursectomy +/− acromioplasty+/− repair of associated rotator cuff tears+/− calcific deposit excision

Learning Pearls

- It is not usually possible to distinguish between isolated subacromial bursitis, rotator cuff tendinopathy or small rotator cuff tears simply based on clinical findings
- Although adhesive capsulitis is thought to affect predominantly the glenohumeral joint in many cases of arthroscopic surgery for this condition, the bursa is found to be inflamed and thickened, suggesting a wider involvement of the shoulder's soft tissues
- Subacromial calcific deposits are usually located within the rotator cuff tendons, but on occasions they may be found in the subacromial bursa

References

1. Caldwell GA, Unkauf BM. Results of treatment of subacromial bursitis in three hundred forty cases. Ann Surg. 1950;132(3):432–42.
2. Blaine TA, Kim YS, Voloshin I, Chen D, Murakami K, Chang SS, Winchester R, Lee FY, O'keefe RJ, Bigliani LU. The molecular pathophysiology of subacromial bursitis in rotator cuff disease. J Shoulder Elbow Surg. 2005;14(1 Suppl S):84S–9S.
3. Voloshin I, Gelinas J, Maloney MD, O'Keefe RJ, Bigliani LU, Blaine TA. Proinflammatory cytokines and metalloproteases are expressed in the subacromial bursa in patients with rotator cuff disease. Arthroscopy. 2005;21(9):1076.e1–9.
4. Gotoh M, Hamada K, Yamakawa H, Inoue A, Fukuda H. Increased substance P in subacromial bursa and shoulder pain in rotator cuff diseases. J Orthop Res. 1998;16(5):618–21.
5. Ishii H, Brunet JA, Welsh RP, Uhthoff HK. "Bursal reactions" in rotator cuff tearing, the impingement syndrome, and calcifying tendinitis. J Shoulder Elbow Surg. 1997;6(2):131–6.
6. Subramaniam R, Tan JW, Chau CY, Lee KT. Subacromial bursitis with giant rice bodies as initial presentation of rheumatoid arthritis. J Clin Rheumatol. 2012;18(7):352–5.
7. Thevenon A, Cocheteux P, Duquesnoy B, Mestdagh H, Lecomte-Houcke M, Delcambre B. Subacromial bursitis with rice bodies as a presenting feature of seronegative rheumatoid arthritis. Arthritis Rheum. 1987;30(6):715–6.
8. Kang BS, Lee SH, Cho Y, Chung SG. Acute calcific bursitis after ultrasound-guided percutaneous barbotage of rotator cuff calcific tendinopathy: a case report. PM R. 2016;8(8):808–12.
9. Hayeri MR, Keefe DT, Chang EY. Suture slippage in knotless suture anchors resulting in subacromial-subdeltoid bursitis. Skeletal Radiol. 2016;45(5):703–6.
10. Urruela AM, Rapp TB, Egol KA. Massive subacromial-subdeltoid bursitis with rice bodies secondary to an orthopedic implant. Am J Orthop (Belle Mead NJ). 2012;41(9):418–21.
11. Uchida S, Sakai A, Nakamura T. Subacromial bursitis following human papilloma virus vaccine misinjection. Vaccine. 2012;31(1):27–30.
12. Lho YM, Ha E, Cho CH, Song KS, Min BW, Bae KC, Lee KJ, Hwang I, Park HB. Inflammatory cytokines are overexpressed in the subacromial bursa of frozen shoulder. J Shoulder Elbow Surg. 2013;22(5):666–72.
13. Sinha R, Tuckett J, Hide G, Dildey P, Karsandas A. Mycobacterium avium-intracellular: a rare cause of subacromial bursitis. Skeletal Radiol. 2015;44(1):143–6.
14. Mathew SD, Tully CC, Borra H, Berven MD, Arroyo R. Septic subacromial bursitis caused by Mycobacterium kansasii in an immunocompromised host. Mil Med. 2012;177(5):617–20.
15. Pookarnjanamorakot C, Sirikulchayanonta V. Tuberculous bursitis of the subacromial bursa. J Shoulder Elbow Surg. 2004;13(1):105–7.
16. Guido FR. Acute calcified subacromial or subdeltoid bursitis. Cal West Med. 1944;60(2):69–72.
17. Huston KA, Nelson AM, Hunder GG. Shoulder swelling in rheumatoid arthritis secondary to subacromial bursitis. Arthritis Rheum. 1978;21(1):145–7.
18. Yoneda M, Wakitani S, Yamamoto T. Huge tumor-like subacromial bursitis associated with rheumatoid arthritis. Mod Rheumatol. 2001;11(3):255–8.
19. Charalambous CP. Clinical examination of the shoulder. In: Charalambous CP, editor. The shoulder made easy. Springer; 2019. pp. 77–122.
20. Law TC, Chong SF, Lu PP, Mak KH. Bilateral subacromial bursitis with macroscopic rice bodies: ultrasound, CT and MR appearance. Australas Radiol. 1998;42(2):161–3.
21. Griffith JF, Peh WC, Evans NS, Smallman LA, Wong RW, Thomas AM. Multiple rice body formation in chronic subacromial/subdeltoid bursitis: MR appearances. Clin Radiol. 1996;51(7):511–4.
22. Chen A, Wong LY, Sheu CY, Chen BF. Distinguishing multiple rice body formation in chronic subacromial-subdeltoid bursitis from synovial chondromatosis. Skeletal Radiol. 2002;31(2):119–21.
23. Madruga Dias J, Costa MM, Duarte A, Pereira da Silva JA. Localized Pigmented Villonodular Synovitis of the shoulder: a rare presentation of an uncommon pathology. Acta Med Port. 2013;26(4):459–62.

Chapter 25
Os Acromiale

The acromion is formed from multiple ossification centres which fuse between the age of 12 and 25 years. If one of the ossification centres fails to fuse, an accessory ossicle is formed known as os-acromiale. The os-acromiale is named according to the fragment located anterior to the unfused site [1–3]. Hence, three types of os-acromiale are described known as the:

- Pre-acromion
- Meso-acromion
- Met-acromion

25.1 Demographics of Os-Acromiale [3–5]

- Incidence amongst the general population is 1–15%
- Bilateral in 1/3 to 2/3 of cases
- Meso-acromion is the most common

© Springer Nature Switzerland AG 2019

C. Panayiotou Charalambous, *The Shoulder Made Easy*,
https://doi.org/10.1007/978-3-319-98908-2_25

Os-acromiale (top and side views) (a) pre-acromion, (b) meso-acromion, (c) met-acromion

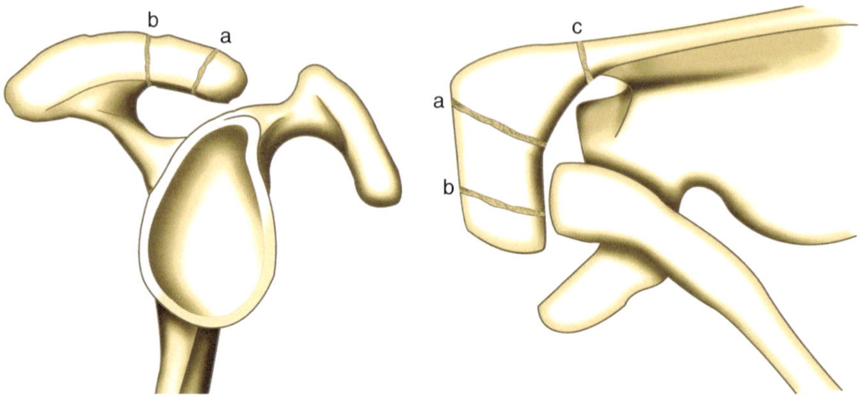

25.2 Clinical Symptoms of Os-Acromiale

- Asymptomatic – often discovered as an incidental finding on radiological imaging of the shoulder
- Pain:
  - Due to subacromial impingement caused by the mobile os-acromiale fragment [6, 7]
  - At the site of non-fusion due to inflammation caused by abnormal movement of the unfused segments [8]
- Clicking
- Weakness – excessive motion of the os-acromiale may predispose to rotator cuff tears [9]

25.3 Clinical Signs of Os-Acromiale

- Acromial or subacromial tenderness
- Subacromial impingement test
- Rotator cuff weakness if associated tears

25.4 Investigations for Os-Acromiale

- Plain radiographs:
  - Anterior-posterior view

    Double density sign suggestive of os-acromiale [10]
  - Axillary view, scapular Y view

    Confirm the presence of os-acromiale
    Define its location
- CT
  - Confirm the presence of os-acromiale
  - Further characterise the size and shape of the os-acromiale in planning surgery
- MRI
  - To identify any associated soft tissue lesions such as rotator cuff tears

Anteroposterior plain radiograph shows double sign (yellow arrow) of the acromion. Axillary view demonstrates an os-acromiale (red arrow)

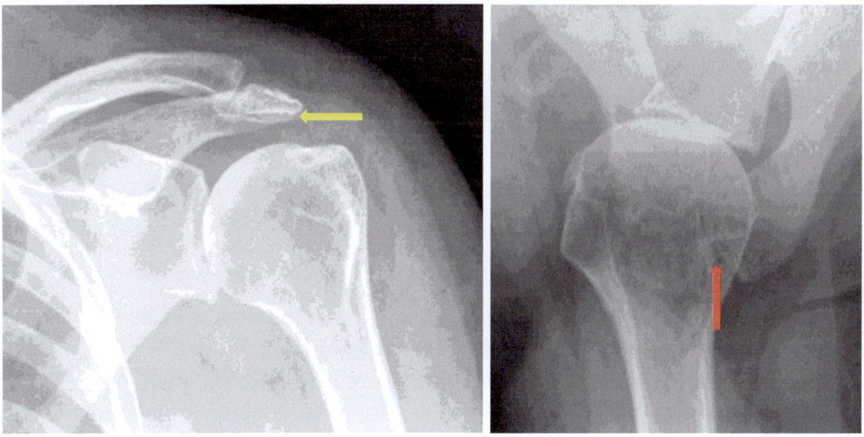

Plain radiograph (axillary view) (a) and CT scan (axial view) (b) showing os-acromiale (red arrows)

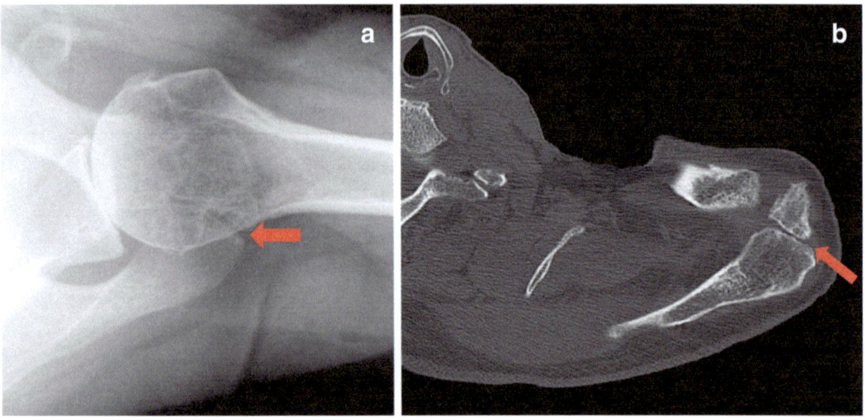

25.5 Management of Os-Acromiale

Nonsurgical

- Leave alone
- Analgesia, anti-inflammatories, local treatment
- Rest, activity modification
- Physiotherapy – eccentric loading to address rotator cuff tendinopathy
- Steroid injections:
  - Subacromial
  - Non-fusion site

Surgical [11–18]

- Arthroscopic subacromial decompression – to thin the os-acromiale fragment
- Arthroscopic or open os-acromiale fragment excision
- Open reduction internal fixation of the os-acromiale fragment plus bone grafting (from acromion, iliac crest, greater tuberosity). Fixation may be achieved with:
  - Tension band wiring
  - Sutures
  - Screws

Os-acromiale fixation (top and side views)

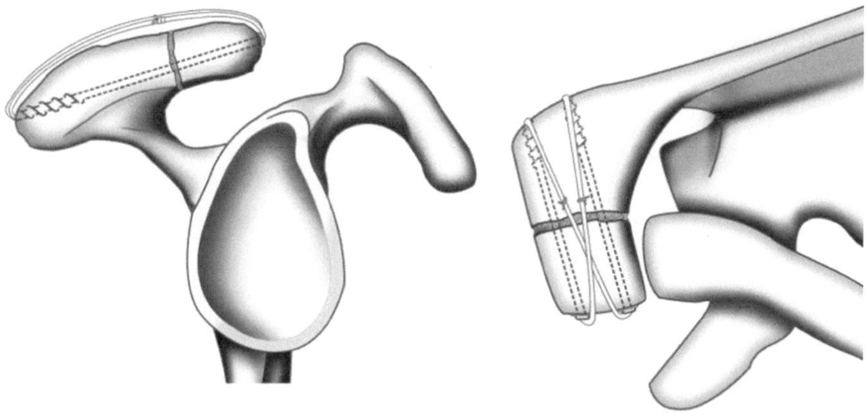

There is controversy as to the exact surgical management of the os-acromiale, with good results reported for surgical excision of small fragments as well as surgical fixation of larger fragments. Surgical excision provides definite removal of the pathological lesion, and the outcome does not rely on bone union. The disadvantage of excision is that, with larger fragments, a substantial part of the deltoid attachment may be lost leading to deltoid dysfunction. Surgical fixation preserves the deltoid attachment, but it is associated with a high rate of non-union as well as pain related to the hardware inserted for the surgical fixation of the os-acromiale. The following may be considered as guidance:

- Pre-acromion—excise
- Meso-acromion—excise or fuse
- Met-acromion—fuse

Excision may lead to deltoid weakness; hence if it is a large fragment, an attempt should be made to save the fragment.

Learning Pearls

- The acromio-clavicular joint stabilises a meso-acromion. Therefore, excision of the distal clavicle could further destabilise the os-acromiale
- If a large fragment is excised, the deltoid attachment must be repaired back to bone to avoid deltoid dysfunction and arm weakness

References

1. Edelson JG, Zuckerman J, Hershkovitz I. Os acromiale: anatomy and surgical implications. J Bone Joint Surg (Br). 1993;75(4):551–5.
2. Kurtz CA, Humble BJ, Rodosky MW, Sekiya JK. Symptomatic os acromiale. J Am Acad Orthop Surg. 2006;14(1):12–9.
3. Sammarco VJ. Os acromiale: frequency, anatomy, and clinical implications. J Bone Joint Surg Am. 2000;82(3):394–400.
4. Yammine K. The prevalence of Os acromiale: a systematic review and meta-analysis. Clin Anat. 2014;27(4):610–21.
5. Rovesta C, Marongiu MC, Corradini A, Torricelli P, Ligabue G. Os acromiale: frequency and a review of 726 shoulder MRI. Musculoskelet Surg. 2017;101(3):201–5.
6. Buss DD, Freehill MQ, Marra G. Typical and atypical shoulder impingement syndrome: diagnosis, treatment, and pitfalls. Instr Course Lect. 2009;58:447–57.
7. Park JG, Lee JK, Phelps CT. Os acromiale associated with rotator cuff impingement: MR imaging of the shoulder. Radiology. 1994;193(1):255–7.
8. Barbier O, Block D, Dezaly C, Sirveaux F, Mole D. Os acromiale, a cause of shoulder pain, not to be overlooked. Orthop Traumatol Surg Res. 2013;99(4):465–72.
9. Ouellette H, Thomas BJ, Kassarjian A, Fritz B, Tétreault P, Palmer WE, Torriani M. Re-examining the association of os acromiale with supraspinatus and infraspinatus tears. Skelet Radiol. 2007;36(9):835–9.
10. Lee DH, Lee KH, Lopez-Ben R, Bradley EL. The double-density sign: a radiographic finding suggestive of an os acromiale. J Bone Joint Surg Am. 2004;86-A(12):2666–70.
11. Harris JD, Griesser MJ, Jones GL. Systematic review of the surgical treatment for symptomatic os acromiale. Int J Shoulder Surg. 2011;5(1):9–16.
12. Hutchinson MR, Veenstra MA. Arthroscopic decompression of shoulder impingement secondary to Os acromiale. Arthroscopy. 1993;9(1):28–32.
13. Wright RW, Heller MA, Quick DC, Buss DD. Arthroscopic decompression for impingement syndrome secondary to an unstable os acromiale. Arthroscopy. 2000;16(6):595–9.
14. Campbell PT, Nizlan NM, Skirving AP. Arthroscopic excision of os acromiale: effects on deltoid function and strength. Orthopedics. 2012;35(11):e1601–5.
15. Abboud JA, Silverberg D, Pepe M, Beredjiklian PK, Iannotti JP, Williams GR, Ramsey ML. Surgical treatment of os acromiale with and without associated rotator cuff tears. J Shoulder Elb Surg. 2006;15(3):265–70.
16. Peckett WR, Gunther SB, Harper GD, Hughes JS, Sonnabend DH. Internal fixation of symptomatic os acromiale: a series of twenty-six cases. J Shoulder Elb Surg. 2004;13(4):381–5.
17. Atoun E, van Tongel A, Narvani A, Rath E, Sforza G, Levy O. Arthroscopically assisted internal fixation of the symptomatic unstable os acromiale with absorbable screws. J Shoulder Elb Surg. 2012;21(12):1740–5.
18. Spiegl UJ, Smith SD, Todd JN, Wijdicks CA, Millett PJ. Biomechanical evaluation of internal fixation techniques for unstable meso-type os acromiale. J Shoulder Elb Surg. 2015;24(4):520–6.

Chapter 26
Long Head of the Biceps Tendon Disease

Long head of the biceps (LHB) tendon disease may be considered as a spectrum of disorders ranging from tenosynovitis to tendinopathy to partial tears or total rupture. The LHB tendon may also show instability in relation to the bicipital groove [1–4].

26.1 Long Head of the Biceps Tendon Pathology

- *Tenosynovitis*—synovial inflammation, increased vascularity and fluid around the tendon, adhesions of the tendon to the groove
- *Tendinopathy*—acute tendon inflammation or chronic degeneration
- *Biceps tear*—tear of the LHB tendon. This may be:
  - Partial
  - Complete

The LHB tendon is a tubular tendon, almost looking like a string. A tear may be described in terms of the extent of tendon involvement:

- Length
- Cross-sectional area

© Springer Nature Switzerland AG 2019

C. Panayiotou Charalambous, *The Shoulder Made Easy*,
https://doi.org/10.1007/978-3-319-98908-2_26

In tendinopathy the tendon may appear macroscopically:

- Normal/smooth or degenerate, frayed, delaminated
- Tubular or flattened and thickened. An hour-glass deformity may develop, whereby the intra-articular part of the tendon hypertrophies and cannot slide in the bicipital groove with arm motion. Hence, on arm elevation the tendon may buckle and get caught between the humeral head and glenoid

Intra-articular part of the long head of the biceps tendon – (a, b) intact, (c, d) frayed and degenerate

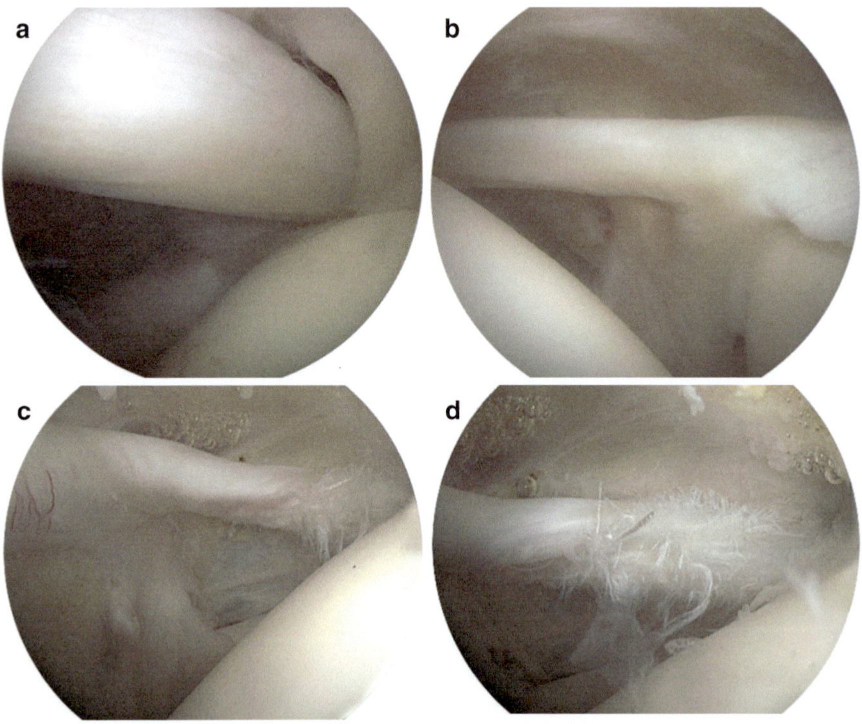

In tendinopathy the tendon may microscopically show [5, 6]:

- Inflammatory cell infiltration—acute or chronic
- Degenerative changes—tenocyte enlargement and proliferation, myxoid changes

Insertion of the long and short heads of biceps tendons. Note the close relation of the long head tendon to the subacromial space

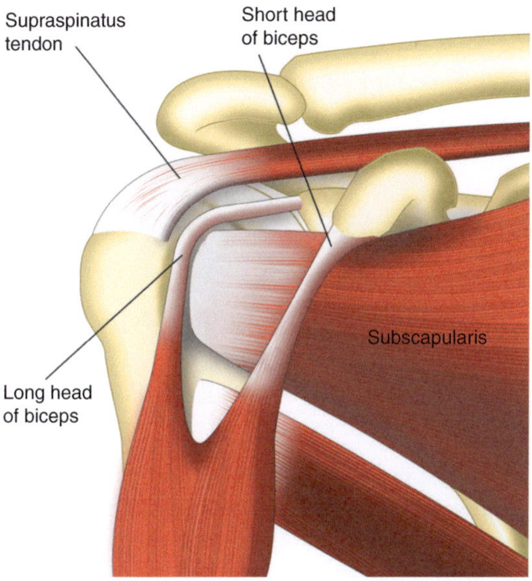

26.1.1 LHB Tendon Instability

This is a condition whereby the LHB tendon moves out of its normal position in the bicipital groove due to disruption of the structures which maintain this position.

The LHB tendon may:

- Sublux—whereby there is partial loss of conduct between the tendon and the groove
- Dislocate—whereby there is complete loss of conduct between the tendon and the groove

LHB tendon displacement may be:

- Static (whereby the tendon does not return back into the groove)
- Dynamic (whereby the tendon flips in and out of the groove as the arm rotates)

26.2 Causes of Long Head of Biceps Tendon Disease

LHB tendinopathy and instability may be:

- Primary
  - Chronic overuse or overloading (swimmers, throwing athletes)
  - Degenerative

- Secondary
  - Traumatic
  - Inflammatory
  - Associated with rotator cuff tears
  - Associated with Superior labrum anterior posterior (SLAP) tears
  - Impingement
    - Subacromial
    - Osteoarthritic spurs in the bicipital groove
    - Bony exostoses from proximal humerus

26.3 Demographics of Long Head of Biceps Tendon Disease

Primary LHB tendon lesions account for less than 5% of cases with the vast majority being secondary to an extrinsic cause:

- Gill et al. [7] reported a prevalence of 5% of partial tears of the LHB tendon in 847 shoulder arthroscopies with 85% of these associated with rotator cuff tears
- Chen et al. [8] looked at 176 cases of complete rotator cuff tears having surgery and reported the following LHB tendon lesions:
  - 33% tendinopathy
  - 11% subluxation
  - 9% dislocation
  - 16% partial tear
  - 7% complete rupture
  - 6% SLAP tears

A cadaveric study [9] found that degenerative changes in the LHB tendon involve mainly the distal part of the bicipital groove or the proximal part of the tendon close to its insertion on the superior part of the glenoid labrum. Hence, these are the sites most often subjected to tendon rupture.

26.4 Clinical Symptoms of Long Head of Biceps Tendon Disease

- Pain
  - In the anterior part of the shoulder, often in the bicipital groove which may be aggravated by rotation of the shoulder. The pain may radiate down the arm and the biceps muscle belly and may be associated with paraesthesia
  - Deep seated in the glenohumeral joint in cases of LHB tendon instability secondary to a rotator cuff tear
- Palpable or audible snap may be present in LHB tendon instability
- In LHB total rupture, the patient may describe an audible or painful snap occurring at the time of rupture. This may be followed by relief of the chronic pain that had been experienced up to that point due to LHB tendinopathy

Partial continuity of a tubular tendon (equivalent to a rope) (b) may allow function similar to the intact tendon (a) until the tendon completely snaps (c)

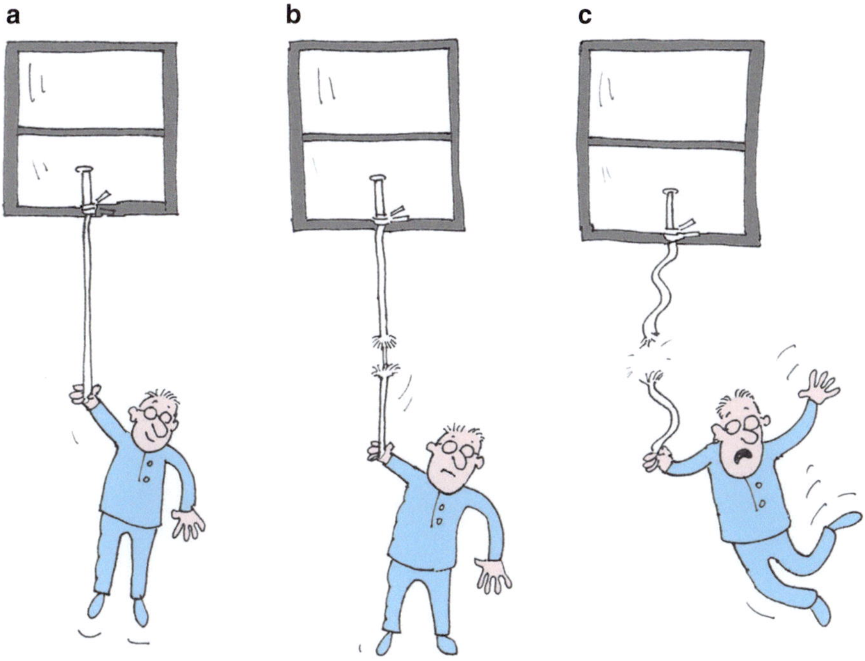

26.5 Clinical Signs of Long Head of Biceps Tendon Disease [10]

These will depend on the underlying pathology and include:

- Tenderness in the bicipital groove. Palpation of the bicipital groove is most easily done with the arm on the side, in 10° of internal rotation, because in this position the bicipital groove faces forwards. External rotation puts the bicipital groove in a more posterior-lateral position. If the arm is taken from external to internal rotation whilst palpating the bicipital groove, the biceps tendon may be felt rolling under the examiner's fingers
- Palpable subluxation of the LHB tendon from the bicipital groove with passive internal and external ration of the arm
- Clinical deformity:
  - Partial tears may lead to pain, but, as there is continuity of part of the tendon, there is no clinical deformity
  - Complete tears may lead to acute bruising in the anterior aspect of the shoulder and a muscle bulge in the lower part of the arm (distal Popeye sign) as the muscle belly retracts distally. However, degenerate LHB tendons are often flattened and thickened; hence, it is possible that upon rupture the LHB

tendon gets stuck in the bicipital groove where it subsequently heals without causing a Popeye sign

Long head of the biceps tendon—(a) intact, (b) divided and reattached (tenodesis) surgically to the humeral head under tension, (c) divided and reattached (tenodesis) surgically to the bicipital groove under tension, (d) spontaneously ruptured or surgically divided and self-attached to the bicipital groove (auto-tenodesis) with loss of tension (giving a Popeye sign), (e) spontaneously ruptured or surgically divided and retracts distally without reattaching with loss of tension (giving a Popeye sign)

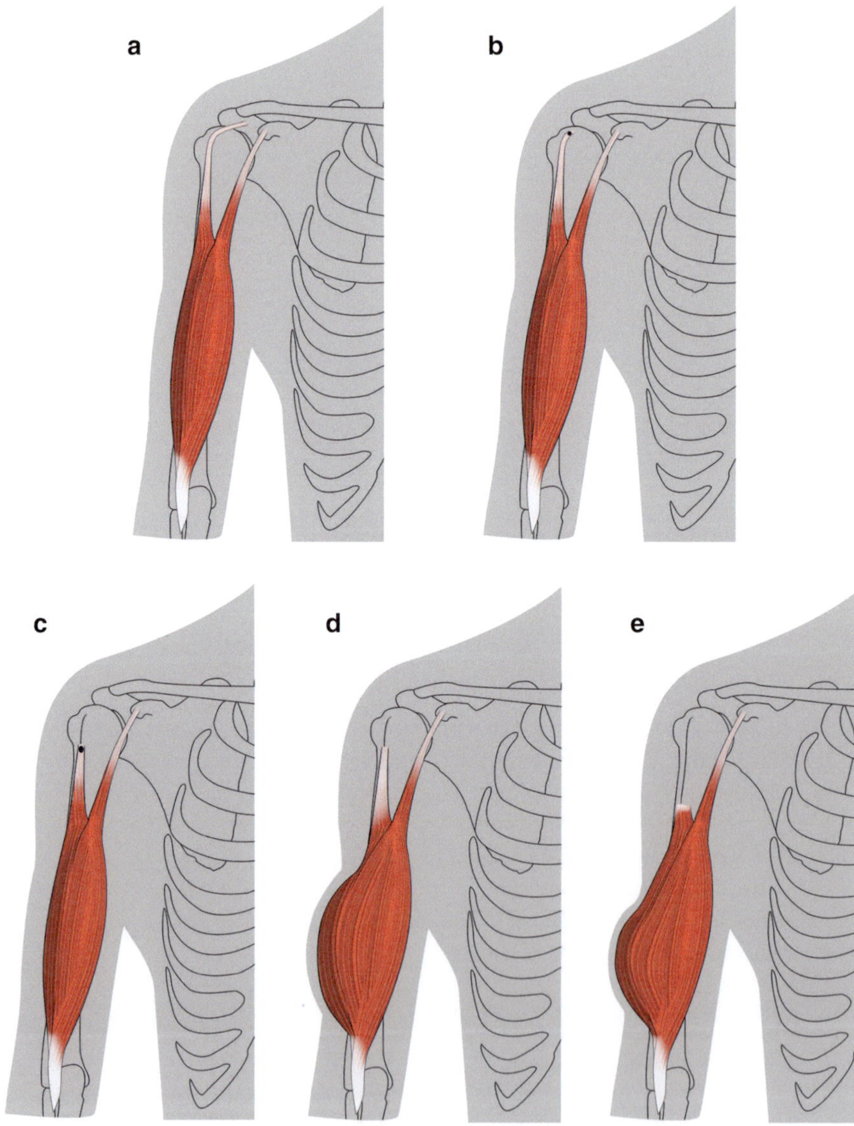

Rupture of the long head of the biceps tendon with distal migration of the muscle belly (distal Popeye sign)

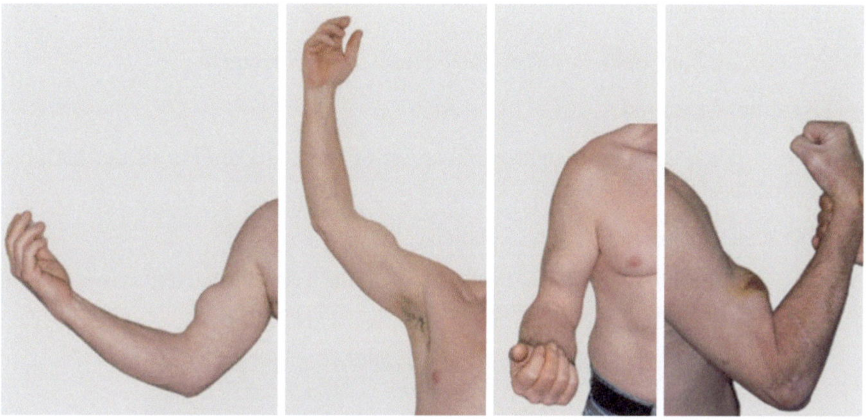

Distal biceps tendon rupture left arm with proximal migration of the muscle belly (proximal Popeye sign)

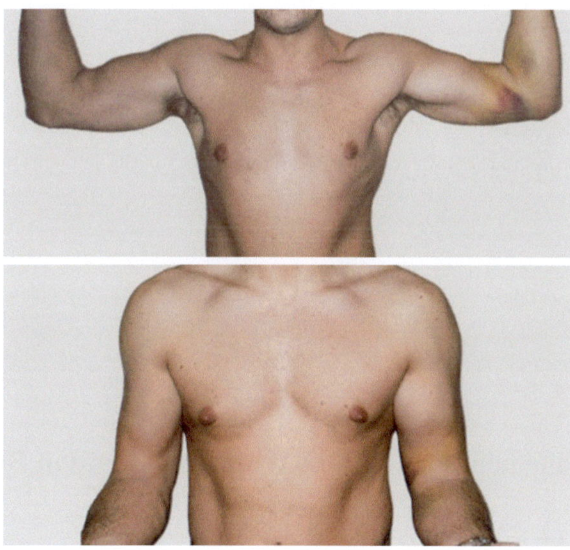

- Positive Speed's test
- Positive Yergason's test

Dislocation of the LHB tendon is usually associated with a tear of the upper part of the subscapularis tendon or the supraspinatus tendon [11–13]. LHB instability is more common in an anterior direction but may also occur in a posterior or combined anterior/posterior direction. Anterior instability is associated with a subscapularis tear and posterior instability with a supraspinatus tear.

26.6 Investigations for Long Head of Biceps Tendon Disease

- Plain radiographs
  - Look for bony spurs or other bony causes of impingement
- Dynamic ultrasound
  - May demonstrate transient subluxation of the LHB tendon in the bicipital groove with arm motion
- MRI scan—the investigation of choice

MRI showing anterior dislocation of the long head of the biceps tendon (red arrow) leaving an empty bicipital groove (yellow arrow)

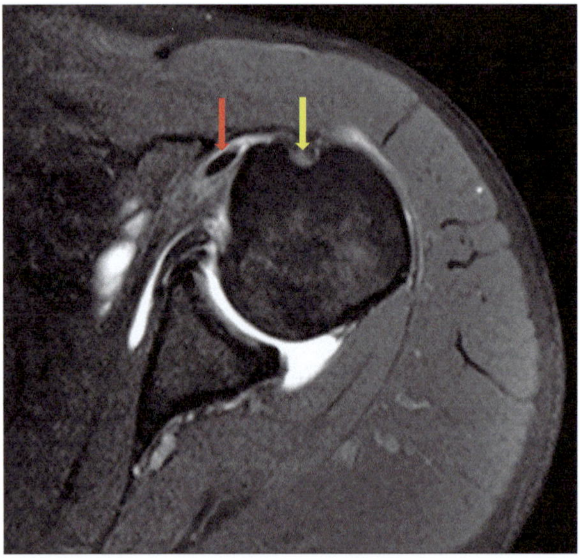

26.7 Management of Long Head of Biceps Tendon Disease

Non-surgical [14, 15]

- Leave alone
- Analgesia, anti-inflammatories, local treatment
- Rest, activity modification
- Physiotherapy—eccentric loading
- Steroid injections:
  - Subacromial—does not reach the bicipital groove if intact rotator cuff
  - Glenohumeral—communicates with the bicipital groove
  - Bicipital groove—better performed under ultrasound guidance to improve accuracy and avoid injection into the LHB tendon

Surgical [16–21]

- LHB tendon debridement
- Acromioplasty, coracoplasty
- Tenotomy
- Tenodesis
- Repair of SLAP lesions

26.7.1 Tenotomy

This is division of the LHB tendon with the stump left free to retract into the arm. This may be performed arthroscopically or via an open approach. Ultrasound-guided percutaneous LHB tenotomy has also been described.

26.7.2 Tenodesis

This is division of the LHB tendon and fixation of the tendon stump into the bone (humerus) to maintain a proximal attachment of the LHB tendon (thus keeping the biceps muscle under tension). Fixation of the tendon stump may be achieved with:

- Suture anchors
- Interference screws
- Suture to adjacent soft tissue such as the pectoralis major tendon (soft tissue tenodesis)

The location of tenodesis may be:

1. Supra-bicipital—tendon is sutured to the humeral head
2. Bicipital—tendon sutured into the groove
3. Subpectoral—tendon sutured distal to the groove, deep to the insertion of the pectoralis major tendon

The choice of location of tenodesis may be guided by the site of LHB tendon disease:

- Symptoms originating from the intra-articular part—tenodesis to the humeral head
- Symptoms originating from the bicipital groove—subpectoral tenodesis with excision of the diseased tendon segment

26.7.3 Tenodesis vs. Tenotomy [22–25]

In the surgical treatment of LHB tendon disease, it is essential to consider the pros and cons of tenotomy and tenodesis, and these are described next.

26.7.3.1 Tenotomy

Some patients who complain of shoulder pain may notice that their pain improves following spontaneous rupture of the LHB tendon which suggests a role for surgical tenotomy as a pain management procedure.

Pros:

- Faster to perform
- Easier postsurgical rehabilitation
- Less costly (does not require fixation implants such as suture anchors or interference screws)
- Good reported outcomes with minimal functional loss

Cons:

- Higher reported incidence of arm cramp/fatigue pain involving the belly of the biceps muscle
- May lead to cosmetic deformity of the arm (Popeye sign) as the biceps stump migrates distally. It should be noted however that tenotomy does not always lead to a Popeye sign due to the auto-tenodesis phenomenon whereby the tendon adheres and fixes itself to the bicipital groove under tension [23]. Nevertheless, if auto-tenodesis occurs with the tendon in a slack position, this can still give rise to a Popeye sign
- Loss of elbow strength—about 20% of forearm supination and about 8% of elbow flexion strength loss has been reported [24]—loss in these parameters may, however, may be similar in tenotomy and tenodesis cases [22]

It is important to discuss these complications with an individual as some patients may highly value their biceps (including its cosmetic appearance), and they may be reluctant to risk its loss.

26.7.3.2 Tenodesis

Pros:

- Minimises cosmetic deformity
- Preserves the length-tension relationship of the muscle
- Associated with lower incidence of cramp pain

Cons:

- Longer surgical time
- More costly
- Higher risk of complications due to a more extensive surgical procedure

Learning Pearls

- Rotator cuff tears are associated with LHB tendon disease. Hence, successful rotator cuff surgery may be influenced by whether simultaneous LHB tendon lesions are addressed
- Intra-articular tenodesis (proximal to the bicipital groove) may lead to residual postoperative pain due to persistent tenosynovitis within the biceps sheath or lesions of the extra-articular part of the tendon not visible on arthroscopy [26]. Hence, the location of surgical tenodesis must be considered based on the possible site of tendon disease
- If a tenotomy is performed, the residual tendon stump could cause ongoing symptoms, especially if it undergoes auto-tenodesis in the bicipital groove. This must be considered in the evaluation of postsurgical tenotomy residual pain
- Congenital variants of the LHB tendon may exist (congenital absence, bifurcate), and these must be distinguished from pathological conditions
- The macroscopic appearance of the tendon may not accurately reflect the underlying tendinopathy [27]

References

1. Ahrens PM, Boileau P. The long head of biceps and associated tendinopathy. J Bone Joint Surg Br. 2007;89(8):1001.
2. Boileau P, Ahrens PM, Hatzidakis AM. Entrapment of the long head of the biceps tendon: the hourglass biceps—a cause of pain and locking of the shoulder. J Shoulder Elbow Surg. 2004;13(3):249–5.
3. Nuelle CW, Stokes DC, Kuroki K, Crim JR, Sherman SL. Radiologic and histologic evaluation of proximal bicep pathology in patients with chronic biceps tendinopathy undergoing open subpectoral biceps tenodesis. Arthroscopy. 2018;34:1790. https://doi.org/10.1016/j.arthro.2018.01.021.
4. Mellano CR, Shin JJ, Yanke AB, Verma NN. Disorders of the long head of the biceps tendon. Instr Course Lect. 2015;64:567–76.
5. Joseph M, Maresh CM, McCarthy MB, Kraemer WJ, Ledgard F, Arciero CL, Anderson JM, Nindl BC, Mazzocca AD. Histological and molecular analysis of the biceps tendon long head post-tenotomy. J Orthop Res. 2009;27(10):1379–85.
6. Mazzocca AD, McCarthy MB, Ledgard FA, Chowaniec DM, McKinnon WJ Jr, Delaronde S, Rubino LJ, Apolostakos J, Romeo AA, Arciero RA, Beitzel K. Histomorphologic changes of the long head of the biceps tendon in common shoulder pathologies. Arthroscopy. 2013;29(6):972–81.
7. Gill HS, El Rassi G, Bahk MS, Castillo RC, McFarland EG. Physical examination for partial tears of the biceps tendon. Am J Sports Med. 2007;35(8):1334–40.
8. Chen CH, Chen CH, Chang CH, Su CI, Wang KC, Wang IC, Liu HT, Yu CM, Hsu KY. Classification and analysis of pathology of the long head of the biceps tendon in complete rotator cuff tears. Chang Gung Med J. 2012;35(3):263–70.
9. Refior HJ, Sowa D. Long tendon of the biceps brachii: sites of predilection for degenerative lesions. J Shoulder Elbow Surg. 1995;4:436–40.

10. Charalambous CP. Clinical examination of the shoulder. In: Charalambous CP, editor. The shoulder made easy. Basel: Springer; 2019.
11. Braun S, Horan MP, Elser F, Millett PJ. Lesions of the biceps pulley. Am J Sports Med. 2011;39(4):790–5.
12. Walch G, Nové-Josserand L, Boileau P, Levigne C. Subluxations and dislocations of the tendon of the long head of the biceps. J Shoulder Elbow Surg. 1998;7(2):100–8.
13. Slätis P, Aalto K. Medial dislocation of the tendon of the long head of the biceps brachii. Acta Orthop Scand. 1979;50(1):73–7.
14. Wilk KE, Hooks TR. The painful long head of the biceps brachii: nonoperative treatment approaches. Clin Sports Med. 2016;35(1):75–92.
15. Messina C, Banfi G, Orlandi D, Lacelli F, Serafini G, Mauri G, Secchi F, Silvestri E, Sconfienza LM. Ultrasound-guided interventional procedures around the shoulder. Br J Radiol. 2016;89(1057):20150372. https://doi.org/10.1259/bjr.20150372.
16. Crenshaw AH, Kilgore WE. Surgical treatment of bicipital tenosynovitis. J Bone Joint Surg Am. 1966;48(8):1496–502.
17. Levy DM, Meyer ZI, Campbell KA, Bach BR Jr. Subpectoral biceps tenodesis. Am J Orthop. 2016;45(2):68–74.
18. Schoch C, Geyer M, Drews B. Suprapectoral biceps tenodesis using a suture plate: clinical results after 2 years. Arch Orthop Trauma Surg. 2017;137(6):829–35.
19. Werner BC, Brockmeier SF, Gwathmey FW. Trends in long head biceps tenodesis. Am J Sports Med. 2015;43(3):570–8.
20. Ge H, Zhang Q, Sun Y, Li J, Sun L, Cheng B. Tenotomy or tenodesis for the long head of biceps lesions in shoulders: a systematic review and meta-analysis. PLoS One. 2015;10(3):e0121286. https://doi.org/10.1371/journal.pone.
21. Boileau P, Baqué F, Valerio L, Ahrens P, Chuinard C, Trojani C. Isolated arthroscopic biceps tenotomy or tenodesis improves symptoms in patients with massive irreparable rotator cuff tears. J Bone Joint Surg Am. 2007;89(4):747–57.
22. Shank JR, Singleton SB, Braun S, Kissenberth MJ, Ramappa A, Ellis H, Decker MJ, Hawkins RJ, Torry MR. A comparison of forearm supination and elbow flexion strength in patients with long head of the biceps tenotomy or tenodesis. Arthroscopy. 2011;27(1):9–16.
23. Karataglis D, Papadopoulos P, Boutsiadis A, Fotiadou A, Ditsios K, Hatzokos I, Christodoulou A. Ultrasound evaluation of the distal migration of the long head of biceps tendon following tenotomy in patients undergoing arthroscopic repair of tears of the rotator cuff. J Bone Joint Surg Br. 2012;94(11):1534–9.
24. Mariani EM, Cofield RH, Askew LJ, Li GP, Chao EY. Rupture of the tendon of the long head of the biceps brachii. Surgical versus nonsurgical treatment. Clin Orthop Relat Res. 1988;228:233–9.
25. Gurnani N, van Deurzen DF, Janmaat VT, van den Bekerom MP. Tenotomy or tenodesis for pathology of the long head of the biceps brachii: a systematic review and meta-analysis. Knee Surg Sports Traumatol Arthrosc. 2016;24(12):3765–71.
26. Saithna A, Longo A, Leiter J, Old J, MacDonald PM. Shoulder arthroscopy does not adequately visualize pathology of the long head of biceps tendon. Orthop J Sports Med. 2016;4(1):2325967115623944. https://doi.org/10.1177/2325967115623944.
27. Wu PT, Jou IM, Yang CC, Lin CJ, Yang CY, Su FC, Su WR. The severity of the long head biceps tendinopathy in patients with chronic rotator cuff tears: macroscopic versus microscopic results. J Shoulder Elbow Surg. 2014;23(8):1099–106.

Chapter 27
Superior Labrum Tears of the Shoulder

It is a condition whereby the superior labrum and its associated long head of the biceps (LHB) tendon insertion detach from the glenoid. Such lesions of the superior part of the labrum may extend anterior and posterior to the biceps tendon insertion, hence their designation as SLAP (superior labrum anterior and posterior) tears [1–7].

27.1 Causes of Superior Labrum Tears

- Traumatic
  - Fall on the outer-stretched arm that forces the humeral head upwards against the superior labrum
  - Pull on the arm (traction injury)
  - Direct force on the abducted shoulder
- Chronic degeneration
  - Repetitive loading
  - Overhead throwing sports
  - Overhead work related activities

Burkhart and Morgan [3] suggested that superior labrum tears may also occur when the biceps insertion is twisted as the arm is brought into abduction and external rotation (peel back mechanism).

© Springer Nature Switzerland AG 2019

C. Panayiotou Charalambous, *The Shoulder Made Easy*,
https://doi.org/10.1007/978-3-319-98908-2_27

27.2 Classification of Superior Labrum Tears

Four types were initially described by Snyder [1, 2] as below:

Type 1—degenerative fraying with no detachment of the LHB tendon insertion

Type 2—detachment of the LHB tendon insertion

Type 3—bucket handle tear of the superior part of the labrum with an intact LHB tendon insertion to the bone

Type 4—intra-substance tear of the LHB tendon with a bucket handle tear of the superior part of the labrum

Types of SLAP tears. In type 2 tear the detached labrum may stay in situ on top of the glenoid (2a), or may fall in front of the glenoid covering the superior part of the glenoid face (beret like appearance) (2b)

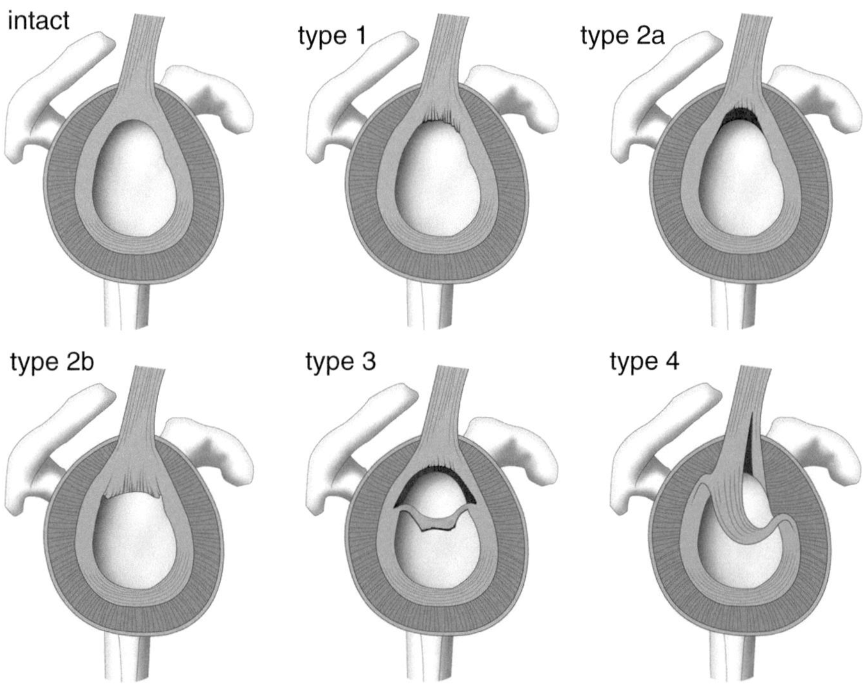

However, since the initial description by Snyder, several other subtypes have been described, some based on whether the superior labrum tear extends to involve the anterior or posterior part of the labrum or both.

Type 2 SLAP tear, with detachment, more evident on probing. Labrum stays on top of the glenoid

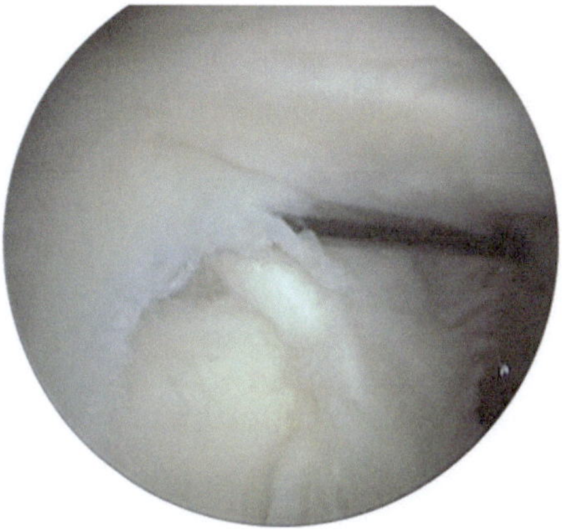

Type 2 SLAP tear with labrum falling in front of the glenoid (beret-like appearance) (a) more evident on probing (b)

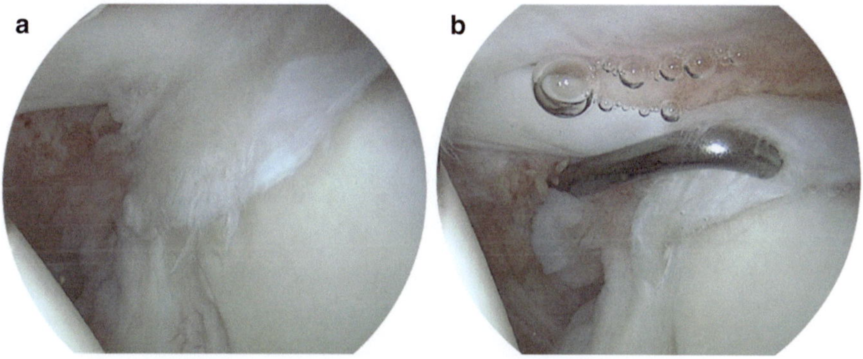

27.3 Demographics of Superior Labrum Tears

Incidence—present in a high proportion of arthroscopies

- In a study [8] reporting on 544 shoulder arthroscopies:
  - 26% had a SLAP lesion of which
    - 74% Type 1
    - 21% Type 2
    - 0.7% Type 3
    - 4% Type 4

27.4 Clinical Symptoms of Superior Labrum Tears

- Pain
- Glenohumeral deep seated pain (constant or activity related)
- Anterior shoulder pain—bicipital pain radiating to the biceps muscle
- Glenohumeral instability
- Clicking, catching, popping, locking
- Neurological symptoms due to para-labrum cysts causing nerve compression
- "Dead arm" sensation

27.5 Clinical Signs of Superior Labrum Tears [9]

- Positive O'Brien's test
- Positive Speed's test
- Positive Yergason's test
- Positive instability apprehension/provocation tests

27.6 Investigations for Superior Labrum Tears

MRI arthrography (sensitivity about 80%, specificity about 91%) [10]

MRI arthrogram showing SLAP tear with escape of contrast between the labrum and superior glenoid (red arrow)

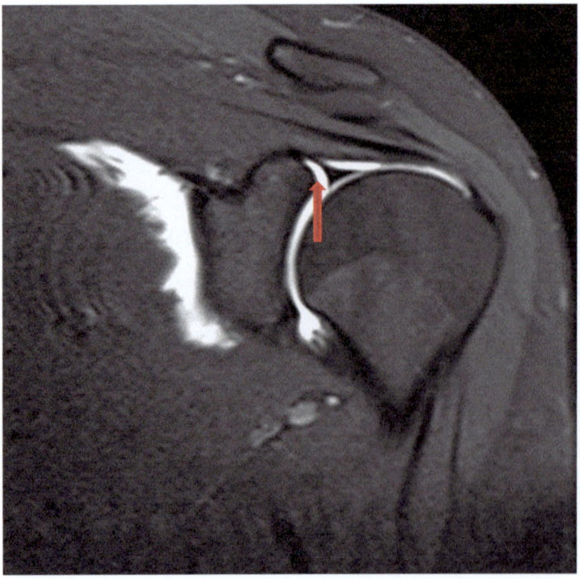

27.7 Management of Superior Labrum Tears

Treatment is directed towards the troubling symptoms:

27.7.1 Treatment for Pain

Non-surgical [11–14]

- Leave alone
- Analgesia, activity modification
- Glenohumeral steroid injections
- Physiotherapy:
  - Posterior capsular stretching to address contractures and regain motion loss
  - Improve scapular muscle strength and neuromuscular control
  - Increase lower extremity strengthening and core strengthening

Surgical [15–17]

- Arthroscopic:
  - Debridement of degenerate labrum tear if biceps anchor is stable
  - Resection of an unstable bucket handle fragment
  - Partial removal of a damaged LHB tendon segment/flap
  - Arthroscopic labrum reattachment
- LHB tendon tenotomy or tenodesis open or arthroscopic (this is preferable in patients over 35–40 years old as the outcomes of arthroscopic labrum repair are inferior to those seen in younger patients) [18, 19]

SLAP tear repair with bone suture anchors. (a) SLAP tear pre-repair (b) post repair

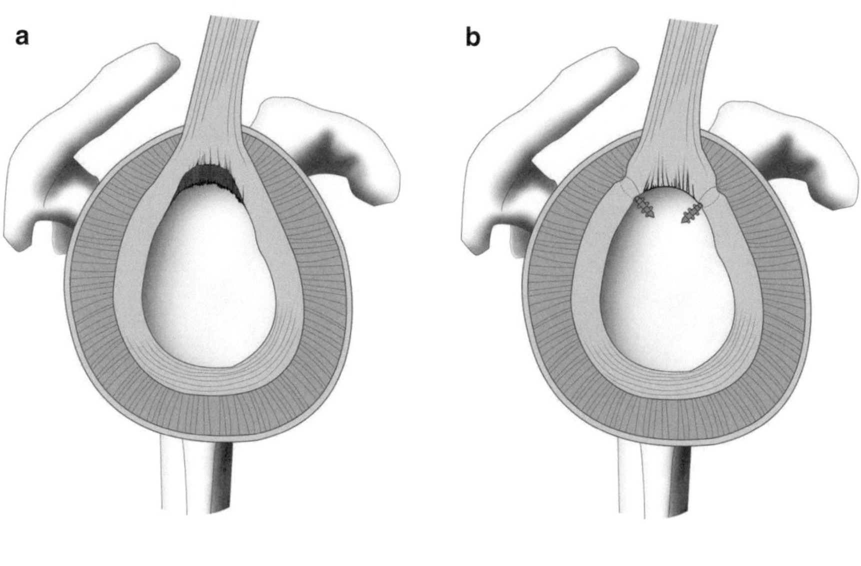

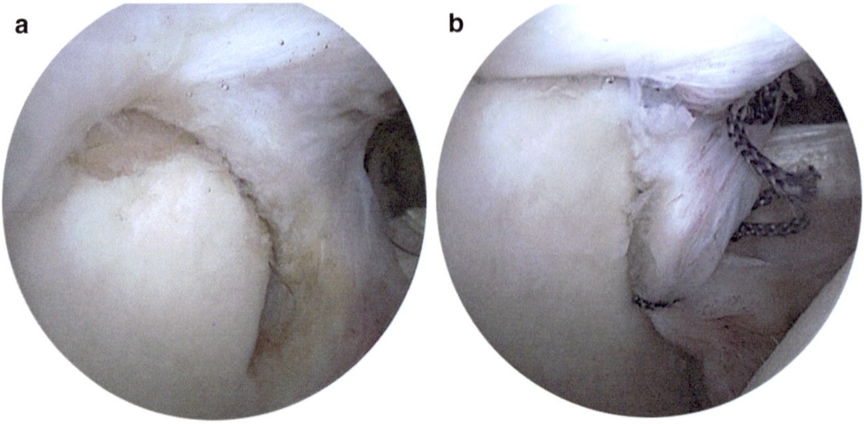

27.7.2 *Treatment for Instability*

Non-surgical

- Leave alone
- Physiotherapy
  - Improve shoulder and scapular muscle strength and neuromuscular control
  - Lower extremity strengthening and core strengthening

Surgical [20, 21]

- Arthroscopic labrum reattachment

Non-surgical treatment of SLAP tears can be successful with reports of up to about 70% returning to sports with improvement in pain and function [13]. Hence, a trial of non-surgical treatment may be appropriate.

Outcomes of SLAP repair vary with some authors reporting 88% of professional athletes returning to pre-injury levels within a year [22]. Others, however, reported more inferior outcomes with resolution of pain in only 26% and restoration of normal function in only 13% [23].

Learning Pearls

- A sub-labrum recess is a sulcus (anatomical variant) located between the superior glenoid cartilage and the labrum. It has smooth edges and is found at a 12 o 'clock position where the biceps inserts onto the glenoid. This may be mistaken for a SLAP tear [24–26]
- Not every SLAP tear needs repair. Many tears are incidental findings on radiological investigations or arthroscopic evaluation of the shoulder, and their presence needs to be correlated with clinical symptoms

- Although the debilitating effect of SLAP tears in some high-level athletes is recognised [27], the overall beneficial effect of SLAP surgery has recently been questioned by a randomised trial that failed to show a difference in outcomes between those treated with SLAP repair, tenodesis or sham surgery [28]

References

1. Snyder SJ, Karzel RP, Del Pizzo W, Ferkel RD, Friedman MJ. SLAP lesions of the shoulder. Arthroscopy. 1990;6(4):274–9.
2. Snyder SJ, Banas MP, Karzel RP. An analysis of 140 injuries to the superior glenoid labrum. J Shoulder Elb Surg. 1995;4(4):243–8.
3. Burkhart SS, Morgan CD. The peel-back mechanism: its role in producing and extending posterior type II SLAP lesions and its effect on SLAP repair rehabilitation. Arthroscopy. 1998;14(6):637–40.
4. Maffet MW, Gartsman GM, Moseley B. Superior labrum-biceps tendon complex lesions of the shoulder. Am J Sports Med. 1995;23(1):93–8.
5. Powell SE, Nord KD, Ryu RKN. The diagnosis, classification and treatment of SLAP lesions. Oper Tech Sports Med. 2004;12:99–110.
6. Morgan CD, Burkhart SS, Palmeri M, Gillespie M. Type II SLAP lesions: three subtypes and their relationships to superior instability and rotator cuff tears. Arthroscopy. 1998;14(6):553–65.
7. Choi NH, Kim SJ. Avulsion of the superior labrum. Arthroscopy. 2004;20(8):872–4.
8. Kim TK, Queale WS, Cosgarea AJ, McFarland EG. Clinical features of the different types of SLAP lesions: an analysis of one hundred and thirty-nine cases. J Bone Joint Surg Am. 2003;85-A(1):66–71.
9. Charalambous CP. Clinical examination of the shoulder. In: Charalambous CP, editor. The shoulder made easy. Basel: Springer; 2019.
10. Symanski JS, Subhas N, Babb J, Nicholson J, Gyftopoulos S. Diagnosis of superior labrum anterior-to-posterior tears by using MR imaging and MR arthrography: a systematic review and meta-analysis. Radiology. 2017;285(1):101–13.
11. Fedoriw WW, Ramkumar P, McCulloch PC, Lintner DM. Return to play after treatment of superior labral tears in professional baseball players. Am J Sports Med. 2014;42(5):1155–60.
12. Lintner DM. Superior labrum anterior to posterior tears in throwing athletes. Instr Course Lect. 2013;62:491–500.
13. Jang SH, Seo JG, Jang HS, Jung JE, Kim JG. Predictive factors associated with failure of nonoperative treatment of superior labrum anterior-posterior tears. J Shoulder Elb Surg. 2016;25(3):428–34.
14. Edwards SL, Lee JA, Bell JE, Packer JD, Ahmad CS, Levine WN, Bigliani LU, Blaine TA. Nonoperative treatment of superior labrum anterior posterior tears: improvements in pain, function, and quality of life. Am J Sports Med. 2010;38(7):1456–61.
15. Friel NA, Karas V, Slabaugh MA, Cole BJ. Outcomes of type II superior labrum, anterior to posterior (SLAP) repair: prospective evaluation at a minimum two-year follow-up. J Shoulder Elb Surg. 2010;19(6):859–67.
16. Ek ET, Shi LL, Tompson JD, Freehill MT, Warner JJ. Surgical treatment of isolated type II superior labrum anterior-posterior (SLAP) lesions: repair versus biceps tenodesis. J Shoulder Elb Surg. 2014;23(7):1059–65.
17. Field LD, Savoie FH. Arthroscopic suture repair of superior labral detachment lesions of the shoulder. Am J Sports Med. 1993;21(6):783–90.

18. Denard PJ, Lädermann A, Parsley BK, Burkhart SS. Arthroscopic biceps tenodesis compared with repair of isolated type II SLAP lesions in patients older than 35 years. Orthopedics. 2014;37(3):e292–7.
19. Erickson J, Lavery K, Monica J, Gatt C, Dhawan A. Surgical treatment of symptomatic superior labrum anterior-posterior tears in patients older than 40 years: a systematic review. Am J Sports Med. 2015;43(5):1274–82.
20. Virk MS, Arciero RA. Superior labrum anterior to posterior tears and glenohumeral instability. Instr Course Lect. 2013;62:501–14.
21. Kessler MA, Burkart A, Weiss M, Imhoff AB. SLAP lesions as a cause of posterior instability. Orthopade. 2003;32(7):642–6.
22. Beyzadeoglu T, Circi E. Superior labrum anterior posterior lesions and associated injuries: return to play in elite athletes. Orthop J Sports Med. 2015;3(4):2325967115577359. https://doi.org/10.1177/2325967115577359.
23. Weber SC, Martin DF, Seiler JG 3rd, Harrast JJ. Superior labrum anterior and posterior lesions of the shoulder: incidence rates, complications, and outcomes as reported by American Board of Orthopedic Surgery. Part II candidates. Am J Sports Med. 2012;40(7):1538–43.
24. Kanatli U, Ozturk BY, Bolukbasi S. Anatomical variations of the anterosuperior labrum: prevalence and association with type II superior labrum anterior-posterior (SLAP) lesions. J Shoulder Elb Surg. 2010;19(8):1199–203.
25. Jin W, Ryu KN, Kwon SH, Rhee YG, Yang DM. MR arthrography in the differential diagnosis of type II superior labral anteroposterior lesion and sublabral recess. AJR Am J Roentgenol. 2006;187(4):887–93.
26. Smith DK, Chopp TM, Aufdemorte TB, Witkowski EG, Jones RC. Sublabral recess of the superior glenoid labrum: study of cadavers with conventional nonenhanced MR imaging, MR arthrography, anatomic dissection, and limited histologic examination. Radiology. 1996;201(1):251–6.
27. Chambers CC, Lynch TS, Gibbs DB, Ghodasra JH, Sahota S, Franke K, Mack CD, Nuber GW. Superior labrum anterior-posterior tears in the National Football League. Am J Sports Med. 2017;45(1):167–72.
28. Schrøder CP, Skare Ø, Reikerås O, Mowinckel P, Brox JI. Sham surgery versus labral repair or biceps tenodesis for type II SLAP lesions of the shoulder: a three-armed randomised clinical trial. Br J Sports Med. 2017;51(24):1759–66.

Chapter 28
Para-labrum Cysts of the Shoulder

This is a condition whereby a ganglion-like cyst develops adjacent to the glenoid or labrum. These are often the result of a labrum tear which acts as a one-way valve allowing synovial fluid to get into the cyst but not escape. The cyst may vary in size (from tiny to very large) and may consist of one or multiple locules. Such cysts are located more frequently in relation to the posterior-superior and anterior labrum as compared to the inferior labrum [1, 2].

28.1 Clinical Symptoms of Para-Labrum Cysts

- None—incidental findings on radiological evaluation of the shoulder
- Pain—dull and difficult to localise
- Neurological symptoms (neurogenic pain, weakness, loss of muscle bulk) due to nerve compression (of the suprascapular nerve at the suprascapular or spino-glenoid notch [3–6] or the axillary nerve [7])
- Symptoms arising from an associated labrum tear—clicking, glenohumeral pain, instability
- Mass lesion, if very large [8]

© Springer Nature Switzerland AG 2019

C. Panayiotou Charalambous, *The Shoulder Made Easy*,
https://doi.org/10.1007/978-3-319-98908-2_28

Para-labrum cyst compressing the suprascapular nerve

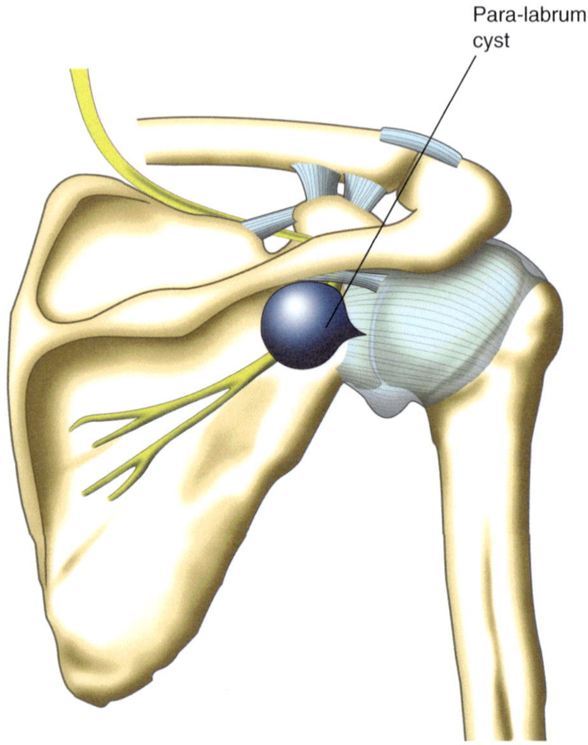

28.2 Clinical Signs of Para-Labrum Cysts

- Signs of a labrum tear
- Neurological dysfunction—altered sensation, muscle weakness, muscle wasting

28.3 Investigations for Para-Labrum Cysts

- MRI arthrogram [9, 10]

MRI arthrogram demonstrating a para-labrum cyst (yellow arrows) in relation to the posterior labrum

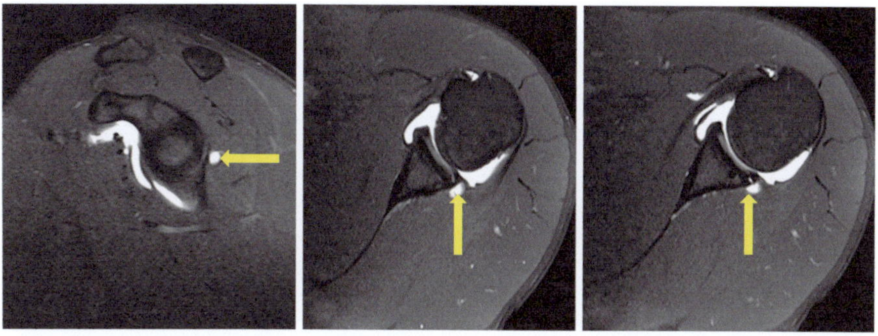

MRI showing para-labrum cyst closely related to the posterior labrum and infraspinatus muscle (red arrows)

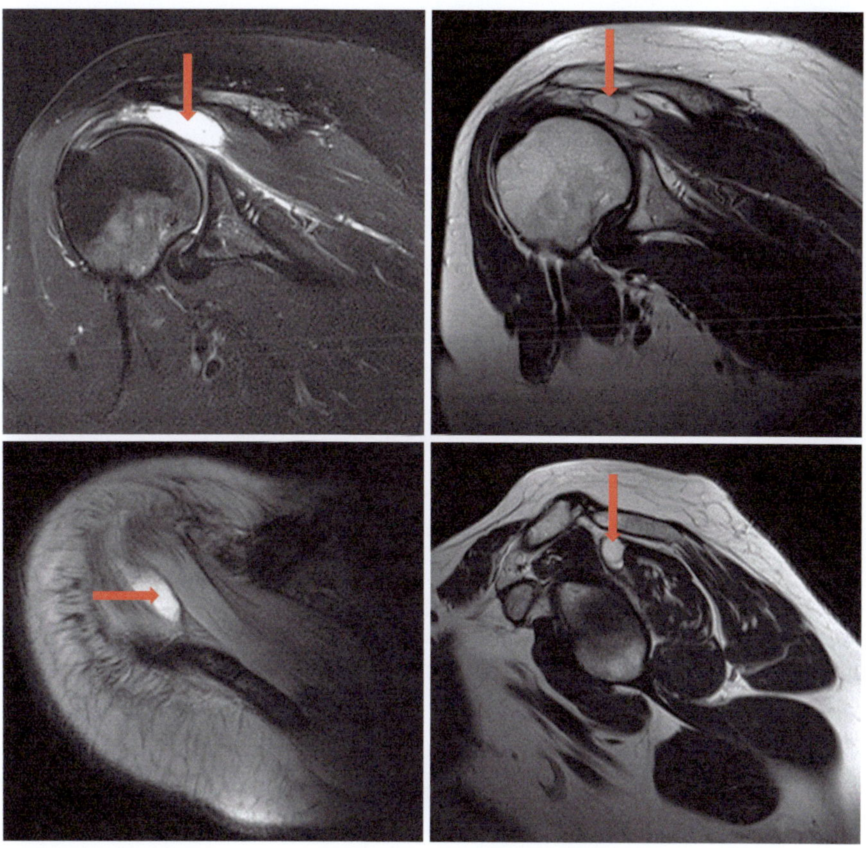

MRI showing para-labrum cyst related to the anterior-inferior labrum (yellow arrows)

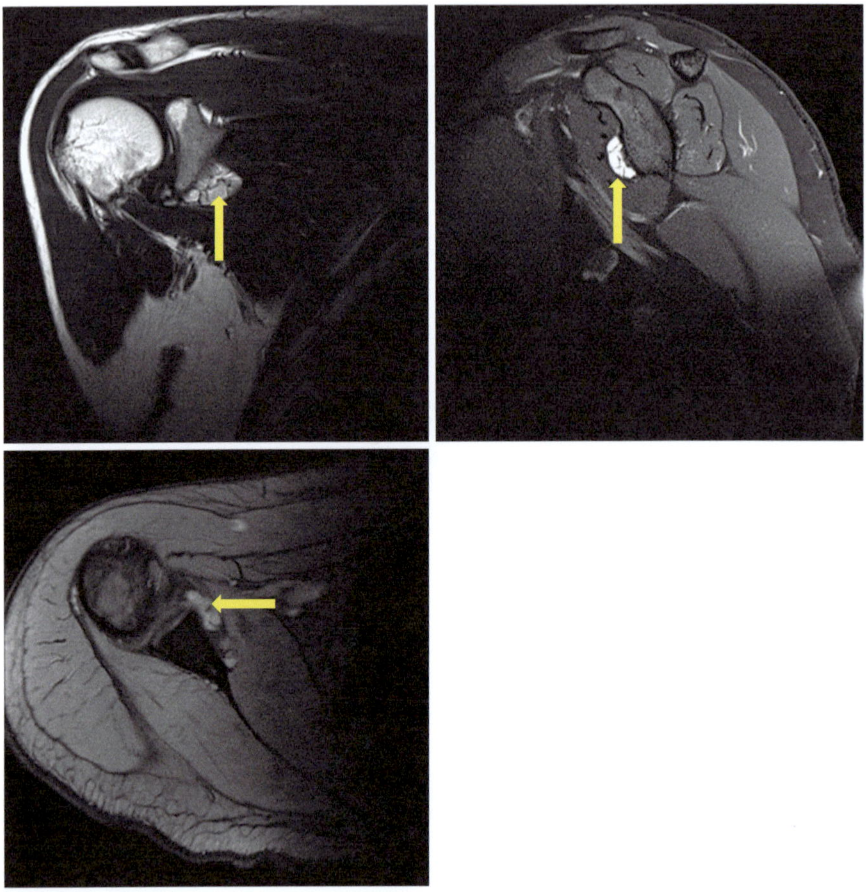

28.4 Management of Para-Labrum Cysts

In dealing with para-labrum cysts, it is important to determine if they are contributing to any of the patient's symptoms or whether they are nonsymptomatic. If nonsymptomatic they are left alone. If symptomatic then options for treatment are as below:

Non-surgical [11–13]

- Leave alone if symptoms are not troublesome enough to warrant intervention
- Activity modification
- Glenohumeral steroid injection
- Aspiration of the cyst under ultrasound guidance and cyst steroid injection

Surgical [14–19]

- Arthroscopic cyst excision with or without labrum tear repair
  - If there is a labrum tear, the cyst is decompressed through the tear
- Open cyst excision
- Labrum repair without cyst excision

There is evidence to suggest that labrum repair along with cyst excision confers better outcomes as compared to isolated labrum repair [19].

Spino-glenoid notch cysts may be seen between the supraspinatus and infraspinatus muscles at the base of the scapular spine. These cysts may be decompressed via the subacromial space by inserting a shaver device through the posterior portal with visualisation through a lateral portal.

Learning Pearls

- Many of the para-labrum cysts detected radiologically are incidental findings and may co-exist with other shoulder disorders. Hence, the presence of a para-labrum cyst should be correlated with patient's symptoms prior to planning any intervention

References

1. Ji JH, Shafi M, Lee YS, Kim DJ. Inferior paralabral ganglion cyst of the shoulder with labral tear—a rare cause of shoulder pain. Orthop Traumatol Surg Res. 2012;98(2):193–8.
2. Kessler MA, Stoffel K, Oswald A, Stutz G, Gaechter A. The SLAP lesion as a reason for glenolabral cysts: a report of five cases and review of the literature. Arch Orthop Trauma Surg. 2007;127(4):287–92.
3. Skirving AP, Kozak TK, Davis SJ. Infraspinatus paralysis due to spinoglenoid notch ganglion. J Bone Joint Surg Br. 1994;76(4):588–91.
4. Bilsel K, Erdil M, Elmadag M, Ozden VE, Celik D, Tuncay I. The effect of infraspinatus hypotrophy and weakness on the arthroscopic treatment of spinoglenoid notch cyst associated with superior labrum anterior-to-posterior lesions. Knee Surg Sports Traumatol Arthrosc. 2014;22(9):2209–15.
5. Lichtenberg S, Magosch P, Habermeyer P. Compression of the suprascapular nerve by a ganglion cyst of the spinoglenoid notch: the arthroscopic solution. Knee Surg Sports Traumatol Arthrosc. 2004;12(1):72–9.
6. Fehrman DA, Orwin JF, Jennings RM. Suprascapular nerve entrapment by ganglion cysts: a report of six cases with arthroscopic findings and review of the literature. Arthroscopy. 1995;11(6):727–34.
7. Sanders TG, Tirman PFJ. Paralabral cyst: an unusual cause of quadrilateral space syndrome. Arthroscopy. 1999;15:632–7.
8. Ho JC, Iannotti JP. Glenoid labral tear associated paralabral ganglion cyst presenting as a neck mass: a case report. J Shoulder Elb Surg. 2010;19(5):e10–3.
9. Zlatkin MB, Sanders TG. Magnetic resonance imaging of the glenoid labrum. Radiol Clin N Am. 2013;51(2):279–97.
10. Tung GA, Entzian D, Stern JB, Green A. MR imaging and MR arthrography of paraglenoid labral cysts. AJR Am J Roentgenol. 2000;174(6):1707–15.

11. Piatt BE, Hawkins RJ, Fritz RC, Ho CP, Wolf E, Schickendantz M. Clinical evaluation and treatment of spinoglenoid notch ganglion cysts. J Shoulder Elb Surg. 2002;11(6):600–4.
12. Davidge CM, Walker R, Brett K, Boorman RS. Spontaneous resolution of a spinoglenoid notch cyst and associated suprascapular nerve palsy: a case report. J Shoulder Elb Surg. 2007;16(3):e4–7.
13. Leitschuh PH, Bone CM, Bouska WM. Magnetic resonance imaging diagnosis, sonographically directed percutaneous aspiration, and arthroscopic treatment of a painful shoulder ganglion cyst associated with a SLAP lesion. Arthroscopy. 1999;15(1):85–7.
14. Kim DS, Park HK, Park JH, Yoon WS. Ganglion cyst of the spinoglenoid notch: comparison between SLAP repair alone and SLAP repair with cyst decompression. J Shoulder Elb Surg. 2012;21(11):1456–63.
15. Shon MS, Jung SW, Kim JW, Yoo JC. Arthroscopic all-intra-articular decompression and labral repair of paralabral cyst in the shoulder. J Shoulder Elb Surg. 2015;24(1):e7–e14.
16. Kim SJ, Choi YR, Jung M, Park JY, Chun YM. Outcomes of arthroscopic decompression of spinoglenoid cysts through a subacromial approach. Arthroscopy. 2017;33(1):62–7.
17. Jeong JJ, Panchal K, Park SE, Kim YY, Lee JM, Lee JK, Ji JH. Outcome after arthroscopic decompression of inferior labral cysts combined with labral repair. Arthroscopy. 2015;31(6):1060–8.
18. Schrøder CP, Lundgreen K, Kvakestad R. Paralabral cysts of the shoulder treated with isolated labral repair: effect on pain and radiologic findings. J Shoulder Elb Surg. 2018;27:1283. https://doi.org/10.1016/j.jse.2017.12.022.
19. Pillai G, Baynes JR, Gladstone J, Flatow EL. Greater strength increase with cyst decompression and SLAP repair than SLAP repair alone. Clin Orthop Relat Res. 2011;469(4):1056–60.

Chapter 29
Avascular Necrosis of the Humeral Head

This is a condition whereby there is interruption of the blood supply to the humeral head. As a result, the humeral head bone undergoes necrosis. The superior central part of the humeral head is most frequently affected [1–7].

29.1 Pathogenesis of Avascular Necrosis of the Humeral Head

Disruption of the blood supply may involve the arterial inflow or venous outflow. It may be due to external mechanical factors causing compression or disruption of blood vessels or due to internal occlusion of the vessel lumen.

29.2 Demographics of Avascular Necrosis of the Humeral Head

- The humeral head is the second most common site of avascular necrosis following the femoral head, and in some cases both the humeral and femoral heads may be affected
- More common in men aged 20–50

29.3 Classification of Avascular Necrosis of the Humeral Head

Cruess [6]

© Springer Nature Switzerland AG 2019

C. Panayiotou Charalambous, *The Shoulder Made Easy*,
https://doi.org/10.1007/978-3-319-98908-2_29

Stage 1—No abnormal radiograph findings, but marrow signal changes on MRI

Stage 2—Sclerosis of the involved part of the humeral head (due to subchondral microfracture) but no collapse of the overlying articular surface. Histologically, there is bone cell death but no substantial resorption or healing

Stage 3—Crescent sign (indicative of subchondral bone collapse)

Stage 4—Extensive humeral head collapse and degeneration without glenoid involvement

Stage 5—Degenerative changes involve both the humeral head and glenoid

Cruess classification of avascular necrosis of the humeral head

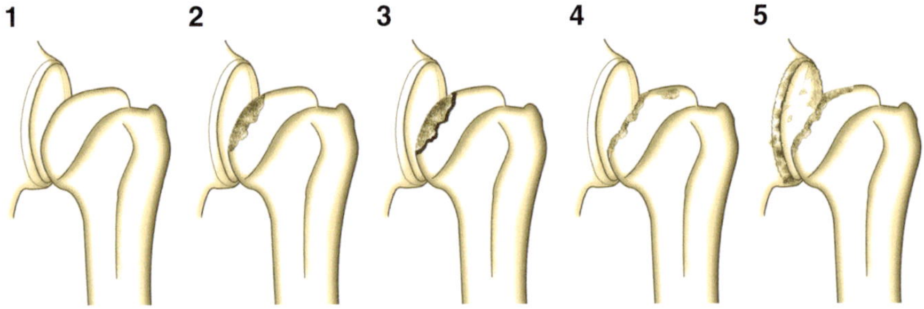

29.4 Causes of Avascular Necrosis of the Humeral Head [7–21]

- Idiopathic
- Trauma
  - Humeral head dislocation
  - Proximal humeral fracture—incidence of 15–30% in three- and four-part proximal humeral fractures
- Surgery
  - Post-rotator cuff repair—possibly due to insertion of multiple bone suture anchors
  - Open surgical approaches disrupting blood supply
- Steroid use—including intra-articular injections
- Alcohol abuse
- Metabolic—Gaucher's disease
- Haematological—haemoglobinopathies (sickle cell disease)
- Connective tissue disorders—lupus
- Inflammatory arthritis—rheumatoid arthritis
- Infective—bacterial or nonbacterial
- Dysbaric—caisson disease
- Other—influenza vaccination

29.5 Clinical Symptoms of Avascular Necrosis of the Humeral Head

- Glenohumeral pain
  - At rest and on activity
  - Night pain, disturbing sleep
- Stiffness
- Apparent weakness
- Clicking/clunking if collapsed or arthritic humeral head
- Locking or popping due to loose osteochondral fragments

29.6 Clinical Signs of Avascular Necrosis of the Humeral Head

- Painful glenohumeral motion
- Loss of glenohumeral motion
  - Apparent due to pain
  - True stiffness

29.7 Investigations for Avascular Necrosis of the Humeral Head

- Radiological [7, 22]
- Plain radiographs
- MRI scan
- Bone scan (may demonstrate other joint involvement)

Plain radiographs and MRI showing avascular necrosis of the humeral head with subchondral collapse (red arrows)

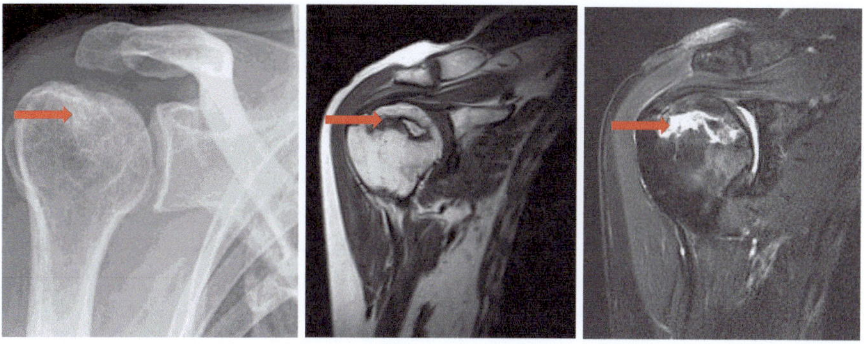

Glenohumeral arthritis with extensive sclerosis (red arrow) of the humeral head, suggestive of avascular necrosis of the humeral head

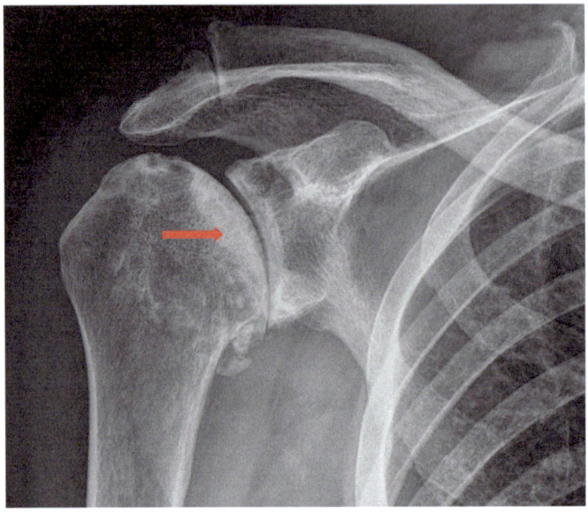

Humeral head sclerosis, loss of joint space and glenoid arthritis, secondary to avascular necrosis (red arrow)

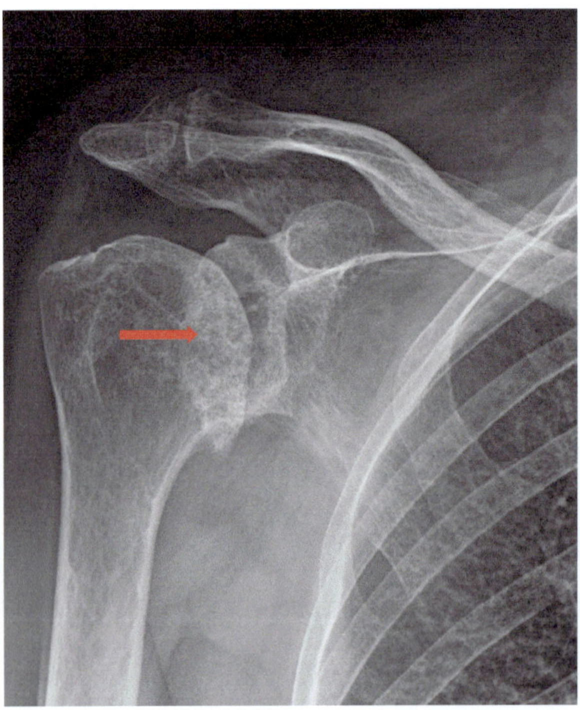

Avascular necrosis of the humeral head with collapse (red arrow), following proximal humeral fracture internal fixation with plate

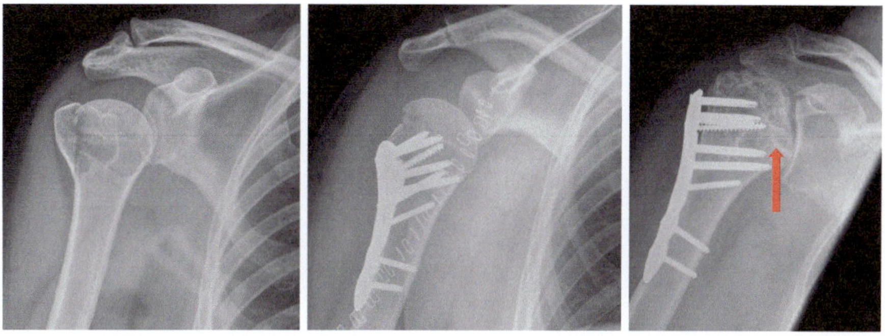

29.8 Management of Avascular Necrosis of the Humeral Head

This will depend on clinical symptoms and disease stage and is described below.

Non-surgical

- Leave alone
- Analgesia
- Eliminate risk factors
- Activity modification to minimise loading of the involved part of the humeral head (such as abduction and forward elevation which brings the superior part of the humeral head in contact with the glenoid)
- Physiotherapy to maintain joint mobility and avoid stiffness

Surgical [23–36]

- Joint preserving
  - Humeral head debridement with removal of chondral flaps and loose bodies
  - Vascularised bone grafting
  - Core decompression ± fibular graft strut
- Joint arthroplasty
  - Interposition arthroplasty involves debridement of the joint and placement of a graft (fascia lata autograft, pyro-carbon) between the articular surfaces. It may be utilised in younger patients where there is concern about the longevity of shoulder replacement implants
  - Hemiarthroplasty replacement
    - Resurfacing
    - Stemmed

- Total shoulder replacement (especially when there is glenoid involvement)
  - Resurfacing
  - Stemmed

29.9 Natural History of Avascular Necrosis of the Humeral Head [37–40]

- There may be a delay between commencing steroid treatment and the development of avascular necrosis (AVN) of 6–24 months
- AVN tends to be a progressive disorder with the development of clinical symptoms even if the precipitating factor (such as steroid use) is stopped
- Although the extent of the necrotic lesion does not usually increase in size, lesions tend to progress to collapse, with only very few recovering (smaller lesions, unilateral, reduced steroid use, nonsymptomatic patients)

Hernigou et al. [38] looked at 215 shoulders with AVN diagnosed by MRI scan as Stage 1 or Stage 2. They reported that pain developed in 74% and collapse in 54% of those previously nonsymptomatic. In contrast, collapse occurred in 82% of those with clinical symptoms. The time between diagnosis and collapse averaged 10 years for those with symptomatic Stage 1 but only 3 years for those with symptomatic Stage 2.

Learning Pearls

- In early stages no specific signs may be apparent, and hence diagnosis may be overlooked
- Late presentation is common as a lot of motion can be compensated by movement at the scapulo-thoracic articulation. Hence, symptoms may not be apparent until the disease has substantially progressed and degenerative changes set in
- AVN should be considered when encountering:
  - Pain in the shoulder of no obvious origin
  - A patient at high risk of AVN (post-proximal humeral fracture, steroid use, alcohol abuse)
  - A young patient presenting with vague shoulder symptoms

References

1. Harreld KL, Marker DR, Wiesler ER, Shafiq B, Mont MA. Osteonecrosis of the humeral head. J Am Acad Orthop Surg. 2009;17(6):345–55.
2. Sarris I, Weiser R, Sotereanos DG. Pathogenesis and treatment of osteonecrosis of the shoulder. Orthop Clin N Am. 2004;35(3):397–404.

3. Gruson KI, Kwon YW. Atraumatic osteonecrosis of the humeral head. Bull NYU Hosp Jt Dis. 2009;67(1):6–14.
4. Kadono M, Kakihana K, Endo I, Kawamura M, Ohashi K, Sakamaki H. Osteonecrosis of the humeral head. Int J Hematol. 2011;94(3):222–3.
5. Cruess RL, Ross D, Crawshaw E. The etiology of steroid-induced avascular necrosis of bone. A laboratory and clinical study. Clin Orthop Relat Res. 1975;(113):178–83.
6. Cruess RL. Steroid-induced avascular necrosis of the head of the humerus. Natural history and management. J Bone Joint Surg Br. 1976;58(3):313–7.
7. Lee JA, Farooki S, Ashman CJ, Yu JS. MR patterns of involvement of humeral head osteonecrosis. J Comput Assist Tomogr. 2002;26(5):839–42.
8. Patel S, Colaco HB, Elvey ME, Lee MH. Post-traumatic osteonecrosis of the proximal humerus. Injury. 2015;46(10):1878–84.
9. Gaudot F, Gregory T, Augereau B, Masmejean EH. Aseptic osteonecrosis of the humeral head after anterior shoulder dislocation. Eur J Trauma Emerg Surg. 2008;34(6):601–5.
10. Kim JK, Jeong HJ, Shin SJ, Yoo JC, Rhie TY, Park KJ, Oh JH. Rapid progressive osteonecrosis of the humeral head after arthroscopic rotator cuff surgery. Arthroscopy. 2018;34(1):41–7.
11. Goto M, Gotoh M, Mitsui Y, Okawa T, Higuchi F, Nagata K. Rapid collapse of the humeral head after arthroscopic rotator cuff repair. Knee Surg Sports Traumatol Arthrosc. 2015;23(2):514–6.
12. Poignard A, Flouzat-Lachaniette CH, Amzallag J, Galacteros F, Hernigou P. The natural progression of symptomatic humeral head osteonecrosis in adults with sickle cell disease. J Bone Joint Surg Am. 2012;94(2):156–62.
13. Hasan SS, Romeo AA. Nontraumatic osteonecrosis of the humeral head. J Shoulder Elb Surg. 2002;11(3):281–98.
14. Usher BW Jr, Friedman RJ. Steroid-induced osteonecrosis of the humeral head. Orthopedics. 1995;18(1):47–51.
15. Laroche M, Arlet J, Mazieres B. Osteonecrosis of the femoral and humeral heads after intraarticular corticosteroid injections. J Rheumatol. 1990;17(4):549–51.
16. Orlić D, Jovanović S, Anticević D, Zecević J. Frequency of idiopathic aseptic necrosis in medically treated alcoholics. Int Orthop. 1990;14(4).383–6.
17. Cruess RL. Corticosteroid-induced osteonecrosis of the humeral head. Orthop Clin N Am. 1985;16(4):789–96.
18. Cruess RL. Steroid-induced osteonecrosis: a review. Can J Surg. 1981;24(6):567–71.
19. Hernigou P, Allain J, Bachir D, Galacteros F. Abnormalities of the adult shoulder due to sickle cell osteonecrosis during childhood. Rev Rhum Engl Ed. 1998;65(1):27–32.
20. Uguen M, Pougnet R, Uguen A, Cornec D, Quintin-Roué I, Dewitte JD, Loddé B. Dysbaric osteonecrosis in professional divers: two case reports. Undersea Hyperb Med. 2015;42(4):363–7.
21. Kuether G, Dietrich B, Smith T, Peter C, Gruessner S. Atraumatic osteonecrosis of the humeral head after influenza A-(H1N1) v-2009 vaccination. Vaccine. 2011;29(40):6830–3.
22. Sakai T, Sugano N, Nishii T, Miki H, Ohzono K, Yoshikawa H. Bone scintigraphy screening for osteonecrosis of the shoulder in patients with non-traumatic osteonecrosis of the femoral head. Skelet Radiol. 2002;31(11):650–5.
23. Makihara T, Yoshioka T, Sugaya H, Yamazaki M, Mishima H. Autologous concentrated bone marrow grafting for the treatment of osteonecrosis of the humeral head: a report of five shoulders in four cases. Case Rep Orthop. 2017;2017:4898057. https://doi.org/10.1155/2017/4898057.
24. Franceschi F, Franceschetti E, Paciotti M, Torre G, Samuelsson K, Papalia R, Karlsson J, Denaro V. Surgical management of osteonecrosis of the humeral head: a systematic review. Knee Surg Sports Traumatol Arthrosc. 2017;25(10):3270–8.
25. Brannon JK. Thorough debridement of the humeral head for osteonecrosis. Orthopedics. 2011;34(1):56. https://doi.org/10.3928/01477447-20101123-21.
26. Kennon JC, Smith JP, Crosby LA. Core decompression and arthroplasty outcomes for atraumatic osteonecrosis of the humeral head. J Shoulder Elb Surg. 2016;25(9):1442–8.
27. Inoue K, Suenaga N, Oizumi N, Tanaka Y, Minami A. A vascularized scapular graft for juvenile osteonecrosis of the humeral head. J Shoulder Elb Surg. 2012;21(4):e9–e13.

28. Sahajpal DT, Zuckerman JD. Core decompression for nontraumatic osteonecrosis of the humeral head: a technique article. Bull NYU Hosp Jt Dis. 2008;66(2):118–9.
29. Chapman C, Mattern C, Levine WN. Arthroscopically assisted core decompression of the proximal humerus for avascular necrosis. Arthroscopy. 2004;20(9):1003–6.
30. LaPorte DM, Mont MA, Mohan V, Pierre-Jacques H, Jones LC, Hungerford DS. Osteonecrosis of the humeral head treated by core decompression. Clin Orthop Relat Res. 1998;355:254–60.
31. Kawamura K, Kawate K, Yajima H, Kobata Y, Takakura Y. Vascularized scapular grafting for treatment of osteonecrosis of the humeral head. J Reconstr Microsurg. 2008;24(8):559–64.
32. Uribe JW, Botto-van Bemden A. Partial humeral head resurfacing for osteonecrosis. J Shoulder Elb Surg. 2009;18(5):711–6.
33. Hudek R, Werner B, Abdelkawi AF, Gohlke F. Pyrocarbon interposition shoulder arthroplasty in advanced collapse of the humeral head. Orthopade. 2017;46(12):1034–44.
34. Garret J, Godeneche A, Boileau P, Molé D, Etzner M, Favard L, Levigne C, Sirveaux F, Gauci MO, Dezaly C, Walch G. Pyrocarbon interposition shoulder arthroplasty: preliminary results from a prospective multicenter study at 2 years of follow-up. J Shoulder Elb Surg. 2017;26(7):1143–51.
35. Schoch BS, Barlow JD, Schleck C, Cofield RH, Sperling JW. Shoulder arthroplasty for post-traumatic osteonecrosis of the humeral head. J Shoulder Elb Surg. 2016;25(3):406–12.
36. Feeley BT, Fealy S, Dines DM, Warren RF, Craig EV. Hemiarthroplasty and total shoulder arthroplasty for avascular necrosis of the humeral head. J Shoulder Elb Surg. 2008;17(5):689–94.
37. L'Insalata JC, Pagnani MJ, Warren RF, Dines DM. Humeral head osteonecrosis: clinical course and radiographic predictors of outcome. J Shoulder Elb Surg. 1996;5(5):355–61.
38. Hernigou P, Flouzat-Lachaniette CH, Roussignol X, Poignard A. The natural progression of shoulder osteonecrosis related to corticosteroid treatment. Clin Orthop Relat Res. 2010;468(7):1809–16.
39. Sakai T, Sugano N, Nishii T, Hananouchi T, Yoshikawa H. Extent of osteonecrosis on MRI predicts humeral head collapse. Clin Orthop Relat Res. 2008;466(5):1074–80.
40. Hattrup SJ, Cofield RH. Osteonecrosis of the humeral head: relationship of disease stage, extent, and cause to natural history. J Shoulder Elb Surg. 1999;8(6):559–64.

Chapter 30
Glenohumeral Arthritis

Several types of arthritis may affect the glenohumeral joint [1–10]. These include:

- Osteoarthritis – condition whereby there is degeneration of the articular cartilage of the glenohumeral joint. This may be limited to the humeral head, glenoid or involve both. Its causes include:
  - Primary
  - Secondary
    - Post-traumatic
    - Avascular necrosis
    - Instability
- Inflammatory arthritis – condition whereby there is destruction of the articular cartilage of the glenohumeral joint due to an inflammatory process. Causes include:
  - Seropositive arthritis – rheumatoid arthritis
  - Seronegative arthritis
  - Crystal arthropathy
  - Infective arthritis
  - Reactive arthritis
- Rotator cuff arthropathy – condition whereby there is degeneration of the articular cartilage of the glenohumeral joint associated with a massive rotator cuff tendon tear

© Springer Nature Switzerland AG 2019

C. Panayiotou Charalambous, *The Shoulder Made Easy*,
https://doi.org/10.1007/978-3-319-98908-2_30

Glenohumeral osteoarthritis with loss of articular cartilage from the humeral head and glenoid. Arthroscopic view of the glenohumeral joint

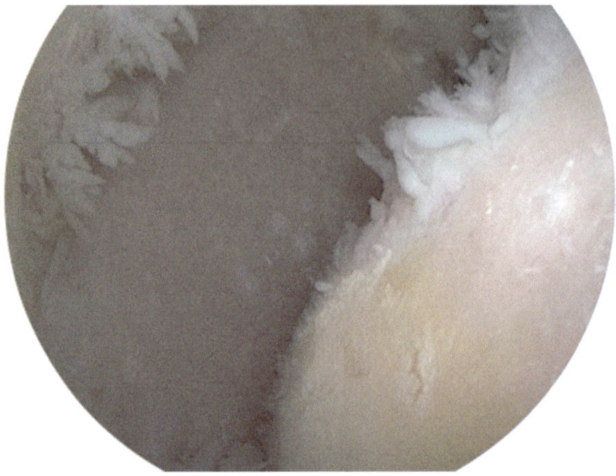

Osteoarthritis, rheumatoid arthritis, and rotator cuff glenohumeral arthropathy are considered next.

30.1 Clinical Symptoms of Glenohumeral Arthritis

- Deep seated glenohumeral pain
- Loss of motion
- Arm weakness

30.2 Clinical Signs of Glenohumeral Arthritis

- Muscle atrophy – related to disuse or tendon tear
- Large, diffuse shoulder swelling – associated with rotator cuff arthropathy
- Painful glenohumeral motion
- Shoulder weakness if associated rotator cuff dysfunction or tear
- Loss of glenohumeral motion
  - Apparent due to pain
  - True stiffness

30.3 Investigations for Glenohumeral Arthritis

- Plain radiographs
  - Osteoarthritis – loss of joint space, subchondral sclerosis, subchondral cysts, osteophyte formation (usually evident in the inferior aspect of the humeral head)
  - Rheumatoid arthritis – joint space narrowing, marginal erosions (that occur in the outer part of the joint), periarticular osteopenia, soft tissue swelling, minimal reactive bone formation
  - Superior migration of the humeral head in rotator cuff arthropathy
- CT – to assess the morphology and extent of glenoid erosion
- MRI – to assess the state of the rotator cuff which, in some instances, may be intact but very thin, degenerate and, hence, dysfunctional

Glenohumeral arthritis with loss of joint space (red arrow) and inferior osteophyte (yellow arrow)

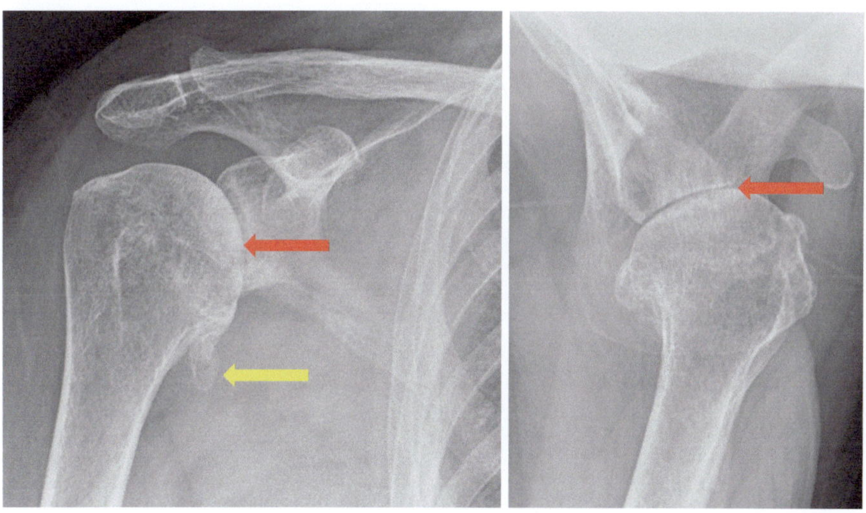

Inflammatory arthritis involving the humeral head, with multiple erosions, humeral head collapse and extensive subchondral cyst formation

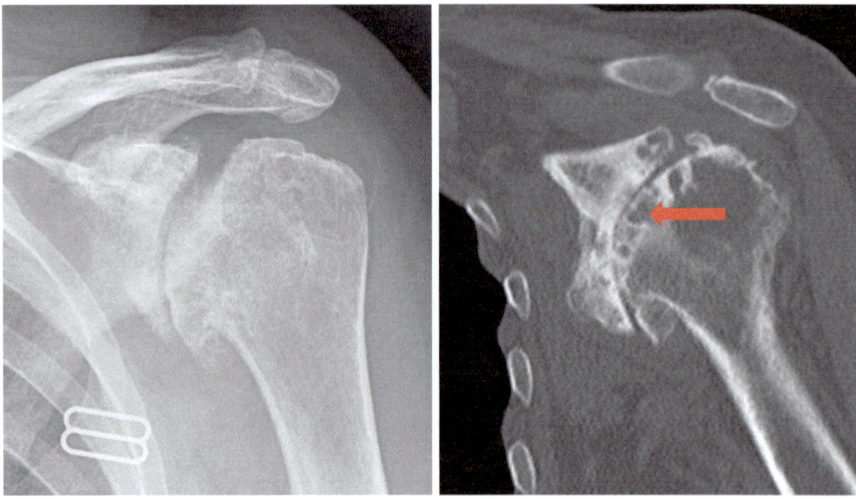

Plain radiograph and MRI showing punched out lesions (red arrows) of the humeral head due to inflammatory (rheumatoid) arthritis

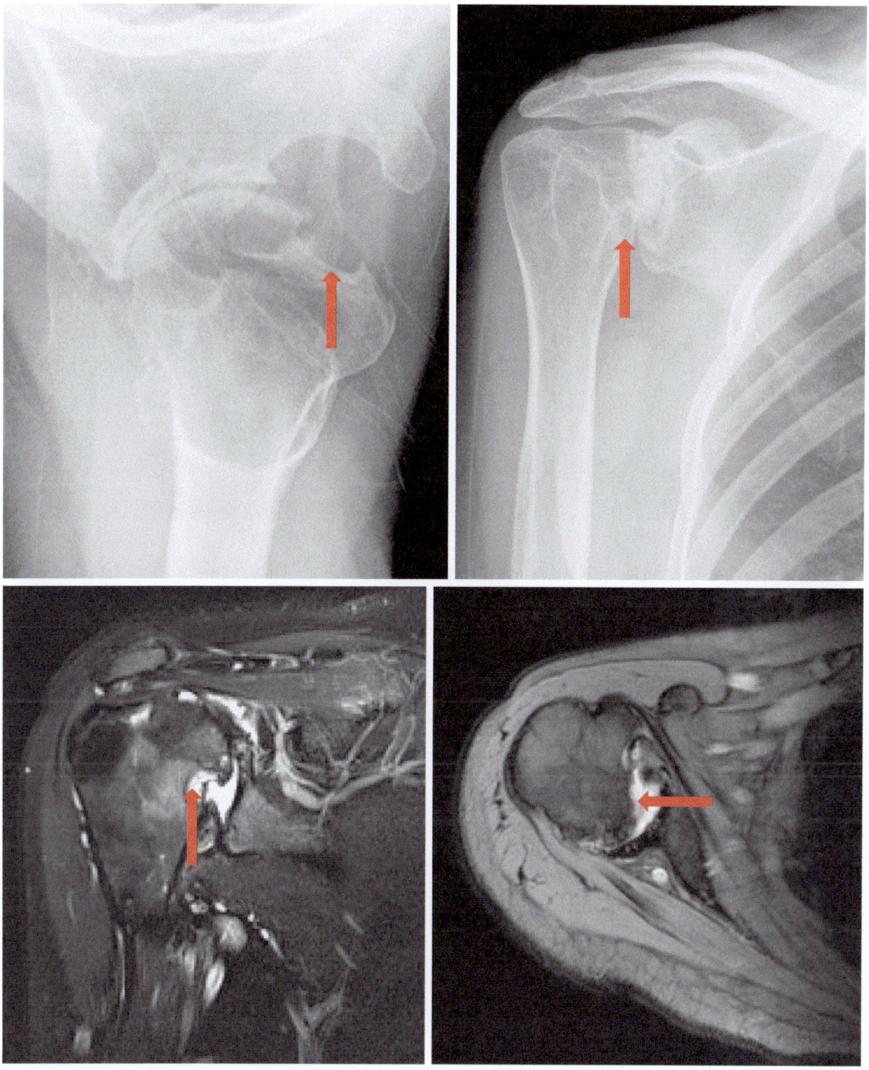

Plain radiograph and MRI showing rotator cuff arthropathy with superior migration of the humeral head, obliteration of the subacromial space (red arrow) and loss of glenohumeral joint space. The superior part of the humeral head is articulating with the under surface of the acromion

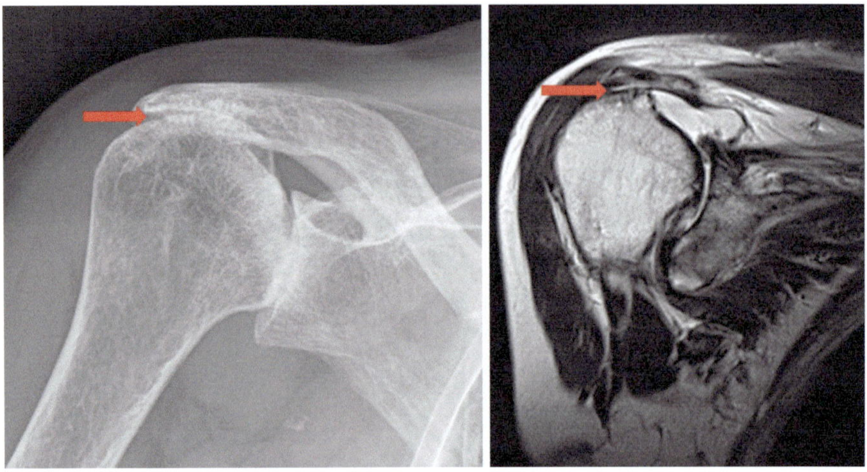

Cystic changes in the humeral head on plain radiographs confirmed with MRI (red arrows) due to tuberculosis involving the humeral head

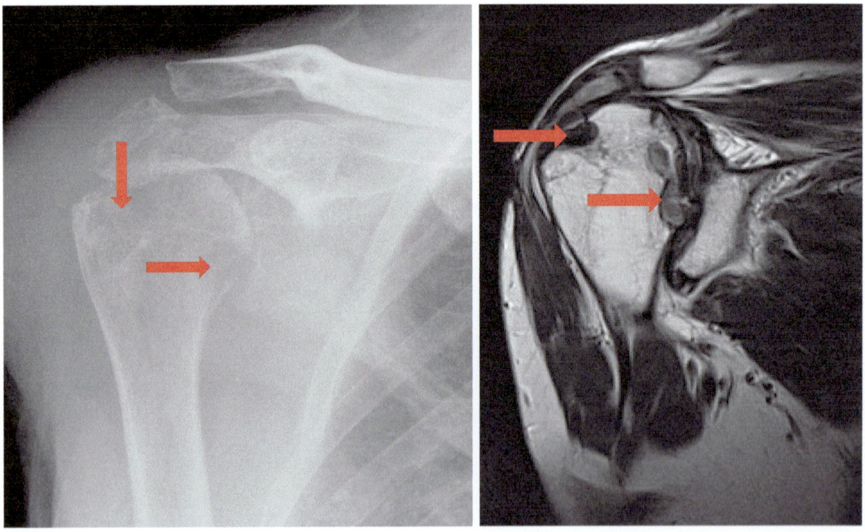

30.4 Management of Glenohumeral Arthritis

Non-surgical

- Leave alone
- Simple analgesia
- Activity modification
- Physiotherapy to:
  - Strengthen the shoulder and peri-scapular muscles
  - Strengthen deltoid to compensate for a dysfunctional rotator cuff
  - Maintain motion
  - Stretch contracted soft tissues to regain motion
- Glenohumeral injections – steroid, hyaluronic acid
- Steroids, disease modifying drugs (for rheumatoid arthritis)

Surgical [11–20]

- Arthroscopic debridement, subacromial decompression, long head of biceps tenotomy or tenodesis, removal of loose bodies
- Shoulder arthroplasty
  - Interposition arthroplasty in younger patients
  - Fusion arthroplasty in:
    - Instability
    - Neuropathy
    - Infection
  - Replacement arthroplasty:
    - Hemi-arthroplasty
      - Humeral head resurfacing
      - Stemmed
    - Total shoulder replacement
      - Humeral head resurfacing
      - Stemmed
      - Anatomic
      - Reverse shoulder replacement

Resurfacing hemi-arthroplasty of the humeral head (green arrow). The anchors have been used to reattach the subscapularis tendon (which was divided as part of the surgical approach) to the proximal humerus (blue arrow)

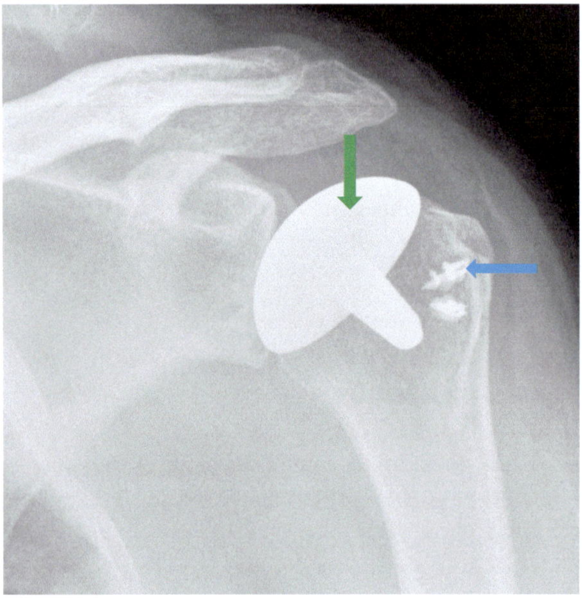

30.5 Shoulder Arthroplasty for Glenohumeral Arthritis

It is important to distinguish between arthritis in the presence of an intact and functional rotator cuff and arthritis in the presence of a massive rotator cuff tear (rotator cuff arthropathy). The former may benefit from a hemi-arthroplasty or anatomic total shoulder replacement, whereas reverse total shoulder replacement is indicated for the latter.

In dealing with glenohumeral arthritis it is vital to determine the state of the rotator cuff

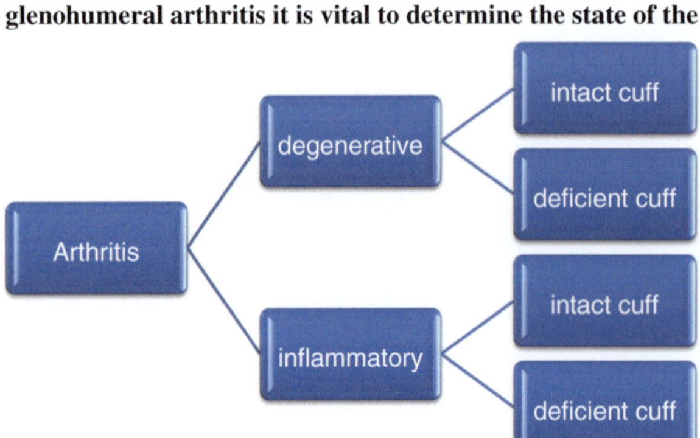

30.5.1 Anatomic Total Shoulder Replacement

In the anatomic total shoulder replacement, the prosthetic components aim to reproduce the native anatomy of the glenohumeral joint, with a ball replacing the humeral head and a socket replacing the glenoid.

The weak points of anatomic shoulder replacement are:

- The glenoid may loosen with time due to eccentric loading by the humeral head component during arm forward elevation or abduction (known as the rocking horse phenomenon)
- The rotator cuff may be intact but dysfunctional or may be initially intact but later tear, due to age related or other degeneration, which can lead to superior humeral component migration and replacement failure

30.5.2 Reverse Total Shoulder Replacement [27–35]

In the reverse shoulder prosthesis, the ball and socket anatomy of the native shoulder is reversed by placing the ball component at the glenoid and the socket at the proximal humerus.

Reverse shoulder designs use either cemented or un-cemented humeral components and cementless glenoid fixation. The glenoid consists of a baseplate with a gleno-sphere placed on top. Reverse shoulder replacement is used in situations where there is deficiency of the rotator cuff or concern about the longevity of the rotator cuff including:

- Rotator cuff deficiency due to extensive degeneration or tear
- Proximal humeral resection, e.g. in neoplasia
- Multi-fragmentary proximal humeral fractures that are better treated by replacement rather than fixation. Dysfunction of the rotator cuff tendon could lead to failure of a prosthesis which relies on an intact rotator cuff such as humeral head hemi-arthroplasty. In such fractures the rotator cuff tendon may dysfunction due to:
  - The fractured tuberosities not healing
  - Vascular compromise
  - Associated rotator cuff tendon tears

The reverse shoulder replacement does not rely on the rotator cuff for shoulder function and motion but on the deltoid, the efficiency of which it aims to enhance through its reverse design [21–23]. This reversal in geometry leads to:

- Lowering of the humerus resulting in increased tension of the deltoid and improved efficiency of this muscle
- Movement of the centre of rotation of the glenohumeral joint medially (to the glenoid bone prosthesis interface) that allows:

- Recruitment of more deltoid fibres with an improvement in its function
- Lengthening of the abduction and forward elevation moment arms of deltoid, which reduces the deltoid effort needed for activities such as lifting
- Reduction of the torque and sheer forces at the gleno-sphere glenoid interface

Reverse total shoulder arthroplasty. The glenoid component (yellow arrow) is spherical, whereas the humeral component (red arrow) is socket shaped (reversal of the normal anatomy)

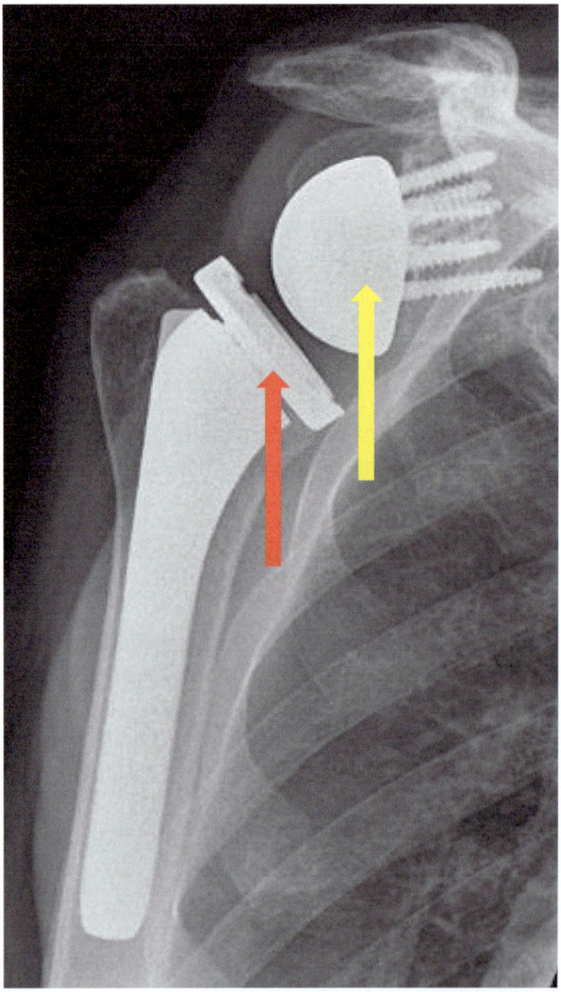

Complications of reverse shoulder arthroplasty [24–26] include:

- Haematoma formation due to the big empty space conferred by the absence of an intact rotator cuff
- Infection
- Nerve injury

- Fractures of the acromion or spine of the scapula
- Glenohumeral dislocation
- Component loosening
- Deltoid weakness and fatigue
- Scapular notching – this refers to the gradual erosion of the scapular neck inferior to the peg of the glenoid component. This is the result of mechanical abutment of the polyethylene in the humeral tray against the scapular neck as the arm is adducted. Such notching may lead to the formation of polyethylene wear debris which can then cause osteolysis. Scapular notching:
  - May occur in up to 80% of cases of reverse shoulder arthroplasty
  - May be graded using the Sirveaux classification:
    - Grade 1 – notch limited to the scapular border
    - Grade 2 – notch reaching the inferior screw of the baseplate
    - Grade 3 – notch extending beyond the inferior screw
    - Grade 4 – notch reaching the central peg of the baseplate
  - May be associated with a pillar spur
  - May be related to decreased shoulder strength, reduced motion and increased incidence of glenoid radiolucent lines
  - May stabilise within the first 2 years or, in some cases, continue to progress
  - May be prevented by placing the baseplate flush with the inferior glenoid edge or overhanging the inferior edge and in a neutral or inferior tilted position (avoiding a superiorly tilted baseplate)

Tips

- Patients with glenohumeral arthritis may experience pain not just from the glenohumeral joint arthritis but also from the subacromial space, the acromioclavicular joint (ACJt) or long head of the biceps tendon due to concomitant disease. Hence:
  - Addressing these associated lesions with non-surgical or surgical means may help improve pain and allow a patient with glenohumeral arthritis to avoid a joint replacement
  - Addressing these associated lesions at the time of shoulder replacement is important, rather than simply replacing the articular surfaces. There is evidence that following a shoulder replacement for arthritis, further reoperations may become necessary if the above lesions are not addressed, as they can continue acting as a source of pain
- Severe joint destruction in the absence of pain raises the possibility of neuropathic arthritis
- Instability arthritis may be seen in instability cases that have been treated surgically or non-surgically

- In the presence of infective arthritis, the initial aim is to treat the infection. Replacement arthroplasty may be considered in joints with previous infective arthritis if the infection has been cured and the inflammatory markers have remained in the normal range for a substantial period of time (more than a year). Nevertheless, the risk of infection recurring may persist even in such cases
- Rheumatoid arthritis may exhibit two phases:
  - Wet phase characterised by active inflammation and sub-articular erosions on radiological imaging
  - Dry phase where the active inflammation has subsided and radiological features similar to osteoarthritis (subchondral sclerosis, loss of joint space, subchondral cysts, osteophytes) are seen
- Inflammatory arthritis may affect the ACJt and subacromial space along with the glenohumeral joint. As a result:
  - It may be more difficult to localise the source of a patient's symptoms
  - All diseased areas may need addressing at the time of surgery, such as during glenohumeral arthroplasty, to minimise the risk of ongoing symptoms

References

1. Parsons IM 4th, Weldon EJ 3rd, Titelman RM, Smith KL. Glenohumeral arthritis and its management. Phys Med Rehabil Clin N Am. 2004;15(2):447–74.
2. Kelley MJ, Ramsey ML. Osteoarthritis and traumatic arthritis of the shoulder. J Hand Ther. 2000;13(2):148–62.
3. Macaulay AA, Greiwe RM, Bigliani LU. Rotator cuff deficient arthritis of the glenohumeral joint. Clin Orthop Surg. 2010;2(4):196–202.
4. Feeley BT, Gallo RA, Craig EV. Cuff tear arthropathy: current trends in diagnosis and surgical management. J Shoulder Elb Surg. 2009;18(3):484–94.
5. Papalia R, Osti L, Del Buono A, Denaro V, Maffulli N. Glenohumeral arthropathy following stabilization for recurrent instability. Br Med Bull. 2010;96:75–92.
6. Brophy RH, Marx RG. Osteoarthritis following shoulder instability. Clin Sports Med. 2005;24(1):47–56.
7. Brown JH, Deluca SA. The radiology of rheumatoid arthritis. Am Fam Physician. 1995;52(5):1372–80.
8. Naranja RJ Jr, Iannotti JP. Surgical options in the treatment of arthritis of the shoulder: alternatives to prosthetic arthroplasty. Semin Arthroplast. 1995;6(4):204–13.
9. Ersoy H, Pomeranz SJ. Milwaukee shoulder syndrome. J Surg Orthop Adv. 2017;26(1):54–7.
10. Namdari S, Skelley N, Keener JD, Galatz LM, Yamaguchi K. What is the role of arthroscopic debridement for glenohumeral arthritis? A critical examination of the literature. Arthroscopy. 2013;29(8):1392–8.
11. Bishop JY, Flatow EL. Management of glenohumeral arthritis: a role for arthroscopy? Orthop Clin N Am. 2003;34(4):559–66.
12. Guyette TM, Bae H, Warren RF, Craig E, Wickiewicz TL. Results of arthroscopic subacromial decompression in patients with subacromial impingement and glenohumeral degenerative joint disease. J Shoulder Elb Surg. 2002;11(4):299–304.

13. Denard PJ, Wirth MA, Orfaly RM. Management of glenohumeral arthritis in the young adult. J Bone Joint Surg Am. 2011;93(9):885–92.
14. Chong PY, Srikumaran U, Kuye IO, Warner JJ. Glenohumeral arthritis in the young patient. J Shoulder Elb Surg. 2011;20(2 Suppl):S30–40.
15. Izquierdo R, Voloshin I, Edwards S, Freehill MQ, Stanwood W, Wiater JM, Watters WC 3rd, Goldberg MJ, Keith M, Turkelson CM, Wies JL, Anderson S, Boyer K, Raymond L, Sluka P, American Academy of Orthopedic Surgeons. Treatment of glenohumeral osteoarthritis. J Am Acad Orthop Surg. 2010;18(6):375–82.
16. Strauss EJ, Roche C, Flurin PH, Wright T, Zuckerman JD. The glenoid in shoulder arthroplasty. J Shoulder Elb Surg. 2009;18(5):819–33.
17. Wiater JM, Fabing MH. Shoulder arthroplasty: prosthetic options and indications. J Am Acad Orthop Surg. 2009;17(7):415–25.
18. Elhassan B, Ozbaydar M, Diller D, Higgins LD, Warner JJ. Soft-tissue resurfacing of the glenoid in the treatment of glenohumeral arthritis in active patients less than fifty years old. J Bone Joint Surg Am. 2009;91(2):419–24.
19. Radnay CS, Setter KJ, Chambers L, Levine WN, Bigliani LU, Ahmad CS. Total shoulder replacement compared with humeral head replacement for the treatment of primary glenohumeral osteoarthritis: a systematic review. J Shoulder Elb Surg. 2007;16(4):396–402.
20. Burkhead WZ Jr, Krishnan SG, Lin KC. Biologic resurfacing of the arthritic glenohumeral joint: Historical review and current applications. J Shoulder Elb Surg. 2007;16(5 Suppl): S248–53.
21. González-Díaz R, Rodríguez-Merchán EC, Gilbert MS. The role of shoulder fusion in the era of arthroplasty. Int Orthop. 1997;21(3):204–9.
22. Schoch B, Werthel JD, Sperling JW, Cofield RH, Sanchez-Sotelo J. Is shoulder arthroplasty an option for charcot arthropathy? Int Orthop. 2016;40(12):2589–95.
23. Urch E, Dines JS, Dines DM. Emerging indications for reverse shoulder arthroplasty. Instr Course Lect. 2016;65:157–69.
24. Walker M, Brooks J, Willis M, Frankle M. How reverse shoulder arthroplasty works. Clin Orthop Relat Res. 2011;469(9):2440–51.
25. Lorenzetti AJ, Stone GP, Simon P, Frankle MA. Biomechanics of reverse shoulder arthroplasty: current concepts. Instr Course Lect. 2016;65:127–43.
26. Berliner JL, Regalado-Magdos A, Ma CB, Feeley BT. Biomechanics of reverse total shoulder arthroplasty. J Shoulder Elb Surg. 2015;24(1):150–60.
27. Boileau P, Watkinson DJ, Hatzidakis AM, Balg F. Grammont reverse prosthesis: design, rationale, and biomechanics. J Shoulder Elb Surg. 2005;14(1 Suppl S):147S–61S.
28. Scalise J, Jaczynski A, Jacofsky M. The effect of glenosphere diameter and eccentricity on deltoid power in reverse shoulder arthroplasty. Bone Joint J. 2016;98-B(2):218–23.
29. Pegreffi F, Pellegrini A, Paladini P, Merolla G, Belli G, Velarde PU, Porcellini G. Deltoid muscle activity in patients with reverse shoulder prosthesis at 2-year follow-up. Musculoskelet Surg. 2017;101(Suppl 2):129–35.
30. Trappey GJ 4th, O'Connor DP, Edwards TB. What are the instability and infection rates after reverse shoulder arthroplasty? Clin Orthop Relat Res. 2011;469(9):2505–11.
31. Lévigne C, Garret J, Boileau P, Alami G, Favard L, Walch G. Scapular notching in reverse shoulder arthroplasty: is it important to avoid it and how? Clin Orthop Relat Res. 2011;469(9):2512–20.
32. Kwaees TA, Charalambous CP. Reverse shoulder arthroplasty—minimum age for surgery, postoperative rehabilitation and long term restrictions. A delphi consensus study. Ortop Traumatol Rehabil. 2014;16(4):435–9.
33. Merolla G, Porcellini G. Reverse shoulder arthroplasty in patients aged sixty years old or younger: are we really doing the best? Transl Med UniSa. 2014;9:66–7.
34. Boileau P. Complications and revision of reverse total shoulder arthroplasty. Orthop Traumatol Surg Res. 2016;102(1 Suppl):S33–43.
35. Alentorn-Geli E, Samitier G, Torrens C, Wright TW. Reverse shoulder arthroplasty. Part 2: systematic review of reoperations, revisions, problems, and complications. Int J Shoulder Surg. 2015;9(2):60–7.

Chapter 31
Synovial Chondromatosis of the Shoulder

This is a condition whereby cartilaginous loose bodies form in a cavity which is lined by synovium [1–3]. This may be:

- Primary – there is primary metaplasia of the synovial membrane to chondrocytes that go on to form cartilage. These cartilaginous bodies increase in size and may become calcified
- Secondary – due to loose bodies arising from osteochondral fractures, degenerative arthritis or avascular necrosis that lead to fragmentation of the joint surface or detachment of osteophytes. These form a central nidus which can then become covered with cartilage and may grow in size. Here, there is proliferation of connective tissue cells and subsequent cartilaginous metaplasia

In primary synovial chondromatosis, there may be three stages to the metaplasia:

1. Confined to the synovium
2. Active synovium with loose bodies
3. Inactive synovium with residual loose bodies

Synovial chondromatosis usually affects one joint and is intra-articular, usually involving the knee. However, it may also involve extra-articular tissues such as tendon sheaths or bursae. In the shoulder this condition has been reported in the glenohumeral joint as well as in the subacromial, sub-coracoid and deltoid bursae [2–8].

© Springer Nature Switzerland AG 2019

C. Panayiotou Charalambous, *The Shoulder Made Easy*,
https://doi.org/10.1007/978-3-319-98908-2_31

Multiple calcified bodies in the subacromial space due to synovial chondromatosis presenting with subacromial pain syndrome

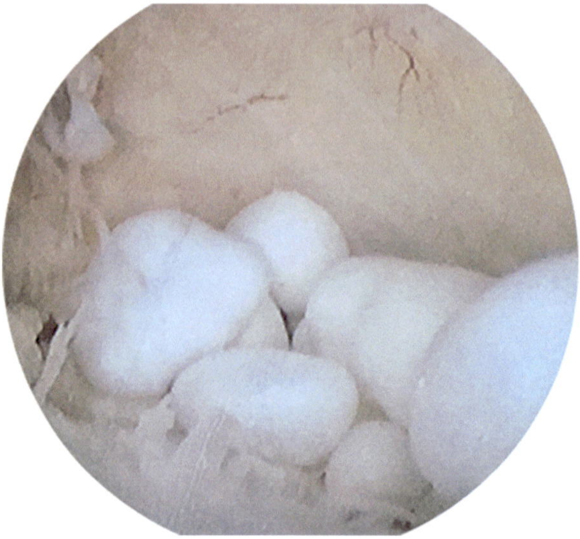

31.1 Clinical Symptoms of Synovial Chondromatosis

- Subacromial pain syndrome or glenohumeral pain
- Clicking/clunking
- Locking
- Stiffness
- Visible or palpable swelling

31.2 Clinical Signs of Synovial Chondromatosis

- Visible swelling
- Localised tenderness
- Positive subacromial impingement test
- Reduced shoulder motion – active and passive

31.3 Investigations for Synovial Chondromatosis [9–11]

- Plain radiographs – popcorn appearance
- MRI – can demonstrate non-calcified loose bodies (that are not visible on plain radiographs)

MRI showing multiple loose bodies in the sub-deltoid area (red arrows) (a,b), not visible on plain radiograph (c)

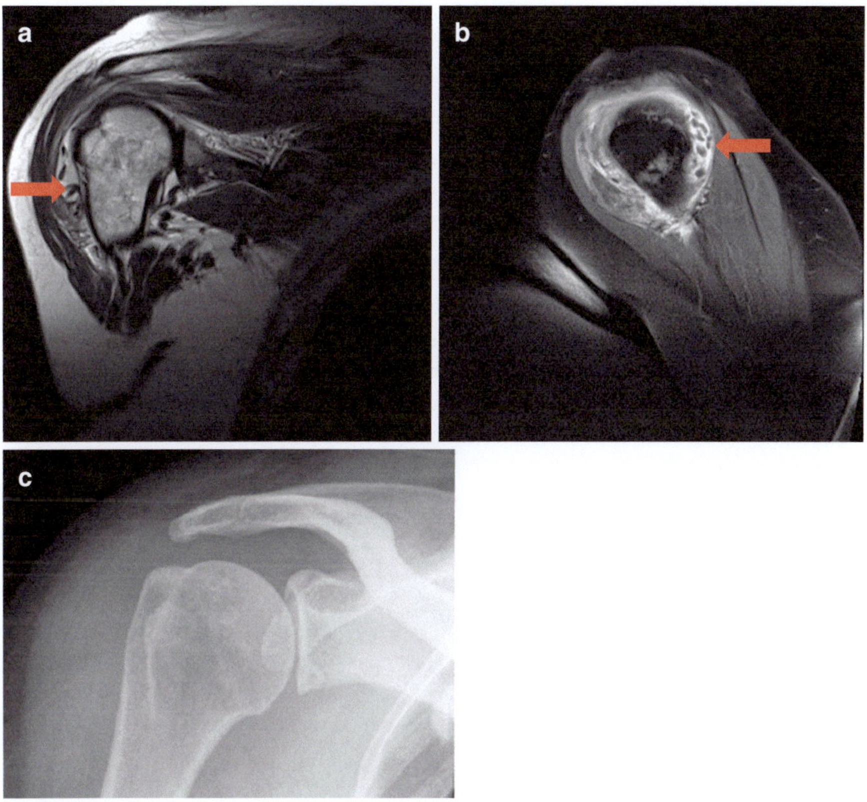

31.4 Differential Diagnosis of Synovial Chondromatosis

- Calcific tendinopathy
- Neoplastic lesions (e.g. synovial sarcoma, periosteal chondroma)

31.5 Management of Synovial Chondromatosis

- Non-surgical
  - Leave alone
  - Activity modification
  - Analgesia
  - Physiotherapy
    - Improve passive motion
- Surgical [12–18]
  - Surgical removal of loose bodies (arthroscopic/open) + synovectomy

    If only loose bodies are removed, there is the potential for the synovium to produce more loose bodies. The aim of surgery is to remove the loose bodies and also carry out a synovectomy to prevent the formation of further loose bodies. However, progression may not occur if the synovium becomes inactive
  - In cases of synovial chondromatosis associated with glenohumeral degeneration or arthritis, the latter may be the main focus of intervention (with arthroplasty), rather than the chondromatosis per se [18]

Tips

- Intra-articular loose bodies may lead to secondary arthritis due to third-body wear
- Loose bodies in the bicipital groove may cause attrition or inflammation of the long head of the biceps tendon, whilst those in the subacromial bursa may lead to rotator cuff tears
- In the absence of obvious degenerative changes, a history of injury should be sought as what appears as primary synovial chondromatosis may be a secondary condition
- Malignant transformation is a very rare but a recognised complication and needs to be considered when aggressive clinical or radiological features are encountered (such as periarticular soft tissue involvement or bone infiltration by a cartilaginous mass). Such neoplasms tend to be locally aggressive neoplasms [19]

References

1. Crotty JM, Monu JU, Pope TL Jr. Synovial osteochondromatosis. Radiol Clin N Am. 1996;34(2):327–42.
2. Chillemi C, Marinelli M, de Cupis V. Primary synovial chondromatosis of the shoulder: clinical, arthroscopic and histopathological aspects. Knee Surg Sports Traumatol Arthrosc. 2005;13(6):483–8.

3. Ji JH, Shafi M, Jeong DS. Secondary synovial chondromatosis of the shoulder. Knee Surg Sports Traumatol Arthrosc. 2015;23(9):2624–7.
4. Neumann JA, Garrigues GE. Synovial chondromatosis of the subacromial bursa causing a bursal-sided rotator cuff tear. Case Rep Orthop. 2015;2015:259483. https://doi.org/10.1155/2015/259483.
5. Horii M, Tamai M, Kido K, Kusuzaki K, Kubo T, Hirasawa Y. Two cases of synovial chondromatosis of the subacromial bursa. J Shoulder Elb Surg. 2001;10(2):186–9.
6. Demirhan M, Eralp L, Atalar AC. Synovial chondromatosis of the subcoracoid bursa. Int Orthop. 1999;23(6):358–60.
7. Dwidmuthe SC, Nemade AS, Agrawal S, Pathak A. Rare case of extra-articular synovial chondromatosis of biceps tendon sheath in 8 years male child. J Orthop Case Rep. 2014;4(4):33–6.
8. Aydogan NH, Kocadal O, Ozmeric A, Aktekin CN. Arthroscopic treatment of a case with concomitant subacromial and subdeltoid synovial chondromatosis and labrum tear. Case Rep Orthop. 2013;2013:636747. https://doi.org/10.1155/2013/636747.
9. McKenzie G, Raby N, Ritchie D. A pictorial review of primary synovial osteochondromatosis. Eur Radiol. 2008;18(11):2662–9.
10. Chen A, Wong LY, Sheu CY, Chen BF. Distinguishing multiple rice body formation in chronic subacromial-subdeltoid bursitis from synovial chondromatosis. Skelet Radiol. 2002;31(2):119–21.
11. Walker EA, Murphey MD, Fetsch JF. Imaging characteristics of tenosynovial and bursal chondromatosis. Skelet Radiol. 2011;40(3):317–25.
12. Ranalletta M, Bongiovanni S, Calvo JM, Gallucci G, Maignon G. Arthroscopic treatment of synovial chondromatosis of the shoulder: report of three patients. J Shoulder Elb Surg. 2009;18(3):e4–8.
13. Urbach D, McGuigan FX, John M, Neumann W, Ender SA. Long-term results after arthroscopic treatment of synovial chondromatosis of the shoulder. Arthroscopy. 2008;24(3):318–23.
14. Lunn JV, Castellanos-Rosas J, Walch G. Arthroscopic synovectomy, removal of loose bodies and selective biceps tenodesis for synovial chondromatosis of the shoulder. J Bone Joint Surg Br. 2007;89:1329.
15. Tokis AV, Andrikoula SI, Chouliaras VT, Vasiliadis HS, Georgoulis AD. Diagnosis and arthroscopic treatment of primary synovial chondromatosis of the shoulder. Arthroscopy. 2007;23(9):1023.e1–5.
16. Jung KA, Kim SJ, Jeong JH. Arthroscopic treatment of synovial chondromatosis that possibly developed after open capsular shift for shoulder instability. Knee Surg Sports Traumatol Arthrosc. 2007;15(12):1499–503.
17. Bruggeman NB, Sperling JW, Shives TC. Arthroscopic technique for treatment of synovial chondromatosis of the glenohumeral joint. Arthroscopy. 2005;21(5):633.
18. Kreines A, McMillan S, Ford E, Dingle A. Reverse total shoulder arthroplasty for the treatment of synovial chondromatosis: a case report and review of the literature. Arch Bone Jt Surg. 2017;5(2):117–20.
19. McCarthy C, Anderson WJ, Vlychou M, Inagaki Y, Whitwell D, Gibbons CL, Athanasou NA. Primary synovial chondromatosis: a reassessment of malignant potential in 155 cases. Skelet Radiol. 2016;45(6):755–62.

Chapter 32
Acromio-Clavicular Joint Arthropathy

This refers to the presence of a diseased acromio-clavicular joint (ACJt). This may be due to multiple causes [1–12] as described below:

- Osteoarthritis—a condition whereby there is degeneration of the articular cartilage of the ACJt
- Degeneration of the joint's fibrocartilaginous disc
- Inflammatory arthritis
- Infective arthritis (bacterial or other)
- Metabolic disorders (e.g. hyperparathyroidism)
- Crystal arthropathy
  - Gout
  - Pseudogout
- Neoplastic causes
- Distal clavicle osteolysis—occurs in repetitive heavy weight lifting (weight trainers, judo players, delivery personnel). Possible causes include:
  - Repetitive micro-trauma giving rise to microfractures of the subchondral bone which the body then tries to repair
  - Disruption of the articular cartilage of the lateral end of the clavicle may lead to synovial invasion of the subchondral bone and osteolysis

32.1 Clinical Symptoms of ACJt Arthropathy

ACJt disease often causes similar clinical symptoms despite the underlying causative disorder:

© Springer Nature Switzerland AG 2019

C. Panayiotou Charalambous, *The Shoulder Made Easy*,
https://doi.org/10.1007/978-3-319-98908-2_32

- Pain over or in the ACJt:
  - Worse in overhead and cross-body activities of the arm
  - Worse during weight lifting or weight training
- Subacromial pain syndrome due to inferior osteophytes abutting the rotator cuff

32.2 Clinical Signs of ACJt Arthropathy [13]

ACJt disease often causes similar clinical signs despite the underlying causative disorder:

- Tenderness localised to the ACJt
- ACJt crepitus
- Paxinos test positive
- Cross body adduction test positive
- Pain over the ACJt with O'Brien's test
- Subacromial impingement test positive

32.3 Investigations for ACJt Arthropathy

- Radiographs—AP and AP 15° cephalad
  - The radiological futures of osteoarthritis include sclerosis, subchondral cysts, superior/inferior or anterior/posterior osteophytes which may involve the medial acromion or the lateral end of the clavicle. Lateral end of the clavicle radiolucency in osteolysis
  - Incidental osteoarthritis radiological futures increase with advancing age and may not correlate with ACJt or subacromial impingement symptoms
- MRI
  - Increased signal intensity with bone marrow oedema in lateral end of clavicle osteolysis
  - Osseous fragments
  - Osseous irregularity
  - Fluid in the ACJt (effusion)

ACJt arthropathy with sclerosis of the lateral end of the clavicle and medial part of the acromion, along with cystic changes (yellow arrow)

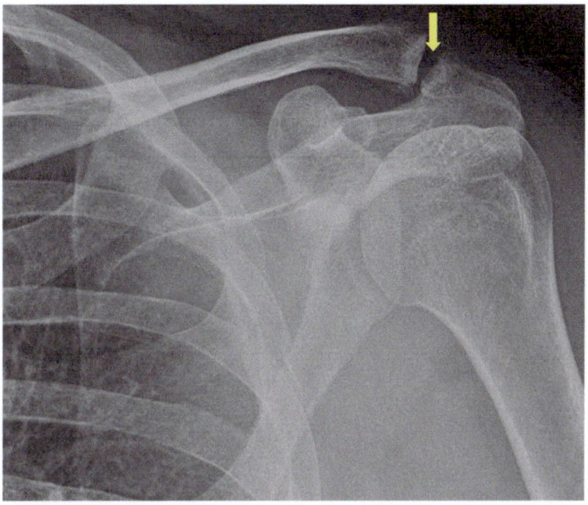

Plain radiograph showing ACJt arthropathy with reduction of joint space. CT scan shows loss of joint space and osteophyte formation (yellow arrows)

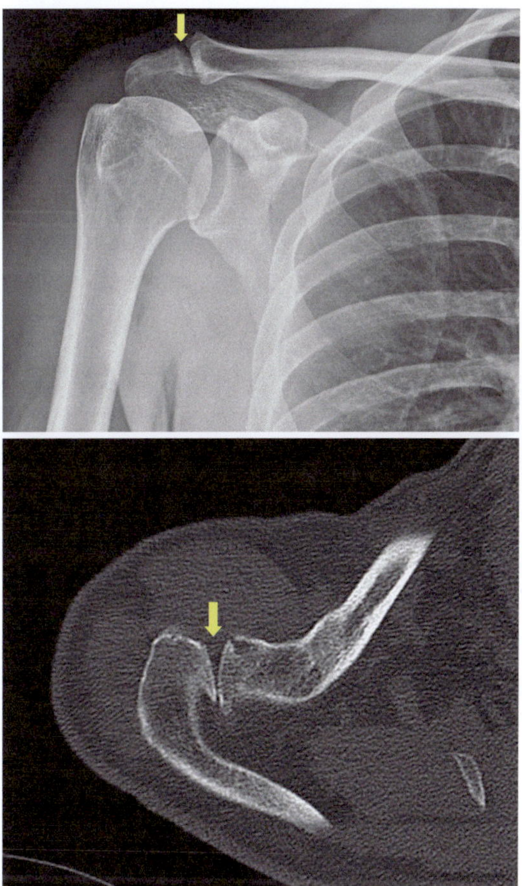

ACJoint arthritis (red arrow)

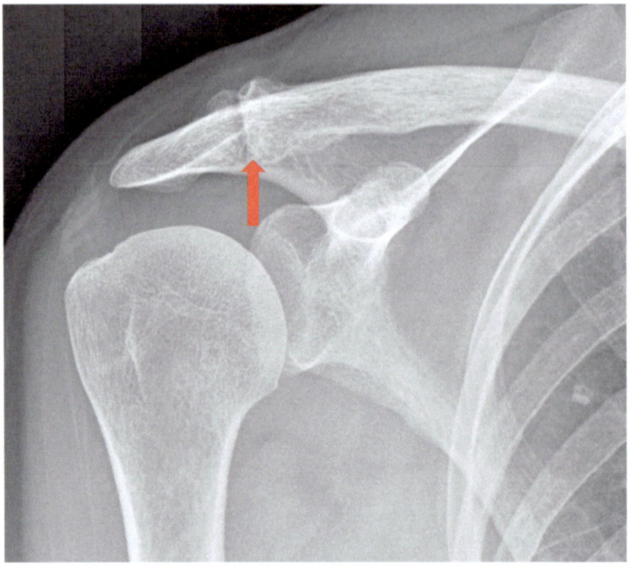

Osteolysis of the lateral end of the clavicle (red arrow)

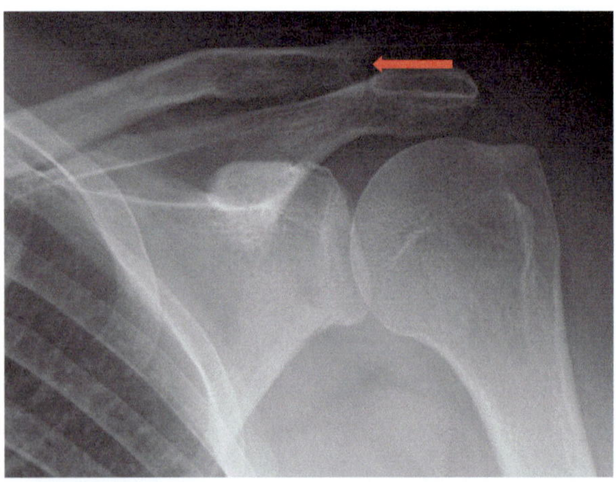

32.4 Management of ACJt Arthropathy

Non-surgical [14–16]

- Leave alone
- Activity modification
- Analgesia
- Physiotherapy
  - Local treatment—cold or heat therapy
  - Passive joint mobilisation—ACJt glides
  - Shoulder and peri-scapular muscle strengthening
  - Addressing motion deficits in glenohumeral joint, sterno-clavicular joint, cervical and thoracic spine
- ACJt intra-articular steroid injections

Surgical [17–20]

- ACJt excision (open or arthroscopic)

ACJt arthropathy (red arrow) treated with surgical excision (green arrow)

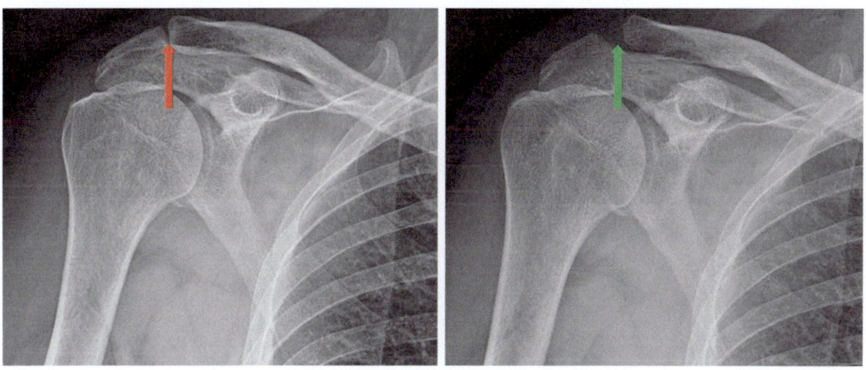

References

1. Mall NA, Foley E, Chalmers PN, Cole BJ, Romeo AA, Bach BR Jr. Degenerative joint disease of the acromioclavicular joint: a review. Am J Sports Med. 2013;41(11):2684–92.
2. Menge TJ, Boykin RE, Bushnell BD, Byram IR. Acromioclavicular osteoarthritis: a common cause of shoulder pain. South Med J. 2014;107(5):324–9.
3. Mcdonald S, Hopper MA. Acromioclavicular joint disease. Semin Musculoskelet Radiol. 2015;19(3):300–6.
4. Buttaci CJ, Stitik TP, Yonclas PP, Foye PM. Osteoarthritis of the acromioclavicular joint: a review of anatomy, biomechanics, diagnosis, and treatment. Am J Phys Med Rehabil. 2004;83(10):791–7.

5. Williams M. Diagnostic challenges in acromioclavicular septic arthritis. BMJ Case Rep. 2016. https://doi.org/10.1136/bcr-2016-216034.
6. Agarwal A, Bhandari A, Maheshwari R. Tuberculosis of Acromioclavicular Joint. J Clin Diagn Res. 2017;11(3):RD03–4.
7. Bossert M, Prati C, Bertolini E, Toussirot E, Wendling D. Septic arthritis of the acromioclavicular joint. Joint Bone Spine. 2010;77(5):466–9.
8. Hakozaki M, Kikuchi S, Otani K, Tajino T, Konno S. Pseudogout of the acromioclavicular joint: report of two cases and review of the literature. Mod Rheumatol. 2011;21(4):440–3.
9. Petersson CJ. Degeneration of the acromioclavicular joint. A morphological study. Acta Orthop Scand. 1983;54(3):434–8.
10. Scavenius M, Iversen BF. Nontraumatic clavicular osteolysis in weight lifters. Am J Sports Med. 1992;20(4):463–7.
11. Cahill BR. Osteolysis of the distal part of the clavicle in male athletes. J Bone Joint Surg Am. 1982;64(7):1053–8.
12. Schwarzkopf R, Ishak C, Elman M, Gelber J, Strauss DN, Jazrawi LM. Distal clavicular osteolysis: a review of the literature. Bull NYU Hosp Jt Dis. 2008;66(2):94–101.
13. Charalambous CP. Clinical Examination of the Shoulder. In: Charalambous CP, editor. The shoulder made easy. Basel: Springer; 2019.
14. Harris KD, Deyle GD, Gill NW, Howes RR. Manual physical therapy for injection-confirmed nonacute acromioclavicular joint pain. J Orthop Sports Phys Ther. 2012;42(2):66–80.
15. Aly AR, Rajasekaran S, Ashworth N. Ultrasound-guided shoulder girdle injections are more accurate and more effective than landmark-guided injections: a systematic review and meta-analysis. Br J Sports Med. 2015;49(16):1042–9.
16. van Riet RP, Goehre T, Bell SN. The long term effect of an intra-articular injection of corticosteroids in the acromioclavicular joint. J Shoulder Elbow Surg. 2012;21(3):376–9.
17. Scavenius M, Iversen BF, Stürup J. Resection of the lateral end of the clavicle following osteolysis, with emphasis on non-traumatic osteolysis of the acromial end of the clavicle in athletes. Injury. 1987;18(4):261–3.
18. Auge WK 2nd, Fischer RA. Arthroscopic distal clavicle resection for isolated atraumatic osteolysis in weight lifters. Am J Sports Med. 1998;26(2):189–92.
19. Robertson WJ, Griffith MH, Carroll K, O'Donnell T, Gill TJ. Arthroscopic versus open distal clavicle excision: a comparative assessment at intermediate-term follow-up. Am J Sports Med. 2011;39(11):2415–20.
20. Freedman BA, Javernick MA, O'Brien FP, Ross AE, Doukas WC. Arthroscopic versus open distal clavicle excision: comparative results at six months and one year from a randomized, prospective clinical trial. J Shoulder Elbow Surg. 2007;16(4):413–8.

Chapter 33
Sterno-clavicular Joint Arthropathy

Sterno-clavicular arthropathy refers to disease of the sterno-clavicular joint. Causes of sterno-clavicular arthropathy include osteoarthritis, degenerative intra-articular disc tears and inflammatory and infective arthritis. It also refers to various other conditions including SAPHO, Friedrich's disease and medial clavicle condensing osteitis [1–23].

33.1 Osteoarthritis of the Sterno-clavicular Joint

This is a condition where there is degeneration of the articular cartilage of the sterno-clavicular joint, often in association with degeneration of the intra-articular cartilaginous disc. It may be primary, occurring in the absence of any precipitating event, or secondary to trauma.

33.2 Intra-articular Disc Tears of the Sterno-clavicular Joint

This is a condition where the intra-articular disc tears as a result of:

- Acute trauma
- Chronic degeneration

33.3 Inflammatory Arthritis of the Sterno-clavicular Joint

This is a group of conditions whereby the sterno-clavicular joint is affected by an underlying inflammatory process. This may lead to inflammation of the soft

© Springer Nature Switzerland AG 2019

C. Panayiotou Charalambous, *The Shoulder Made Easy*,
https://doi.org/10.1007/978-3-319-98908-2_33

tissues or destruction of the articular cartilage. Such inflammatory processes include:

- Rheumatoid arthritis
- Seronegative arthritides—ankylosing spondylitis, Reiter's syndrome, psoriatic arthritis
- Crystal arthropathies—due to deposition of uric acid (gout) or calcium pyrophosphate crystals (pseudogout)

Sterno-clavicular joint osteoarthritis, inflammatory arthritis, and intra-articular disc tears may present with similar symptoms and signs, and their management is similar; hence, they are discussed together below.

33.4 Clinical Symptoms of Sterno-clavicular Joint Arthritis/Disc Tears

- Pain
- Swelling
- Clicking

33.5 Clinical Signs of Sterno-clavicular Joint Arthritis/Disc Tears

- Visible swelling
- Tenderness
- Palpable crepitus on arm motion

33.6 Investigations for Sterno-clavicular Joint Arthritis/Disc Tears

- Plain radiographs
- MRI scan
- Serological
  - Inflammatory markers
  - Rheumatoid screen
- Joint aspiration—culture and sensitivity, microscopy for crystals

33.7 Management of Sterno-clavicular Joint Arthritis/Disc Tears

Management of osteoarthritis, inflammatory arthritis and disc tears may be:

Non-surgical

- Leave alone
- Activity modification
- Analgesia, anti-inflammatories
- Local treatment—cold or heat therapy
- Intra-articular steroid injections
- Steroids, disease-modifying drugs for inflammatory arthritis

Surgical [3, 4]

- Arthroscopic debridement—of disc tears
- Medial end of clavicle excision (open or arthroscopic)—for arthritis

33.8 Infective Arthritis of the Sterno-clavicular Joint

This is a condition whereby there is infection of the sterno-clavicular joint [15–19]. This may be limited to the soft tissues or lead to destruction of the articular cartilage.

Commonly involved organisms include *Staphylococcus aureus*, *Pseudomonas aeruginosa*, *Escherichia coli* and *Brucella melitensis*. Tuberculosis of the sterno-clavicular joint has also been described.

33.8.1 Clinical Symptoms of Infective Arthritis of the Sterno-clavicular Joint

May present with acute or chronic symptoms:

- Pain
- Swelling
- Systemic symptoms—shivers, rigours

33.8.2 Clinical Signs of Infective Arthritis of the Sterno-clavicular Joint

- Tenderness
- Visible swelling
- Hot, red joint
- Pyrexia

33.8.3 Investigations for Infective Arthritis of the Sterno-clavicular Joint

- Plain radiographs
- MRI scan
- Inflammatory markers
- Joint aspiration—microscopy (Gram stain), culture and sensitivity

33.8.4 Management of Infective Arthritis of the Sterno-clavicular Joint

- Antibiotics
- Joint washout

33.9 Synovitis, Acne, Pustulosis, Hyperostosis and Osteitis (SAPHO) Syndrome

This is a condition whereby there is joint arthritis along with bone and skin lesions [2, 11–14]. It may involve several bones or joints, most often involving the sterno-clavicular joint. The spine, pelvis, long bones and mandible may also be involved.

It usually appears between childhood and middle age and may have remissions and relapses. Bone and skin lesions may not appear at the same time, and on occasions skin lesions may precede or follow the bone lesions by several years or may co-exist.

The pathogenesis of SAPHO is uncertain, and several theories have been proposed including low-grade infection, an autoimmune response triggered by a bacterial or viral infection or a subtype of seronegative spondylo-arthropathies. It is characterised by:

- Joint synovitis
- Acne

- Pustulosis of the palms of the hands and soles of feet
- Hyperostosis—cortical thickening, narrowing of the medullary canal and periosteal new bone formation leading to bone hypertrophy. The bone appears enlarged and irregular
- Osteitis—bone sclerosis due to inflammation of the bone with infiltration of inflammatory cells

33.9.1 Clinical Symptoms of SAPHO

- Pain
- Swelling

33.9.2 Clinical Signs of SAPHO

- Tenderness
- Visible swelling
- Acne
- Pustulosis of the palms of the hands and soles of feet

33.9.3 Investigations for SAPHO

- Plain radiographs:
  - Hyperostosis
  - Osteitis—bone sclerosis
- MRI scan
- Bone scan may show other, synchronous, lesions demonstrating increased uptake
- ESR, CRP
- Open biopsy—histological examination, culture and sensitivity—to exclude infection and neoplastic cause. *Propionibacterium acnes* (*P. acnes*) and *Staph aureus* have been isolated in some cases

Diagnosis is clinically based on symptoms and signs as well as on exclusion of infective or neoplastic process or other conditions such as Paget's.

33.9.4 Management of SAPHO [2, 11–14]

- Antibiotics against *P. acnes* and *Staph aureus*
- Anti-inflammatories

- Bisphosphonates
- Steroids
- Disease-modifying drugs—methotrexate, sulfasalazine

33.10 Avascular Necrosis of the Medial End of Clavicle-Friedrich's Disease

This is a condition whereby there is necrosis of the medial end of the clavicle [20–23].

33.10.1 Clinical Symptoms of Medial Clavicle Necrosis

- Pain
- Swelling
- Clicking

33.10.2 Clinical Signs of Medial Clavicle Necrosis

- Tenderness
- Visible swelling
- Palpable crepitus

33.10.3 Investigations for Medial Clavicle Necrosis

- Plain radiographs—sclerosis, fragmentation of the medial end of the clavicle
- MRI
- Bone scan

33.10.4 Management of Medial Clavicle Necrosis

- Leave alone
- Activity modification
- Analgesia, anti-inflammatories
- May lead to osteoarthritis which is then treated as described previously

33.11 Medial Clavicle Condensing Osteitis

This a condition characterised by sclerosis and expansion of the medial and inferior end of the clavicle [6–9]. It is usually unilateral and more common in women of child-bearing age.

Its pathogenesis is uncertain with several theories proposed including inflammation due to abnormal loading (by heavy weight lifting or trauma), osteonecrosis or marrow fibrosis.

33.11.1 Clinical Symptoms of Clavicle Condensing Osteitis

- Pain
- Swelling

33.11.2 Clinical Signs of Clavicle Condensing Osteitis

- Visible swelling
- Tenderness

33.11.3 Investigations for Clavicle Condensing Osteitis

- Plain radiographs—sclerosis, expansion of the medial part of the clavicle
- Bone scan—increased uptake
- CT scan—obliteration of the bone marrow space with new bone formation
- MRI—bone oedema
- Biopsy—in rare cases where diagnosis cannot be made by imaging

33.11.4 Management of Clavicle Condensing Osteitis

- Leave alone—pain may improve with time, although swelling tends to persist
- Analgesia
- Steroid injection of the sterno-clavicular joint
- Excision of the medial end of the clavicle

References

1. Robinson CM, Jenkins PJ, Markham PE, Beggs I. Disorders of the sternoclavicular joint. J Bone Joint Surg Br. 2008;90(6):685–96.
2. Lawrence CR, East B, Rashid A, Tytherleigh-Strong GM. The prevalence of osteoarthritis of the sternoclavicular joint on computed tomography. J Shoulder Elbow Surg. 2017;26(1):e18–22.
3. Tytherleigh-Strong G, Rashid A, Lawrence C, Morrissey D. Arthroscopic sternoclavicular joint diskectomy for acute and chronic tears. Arthroscopy. 2017;33(11):1965–70.
4. Katthagen JC, Tahal DS, Menge TJ, Horan MP, Millett PJ. Minimum 2-year outcomes and return to sport following resection arthroplasty for the treatment of sternoclavicular osteoarthritis. J Shoulder Elbow Surg. 2017;26(2):e37–43.
5. Borowski A, Heikaus S, Kurt M. Calcium pyrophosphate dihydrate crystal deposition disease of the sternoclavicular joint. Thorac Cardiovasc Surg Rep. 2015;4(1):46–8.
6. Vierboom MA, Steinberg JD, Mooyaart EL, van Rijswijk MH. Condensing osteitis of the clavicle: magnetic resonance imaging as an adjunct method for differential diagnosis. Ann Rheum Dis. 1992;51(4):539–41.
7. Kruger GD, Rock MG, Munro TG. Condensing osteitis of the clavicle. A review of the literature and report of three cases. J Bone Joint Surg Am. 1987;69(4):550–7.
8. Harden SP, Argent JD, Blaquiere RM. Painful sclerosis of the medial end of the clavicle. Clin Radiol. 2004;59(11):992–9.
9. Shiv Shanker V, Paterson JM, Dodd S. Hypertrophic osteitis of the medial end of the clavicle. J Pediatr Orthop B. 1999;8(1):48–9.
10. Galla R, Basava V, Conermann T, Kabazie AJ. Sternoclavicular steroid injection for treatment of pain in a patient with Osteitis condensans of the clavicle. Pain Physician. 2009;12(6):987–90.
11. Sallés M, Olivé A, Perez-Andres R, Holgado S, Mateo L, Riera E, Tena X. The SAPHO syndrome: a clinical and imaging study. Clin Rheumatol. 2011;30(2):245–9.
12. Kahn MF, Bouvier M, Palazzo E, Tebib JG, Colson F. Sternoclavicular pustulotic osteitis (SAPHO). 20-year interval between skin and bone lesions. J Rheumatol. 1991;18(7):1104–8.
13. Berenguer Francés MÁ, Lafaurie Acevedo A, Tormo Ferrero V, Cardenal Macia R, Andreu Martínez FJ. SAPHO syndrome in the differential diagnosis of metastasis. Reumatol Clin. 2016;12(5):288–91.
14. Jung J, Molinger M, Kohn D, Schreiber M, Pfreundschuh M, Assmann G. Intra-articular glucocorticosteroid injection into sternocostoclavicular joints in patients with SAPHO syndrome. Semin Arthritis Rheum. 2012;42(3):266–70.
15. Rodchuae M, Ruangpin C, Katchamart W. Clinical manifestations, treatment outcomes, and risk factors for sternoclavicular septic arthritis. Rheumatol Int. 2017;37(5):819–24.
16. Ross JJ, Shamsuddin H. Sternoclavicular septic arthritis: review of 180 cases. Medicine (Baltimore). 2004;83(3):139–48.
17. Murga A, Copeland H, Hargrove R, Wallen JM, Zaheer S. Treatment for sternoclavicular joint infections: a multi-institutional study. J Thorac Dis. 2017;9(6):1503–8.
18. Kachala SS, D'Souza DM, Teixeira-Johnson L, Murthy SC, Raja S, Blackstone EH, Raymond DP. Surgical management of sternoclavicular joint infections. Ann Thorac Surg. 2016;101(6):2155–60.
19. Takiguchi J, Sakamoto H. Tuberculosis of the sternoclavicular joint. Intern Med. 2017;56(18):2543–4.
20. Christensen PB, Christensen I. A case of Friedrich's disease of the clavicle. Acta Orthop Scand. 1987;58(5):585–6.
21. Macule F, Ferreres A, Palliso F, Prat S, Ramon R. Aseptic necrosis of the sternal end of the clavicle Friedrich's disease. Acta Orthop Belg. 1990;56(3–4):613–5.
22. Levy M, Goldberg I, Fischel RE, Frisch E, Maor P. Friedrich's disease. Aseptic necrosis of the sternal end of the clavicle. J Bone Joint Surg Br. 1981;63B(4):539–41.
23. Heinemeier G, Torklus D. Resection arthroplasty of the clavicle in Friedrich's disease. Z Orthop Ihre Grenzgeb. 1979;117(5):849–51.

Chapter 34
Adhesive Capsulitis of the Shoulder (Frozen Shoulder)

Adhesive capsulitis (frozen shoulder) is a condition whereby the shoulder becomes painful, loses movement and stiffens. The stiffness is due to the capsule and ligaments of the glenohumeral joint becoming inflamed, contracted and shrunk. The bone and articular surfaces are normal. The rotator interval, coraco-humeral and anterior glenohumeral ligaments and capsule are mainly involved, but posterior and superior capsule involvement are often present.

34.1 Demographics [1–3]

- Affects 2–8% of the population
- More common between the age of 40 and 60
- More common in females

Adhesive capsulitis may occur in the absence of known risk factors or in the presence of recognised risk factors:

- Diabetes
- Hypothyroidism
- Cardiovascular disease
- Hemiparesis

It is estimated that 30% of those presenting with adhesive capsulitis have diabetes and 10% of diabetics go on to develop adhesive capsulitis. Adhesive capsulitis in diabetics is often a more aggressive and resistant to treatment condition, as compared to adhesive capsulitis in nondiabetics. There may also be a genetic predisposition to adhesive capsulitis.

Adhesive capsulitis is divided into three phases, but clear distinction between these is not always possible:

© Springer Nature Switzerland AG 2019

C. Panayiotou Charalambous, *The Shoulder Made Easy*,
https://doi.org/10.1007/978-3-319-98908-2_34

- Freezing phase (pain main complaint)
- Frozen phase (stiffness main complaint)
- Thawing phase (movements return)

34.2 Clinical Symptoms of Adhesive Capsulitis

- Diffuse shoulder pain
- Pain may be worse in the anterior part of the shoulder
- Stiffness
- Substantial functional loss, impaired activities of daily living and ability to work

Typical presentation is that of initial severe pain which gradually improves leaving persisting stiffness. Onset is usually with no precipitating event but may follow a trivial upper limb injury, myocardial infarction or cerebrovascular accident.

34.3 Clinical Signs of Adhesive Capsulitis

- Complete loss or reduction of shoulder motion in multiple directions
- External rotation is the movement predominantly affected
- Both active and passive movements are reduced

Loss of passive movements implies a mechanical block to motion, in this case the contracted, shrunk capsule and ligaments. In assessing passive movements, the examiner must stabilise the scapula, to distinguish between glenohumeral motion (reduced in frozen shoulder) and scapulo-thoracic motion (preserved).

34.4 Investigations for Adhesive Capsulitis

- Plain radiographs (shoulder anterior-posterior and axillary views) are normal in adhesive capsulitis (apart from the possible presence of calcific tendinopathy) but are taken to exclude alternative diagnoses
- MRI to look for associated soft tissue injuries (rotator cuff or labrum tears) in post-traumatic adhesive capsulitis
- HgA1C, thyroid function tests

34.5 Differential Diagnosis of Adhesive Capsulitis

- Glenohumeral arthritis—arthritic distortion of the articular surfaces and soft tissue contracture limit motion. Patients are usually older and plain radiographs are diagnostic of this condition

- Chronic posterior shoulder dislocation—the humeral head is locked out of joint and cannot rotate causing motion loss, mainly external rotation. History of old trauma or epileptic fits. Plain radiographs (axillary view) are diagnostic
- Post-traumatic stiffness—in this case the shoulder loses movement following a specific and usually substantial shoulder injury

34.6 Management of Adhesive Capsulitis

Adhesive capsulitis is a self-limiting condition, improving over 2–3 years, but some motion loss may persist in the longer term [4–6]. Hence, expectant management with no medical intervention, giving time for the natural history to evolve, is an acceptable option. Treatment is initiated to speed recovery and help those struggling with daily activities and working.

Non-surgical [6–9]

Treatment is guided by symptoms:

Pain:

- Analgesics, non-steroidal anti-inflammatories (oral, topical)
- Glenohumeral steroid injection
- Physiotherapy localised ultrasound, mega-pulse, acupuncture

Stiffness:

- Physiotherapy—stretching exercises that aim to elongate the contracted, shrunk capsule and ligaments

Adequate pain control is essential for stretching exercises to be performed.

Interventional/Surgical [8, 10–14]

Persistent stiffness may be treated with hydrodilatation or surgery:

- Hydrodilatation—under local anaesthesia and ultrasound or X-ray guidance, normal saline is injected into the glenohumeral joint to distend and tear the contracted capsule to regain movement
- Manipulation—under general anaesthesia the shoulder is moved by the surgeon and stretched, to tear the contracted tissue and regain movement
- Arthroscopic release—the contracted tissue is visualised and divided. The rotator interval and anterior glenohumeral ligaments and capsule as well as the posterior and superior capsule are released. It may be combined with manipulation to achieve tearing of any contracted inferior capsule
- Open arthrolysis—open surgery. The rotator interval is released and contracted tissue is divided

Inflamed and thickened rotator interval and anterior glenohumeral ligaments (a, b) which are released using an arthroscopic vapour (c, d, e). Additional manipulation tears the capsule down to the inferior sulcus (f)

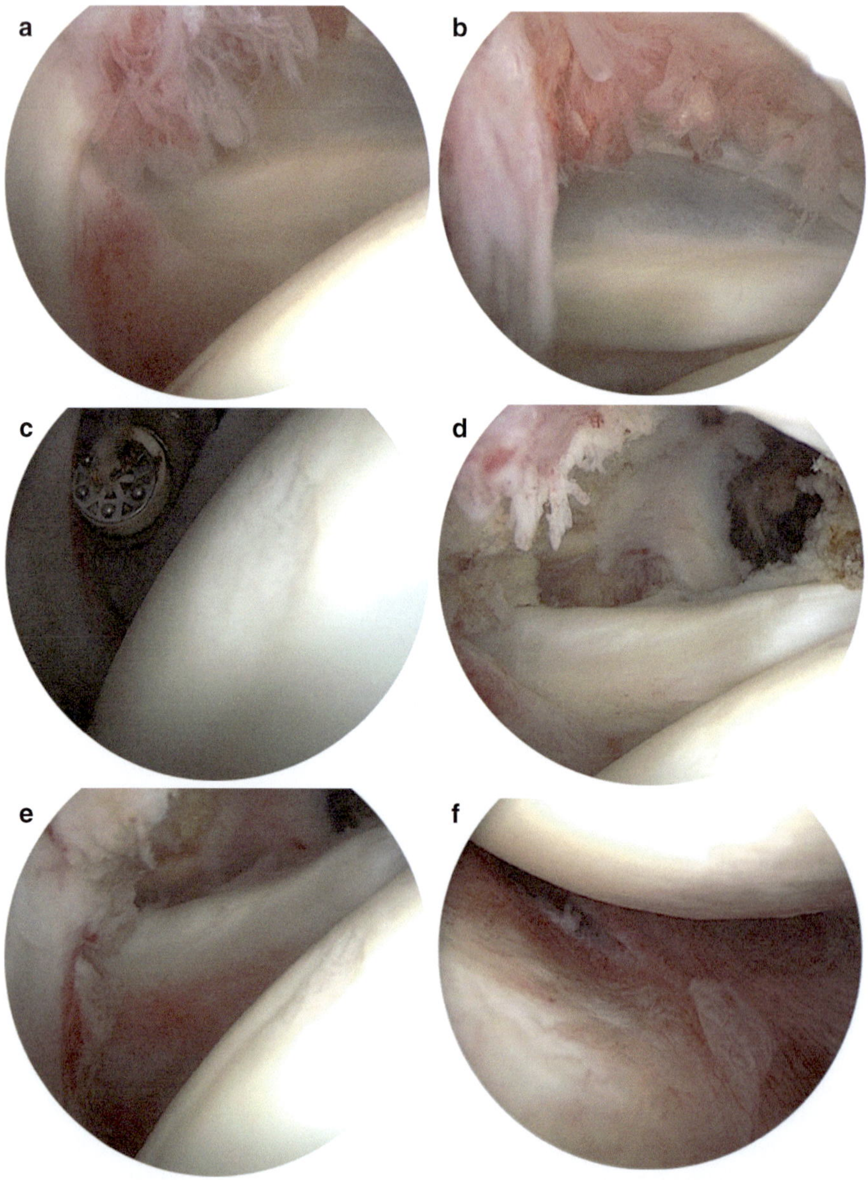

References

1. Wang K, Ho V, Hunter-Smith DJ, Beh PS, Smith KM, Weber AB. Risk factors in idiopathic adhesive capsulitis: a case control study. J Shoulder Elb Surg. 2013;22(7):e24–9.
2. Zreik NH, Malik RA, Charalambous CP. Adhesive capsulitis of the shoulder and diabetes: a meta-analysis of prevalence. Muscles Ligaments Tendons J. 2016;6(1):26–34.
3. Prodromidis AD, Charalambous CP. Is there a genetic predisposition to frozen shoulder? A systematic review and meta-analysis. JBJS Rev. 2016;4(2) https://doi.org/10.2106/JBJS.RVW.O.00007.
4. Vastamäki H, Kettunen J, Vastamäki M. The natural history of idiopathic frozen shoulder: a 2- to 27-year followup study. Clin Orthop Relat Res. 2012;470(4):1133–43.
5. Reeves B. The natural history of the frozen shoulder syndrome. Scand J Rheumatol. 1975;4(4):193–6.
6. Levine WN, Kashyap CP, Bak SF, Ahmad CS, Blaine TA, Bigliani LU. Nonoperative management of idiopathic adhesive capsulitis. J Shoulder Elb Surg. 2007;16(5):569–73.
7. Sun Y, Liu S, Chen S, Chen J. The effect of corticosteroid injection into rotator interval for early frozen shoulder: a randomized controlled trial. Am J Sports Med. 2018;46(3):663–70. https://doi.org/10.1177/0363546517744171.
8. Kwaees TA, Charalambous CP. Surgical and non-surgical treatment of frozen shoulder. Survey on surgeons treatment preferences. Muscles Ligaments Tendons J. 2015;4(4):420–4.
9. Wang W, Shi M, Zhou C, Shi Z, Cai X, Lin T, Yan S. Effectiveness of corticosteroid injections in adhesive capsulitis of shoulder: a meta-analysis. Medicine (Baltimore). 2017;96(28):e7529. https://doi.org/10.1097/MD.0000000000007529.
10. Gallacher S, Beazley JC, Evans J, Anaspure R, Silver D, Redfern A, Thomas W, Kitson J, Smith C. A randomized controlled trial of arthroscopic capsular release versus hydrodilatation in the treatment of primary frozen shoulder. J Shoulder Elb Surg. 2018;27(8):1401–6. https://doi.org/10.1016/j.jse.2018.04.002.
11. Kwaees TA, Charalambous CP. Rates of surgery for frozen shoulder: an experience in England. Muscles Ligaments Tendons J. 2016;5(4):276–9.
12. Saltychev M, Laimi K, Virolainen P, Fredericson M. Effectiveness of hydrodilatation in adhesive capsulitis of shoulder: a systematic review and meta-analysis. Scand J Surg. 2018;1:1457496918772367. https://doi.org/10.1177/1457496918772367.
13. Le Lievre HM, Murrell GA. Long-term outcomes after arthroscopic capsular release for idiopathic adhesive capsulitis. J Bone Joint Surg Am. 2012;94(13):1208–16.
14. D'Orsi GM, Via AG, Frizziero A, Oliva F. Treatment of adhesive capsulitis: a review. Muscles Ligaments Tendons J. 2012;2(2):70–8.

Chapter 35
Shoulder Post-traumatic Stiffness

This is a condition whereby the shoulder loses movement following a specific and usually substantial shoulder injury. It may have a pure soft tissue component, a bony component or a combination of both. It is often seen following a fracture of the proximal humerus or glenoid. Patients may have had surgery to stabilise their fracture but still develop stiffness.

The mechanical block to motion accounting for the loss of motion may be due to several causes including:

- A contracted, shrunk capsule and ligaments. A substantial injury force going through the soft tissues may sprain these tissues, leading to their inflammation and contracture
- Intra-articular or subacromial adhesions—adhesions between the articulating surfaces or between the superior surface of the rotator cuff and deltoid may limit motion
- Displaced bony fragments that impinge on surrounding parts of the joint or soft tissues limiting motion
- Glenohumeral joint dislocation

35.1 Clinical Symptoms of Post-traumatic Stiffness

- Stiffness that confers substantial functional loss
- Pain—in some cases the acute pain experienced following the injury settles leaving residual stiffness

© Springer Nature Switzerland AG 2019

C. Panayiotou Charalambous, *The Shoulder Made Easy*,
https://doi.org/10.1007/978-3-319-98908-2_35

35.2 Clinical Signs of Post-traumatic Stiffness

- Loss or reduction of shoulder motion in one or more directions
- Both active and passive movements are affected

In assessing passive movements, the examiner must stabilise the scapula, to distinguish between glenohumeral motion and scapulo-thoracic motion. The latter may compensate for loss in the former, masking the true loss of joint motion.

35.3 Investigations for Post-traumatic Stiffness

- Plain radiographs (shoulder anterior-posterior and axillary views) to assess the bony morphology and relation of articulating surfaces
- CT scan with 3D reconstruction to assess the bony morphology and look for displaced/mal-united fragments
- MRI to look for associated soft tissue injuries (rotator cuff or labrum tears) in post-traumatic capsular contracture and loss of the inferior capsular fold

35.4 Differential Diagnosis of Post-traumatic Stiffness

- Glenohumeral arthritis
- Adhesive capsulitis

35.5 Management of Post-traumatic Stiffness

Non-surgical

Treatment is guided by symptoms:

Pain

- Analgesics, non-steroidal anti-inflammatories (oral, topical)
- Glenohumeral steroid injection
- Physiotherapy (localised ultrasound, mega-pulse, acupuncture)

Stiffness

- Physiotherapy—stretching exercises that aim to elongate the contracted, shrunk capsule and ligaments

Adequate pain control is essential for stretching exercises to be performed. Even in cases where there is obvious displacement of bony fragments, stretching the soft tissues may improve joint motion, by compensating for the bony block.

Surgical [1–5]

Persistent stiffness may be treated with surgery

- Manipulation—under general anaesthesia the shoulder is moved by the surgeon and stretched, to tear the contracted tissue and regain movement. This is performed once union of the fracture is confirmed
- Arthroscopic release—the contracted tissue is visualised and divided; adhesions are excised
- Open arthrolysis—open surgery. The contracted tissue is divided. Hardware used for fracture fixation and which may be providing a mechanical block to movement is removed
- Osteotomy and realignment of displaced bony fragments—to address mechanical block due to bony components
- Reduction of a dislocated glenohumeral joint
- Glenohumeral replacement arthroplasty to improve conformity of the articulating surfaces

References

1. Lancaster ST, Grove TN, Woods DA. Management of post-traumatic stiffness of the shoulder following upper limb trauma with manipulation under anaesthetic. Shoulder Elbow. 2017;9(4):258–65.
2. Elhassan B, Ozbaydar M, Massimini D, Higgins L, Warner JJ. Arthroscopic capsular release for refractory shoulder stiffness: a critical analysis of effectiveness in specific etiologies. J Shoulder Elb Surg. 2010;19(4):580–7.
3. Maroun C, Aliani D, Hass A, Werthel JD, Vidil A, Valenti P. Shoulder arthroscopy combined to hardware removal in proximal humeral fractures: a series of 58 cases with a mean follow-up of 2 years. Eur J Orthop Surg Traumatol. 2017;27(3):317–21.
4. Katthagen JC, Hennecke D, Jensen G, Ellwein A, Voigt C, Lill H. Arthroscopy after locked plating of proximal humeral fractures: implant removal, capsular release, and intra-articular findings. Arthroscopy. 2014;30(9):1061–7.
5. Raiss P, Alami G, Bruckner T, Magosch P, Habermeyer P, Boileau P, Walch G. Reverse shoulder arthroplasty for type 1 sequelae of a fracture of the proximal humerus. Bone Joint J. 2018;100-B(3):318–23.

Chapter 36
Anterior Glenohumeral Instability

Anterior glenohumeral instability is a condition where there is symptomatic anterior (usually along with inferior) translation of the humeral head in relation to the glenoid.

The humeral head may:

- Sublux – displace but with part of the articular cartilage of the humeral head and glenoid remaining in contact
- Dislocate – with loss of all articular contact

The shoulder is mostly unstable anteriorly when the arm is placed in abduction and external rotation.

Although anterior instability may be part of multidimensional instability, isolated anterior instability is considered in this chapter.

36.1 Causes of Anterior Glenohumeral Instability [1–17]

36.1.1 Disruption or Inefficiency of Static Stabilisers

- Soft tissue
  - Excessive anterior capsular laxity

    As part of generalised ligamentous laxity
    Acute trauma
    Micro-trauma

© Springer Nature Switzerland AG 2019

C. Panayiotou Charalambous, *The Shoulder Made Easy*,
https://doi.org/10.1007/978-3-319-98908-2_36

- Labrum tears (detachments)

  Bankart lesion: detachment of the anterior-inferior part of the labrum from the glenoid, usually from 3 to 6 o'clock position in the right shoulder (6–9 o'clock position in the left)

  SLAP lesion: detachment of the superior labrum with extension into the anterior labrum

- Humeral avulsion glenohumeral ligament (HAGL) lesion – avulsion of the inferior glenohumeral ligament from its humeral attachment. Here the humeral rather than the glenoid end of the ligament is detached
- Mid-substance tear of the anterior glenohumeral ligaments and capsule

Soft tissue (b) and bony (c) anterior-inferior labrum detachment (soft-tissue and bony Bankart lesion)

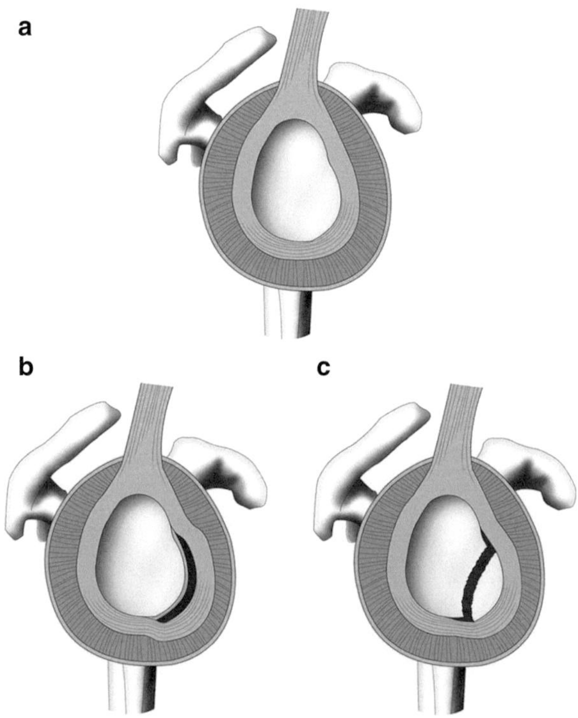

Types of SLAP tears. In type 2 tear the detached labrum may stay in situ on top of the glenoid (2a), or may fall in front of the glenoid covering the superior part of the glenoid face (beret like appearance) (2b)

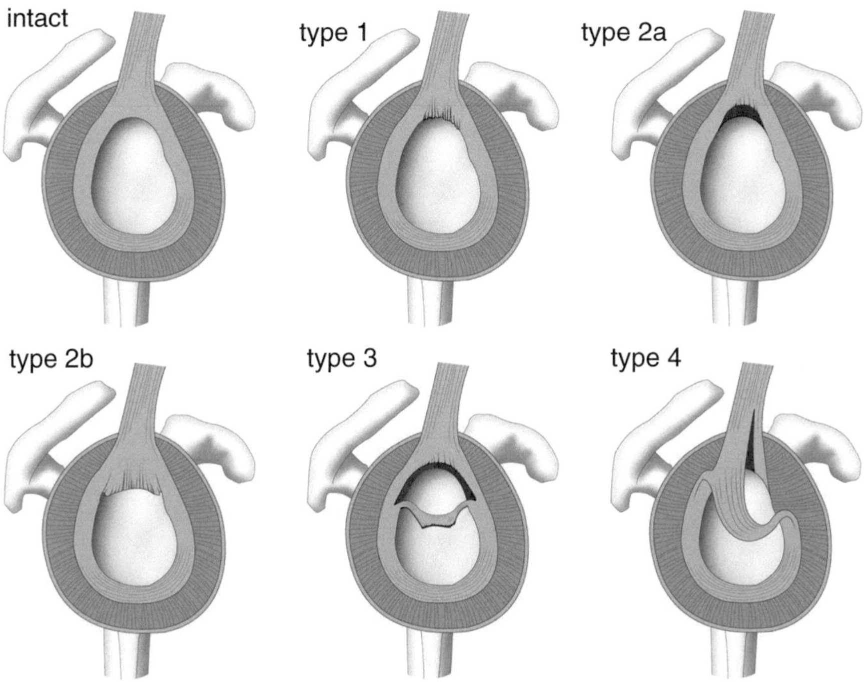

Superior labrum tear extending onto anterior labrum, apparent on probing

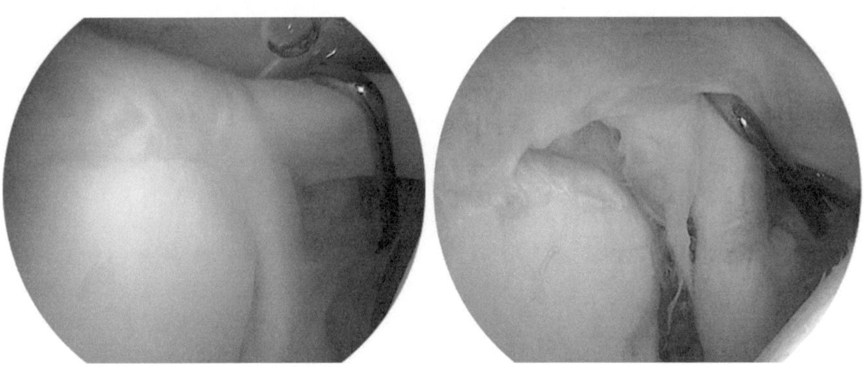

A ligament is taut only when it is firmly attached at its two ends. This is analogous to a hammock suspended by two ropes. If one rope loses its attachment, then the hammock cannot sustain any weight. Similarly, for the hammock to sustain weight, the two ropes must be attached to such a position, so they are taut. If one rope becomes slack, the hammock cannot sustain much weight.

- Rotator cuff tears (with loss of the buttress/checkrein effect of the tendon in addition to loss of the dynamic effect of the muscle)

  Subscapularis tear
  Supraspinatus tear

- Bony

  - Glenoid

    Dysplastic
    Reduced retroversion
    Anterior bone loss
    Avulsion fracture
    Impaction fracture

An intact glenoid is pear shaped (a). Avulsion fracture and bone loss from the anterior-inferior part of the glenoid (bony Bankart lesion) leads to a bitten pear appearance (b)

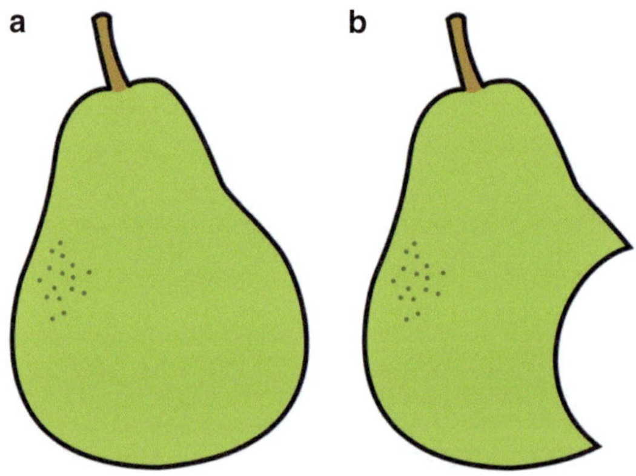

- Humeral head

  Dysplastic
  Reduced retroversion
  Fracture: Hill-Sachs lesion – this is a compression fracture of the humeral head. As the humeral head dislocates, the anterior glenoid edge may dig into the humeral head. A Hill-Sachs lesion is located on the superior and lateral aspect of the humeral head. A Hill-Sachs lesion may subsequently engage with the anterior edge of the glenoid during arm abduction and external rotation levering it out of the joint and causing re-dislocation (this is described as an engaging Hill-Sachs lesion). The size, orientation and location of the Hill-Sachs lesion determine whether it engages the glenoid edge and at what arm position it does so. A lesion parallel to the glenoid edge and involving more than 20% of the articular surface is more likely to engage and hence influence shoulder stability

Hill-Sachs lesion of the humeral head (b)—upon external rotation of the arm, the Hill-Sachs lesion engages on the edge of the glenoid (c), levering out and dislocating the humeral head in an anterior direction (d)

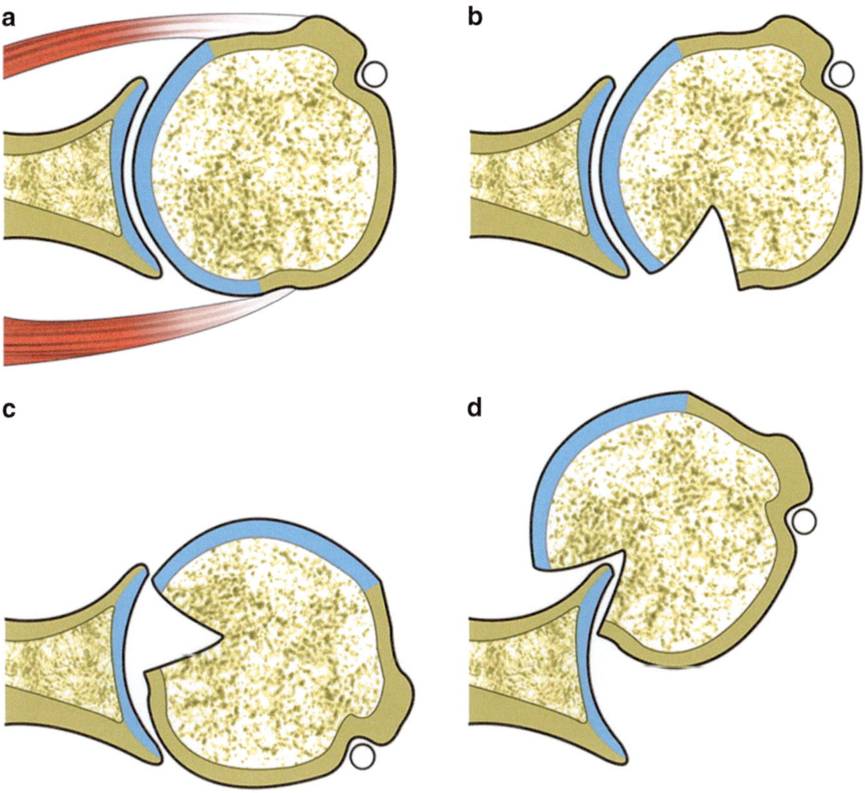

Hill-Sachs lesion engaging with the anterior edge of the glenoid with the arm in abduction and external rotation

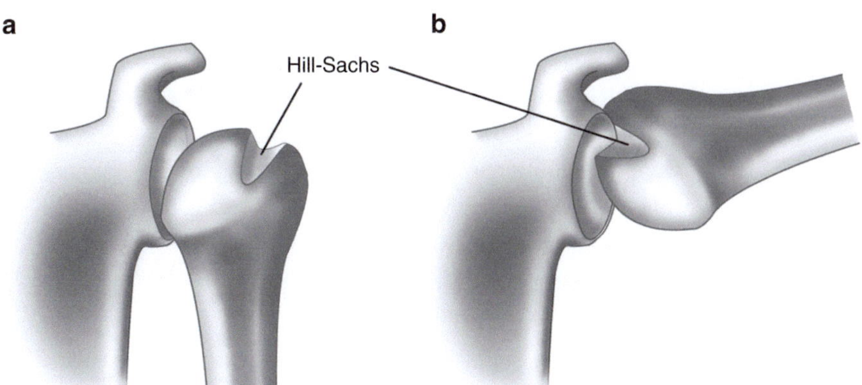

Disruption of static restraints to anterior instability may be:

- Congenital/developmental – capsular laxity, bony dysplasia/anteversion
- Acquired
  - Chronic repetitive micro-trauma – capsular/ligamentous laxity, labrum tears. This may be seen in athletes that repetitively stretch the anterior soft tissue stabilisers – overhead throwers
  - Acute substantial trauma – soft tissue tears/avulsions, bony fractures

36.1.2 Disruption or Inefficiency of Dynamic Stabilisers

This may occur in isolation or in association with deficient static stabilisers and may include:

- Shoulder muscle weakness (rotator cuff, deltoid)
- Dis-coordinated muscle activity (muscle patterning) – over- or underactivity of rotator cuff muscles, deltoid, pectoralis major and latissimus dorsi:
  - With the arm in abduction and external rotation excess activity of the pectoralis major pulls the humeral head anteriorly in relation to the glenoid predisposing to anterior instability
  - With the arm in abduction and external rotation excess activity of the latissimus dorsi pulls the proximal humerus inferiorly predisposing the shoulder to anterior/inferior instability
- Lack of stable platform to act upon
  - Poor scapular dynamics
  - Poor core control
- Defective proprioception – leading to uncoordinated muscle response to joint motion or forces applied on the joint

36.2 Classification of Anterior Glenohumeral Instability

Anterior glenohumeral instability may be classified according to the Stanmore triangle [18], based on its underlying pathological findings:

- Structural defects secondary to substantial trauma
- Structural defects but with no trauma
- Nonstructural – abnormal muscle patterning
- Combination of the above

It is important to recognise that in this triangle many patients are somewhere between the extreme corners. It is also important to recognise that the cause of instability is not static but may progress over time such as a patient starting with a structural cause only to develop abnormal muscle patterning as a compensatory mechanism at a later stage.

Stanmore triangle of instability. In anterior glenohumeral instability cases tend to be structural traumatic or non-structural

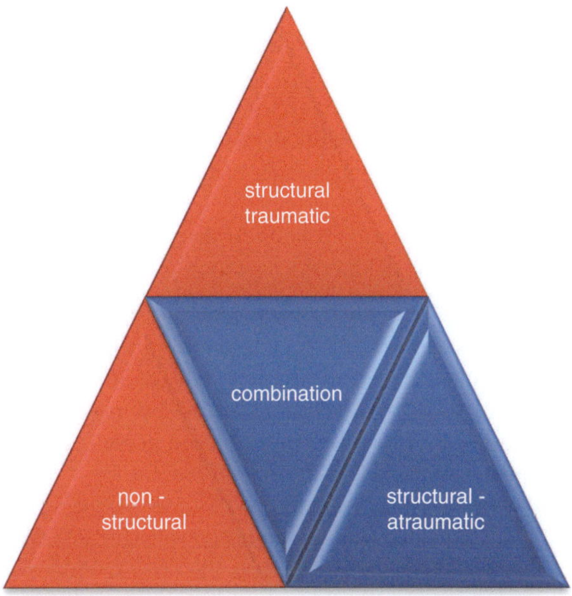

36.3 Clinical Symptoms of Anterior Glenohumeral Instability

- Vague pain
- Dead arm syndrome, heavy arm, paraesthesia
- Clicking, clunking
- Feeling of abnormal displacement – feeling "wobbly" to "popping in and out" to "popping out and can't go back", "coming out to the edge" to "coming out fully"

- Apprehension in placing the arm in abduction and external rotation (scared that the shoulder may come out)
- Patients may present with episodes of frank dislocation where the humeral head comes out of joint. The shoulder may then spontaneously reduce or the patient may be able to reduce it themselves. Alternatively, the patient may need to present to hospital to have the shoulder reduced under sedation or general anaesthesia

The onset of anterior instability may be:

- Occasionally atraumatic – gradual onset with vague pain, arm feeling heavy and then symptoms of abnormal glenohumeral translation without an obvious precipitating event
- Often precipitated by minor trauma (which involves much lower forces that those required under normal conditions to cause glenohumeral dislocation) – such as carrying a bag, throwing a ball, reaching out and standing up from a chair using arms
- Often precipitated by substantial trauma to the shoulder that causes extensive disruption to combinations of anterior, posterior or inferior static stabilisers

At the initial dislocation, the shoulder may spontaneously relocate, or the patient may manage to reduce it themselves, and this is often the case in those with atraumatic or minor injury first dislocations. In those that sustain first-time anterior dislocation secondary to substantial trauma, reduction by medical means (closed or open) is usually necessary. This may also be needed in some cases where the first dislocation is atraumatic or the result of minimal trauma.

Following this first dislocation episode, the shoulder may start to show recurrent subluxations or dislocations that occur with further substantial trauma or with minimal or no further trauma (such as by putting the arm in abduction and external rotation).

Anterior glenohumeral instability may be:

- Voluntary – the patient can dislocate the shoulder at will by influencing muscular contraction or by placing the shoulder in a particular position
- Involuntary – the patient cannot achieve the above

One may start with voluntary instability and progress to involuntary instability or vice versa.

Hence, it is important to get a clear history and define the mechanism of the first dislocation as well as subsequent instability episodes.

Progression of severity of symptoms in anterior glenohumeral instability

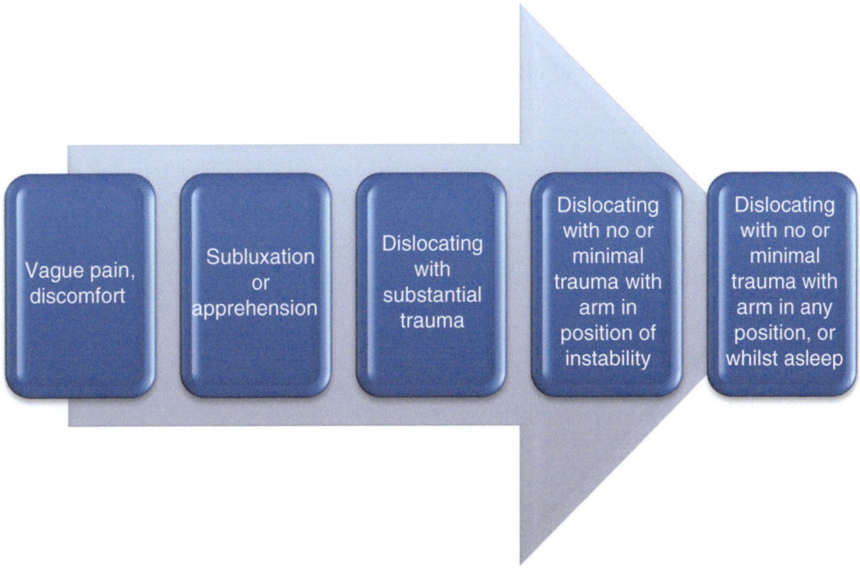

Progression of severity of symptoms in anterior glenohumeral instability according to the intervention needed to relocate the joint

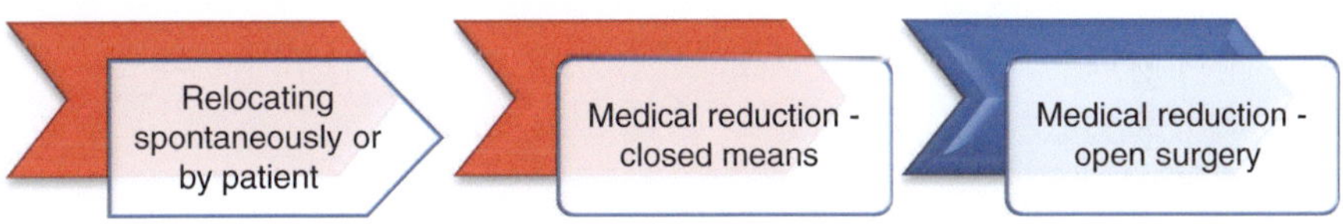

36.4 Clinical Signs of Anterior Glenohumeral Instability [19, 20]

- Anterior glenohumeral laxity
- Positive anterior apprehension/relocation/release tests
- Patient may be able to demonstrate the subluxation/dislocation
- Patient may be able to voluntarily make the shoulder sublux or dislocate
- Hyper-laxity:
  - Localised to the shoulder, in one or more directions
  - Generalised ligamentous laxity with high Beighton score

36.5 Investigations for Anterior Glenohumeral Instability

Investigations for the unstable shoulder aim to confirm the presence of instability, determine its likely cause and identify any structural lesions that may be amenable to surgical intervention. These include:

- Radiological:
  - Plain radiographs
  - MRI/MRI arthrogram/CT scan
- Neurophysiological:
  - Nerve conduction studies
  - Electromyography
- Examination under general anaesthesia – joint translation and laxity are assessed with the patient under general anaesthesia to abolish pain and allow muscle relaxation
- Arthroscopic evaluation

Plain radiograph showing antero-inferior dislocation of the humeral head (red arrow) in relation to the glenoid (yellow arrow)

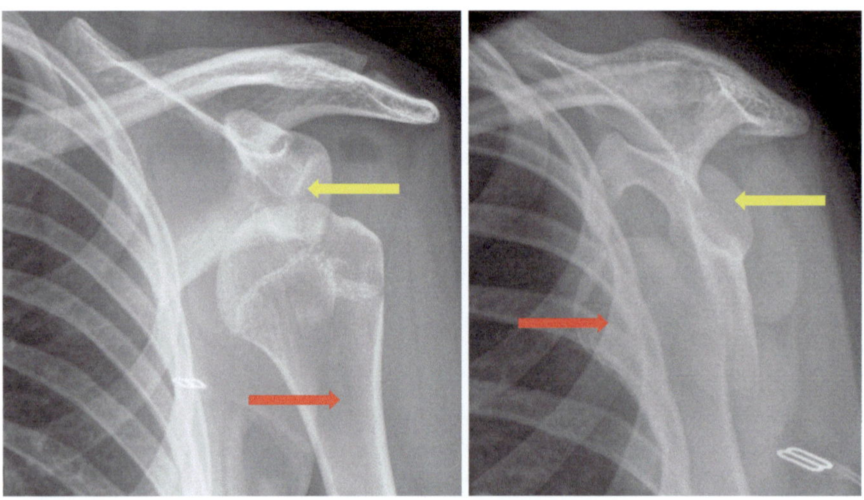

Plain radiograph and MRI scan showing Hill-Sachs lesion (red arrow)

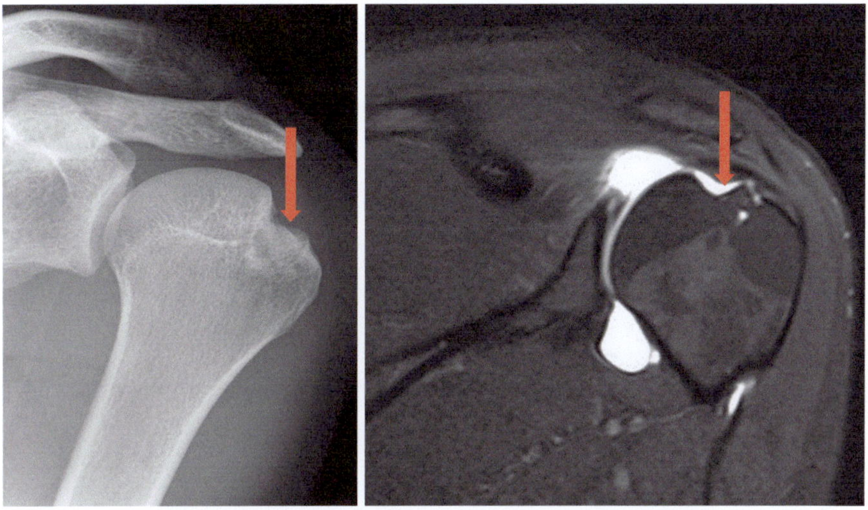

MRI arthrogram showing detachment of the anterior labrum (red arrow)

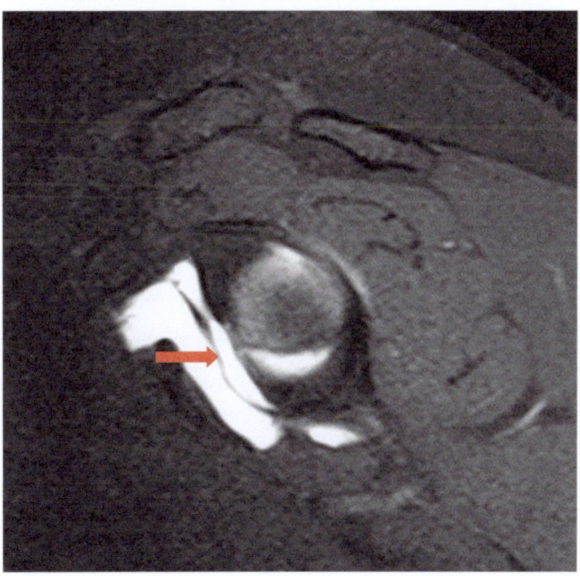

36.6 Management of Anterior Glenohumeral Instability

Initial management involves relocating a dislocated joint. Once the joint is relocated further management aims at improving stability and reducing the risk of subsequent instability episodes. Management of recurrent instability depends on:

- Symptoms – severity, frequency
- Underlying cause

Management of anterior glenohumeral instability

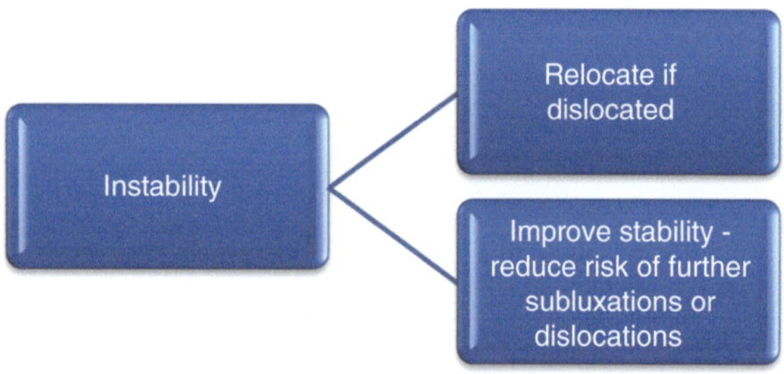

Non-surgical [21–25]

- Leave alone
- Activity modification, avoiding unstable positions
- Physiotherapy to address:
  - Core imbalance – core strengthening
  - Scapular dysrhythmia – strengthening of scapular muscles
  - Proprioception – proprioceptive training
  - Abnormal muscle patterning – biofeedback, inhibit overactive and enhance underactive muscles, improve neuromuscular control
  - Rotator cuff weakness – rotator cuff muscle strengthening, balance

It should be noted that non-surgical management does not specifically address any damaged or stretched static joint restraints but aims to improve stability by enhancing the function of dynamic stabilisers (through strengthening, better control and coordination).

Surgical [25–54]

If symptoms do not improve with non-surgical intervention and patient has structural lesions that are amenable to surgery, then surgery may be considered. Structural derangements are corrected either directly or indirectly:

- Directly – correct the structural defect itself
- Indirectly – compensate for the structural defect

Directly – correcting the structural defect itself

- Labrum avulsion – reattach (surge anchors, bone tunnels)
- Glenoid avulsion fracture:

- Reattach anchors or screws according to bony fragment size
- Glenoid osteochondral allograft

- Hill-Sachs:
  - Elevate defect
  - Fill defect to stop it engaging using:
    - Tendon/capsule – Remplissage
    - Allograft reconstruction of segmental defects
    - Humeral head arthroplasty – for large Hill-Sachs lesions
- Abnormal version:
  - Humeral head – rotational osteotomy
  - Glenoid – osteotomy
- HAGL lesion – reattachment to humerus (anchors, bone tunnels)
- Mid-substance ligamentous rupture – capsular plication
- Excessive redundancy of the joint capsule:
  - Plication, open or arthroscopic
  - Capsular shift
  - Thermal shrinkage

Indirectly – compensate for the structural defect

- Bone block procedure – adding an extension to the anterior border of the glenoid increases the amount of external rotation that can occur before the Hill-Sachs lesion engages on the edge of the glenoid and levers out
  - Latarjet
  - Tri-cortical graft bone block – anterior
    - Autograft
    - Allograft
- Humeral rotational osteotomy – to translate the Hill-Sachs posteriorly and hence allow more external rotation prior to engagement with the anterior glenoid rim
- Glenohumeral fusion:
  - When stability cannot be achieved by other means
  - Patients that cannot comply with restrictions of postoperative stabilisation by other means

The following describes three of the stabilisation procedures in more detail:

Latarjet Procedure

This is the transfer of the distal part of the coracoid along with its attached conjoined tendon to the anterior surface of the glenoid to which it is fixed (with two screws or other means). The coracoid is transferred through a horizontal split in the subscapularis tendon. The Latarjet procedure is believed to improve stability by [55]:

1. Increasing the posterior to anterior dimensions of the glenoid, therefore increasing the arc of rotation that the humeral head may achieve before dislocating. In particular, it increases the arc of rotation before a Hill-Sachs lesion engages the glenoid edge
2. Transfer of the conjoined tendon to the front of the shoulder provides a thick soft tissue constraint which becomes taught upon external rotation and abduction, limiting the anterior translation of the humeral head
3. Transfer of the conjoined tendon through a subscapularis split tensions the inferior part of subscapularis during abduction and external rotation. This provides a further passive constraint to the anterior translation of the humeral head

Latarjet procedure involves transfer of the coracoid to the anterior-inferior part of the glenoid and fixation with screws or other means (yellow arrows)

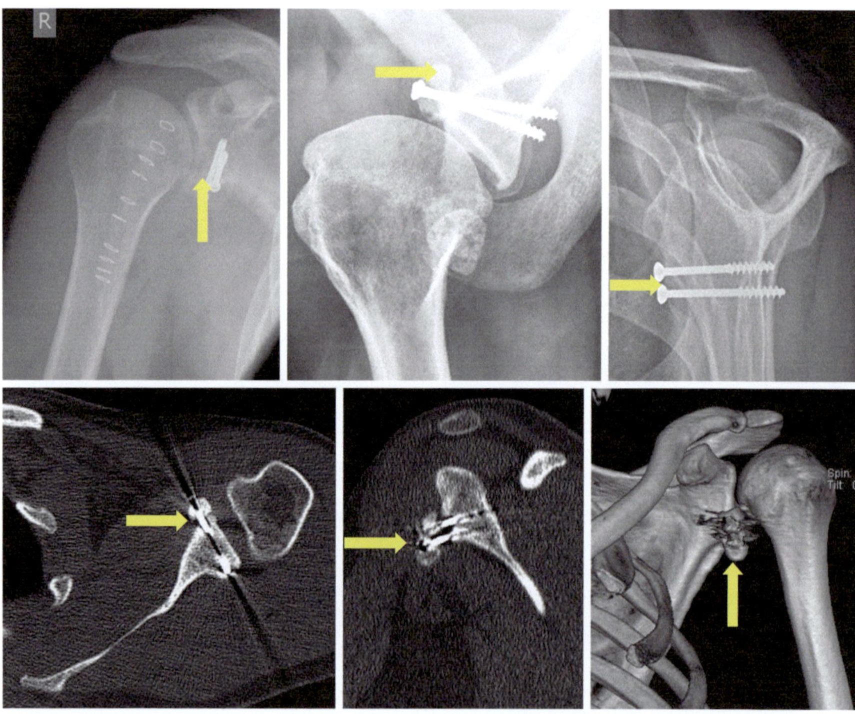

Bone Block Procedure

A cortical graft is transferred to the anterior surface of the glenoid to increase its anterior posterior dimension. Autografts from the iliac crest or acromion and distal tibial allografts have been described. Increasing the posterior to anterior dimension of the glenoid increases the arc of rotation that the humeral head may achieve before dislocating.

Transfer of the tip of the coracoid or a free bone block to the anterior edge of the glenoid increases the amount of external rotation that can be achieved prior to the Hill-Sachs lesion engaging and dislocating the humeral head

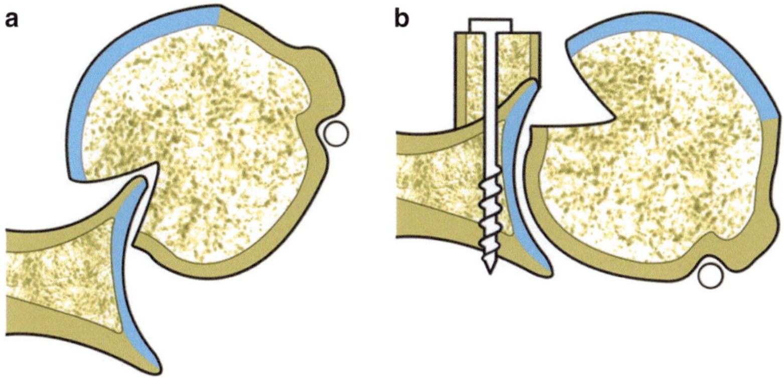

Remplissage

This term means to fill a defect, and the procedure involves the suturing of a tendon (infraspinatus) or capsule into the Hill-Sachs lesion. This attempts to remove the Hill-Sachs from the articulation so that it does not catch on the glenoid edge and lever out the humeral head.

Ramplissage- the infraspinatus tendon is sutured into the Hill-Sachs lesion, filling the humeral head defect and stopping it from engaging on the edge of glenoid upon external rotation of the arm, reducing the risk of dislocation

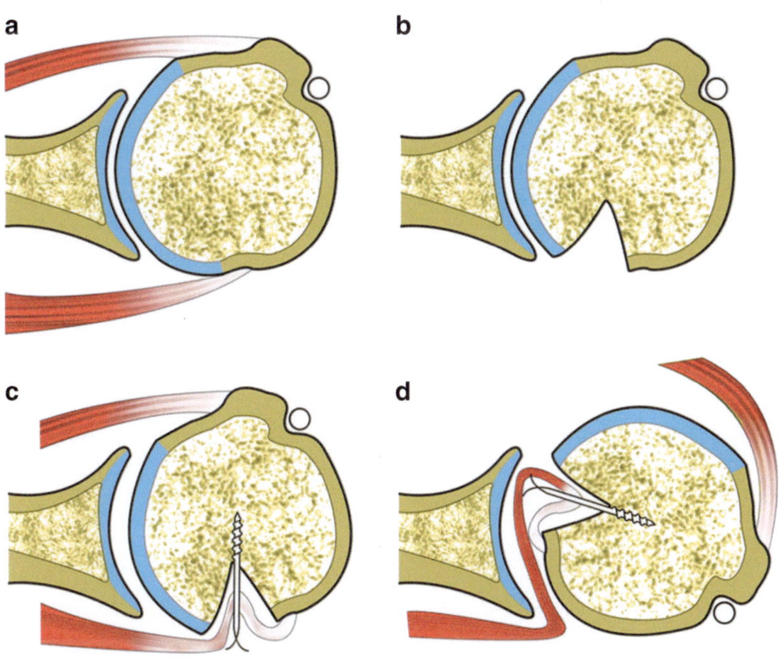

(a) Large Hill-Sachs lesion – (articular cartilage on either side of the lesion distinguishes it from the normal base area of the humeral head) (b) Suture anchors inserted into the Hill-Sachs lesion with sutures traversing the overlying tendon and capsule (c) Following tying of the sutures the Hill-Sachs lesion is covered by soft tissue (tendon and capsule)

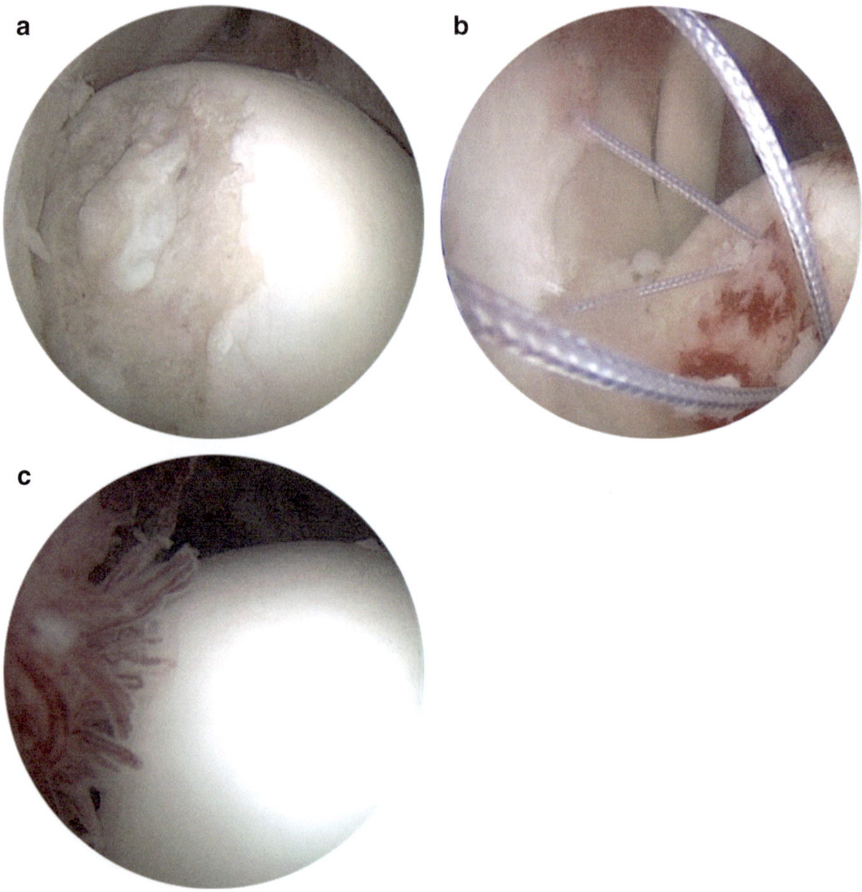

Hill-Sachs lesion engages with the anterior edge of the glenoid upon external rotation of the arm, levering out and dislocating the humeral head in an anterior direction. Derotation osteotomy increases the amount of external rotation that can be achieved prior to engagement of the Hill-Sachs lesion

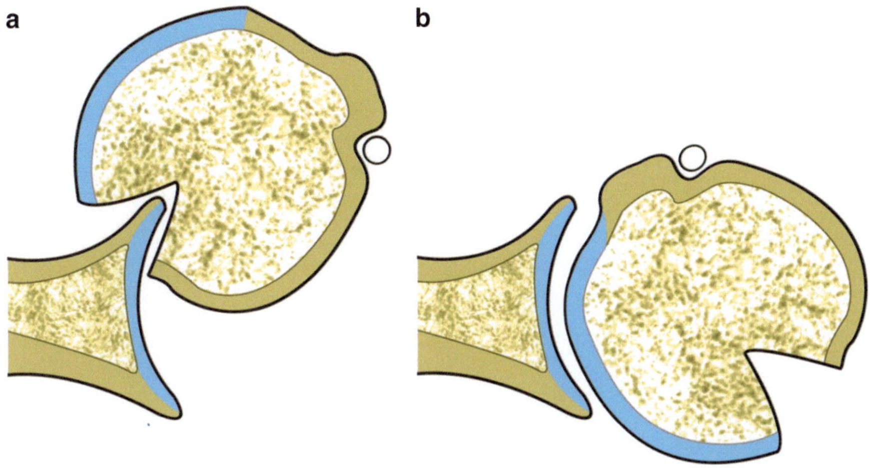

36.7 Primary Surgical Stabilisation Following First-Time Anterior Glenohumeral Dislocation

An initial anterior dislocation secondary to substantial trauma increases the risk of subsequent recurrent instability. This risk is higher with younger age [56]:

- Fifty percent in those aged 15–30
- Thirty-six percent in those aged 21–40
- Eleven percent in those older than 40
- Ten percent in those older than 60

Some clinicians recommend that following a first-time dislocation, those at higher risk of sustaining further dislocations should be offered primary stabilisation (rather than waiting until recurrent instability develops). This would minimise any further damage to the shoulder sustained by further instability. High-quality clinical evidence supporting such recommendation is awaited, and it is recognised that a substantial proportion of non-surgically treated patients do well [57–59].

36.8 Shoulder Instability in Older Age

The structural deficits that may occur following a shoulder dislocation may differ in older as compared to younger patients. In particular, there is an increased risk of rotator cuff tears encountered in the older age group, although labrum lesions are still prevalent. Robinson et al. [60] looked at patients older than 35 presenting following an anterior shoulder dislocation and found the following lesions:

- Sixty-four percent – rotator cuff tear
- Sixty-four percent – Bankart lesion
- Ten percent – HAGL lesion
- Seven percent – SLAP tear
- Hundred percent – Hill-Sachs lesion

Hence, in such groups surgical repair of a rotator cuff tear may also be needed.

If faced with a patient having a shoulder dislocation (especially when older than 40), it is important (following relocation of the joint) to evaluate clinically the integrity of the rotator cuff by examining strength. This may not be possible in the acute setting due to pain; hence repeating clinical assessment at 4–6 weeks post-injury may be necessary. If there is any doubt about the integrity of the rotator cuff, radiological imaging should be obtained.

Learning Pearls

Following an acute traumatic anterior shoulder dislocation:

- Immobilisation in a sling (with the arm in internal rotation) is utilised. There have been studies suggesting that immobilisation with the arm in external rotation may facilitate apposition of the detached labrum to the glenoid and healing in a more optimal position, but this has not been supported by further investigations [61]
- Careful examination of the neurovascular status of the arm (particularly the axillary nerve) prior and post relocation is essential

- Clinical and radiological examination of the shoulder is performed within a week to check for recurrent dislocation. Some patients re-disclocate early with the following factors increasing the risk of an early re-dislocation (within 6 weeks of the initial dislocation) [62]:
  - High-energy injury
  - Associated neurological deficit
  - Associated large rotator cuff tear
  - Glenoid rim fracture
  - Combined glenoid rim and greater tuberosity fracture
- Mobilisation is commenced guided by pain and by the ability of the patient to control the arm through range of motion

References

1. Kraeutler MJ, McCarty EC, Belk JW, Wolf BR, Hettrich CM, Ortiz SF, MOON Shoulder Instability Group, Bravman JT, Baumgarten KM, Bishop JY, Bollier MJ, Brophy RH, Carey JL, Carpenter JE, Cox CL, Feeley BT, Grant JA, Jones GL, Kuhn JE, Kelly JD, Ma CB, Marx RG, Miller BS, Sennett BJ, Smith MV, Wright RW, Zhang AL. Descriptive epidemiology of the MOON shoulder instability cohort. Am J Sports Med. 2018;46(5):1064–9.
2. Yiannakopoulos CK, Mataragas E, Antonogiannakis E. A comparison of the spectrum of intra-articular lesions in acute and chronic anterior shoulder instability. Arthroscopy. 2007;23(9):985–90.
3. Bankart AS. Recurrent or habitual dislocation of the shoulder joint. Br Med J. 1923;2(3285):1132–3.
4. McMahon PJ, Burkart A, Musahl V, Debski RE. Glenohumeral translations are increased after a type II superior labrum anterior-posterior lesion: a cadaveric study of severity of passive stabilizer injury. J Shoulder Elb Surg. 2004;13(1):39–44.
5. Longo UG, Rizzello G, Ciuffreda M, Locher J, Berton A, Salvatore G, Denaro V. Humeral avulsion of the glenohumeral ligaments: a systematic review. Arthroscopy. 2016;32(9):1868–76.
6. Shin SJ, Kim RG, Jeon YS, Kwon TH. Critical value of anterior glenoid bone loss that leads to recurrent glenohumeral instability after arthroscopic bankart repair. Am J Sports Med. 2017;45(9):1975–81.
7. Yamamoto N, Itoi E, Abe H, Kikuchi K, Seki N, Minagawa H, Tuoheti Y. Effect of an anterior glenoid defect on anterior shoulder stability: a cadaveric study. Am J Sports Med. 2009;37(5):949–54.
8. Kurokawa D, Yamamoto N, Nagamoto H, Omori Y, Tanaka M, Sano H, Itoi E. The prevalence of a large Hill-Sachs lesion that needs to be treated. J Shoulder Elb Surg. 2013;22(9):1285–9.
9. Hill HA, Sachs MD. The grooved defect of the humeral head: a frequently unrecognized complication of dislocations of the shoulder joint. Radiology. 1940;35:690–700.
10. Johnson SM, Robinson CM. Shoulder instability in patients with joint hyperlaxity. J Bone Joint Surg Am. 2010;92(6):1545–57.
11. Emery RJ, Mullaji AB. Glenohumeral joint instability in normal adolescents. Incidence and significance. J Bone Joint Surg Br. 1991;73(3):406–8.

12. Jia X, Ji JH, Petersen SA, Freehill MT, McFarland EG. An analysis of shoulder laxity in patients undergoing shoulder surgery. J Bone Joint Surg Am. 2009;91(9):2144–50.
13. Lephart SM, Warner JJ, Borsa PA, Fu FH. Proprioception of the shoulder joint in healthy, unstable, and surgically repaired shoulders. J Shoulder Elb Surg. 1994;3(6):371–80.
14. Gilman S. Joint position sense and vibration sense: anatomical organisation and assessment. J Neurol Neurosurg Psychiatry. 2002;73(5):473–7.
15. Barden JM, Balyk R, Raso VJ, Moreau M, Bagnall K. Atypical shoulder muscle activation in multidirectional instability. Clin Neurophysiol. 2005;116(8):1846–57.
16. Jaggi A, Noorani A, Malone A, Cowan J, Lambert S, Bayley I. Muscle activation patterns in patients with recurrent shoulder instability. Int J Shoulder Surg. 2012;6(4):101–7.
17. Kibler WB, Press J, Sciascia A. The role of core stability in athletic function. Sports Med. 2006;36(3):189–98.
18. Lewis A, Kitamura T, Bayley JIL. The classification of shoulder instability: new light through old windows! Curr Orthop. 2004;18:97–108.
19. Valencia Mora M, Ibán MÁR, Heredia JD, Gutiérrez-Gómez JC, Diaz RR, Aramberri M, Cobiella C. Physical exam and evaluation of the unstable shoulder. Open Orthop J. 2017;11:946–56.
20. Charalambous CP. Clinical examination of the shoulder. In: Charalambous CP, editor. The shoulder made easy. Basel: Springer; 2019.
21. Jaggi A, Lambert S. Rehabilitation for shoulder instability. Br J Sports Med. 2010; 44(5):333–40.
22. Burkhead WZ Jr, Rockwood CA Jr. Treatment of instability of the shoulder with an exercise program. J Bone Joint Surg Am. 1992;74(6):890–6.
23. Buss DD, Lynch GP, Meyer CP, Huber SM, Freehill MQ. Nonoperative management for in-season athletes with anterior shoulder instability. Am J Sports Med. 2004;32(6):1430–3.
24. Huxel Bliven KC, Anderson BE. Core stability training for injury prevention. Sports Health. 2013;5(6):514–22.
25. Dickens JF, Rue JP, Cameron KL, Tokish JM, Peck KY, Allred CD, Svoboda SJ, Sullivan R, Kilcoyne KG, Owens BD. Successful return to sport after arthroscopic shoulder stabilization versus nonoperative management in contact athletes with anterior shoulder instability: a prospective multicenter study. Am J Sports Med. 2017;45(11):2540–6.
26. Rowe CR, Patel D, Southmayd WW. The Bankart procedure: a long-term end-result study. J Bone Joint Surg Am. 1978;60(1):1–16.
27. Harris JD, Gupta AK, Mall NA, Abrams GD, McCormick FM, Cole BJ, Bach BR Jr, Romeo AA, Verma NN. Long-term outcomes after Bankart shoulder stabilization. Arthroscopy. 2013;29(5):920–33.
28. An VV, Sivakumar BS, Phan K, Trantalis J. A systematic review and meta-analysis of clinical and patient-reported outcomes following two procedures for recurrent traumatic anterior instability of the shoulder: Latarjet procedure vs. Bankart repair. J Shoulder Elb Surg. 2016;25(5):853–63.
29. Blonna D, Bellato E, Caranzano F, Assom M, Rossi R, Castoldi F. Arthroscopic Bankart repair versus open Bristow-Latarjet for shoulder instability: a matched-pair multicenter study focused on return to sport. Am J Sports Med. 2016;44(12):3198–205.
30. Bozzo A, Oitment C, Thornley P, Yan J, Habib A, Hoppe DJ, Athwal GS, Ayeni OR. Humeral avulsion of the glenohumeral ligament: indications for surgical treatment and outcomes-a systematic review. Orthop J Sports Med. 2017;5(8):2325967117723329. https://doi.org/10.1177/2325967117723329.
31. Flury M, Rickenbacher D, Audigé L. Arthroscopic treatment of anterior shoulder instability associated with a HAGL lesion-a case series. J Shoulder Elb Surg. 2016;25(12): 1989–96.
32. Longo UG, Loppini M, Rizzello G, Ciuffreda M, Berton A, Maffulli N, Denaro V. Remplissage, humeral osteochondral grafts, weber osteotomy, and shoulder arthroplasty for the management of humeral bone defects in shoulder instability: systematic review and quantitative synthesis of the literature. Arthroscopy. 2014;30(12):1650–66.

33. Provencher MT, McCormick F, LeClere L, Sanchez G, Golijanin P, Anthony S, Dewing CB. Prospective evaluation of surgical treatment of humeral avulsions of the glenohumeral ligament. Am J Sports Med. 2017;45(5):1134–40.
34. Arciero RA, Mazzocca AD. Mini-open repair technique of HAGL (humeral avulsion of the glenohumeral ligament) lesion. Arthroscopy. 2005;21(9):1152.
35. Bokor DJ, Conboy VB, Olson C. Anterior instability of the glenohumeral joint with humeral avulsion of the glenohumeral ligament. A review of 41 cases. J Bone Joint Surg Br. 1999;81(1):93–6.
36. Wolf EM, Cheng JC, Dickson K. Humeral avulsion of glenohumeral ligaments as a cause of anterior shoulder instability. Arthroscopy. 1995;11(5):600–7.
37. Aboalata M, Plath JE, Seppel G, Juretzko J, Vogt S, Imhoff AB. Results of arthroscopic Bankart repair for anterior-inferior shoulder instability at 13-year follow-up. Am J Sports Med. 2017;45(4):782–7.
38. Frank RM, Romeo AA, Richardson C, Sumner S, Verma NN, Cole BJ, Nicholson GP, Provencher MT. Outcomes of Latarjet versus distal tibia allograft for anterior shoulder instability repair: a matched cohort analysis. Am J Sports Med. 2018;46(5):1030–8.
39. Hurley ET, Lim Fat D, Farrington SK, Mullett H. Open versus arthroscopic Latarjet procedure for anterior shoulder instability: a systematic review and meta-analysis. Am J Sports Med. 2018;1:363546518759540. https://doi.org/10.1177/0363546518759540.
40. Baverel L, Colle PE, Saffarini M, Anthony Odri G, Barth J. Open Latarjet procedures produce better outcomes in competitive athletes compared with recreational athletes: a clinical comparative study of 106 athletes aged under 30 years. Am J Sports Med. 2018;1:363546518759730. https://doi.org/10.1177/0363546518759730.
41. Bonnevialle N, Thélu CE, Bouju Y, Vogels J, Agout C, Duriez P, Azoulay V. Arthroscopic Latarjet procedure with double-button fixation: short-term complications and learning curve analysis. J Shoulder Elb Surg. 2018;27(6):e189–95. https://doi.org/10.1016/j.jse.2017.12.007.
42. Provencher MT, Frank RM, Golijanin P, Gross D, Cole BJ, Verma NN, Romeo AA. Distal tibia allograft glenoid reconstruction in recurrent anterior shoulder instability: clinical and radiographic outcomes. Arthroscopy. 2017;33(5):891–7.
43. Sanchez M, Klouche S, Faivre B, Bauer T, Hardy P. Acromial J-bone graft on the acromion for surgical treatment of glenohumeral instability: an anatomical study. Shoulder Elbow. 2017;9(4):272–8.
44. Rashid MS, Crichton J, Butt U, Akimau PI, Charalambous CP. Arthroscopic "Remplissage" for shoulder instability: a systematic review. Knee Surg Sports Traumatol Arthrosc. 2016;24(2):578–84.
45. Cho NS, Yoo JH, Juh HS, Rhee YG. Anterior shoulder instability with engaging Hill-Sachs defects: a comparison of arthroscopic Bankart repair with and without posterior capsulodesis. Knee Surg Sports Traumatol Arthrosc. 2016;24(12):3801–8.
46. Lädermann A, Arrigoni P, Barth J, Narbona P, Hanypsiak B, Burkhart SS, Denard PJ. Is arthroscopic remplissage a tenodesis or capsulomyodesis? An anatomic study. Knee Surg Sports Traumatol Arthrosc. 2016;24(2):573–7.
47. Provencher MT, Frank RM, Leclere LE, Metzger PD, Ryu JJ, Bernhardson A, Romeo AA. The Hill-Sachs lesion: diagnosis, classification, and management. J Am Acad Orthop Surg. 2012;20(4):242–52.
48. Brooks-Hill AL, Forster BB, van Wyngaarden C, Hawkins R, Regan WD. Weber osteotomy for large Hill-Sachs defects: clinical and CT assessments. Clin Orthop Relat Res. 2013;471(8):2548–55.
49. Statz JM, Schoch BS, Sanchez-Sotelo J, Sperling JW, Cofield RH. Shoulder arthroplasty for locked anterior shoulder dislocation: a role for the reversed design. Int Orthop. 2017;41(6):1227–34.
50. Hohmann E, Tetsworth K, Glatt V. Open versus arthroscopic surgical treatment for anterior shoulder dislocation: a comparative systematic review and meta-analysis over the past 20 years. J Shoulder Elb Surg. 2017;26(10):1873–80.

51. Fritz EM, Pogorzelski J, Hussain ZB, Godin JA, Millett PJ. Arthroscopic repair of humeral avulsion of the glenohumeral ligament lesion. Arthrosc Tech. 2017;6(4):e1195–200.
52. Patel RM, Amin NH, Lynch TS, Miniaci A. Management of bone loss in glenohumeral instability. Orthop Clin North Am. 2014;45(4):523–39.
53. Neer CS 2nd, Foster CR. Inferior capsular shift for involuntary inferior and multidirectional instability of the shoulder. A preliminary report. J Bone Joint Surg Am. 1980;62(6):897–908.
54. Bessette MC, Frisch NC, Kodali P, Jones MH, Miniaci A. Partial resurfacing for humeral head defects associated with recurrent shoulder instability. Orthopedics. 2017;40(6):e996–e1003.
55. Yamamoto N, Muraki T, An KN, Sperling JW, Cofield RH, Itoi E, Walch G, Steinmann SP. The stabilizing mechanism of the Latarjet procedure: a cadaveric study. J Bone Joint Surg Am. 2013;95(15):1390–7.
56. Olds M, Ellis R, Donaldson K, Parmar P, Kersten P. Risk factors which predispose first-time traumatic anterior shoulder dislocations to recurrent instability in adults: a systematic review and meta-analysis. Br J Sports Med. 2015;49(14):913–22.
57. Chahal J, Marks PH, Macdonald PB, Shah PS, Theodoropoulos J, Ravi B, Whelan DB. Anatomic Bankart repair compared with nonoperative treatment and/or arthroscopic lavage for first-time traumatic shoulder dislocation. Arthroscopy. 2012;28(4):565–75.
58. Crall TS, Bishop JA, Guttman D, Kocher M, Bozic K, Lubowitz JH. Cost-effectiveness analysis of primary arthroscopic stabilization versus nonoperative treatment for first-time anterior glenohumeral dislocations. Arthroscopy. 2012;28(12):1755–65.
59. Bishop JA, Crall TS, Kocher MS. Operative versus nonoperative treatment after primary traumatic anterior glenohumeral dislocation: expected-value decision analysis. J Shoulder Elb Surg. 2011;20(7):1087–94.
60. Robinson EC, Thangamani VB, Kuhn MA, Ross G. Arthroscopic findings after traumatic shoulder instability in patients older than 35 years. Orthop J Sports Med. 2015;3(5):2325967115584318. https://doi.org/10.1177/2325967115584318.
61. Whelan DB, Kletke SN, Schemitsch G, Chahal J. Immobilization in external rotation versus internal rotation after primary anterior shoulder dislocation: a meta-analysis of randomized controlled trials. Am J Sports Med. 2016;44(2):521–32.
62. Robinson CM, Kelly M, Wakefield AE. Redislocation of the shoulder during the first six weeks after a primary anterior dislocation: risk factors and results of treatment. J Bone Joint Surg Am. 2002;84-A(9):1552–9.

Chapter 37
Posterior Glenohumeral Instability

Posterior glenohumeral instability is a condition where there is symptomatic posterior translation of the humeral head in relation to the glenoid.

The humeral head may:

- Sublux – displace but part of the articular cartilage of the humeral head and glenoid remaining in contact
- Dislocate – with loss of all articular contact

The shoulder is posteriorly unstable mostly with the arm in forward elevation, adduction and internal rotation.

Although posterior instability may be part of multidirectional instability, isolated posterior instability is considered in this chapter.

37.1 Causes of Posterior Glenohumeral Instability [1–17]

37.1.1 Disruption or Inefficiency of Static Stabilisers

Soft tissue:

- Excessive posterior capsular laxity
  - As part of generalised ligamentous laxity
  - Acute trauma
  - Chronic trauma
- Labrum tears (detachments) – detachment of the posterior/inferior part of the labrum from the glenoid, detachment of the posterior part of the glenohumeral ligament from the humerus (reverse humeral avulsion glenohumeral ligament lesion – reverse HAGL)
- Rotator cuff tears (losing static tendon effect in addition to dynamic muscle effect)

© Springer Nature Switzerland AG 2019

C. Panayiotou Charalambous, *The Shoulder Made Easy*,
https://doi.org/10.1007/978-3-319-98908-2_37

Bony:

- Glenoid
  - Dysplastic
  - Excessive retroversion
  - Posterior bone loss:

    Avulsion fracture
    Impaction fracture

- Humeral head
  - Dysplastic
  - Excessive retroversion
  - Fractured – reverse Hill-Sachs lesion – a compression fracture of the humeral head. As the humeral head dislocates, the posterior glenoid edge may dig into the humeral head. A reverse Hill-Sachs lesion is located on the anterior and medial aspect of the humeral head. A reverse Hill-Sachs lesion may subsequently engage with the posterior edge of the glenoid during arm forward elevation, adduction and internal rotation levering it out of the joint and causing re-dislocation (described as engaging lesion). The size, orientation and location of the reverse Hill-Sachs lesion determine whether it engages the glenoid edge and at what arm position it does so

Reverse Hill-Sachs lesion of the humeral head (b) – upon internal rotation of the arm the reverse Hill-Sachs lesion engages on the edge of the glenoid (c), levering out and dislocating the humeral head in a posterior direction (d)

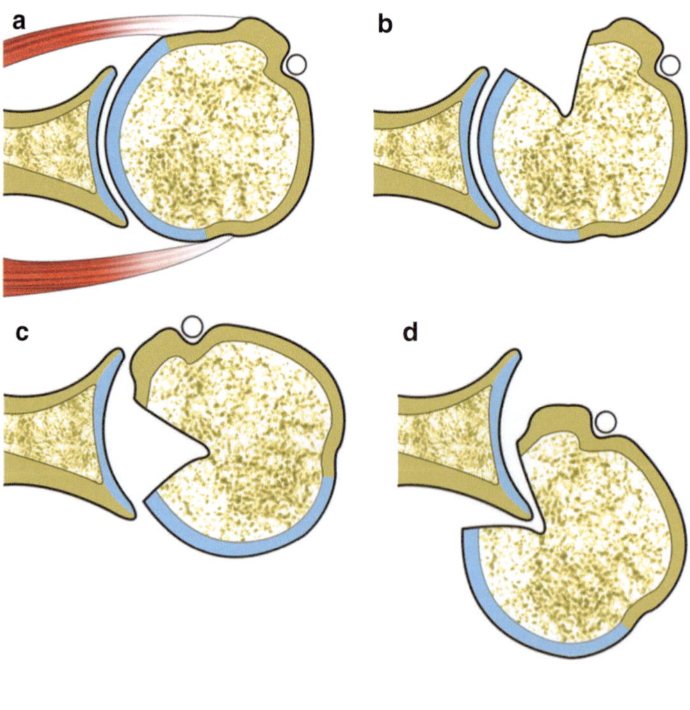

Disruption of static restraints to posterior instability may be:

- Congenital/developmental – capsular laxity, bony dysplasia/retroversion
- Acquired
  - Acute substantial trauma – soft tissue tears/avulsions, bony fractures
  - Chronic repetitive micro-trauma – capsular/ligamentous laxity, labrum tears. This may be seen in athletes (archers) that repetitively stretch the posterior soft tissue stabilisers

37.1.2 Disruption or Inefficiency of Dynamic Stabilisers

These may occur in isolation or in association with deficient static stabilisers and may include:

- Shoulder muscle weakness (rotator cuff, deltoid)
- Dis-coordinated muscle activity (muscle patterning) – over- or underactivity of rotator cuff muscles, deltoid and latissimus dorsi (LD):
  - Increased latissimus dorsi activity – with the arm in adduction and forward elevation, increased LD activity pulls the proximal humerus into internal rotation causing posterior instability
  - Reduced activity of infraspinatus (which acts as external rotator) can lead to unopposed internal rotation activity and posterior instability
- Lack of stable platform to act upon:
  - Poor scapular dynamics
  - Poor core control
- Defective proprioception – leading to uncoordinated muscle response to joint motion or response to forces applied on the joint

37.2 Classification of Posterior Glenohumeral Instability

Posterior glenohumeral instability may be classified according to the Stanmore triangle [18], based on its underlying pathological findings:

- Structural defects secondary to substantial trauma
- Structural defects but with no trauma
- Nonstructural – abnormal muscle patterning
- Combination of the above

It is important to recognise that in this triangle many patients are somewhere between the extreme corners. It is also important to recognise that the cause of instability is not static but may progress over time such as a patient starting with a structural cause only to develop abnormal muscle patterning as a compensatory mechanism at a later stage.

Stanmore triangle of instability—in posterior glenohumeral instability cases tend to be structural atraumatic or non-structural

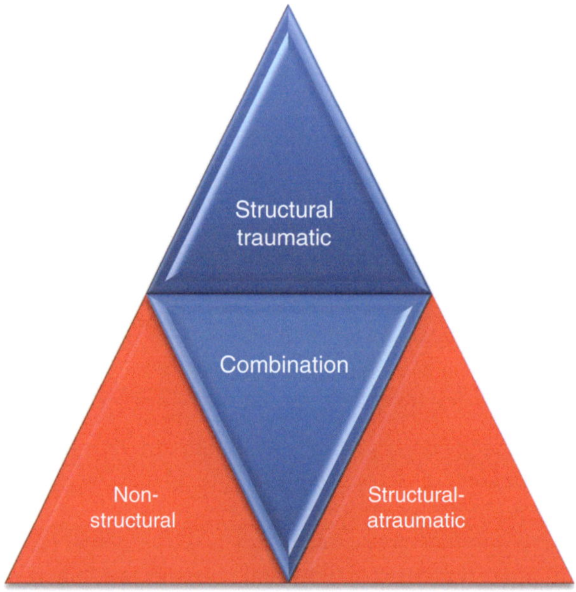

37.3 Clinical Symptoms of Posterior Glenohumeral Instability

- Vague pain
- Dead arm syndrome, paraesthesia
- Clicking
- Feeling of abnormal displacement – feeling "wobbly" to "popping in and out" to "popping out and can't go back", "coming out to the edge" to "coming out fully"
- Apprehension in placing the arm in forward elevation, adduction and internal rotation (scared that the shoulder may come out)
- Patients may present with episodes of frank dislocation where the humeral head comes out of joint. The joint may then spontaneously relocate or the patient may be able to reduce it themselves. Alternatively, the patient may need to present to hospital to have that reduced under sedation or general anaesthesia

The onset of posterior instability may be:

- Often atraumatic – gradual onset with vague pain, arm heaviness and then symptoms of abnormal glenohumeral translation without an obvious precipitating event
- Often precipitated by minor trauma (which involves much lower forces that those required under normal conditions to cause glenohumeral dislocation) – such as carrying a bag, throwing a ball, reaching out
- Occasionally precipitated by substantial trauma to the shoulder that causes extensive disruption to posterior static stabilisers

At the initial dislocation, the shoulder may spontaneously relocate, or the patient may manage to reduce it themselves, and this is often the case in those with atraumatic or minor injury first-time dislocations. Following this first dislocation, the shoulder starts to show recurrent subluxations or dislocations that may occur with further substantial trauma or with minimal or no further trauma (such as placing the arm in forward elevation, adduction and internal rotation or pushing forwards or reaching out on a shelf).

Most cases of recurrent posterior instability present with vague symptoms or recurrent subluxation/recurrent dislocation that spontaneously reduces rather than recurrent dislocations which need to be reduced by medical means.

In those that sustain a first-time posterior dislocation secondary to substantial trauma, reduction by medical means (closed or open) is usually necessary. In those with substantial bone lesions, the shoulder may be unstable following reduction when immobilised in a sling with the arm in internal rotation and may need to be immobilised in an external rotation splint for 4–6 weeks. In some cases primary stabilisation surgery is needed to maintain joint reduction. Close follow-up with serial radiographs for 4–6 weeks is thus essential. Cases of first-time posterior dislocation due to substantial trauma in which the shoulder stabilises post the initial reduction are highly unlikely to go on to develop recurrent episodes of frank dislocation that needs reduction by medical means (in contrast to equivalent cases of anterior instability).

Posterior glenohumeral instability may be:

- Voluntary – the patient can dislocate the shoulder at will by influencing muscular contraction or placing the shoulder in a particular position
- Involuntary – the patient cannot achieve the above

One may start with voluntary posterior instability and progress to involuntary instability or vice versa. Voluntary instability may be associated with psychological symptoms, but in many cases this may not be the case.

Hence, it is important to get a clear history and define the mechanism of the first dislocation as well as subsequent instability episodes.

Progression of severity of symptoms in posterior glenohumeral instability—most cases tend to be subluxations rather than frank dislocations

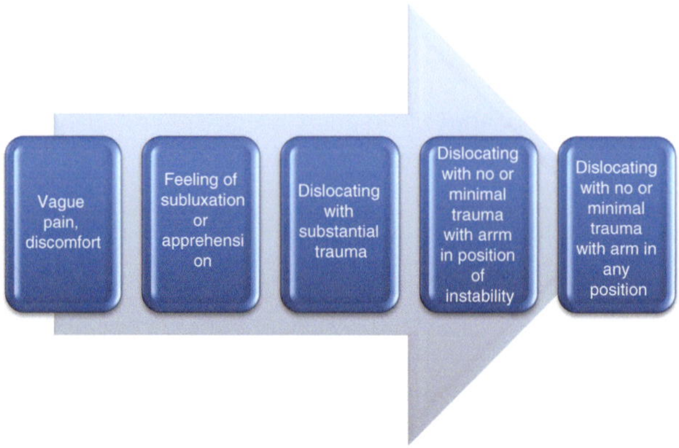

Progression of severity of symptoms in posterior glenohumeral instability according to the intervention needed to relocate the joint—usually relocate spontaneously

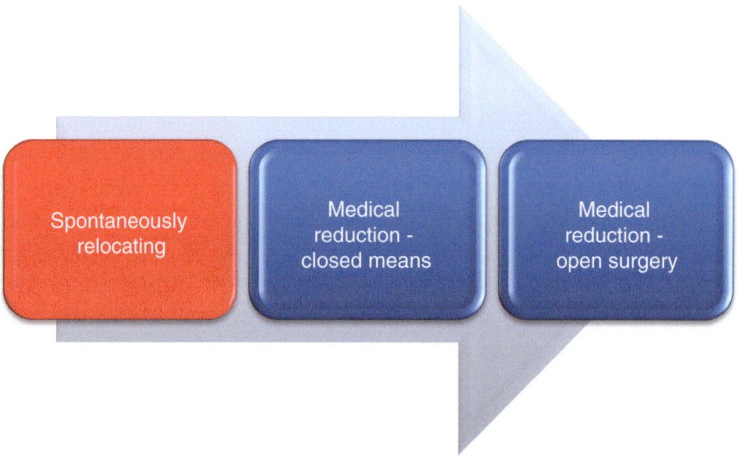

37.4 Clinical Signs of Posterior Glenohumeral Instability [19, 20]

- Posterior glenohumeral laxity on posterior drawer test
- Positive posterior apprehension test
- Positive Kim's test
- Positive Jerk test
- Patient may be able to demonstrate the subluxation/dislocation
- Patient may be able to voluntarily sub-lux or dislocate the shoulder

- Hyper-laxity
  - Localised to the shoulder, in one or more directions
  - Generalised ligamentous laxity with high Beighton score

37.5 Investigations for Posterior Glenohumeral Instability

Investigations of the unstable shoulder aim to confirm the presence of instability, determine its likely cause and identify any structural lesions that may be amenable to surgical intervention. These include:

- Radiological
  - Plain radiographs
  - MRI/MRI arthrogram [21]/CT scan
- Neurophysiological
  - Nerve conduction studies
  - Electromyography
- Examination under general anaesthesia – joint translation and laxity are assessed with the patient under general anaesthesia to abolish pain and allow muscle relaxation
- Arthroscopic evaluation

MRI showing posterior labrum detachment from the glenoid rim (red arrow)

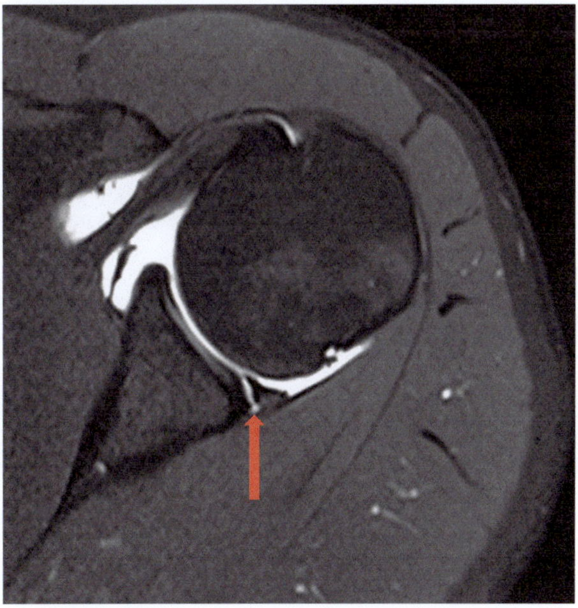

MRI showing a posterior glenoid avulsion fracture (yellow arrows)

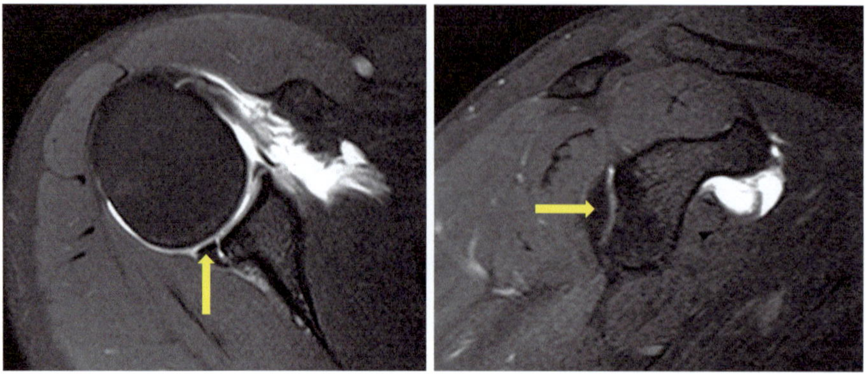

37.6 Management of Posterior Glenohumeral Instability

Initial management involves relocating a dislocated joint. Once the joint is relocated, further management aims at improving stability and reducing the risk of subsequent instability. Management of recurrent instability depends on:

- Symptoms – severity and frequency
- Underlying cause

Management of posterior glenohumeral instability

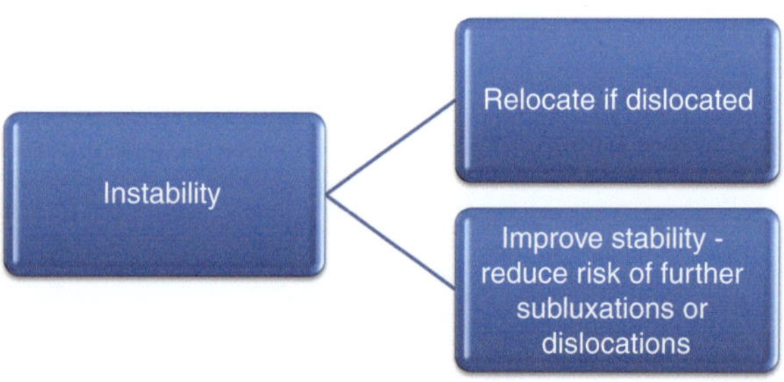

Non-surgical [22–30]

- Activity modification, avoiding unstable positions
- Physiotherapy to address:
  - Core imbalance – core strengthening
  - Scapular dysrhythmia – strengthening of scapular muscles
  - Proprioception – proprioceptive training
  - Abnormal muscle patterning – biofeedback
  - Rotator cuff weakness – rotator cuff muscle strengthening and balance

Non-surgical management does not directly address deficient static stabilisers but aims to improve stability by enhancing the function of dynamic stabilisers.

Surgical [31–61]

If symptoms do not improve with non-surgical intervention and the patient has structural lesions that are amenable to surgery, then surgery may be considered. Structural derangements are corrected either directly or indirectly:

- Directly – correct the structural defect itself
- Indirectly – compensate for the structural defect

- Directly – correct the structural defect itself
  - Labrum avulsion – reattach (suture anchors, bone tunnels)
  - Glenoid avulsion fracture:

    Reattach using anchors or screws according to bony fragment size

  - Reverse Hill-Sachs:

    Elevate defect
    Fill defect to stop it engaging using:

      Tendon/capsule – subscapularis
      Lesser tuberosity with attached subscapularis – McLaughlin procedure
      Allograft reconstruction of segmental defects

  - Abnormal version – osteotomy

    Glenoid – posterior open wedge osteotomy
    Humerus – external rotation osteotomy

  - Reverse HAGL lesion –reattachment to the humerus (using anchors, bone tunnels)
  - Mid substance ligamentous rupture – capsular plication
  - Excessive redundancy of the joint capsule

    Plication, open or arthroscopic
    Capsular shift
    Thermal shrinkage

- Indirectly – compensate for the structural defect
  - Bone block procedure – adding a bone block to the posterior glenoid may increase the amount of internal rotation that can occur before the humeral head dislocates

    Tri-cortical graft bone block:

      Autograft
      Allograft

- Humeral head arthroplasty – for large reverse Hill-Sachs lesions
- Glenohumeral fusion

Learning Pearls

- Acute posterior dislocations may be missed and present as chronic dislocations – beware of the light bulb sign on plain radiographs – obtain axillary views rather than simply relying on anterior-posterior views
- Posterior recurrent instability may be more difficult to diagnose than anterior instability due to subtle clinical symptoms and signs

References

1. Robinson CM, Seah M, Akhtar MA. The epidemiology, risk of recurrence, and functional outcome after an acute traumatic posterior dislocation of the shoulder. J Bone Joint Surg Am. 2011;93(17):1605–13.
2. Rouleau DM, Hebert-Davies J, Robinson CM. Acute traumatic posterior shoulder dislocation. J Am Acad Orthop Surg. 2014;22(3):145–52.
3. Weber SC, Caspari RB. A biochemical evaluation of the restraints to posterior shoulder dislocation. Arthroscopy. 1989;5(2):115–21.
4. McFarland EG, Campbell G, McDowell J. Posterior shoulder laxity in asymptomatic athletes. Am J Sports Med. 1996;24(4):468–71.
5. Richards RR, Delaney J. Syringomyelia presenting as shoulder instability. J Shoulder Elb Surg. 1992;1(3):155–61.
6. Castagna A, Snyder SJ, Conti M, Borroni M, Massazza G, Garofalo R. Posterior humeral avulsion of the glenohumeral ligament: a clinical review of 9 cases. Arthroscopy. 2007;23(8):809–15.
7. Galinat BJ, Howell SM. Excessive retroversion of the glenoid cavity. A cause of non-traumatic posterior instability of the shoulder. J Bone Joint Surg Am. 1987;69(4):632–3.
8. Fukuda H, Neer CS 2nd. Archer's shoulder. Recurrent posterior subluxation and dislocation of the shoulder in two archers. Orthopedics. 1988;11(1):171–4.
9. Pande P, Hawkins R, Peat M. Electromyography in voluntary posterior instability of the shoulder. Am J Sports Med. 1989;17(5):644–8.
10. Pokabla C, Hobgood ER, Field LD. Identification and management of "floating" posterior inferior glenohumeral ligament lesions. J Shoulder Elb Surg. 2010;19(2):314–7.
11. Wellmann M, Blasig H, Bobrowitsch E, Kobbe P, Windhagen H, Petersen W, Bohnsack M. The biomechanical effect of specific labral and capsular lesions on posterior shoulder instability. Arch Orthop Trauma Surg. 2011;131(3):421–7.
12. Shah AA, Butler RB, Fowler R, Higgins LD. Posterior capsular rupture causing posterior shoulder instability: a case report. Arthroscopy. 2011;27(9):1304–7.
13. Rouleau DM, Hebert-Davies J. Incidence of associated injury in posterior shoulder dislocation: systematic review of the literature. J Orthop Trauma. 2012;26(4):246–51.
14. Nacca C, Gil JA, Badida R, Crisco JJ, Owens BD. Critical glenoid bone loss in posterior shoulder instability. Am J Sports Med. 2018;46(5):1058–63.
15. Hines A, Cook JB, Shaha JS, Krul K, Shaha SH, Johnson J, Bottoni CR, Rowles DJ, Tokish JM. Glenoid bone loss in posterior shoulder instability: prevalence and outcomes in arthroscopic treatment. Am J Sports Med. 2018;46(5):1053–7.
16. Jaggi A, Noorani A, Malone A, Cowan J, Lambert S, Bayley I. Muscle activation patterns in patients with recurrent shoulder instability. Int J Shoulder Surg. 2012;6(4):101–7.
17. Lephart SM, Warner JJ, Borsa PA, Fu FH. Proprioception of the shoulder joint in healthy, unstable, and surgically repaired shoulders. J Shoulder Elb Surg. 1994;3(6):371–80.

18. Lewis A, Kitamura T, Bayley JIL. The classification of shoulder instability: new light through old windows! Curr Orthop. 2004;18:97–108.
19. Valencia Mora M, Ibán MÁR, Heredia JD, Gutiérrez-Gómez JC, Diaz RR, Aramberri M, Cobiella C. Physical exam and evaluation of the unstable shoulder. Open Orthop J. 2017;11:946–56.
20. Charalambous CP. Clinical examination of the shoulder. In: Charalambous CP, editor. The shoulder made easy. Basel: Springer; 2019.
21. Galvin JW, Parada SA, Li X, Eichinger JK. Critical findings on magnetic resonance arthrograms in posterior shoulder instability compared with an age-matched controlled cohort. Am J Sports Med. 2016;44(12):3222–9.
22. Frank RM, Romeo AA, Provencher MT. Posterior glenohumeral instability: evidence-based treatment. J Am Acad Orthop Surg. 2017;25(9):610–23.
23. Jaggi A, Lambert S. Rehabilitation for shoulder instability. Br J Sports Med. 2010; 44(5):333–40.
24. Huxel Bliven KC, Anderson BE. Core stability training for injury prevention. Sports Health. 2013;5(6):514–22.
25. Beall MS Jr, Diefenbach G, Allen A. Electromyographic biofeedback in the treatment of voluntary posterior instability of the shoulder. Am J Sports Med. 1987;15(2):175–8.
26. McIntyre K, Bélanger A, Dhir J, Somerville L, Watson L, Willis M, Sadi J. Evidence-based conservative rehabilitation for posterior glenohumeral instability: a systematic review. Phys Ther Sport. 2016;22:94–100.
27. Watson L, Balster S, Warby SA, Sadi J, Hoy G, Pizzari T. A comprehensive rehabilitation program for posterior instability of the shoulder. J Hand Ther. 2017;30(2):182–92.
28. Blacknall J, Mackie A, Wallace WA. Patient-reported outcomes following a physiotherapy rehabilitation programme for atraumatic posterior shoulder subluxation. Shoulder Elbow. 2014;6(2):137–41.
29. Merolla G, De Santis E, Cools AM, Porcellini G. Functional outcome and quality of life after rehabilitation for voluntary posterior shoulder dislocation: a prospective blinded cohort study. Eur J Orthop Surg Traumatol. 2015;25(2):263–72.
30. Burkhead WZ Jr, Rockwood CA Jr. Treatment of instability of the shoulder with an exercise program. J Bone Joint Surg Am. 1992;74(6):890–6.
31. Frank RM, Shin J, Saccomanno MF, Bhatia S, Shewman E, Bach BR Jr, Wang VM, Cole BJ, Provencher MT, Verma NN, Romeo AA. Comparison of glenohumeral contact pressures and contact areas after posterior glenoid reconstruction with an iliac crest bone graft or distal tibial osteochondral allograft. Am J Sports Med. 2014;42(11):2574–82.
32. Leivadiotou D, Ahrens P. Arthroscopic treatment of posterior shoulder instability: a systematic review. Arthroscopy. 2015;31(3):555–60.
33. Cerciello S, Visonà E, Morris BJ, Corona K. Bone block procedures in posterior shoulder instability. Knee Surg Sports Traumatol Arthrosc. 2016;24(2):604–11.
34. DeLong JM, Jiang K, Bradley JP. Posterior instability of the shoulder: a systematic review and meta-analysis of clinical outcomes. Am J Sports Med. 2015;43(7):1805–17.
35. Struck M, Wellmann M, Becher C, Pastor MF, Smith T. Results of an open posterior bone block procedure for recurrent posterior shoulder instability after a short- and long-time follow-up. Knee Surg Sports Traumatol Arthrosc. 2016;24(2):618–24.
36. Wooten C, Klika B, Schleck CD, Harmsen WS, Sperling JW, Cofield RH. Anatomic shoulder arthroplasty as treatment for locked posterior dislocation of the shoulder. J Bone Joint Surg Am. 2014;96(3):e19. https://doi.org/10.2106/JBJS.L.01588.
37. Galvin JW, Morte DR, Grassbaugh JA, Parada SA, Burns SH, Eichinger JK. Arthroscopic treatment of posterior shoulder instability in patients with and without glenoid dysplasia: a comparative outcomes analysis. J Shoulder Elb Surg. 2017;26(12):2103–9.
38. Toth AP, Warren RF, Petrigliano FA, Doward DA, Cordasco FA, Altchek DW, O'Brien SJ. Thermal shrinkage for shoulder instability. HSS J. 2011;7(2):108–14.
39. Charalambous CP, Gullett TK, Ravenscroft MJ. A modification of the McLaughlin procedure for persistent posterior shoulder instability: technical note. Arch Orthop Trauma Surg. 2009;129(6):753–5.
40. Lavender CD, Hanzlik SR, Pearson SE, Caldwell PE 3rd. Arthroscopic reverse remplissage for posterior instability. Arthrosc Tech. 2016;5(1):e43–7.

41. Meuffels DE, Schuit H, van Biezen FC, Reijman M, Verhaar JA. The posterior bone block procedure in posterior shoulder instability: a long-term follow-up study. J Bone Joint Surg Br. 2010;92(5):651–5.
42. Riggenbach MD, Najarian RG, Bishop JY. Recurrent, locked posterior glenohumeral dislocation requiring hemiarthroplasty and posterior bone block with humeral head autograft. Orthopedics. 2012;35(2):e277–82.
43. Diklic ID, Ganic ZD, Blagojevic ZD, Nho SJ, Romeo AA. Treatment of locked chronic posterior dislocation of the shoulder by reconstruction of the defect in the humeral head with an allograft. Bone Joint Surg Br. 2010;92(1):71–6.
44. Bradley JP, Baker CL 3rd, Kline AJ, Armfield DR, Chhabra A. Arthroscopic capsulolabral reconstruction for posterior instability of the shoulder: a prospective study of 100 shoulders. Am J Sports Med. 2006;34(7):1061–71.
45. Misamore GW, Facibene WA. Posterior capsulorrhaphy for the treatment of traumatic recurrent posterior subluxations of the shoulder in athletes. J Shoulder Elb Surg. 2000;9(5):403–8.
46. Wolf EM, Eakin CL. Arthroscopic capsular plication for posterior shoulder instability. Arthroscopy. 1998;14(2):153–63.
47. Fuchs B, Jost B, Gerber C. Posterior-inferior capsular shift for the treatment of recurrent, voluntary posterior subluxation of the shoulder. J Bone Joint Surg Am. 2000;82(1):16–25.
48. Bessems JH, Vegter J. Glenoplasty for recurrent posterior shoulder instability. Good results in 13 cases followed for 1-16 years. Acta Orthop Scand. 1995;66(6):535–7.
49. Metcalf MH, Duckworth DG, Lee SB, Sidles JA, Smith KL, Harryman DT 2nd, Matsen FA 3rd. Posteroinferior glenoplasty can change glenoid shape and increase the mechanical stability of the shoulder. J Shoulder Elb Surg. 1999;8(3):205–13.
50. Bokor DJ, Fritsch BA. Posterior shoulder instability secondary to reverse humeral avulsion of the glenohumeral ligament. J Shoulder Elb Surg. 2010;19(6):853–8.
51. Petrera M, Veillette CJ, Taylor DW, Park SS, Theodoropoulos JS. Use of fresh osteochondral glenoid allograft to treat posteroinferior bone loss in chronic posterior shoulder instability. Am J Orthop (Belle Mead NJ). 2013;42(2):78–82.
52. Schwartz DG, Goebel S, Piper K, Kordasiewicz B, Boyle S, Lafosse L. Arthroscopic posterior bone block augmentation in posterior shoulder instability. J Shoulder Elb Surg. 2013;22(8):1092–101.
53. Martinez AA, Navarro E, Iglesias D, Domingo J, Calvo A, Carbonel I. Long-term follow-up of allograft reconstruction of segmental defects of the humeral head associated with posterior dislocation of the shoulder. Injury. 2013;44(4):488–91.
54. Millett PJ, Schoenahl JY, Register B, Gaskill TR, van Deurzen DF, Martetschläger F. Reconstruction of posterior glenoid deficiency using distal tibial osteoarticular allograft. Knee Surg Sports Traumatol Arthrosc. 2013;21(2):445–9.
55. Inui H, Nobuhara K. Glenoid osteotomy for atraumatic posteroinferior shoulder instability associated with glenoid dysplasia. Bone Joint J. 2018;100-B(3):331–7.
56. Graichen H, Koydl P, Zichner L. Effectiveness of glenoid osteotomy in atraumatic posterior instability of the shoulder associated with excessive retroversion and flatness of the glenoid. Int Orthop. 1999;23(2):95–9.
57. Schliemann B, Muder D, Gessmann J, Schildhauer TA, Seybold D. Locked posterior shoulder dislocation: treatment options and clinical outcomes. Arch Orthop Trauma Surg. 2011;131(8):1127–34.
58. Ziran B, Nourbakhsh A. Proximal humerus derotational osteotomy for internal rotation instability after locked posterior shoulder dislocation: early experience in four patients. Joints. 2014;1(4):171–9.
59. Wellmann M, Pastor MF, Ettinger M, Koester K, Smith T. Arthroscopic posterior bone block stabilization-early results of an effective procedure for the recurrent posterior instability. Knee Surg Sports Traumatol Arthrosc. 2018;26(1):292–8.
60. Katthagen JC, Tahal DS, Montgomery SR, Horan MP, Millett PJ. Association of traumatic and atraumatic posterior shoulder instability with glenoid retroversion and outcomes after arthroscopic capsulolabral repair. Arthroscopy. 2017;33(2):284–90.
61. Bessette MC, Frisch NC, Kodali P, Jones MH, Miniaci A. Partial resurfacing for humeral head defects associated with recurrent shoulder instability. Orthopedics. 2017;40(6):e996–e1003.

Chapter 38
Multidirectional Glenohumeral Instability

Multidirectional instability (MDI) is a symptomatic instability of the glenohumeral joint in more than one direction (anterior, posterior, inferior). Although instability may exist in more than one direction, instability in one of those directions may predominate and be more symptomatic than the rest.

The humeral head may:

- Sublux – displace but part of the articular surfaces of the humeral head and glenoid remain in contact
- Dislocate – with loss of all articular contact

38.1 Causes of Multidirectional Glenohumeral Instability [1–11]

In MDI there is dysfunction of the stabilisers of more than one direction as presented below.

38.1.1 Disruption of Static Stabilisers

MDI is often associated with:

- Lax, stretched capsule and ligaments
- Increased glenohumeral volume

In these cases the ligaments and capsule are not torn but are stretched and hence less effective in providing stability. Such laxity changes in static stabilisers may be:

© Springer Nature Switzerland AG 2019

C. Panayiotou Charalambous, *The Shoulder Made Easy*,
https://doi.org/10.1007/978-3-319-98908-2_38

- Congenital, as a result of connective tissue conditions including:
  - Benign generalized hyper-laxity
  - Ehlers-Danlos
  - Marfan's
- Acquired
  - Micro-traumatic – due to repetitive placement of the arm in positions at the extreme of motion (such as in high level athletes) which leads to stretching of static stabilisers
  - Traumatic – as a result of a well-defined episode of substantial shoulder trauma that stretches but does not tear the static stabilisers

Hence, increased laxity may either involve only the symptomatic shoulder or involve multiple joints.

However, on rare occasions, when there has been substantial trauma, there may be extensive damage of soft tissue or bony stabilisers (with lesions similar to those encountered in unilateral instability- tears and fractures) rather than sole hyper-laxity due to capsule or ligament stretching. In such cases a combination of anterior, posterior and inferior stabilisers may be disrupted, leading to instability in more than one direction. Extensive labrum detachments have been described leading to MDI:

- 180° tear – inferior labrum anterior to posterior (ILAP) tear that involves the inferior part of the glenoid labrum, defunctioning the anterior and posterior bands of the inferior glenohumeral ligament
- 270° tear that extends from just anterior to the superior labrum all the way to the mid-posterior labrum
- 360° tear, involving detachment of the whole labrum

Extensive labrum detachment – (a) 180°, (b) 270°, (c) 360° detachments

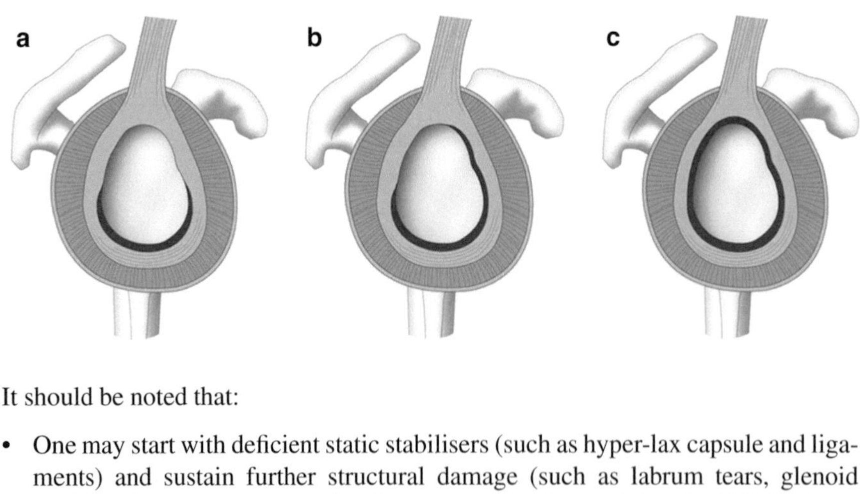

It should be noted that:

- One may start with deficient static stabilisers (such as hyper-lax capsule and ligaments) and sustain further structural damage (such as labrum tears, glenoid avulsion fractures, compression fractures of the humeral head – Hill-Sachs or reverse Hill-Sachs lesions) during:

  - The process of recurrent subluxation or dislocation
  - Further isolated substantial trauma

- One may start with deficient static stabilisers in one direction but then sustain substantial trauma that disrupts stabilisers of a different direction

38.1.2 Disruption of Dynamic Stabilisers

Inadequate dynamic stabilisers may lead to instability in more than one direction. These may occur in isolation or in association with deficient static stabilisers. Such inadequacy of dynamic stability may be due to:

- Shoulder muscle weakness (rotator cuff, deltoid)
- Dis-coordinated muscle activity (muscle patterning) – over- or underactivity of rotator cuff muscles, deltoid, pectoralis major and latissimus dorsi
- Lack of stable platform to act upon:
  - Poor scapular dynamics
  - Poor core control
- Defective proprioception – leading to uncoordinated muscle activity in response to joint motion or in response to forces applied on the joint

38.2 Classification of Multidirectional Glenohumeral Instability

Multidirectional glenohumeral instability may be classified using the Stanmore triangle [12] that takes into consideration underlying pathological findings:

- Structural but with no trauma
- Nonstructural – abnormal muscle patterning
- Structural secondary to substantial trauma
- Combination of the above

Patients with MDI usually fall in the structural atraumatic or nonstructural corners of the triangle, but, on occasions (as explained above), they may be in the structural traumatic group.

Stanmore triangle of instability—in multi-directional glenohumeral instability cases tend to be non-structural or structural atraumatic

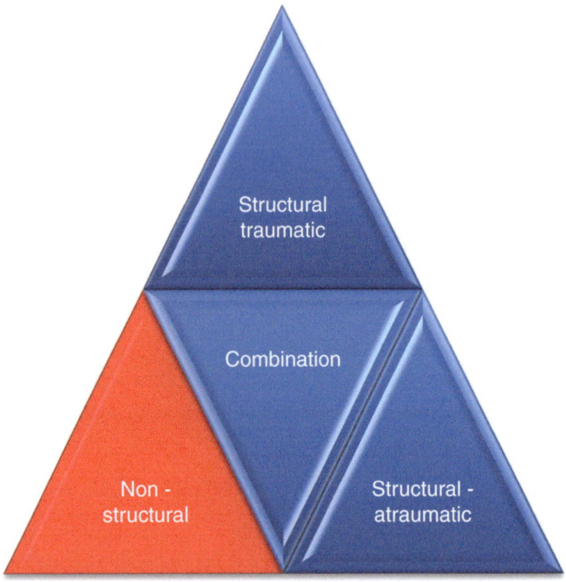

38.3 Clinical Symptoms of Multidirectional Glenohumeral Instability

- Vague shoulder or arm pain
- Arm going "dead", feeling heavy, paraesthesia
- Clicking, clunking of the shoulder
- Feeling of abnormal displacement – feeling "wobbly" to "popping in and out" to "popping out and can't go back", "coming out to the edge" to "coming out fully". The shoulder may feel as subluxing (almost comes out of joint but then spontaneously reduces). Alternatively, patients may present with frank dislocation where the humeral head comes out of joint. The patient may be able to reduce the shoulder themselves or may need medical reduction. In many cases of MDI, the shoulder spontaneously relocates with very few needing medical reduction
- Apprehension in placing the arm in more than one position:
  - Abduction and external rotation (throwing or lifting weights above head)
  - Forward elevation and adduction (pushing, reaching out to a shelf)
  - Carrying weights with the arm by the side

In many cases even though there is instability in more than one direction, symptoms in one direction may predominate.

Onsets of symptoms are:

- *Often* atraumatic – gradual onset with vague pain, arm heaviness and then symptoms of abnormal glenohumeral translation without an obvious precipitating event
- *Occasionally* precipitated by minor trauma (which involves much lower forces that those required under normal conditions to cause glenohumeral dislocation), such as carrying a bag, throwing a ball, reaching out and standing up from a chair using arms
- *Rarely* precipitated by substantial trauma to the shoulder that causes extensive disruption to combinations of anterior, posterior or inferior static stabilisers

At the initial dislocation, the shoulder may spontaneously relocate or the patient may manage to reduce it themselves and this is often the case in those with atraumatic or minor injury first-time dislocations. Infrequently, first-time dislocations in those with MDI may need medical intervention for reduction (this may be often necessary when the first dislocation is the result of substantial trauma but may also be encountered in those cases where first dislocation is atraumatic or the result of minimal trauma).

Following this first dislocation, the shoulder starts to show recurrent subluxations or dislocations that may occur with further substantial trauma or with minimal or no further trauma (such as by putting the arm in certain positions).

Hence, it is important to get a clear history and define the mechanism of the first dislocation, even if seeing the patient for the first time many years after that initial event.

Multidirectional glenohumeral instability may be:

- Voluntary, whereby the patient can sublux/dislocate the shoulder at will by putting the shoulder in a particular position or contracting specific muscles
- Involuntary, whereby the patient cannot sublux/dislocate the shoulder at will

Progression of severity of symptoms in multidirectional glenohumeral instability

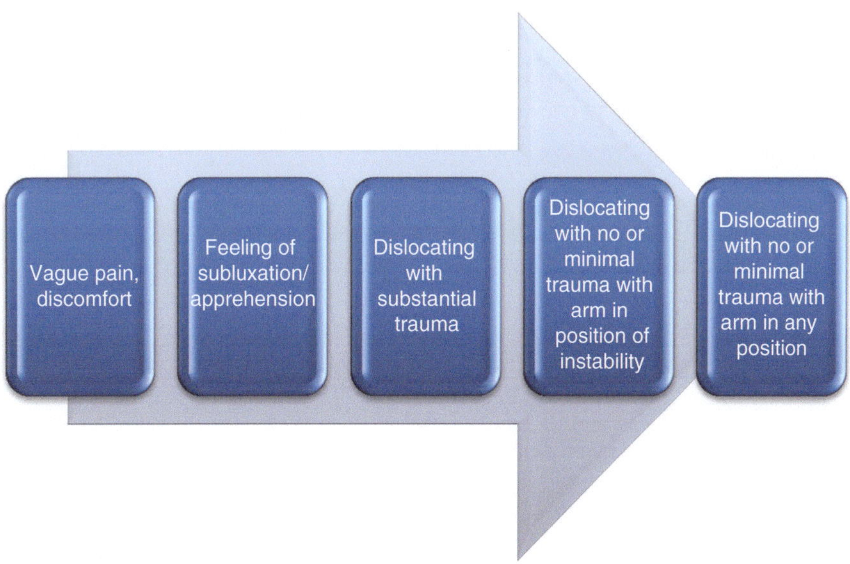

Progression of severity of symptoms in multidirectional glenohuemral instability according to the intervention needed to relocate the joint—usually relocate spontaneously

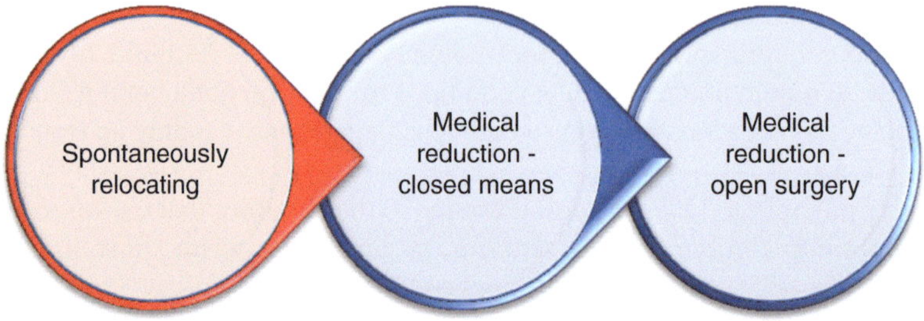

38.4 Clinical Signs of Multidirectional Glenohumeral Instability [13, 14]

- Patient may be able to demonstrate the subluxation/dislocation
- Patient may be able to voluntarily make the shoulder sublux or dislocate
- Hyper-laxity
  - Localised to the shoulder, in one or more directions
  - Generalised ligamentous laxity with high Beighton score
- Apprehension in more than one direction:
  - Anterior apprehension with the arm in abduction and external rotation
  - Posterior apprehension with the arm in forward elevation, adduction and internal rotation
  - Inferior sulcus test causing apprehension rather than simply increased humeral head translation

The diagnosis of MDI is primarily clinical, with clinical symptoms and signs suggestive of instability in two or more directions.

38.5 Investigations for Multidirectional Glenohumeral Instability

Investigations of the unstable shoulder aim to confirm the presence of instability, determine its likely cause and identify any structural lesions that may be amenable to surgical intervention. These include:

- Radiological
  - Plain radiographs
  - MRI/MRI arthrogram [9, 15, 16]/CT scan
- Neurophysiological
  - Nerve conduction studies
  - Electromyography
- Examination undergeneral anaesthesia – joint translation and laxity are assessed with the patient under general anaesthesia to abolish pain and allow muscle relaxation
- Arthroscopic evaluation

38.6 Management of Multidirectional Glenohumeral Instability

Management aims at improving joint stability and in doing so minimises any associated functional loss, apprehension or pain. Initially management involves relocating a dislocated joint. Once the joint is relocated, further management aims at improving stability and reducing the risk of subsequent instability episodes. Further management depends on:

- Symptoms – frequency and severity
- Underlying cause of instability

Management of multidirectional glenohumeral instability

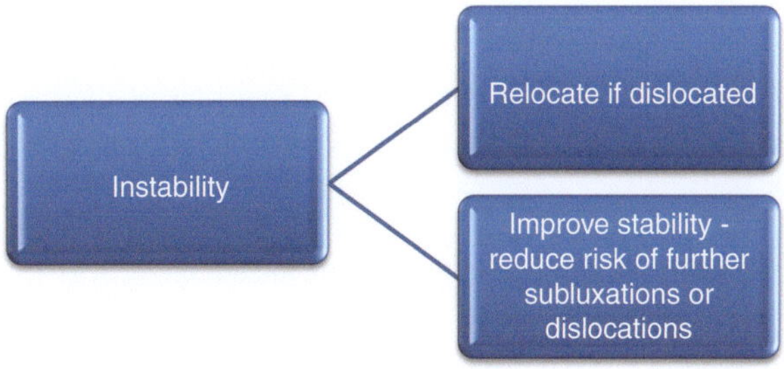

In MDI that is not associated with specific high-energy trauma, the preferred management is non-surgical for a period of at least 6 months. Earlier surgical intervention is warranted for the cases that are secondary to substantial trauma.

Non-surgical [17–24]

Non-surgical management aims to improve stability by enhancing the function of dynamic stabilisers (through strengthening, better control and coordination), to compensate for the deficient static joint constraints.

- Leave alone
- Activity modification, avoiding unstable positions
- Physiotherapy to address:
  - Core imbalance – core strengthening
  - Scapular dysrhythmia – strengthening of scapular muscles
  - Proprioception – proprioceptive training
  - Abnormal muscle patterning – biofeedback, inhibit overactive and enhance underactive muscles, improve neuromuscular control
  - Rotator cuff weakness – rotator cuff muscle strengthening, balance

Surgical [11, 25–33]

If symptoms do not improve with non-surgical intervention, and the patient has structural lesions that are amenable to surgery, then surgery may be considered. Surgery for MDI aims to address any laxity and any structural lesions contributing to the instability. Structural derangements are corrected either directly or indirectly:

- Directly – correct the structural defect itself
- Indirectly – compensate for the structural defect

In MDI there is often lax and redundant capsule which may be addressed by:

- Plication, open or arthroscopic (sutures are passed through the capsule, which are then tied causing a fold in the capsule and hence reducing its effective length, tightening the capsule) [19, 20]
- Capsular shift – the capsule is divided, and one part of the capsule is moved (shifted) over the other, and the two are stitched together, essentially reducing the length of the capsule [21, 22]
- Thermal capsulorrhaphy – thermal energy is applied using an arthroscopic device causing denaturation of collagen and capsule shrinkage [23, 24]
- Rotator interval closure – sutures are passed through the capsule of the rotator interval, which are then tied, causing rotator interval tightness [25, 26]

Soft tissue may be tightened by: (a) dividing the soft tissue and suturing the two ends in an overlapping position (equivalent to capsular shift). (b) passing sutures through the soft tissue which upon tying fold and effectively shorten the tissue (plication)

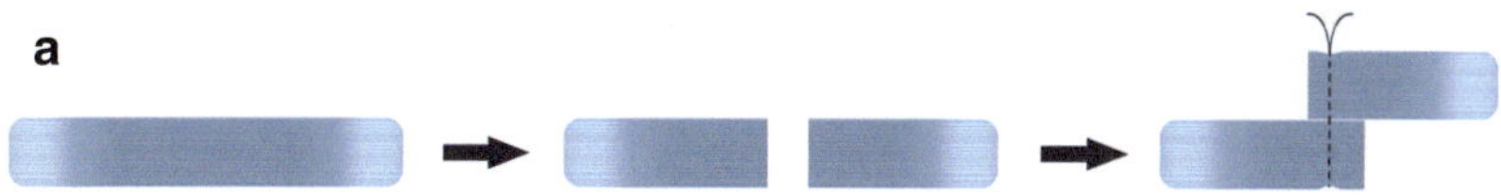

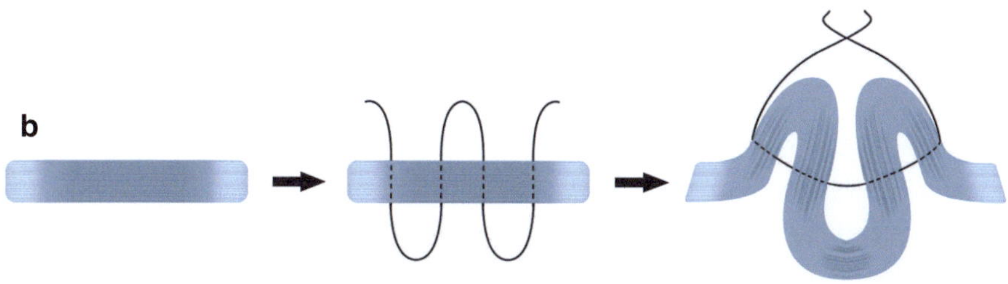

Traditionally, open surgery in the form of capsular shift has been utilised to reduce capsular laxity and glenohumeral joint volume. More recently, arthroscopic techniques have been able to exert the same effect by plication or thermal capsulorrhaphy of the capsule. Thermal capsulorrhaphy has shown high recurrence rates and is less favoured than plication techniques. The exact pattern of shift/plication is planned such as to improve general shoulder tightness or tightness in certain directions.

As described above, occasionally MDI may be associated with other structural defects (due to an initial substantial trauma or due to trauma sustained as a result of repeated subluxations or dislocations). Hence, other direct or indirect surgical procedures may be employed as discussed below to improve stability either directly or indirectly:

- *Directly*
  - Labrum avulsion – reattach (suture anchors, bone tunnels)
  - Glenoid avulsion fracture:

    Reattach using anchors or screws according to fragment size
    Glenoid osteochondral allograft

- Hill-Sachs/Reverse Hill-Sachs

  Elevate defect
  Fill defect to stop it engaging with:

    Tendon/capsule
    Allograft reconstruction of segmental defects

- Abnormal glenoid version – osteotomy
- HAGL/reverse HAGL lesion – reattachment to humerus (anchors, bone tunnels)
- Mid-substance ligamentous rupture – capsular plication

• *Indirectly* – compensate for the structural defect

- Bone block procedure – adding an extension to the glenoid increases the amount of rotation that can occur before the Hill-Sachs or reverse Hill-Sachs engages on the edge of the glenoid and levers out
- Humeral head arthroplasty – for large Hill-Sachs or reverse Hill-Sachs lesions

Surgery may address only structural defects hence other nonstructural contributors to instability (such as abnormal proprioception or abnormal muscle patterning) will still need to be corrected.

References

1. Warby SA, Watson L, Ford JJ, Hahne AJ, Pizzari T. Multidirectional instability of the glenohumeral joint: etiology, classification, assessment, and management. J Hand Ther. 2017;30(2):175–81.
2. Ren H, Bicknell RT. From the unstable painful shoulder to multidirectional instability in the young athlete. Clin Sports Med. 2013;32(4):815–23.
3. Neer CS 2nd. Involuntary inferior and multidirectional instability of the shoulder: etiology, recognition, and treatment. Instr Course Lect. 1985;34:232–8.
4. Jaggi A, Noorani A, Malone A, Cowan J, Lambert S, Bayley I. Muscle activation patterns in patients with recurrent shoulder instability. Int J Shoulder Surg. 2012;6(4):101–7.
5. Barden JM, Balyk R, Raso VJ, Moreau M, Bagnall K. Atypical shoulder muscle activation in multidirectional instability. Clin Neurophysiol. 2005;116(8):1846–57.
6. Jeremiah HM, Alexander CM. Do hypermobile subjects without pain have alteration to the feedback mechanisms controlling the shoulder girdle? Musculoskeletal Care. 2010;8(3):157–63.
7. Lephart SM, Warner JJ, Borsa PA, Fu FH. Proprioception of the shoulder joint in healthy, unstable, and surgically repaired shoulders. J Shoulder Elb Surg. 1994;3(6):371–80.
8. Saccomanno MF, Fodale M, Capasso L, Cazzato G, Milano G. Generalized joint laxity and multidirectional instability of the shoulder. Patient Saf Surg. 2015;9:15. https://doi.org/10.1186/s13037-015-0062-9.
9. Lee HJ, Kim NR, Moon SG, Ko SM, Park JY. Multidirectional instability of the shoulder: rotator interval dimension and capsular laxity evaluation using MR arthrography. Skelet Radiol. 2013;42(2):231–8.
10. Kibler WB, Press J, Sciascia A. The role of core stability in athletic function. Sports Med. 2006;36(3):189–98.
11. Burt DM. Arthroscopic repair of inferior labrum from anterior to posterior lesions associated with multidirectional instability of the shoulder. Arthrosc Tech. 2014;3(6):e727–30.

12. Lewis A, Kitamura T, Bayley JIL. The classification of shoulder instability: new light through old windows! Curr Orthop. 2004;18:97–108.
13. Valencia Mora M, Ibán MÁR, Heredia JD, Gutiérrez-Gómez JC, Diaz RR, Aramberri M, Cobiella C. Physical exam and evaluation of the unstable shoulder. Open Orthop J. 2017;11:946–56.
14. Charalambous CP. Clinical examination of the shoulder. In: Charalambous CP, editor. The shoulder made easy. Basel: Springer; 2019.
15. Macmahon PJ, Palmer WE. Magnetic resonance imaging in glenohumeral instability. Magn Reson Imaging Clin N Am. 2012;20(2):295–312.
16. Lim CO, Park KJ, Cho BK, Kim YM, Chun KA. A new screening method for multidirectional shoulder instability on magnetic resonance arthrography: labro-capsular distance. Skelet Radiol. 2016;45(7):921–7.
17. Jaggi A, Lambert S. Rehabilitation for shoulder instability. Br J Sports Med. 2010;44(5):333–40.
18. Watson L, Balster S, Lenssen R, Hoy G, Pizzari T. The effects of a conservative rehabilitation program for multidirectional instability of the shoulder. J Shoulder Elb Surg. 2018;27(1):104–11.
19. Watson L, Warby S, Balster S, Lenssen R, Pizzari T. The treatment of multidirectional instability of the shoulder with a rehabilitation programme: part 2. Shoulder Elbow. 2017;9(1):46–53.
20. Watson L, Warby S, Balster S, Lenssen R, Pizzari T. The treatment of multidirectional instability of the shoulder with a rehabilitation program: part 1. Shoulder Elbow. 2016;8(4):271–8.
21. Warby SA, Pizzari T, Ford JJ, Hahne AJ, Watson L. Exercise-based management versus surgery for multidirectional instability of the glenohumeral joint: a systematic review. Br J Sports Med. 2016;50(18):1115–23.
22. Warby SA, Ford JJ, Hahne AJ, Watson L, Balster S, Lenssen R, Pizzari T. Comparison of 2 exercise rehabilitation programs for multidirectional instability of the glenohumeral joint: a randomized controlled trial. Am J Sports Med. 2018;46(1):87–97.
23. Burkhead WZ Jr, Rockwood CA Jr. Treatment of instability of the shoulder with an exercise program. J Bone Joint Surg Am. 1992;74(6):890–6.
24. Huxel Bliven KC, Anderson BE. Core stability training for injury prevention. Sports Health. 2013;5(6):514–22.
25. Chen D, Goldberg J, Herald J, Critchley I, Barmare A. Effects of surgical management on multidirectional instability of the shoulder: a meta-analysis. Knee Surg Sports Traumatol Arthrosc. 2016;24(2):630–9.
26. Raynor MB, Horan MP, Greenspoon JA, Katthagen JC, Millett PJ. Outcomes after arthroscopic pancapsular capsulorrhaphy with suture anchors for the treatment of multidirectional glenohumeral instability in athletes. Am J Sports Med. 2016;44(12):3188–97.
27. Duncan R, Savoie FH 3rd. Arthroscopic inferior capsular shift for multidirectional instability of the shoulder: a preliminary report. Arthroscopy. 1993;9(1):24–7.
28. Frangiamore SJ, Mannava S, Godin JA, Anavian J, Fritz EM, Millett PJ. Arthroscopic pancapsular shift with labral repair for multidirectional instability of the shoulder. Arthrosc Tech. 2017;6(4):e1113–7. https://doi.org/10.1016/j.eats.2017.03.032.
29. Witney-Lagen C, Hassan A, Doodson A, Venkateswaran B. Arthroscopic plication for multidirectional instability: 50 patients with a minimum of 2 years of follow-up. J Shoulder Elb Surg. 2017;26(2):e29–36. https://doi.org/10.1016/j.jse.2016.07.015.
30. Neer CS 2nd, Foster CR. Inferior capsular shift for involuntary inferior and multidirectional instability of the shoulder. A preliminary report. J Bone Joint Surg Am. 1980;62(6):897–908.
31. Vavken P, Tepolt FA, Kocher MS. Open inferior capsular shift for multidirectional shoulder instability in adolescents with generalized ligamentous hyperlaxity or Ehlers-Danlos syndrome. J Shoulder Elb Surg. 2016;25(6):907–12.
32. Bankart AS. Recurrent or habitual dislocation of the shoulder-joint. Br Med J. 1923;2(3285):1132–3.
33. Patel RM, Amin NH, Lynch TS, Miniaci A. Management of bone loss in glenohumeral instability. Orthop Clin North Am. 2014;45(4):523–39.

Chapter 39
Acromio-Clavicular Joint Instability

This is a condition whereby there is disruption of the acromio-clavicular joint (ACJt) with resultant abnormal displacement of the lateral end of the clavicle in relation to the acromion.

39.1 Spectrum of ACJt Instability

The ACJt is stabilised by the:

- Coraco-clavicular ligaments (conoid and trapezoid) – limit superior translation of the clavicle
- Acromio-clavicular ligaments – limit anterior-posterior displacement of the clavicle [1, 2]

ACJt instability may be:

- Partial displacement (subluxation)
- Complete displacement (dislocation)

It may also be:

- Static – the clavicle is relatively stabilised in the displaced position
- Dynamic – the clavicle is mobile

39.2 Causes of ACJt Instability [3–6]

ACJt instability may occur secondary to disruption of the stabilising ligaments due to:

© Springer Nature Switzerland AG 2019

C. Panayiotou Charalambous, *The Shoulder Made Easy*,
https://doi.org/10.1007/978-3-319-98908-2_39

- Trauma
  - Direct fall on the shoulder, fall on outstretched arm
  - Iatrogenic – during a Latarjet procedure, harvesting of the coracoid may lead to coraco-clavicular ligament disruption
- Non-traumatic
  - Hyper-laxity
  - Infection
  - Inflammatory arthritis

The most common cause of ACJt instability encountered in clinical practise is post-traumatic.

39.3 Classification of ACJt Instability

The Rockwood classification of ACJt instability [7] describes the degree and direction of clavicular displacement in relation to the acromion at the ACJt joint on plain radiographs:

1. No widening, separation or deformity of the ACJt
2. Distal part of the clavicle slightly elevated, less than 100%
3. Distal part of the clavicle 100% displaced superiorly in relation to the acromion
4. Distal part of the clavicle is displaced posteriorly in relation to the acromion
5. Distal part of the clavicle is markedly displaced superiorly due to extensive soft tissue disruption
6. Distal part of the clavicle is displaced inferiorly, under the acromion or coracoid

39.4 Clinical Symptoms of ACJt Instability

- Pain over the ACJt
- Clicking of the ACJt
- Feeling of exaggerated mobility of the clavicle
- Clinical deformitywith "bump" at the ACJt

39.5 Clinical Signs of ACJt Instability

- Visible and palpable displacement of the lateral end of the clavicle in relation to the acromion at rest or during arm motion
- Superior displacement of the clavicle in relation to the acromion may be reduced by the examiner supporting the arm and applying an upward force on the arm

ACJt dislocation – the lateral end of the clavicle displaces upwards in relation to the acromion, appearing as a lump on top of the shoulder

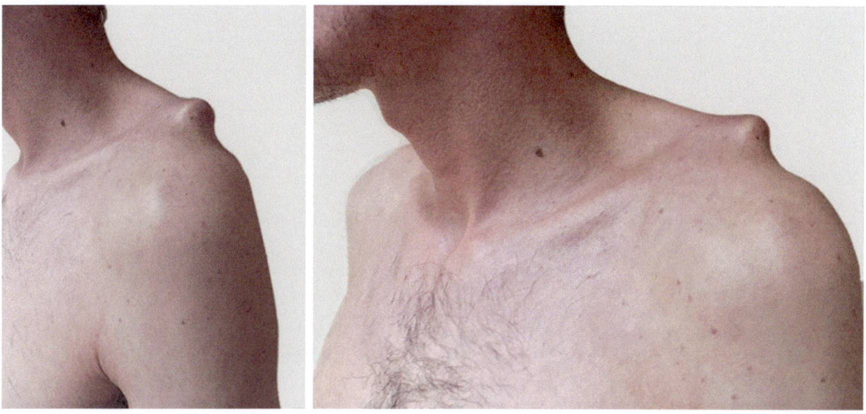

39.6 Investigations for ACJt Instability

- Plain radiographs:
  - AP and axillary views can demonstrate the position of the lateral end of the clavicle in relation to the acromion
  - AP view with 10–15° cephalad angulation of the X-ray beam (Zanca view [8]) is considered highly accurate view for evaluating the AC joint
  - Stress (weight bearing) AP view can demonstrate the position of the lateral end of the clavicle in relation to the acromion [9]
- CT with 3D reconstruction – to provide an accurate evaluation of the position of the clavicle
- MRI – to demonstrate concomitant soft tissue injuries such as rotator cuff or labrum tears [10]

ACJt superior dislocation – lateral end of clavicle (red arrow) displaced superiorly in relation to the acromion

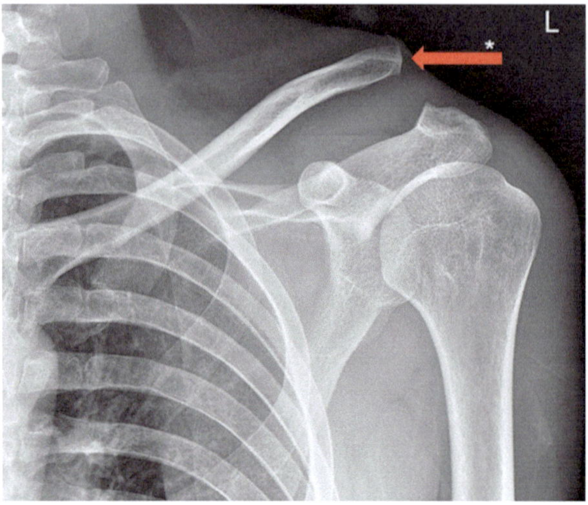

Plain radiograph of ACJt dislocation. ACJt displacement of the clavicle (green arrow) increases with the application of a downwards load to the arm (stress view) (yellow arrow)

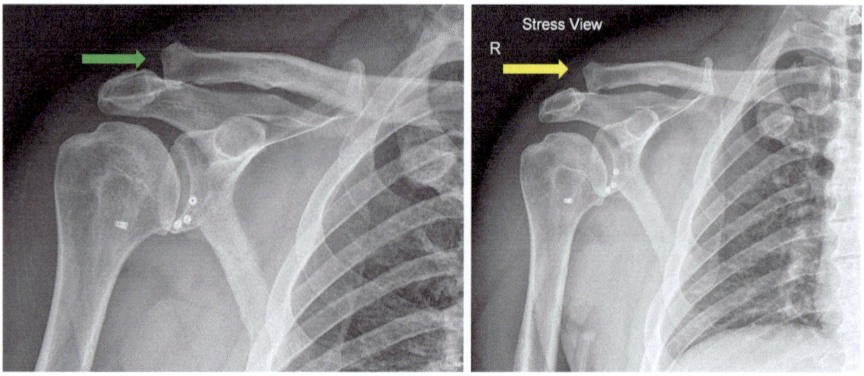

Plain radiograph of ACJt dislocation. Stress application causes inferior displacement of the humeral head (red arrow) but with no change in the relation between the clavicle and acromion (yellow arrow)

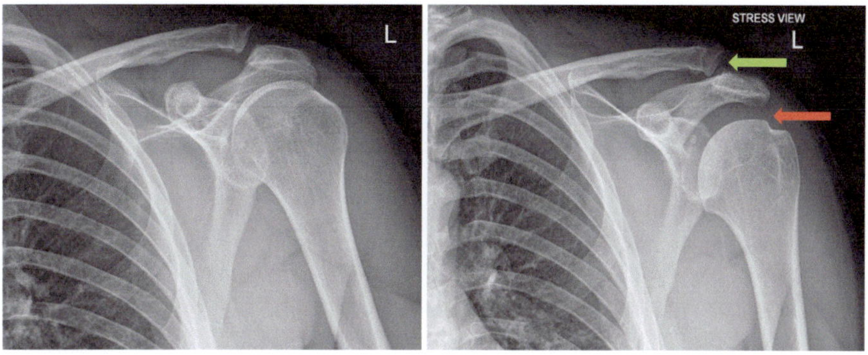

39.7 Management of ACJt Instability

This depends on the patient's symptoms, functional demands and extent of clavicular displacement. Symptoms may be those of:

1. Painful arthropathy
2. Instability
3. Combined painful arthropathy and instability

Non-surgical [11, 12]

- Leave alone
- Analgesia
- Activity modification
- ACJt steroid injection

Surgical [11–18]

- ACJt excision – for ACJt painful arthropathy but no substantial symptoms of instability
- ACJt stabilisation +/– lateral end of clavicle excision – for troublesome instability symptoms

It may be suggested (even though this is not an absolute rule) [3] that:

- Type 1 injuries are treated non-surgically
- Types 4–6 are reduced and stabilised
- Type 2 and 3 injuries are treated either non-surgically or surgically

Various techniques for ACJt stabilisation have been described, both open and arthroscopic. These include:

- Using an autograft, allograft or synthetic ligament passing from the coracoid (or round the coracoid) to the clavicle to hold the clavicle in a reduced position
- Using a local native ligament – in the Weaver-Dunn procedure, the coraco-acromial ligament is detached from the acromion and is sutured via thread holes to the lateral end of the clavicle limiting its superior translation
- Hook plate fixation which aims to hold down the dislocated clavicle to allow healing of the coraco-clavicular ligaments

ACJt dislocation with rupture of the ACJt and coraco – clavicular ligaments (a). Stabilisation of the ACJt may involve lateral end of clavicle excision and transfer of the coraco-acromial ligament to the lateral end of the clavicle (b). Alternatively, an artificial ligament may be utilised to hold the clavicle down (c)

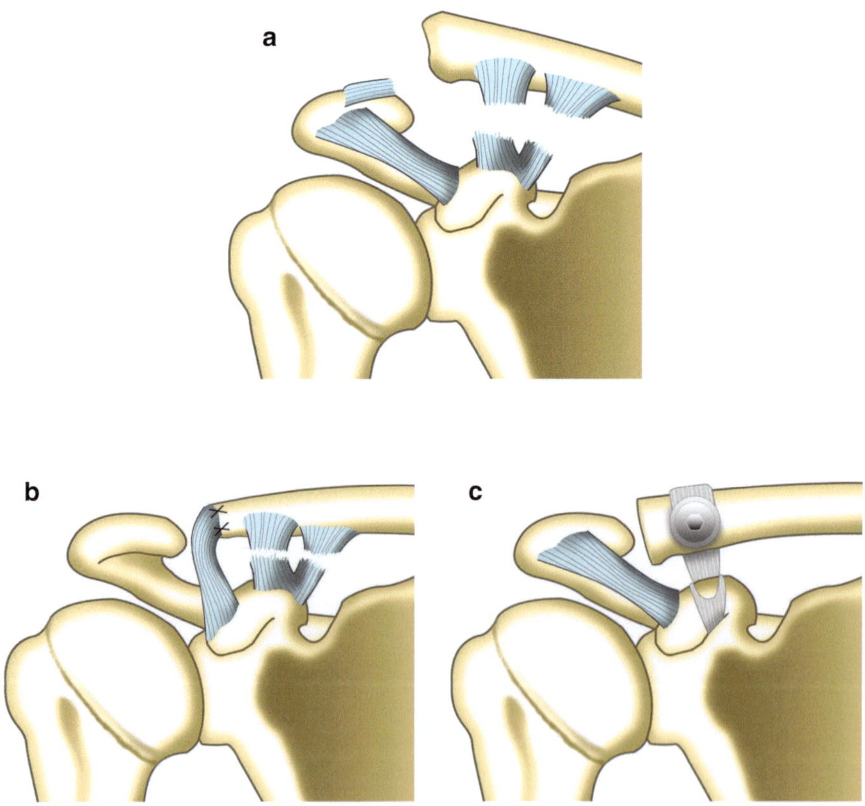

Learning Pearls

- There is a need to distinguish between pain and instability symptoms in the presence of ACJt dislocation or subluxation – the former may improve with less extensive interventions and avoid the need for a stabilisation procedure

References

1. Lee KW, Debski RE, Chen CH, Woo SL, Fu FH. Functional evaluation of the ligaments at the acromioclavicular joint during anteroposterior and superoinferior translation. Am J Sports Med. 1997;25:858–62.
2. Fukuda K, Craig EV, An KN, Cofield RH, Chao EY. Biomechanical study of the ligamentous system of the acromioclavicular joint. J Bone Joint Surg Am. 1986;68:434–40.
3. Simovitch R, Sanders B, Ozbaydar M, Lavery K, Warner JJ. Acromioclavicular joint injuries: diagnosis and management. J Am Acad Orthop Surg. 2009;17(4):207–19.
4. Dolan CM. An anatomic study of the coracoid process as it relates to bone transfer procedures. J Shoulder Elb Surg. 2011;20(3):497–501.
5. Lehtinen JT, Lehto MU, Kaarela K, Belt EA, Kautiainen HJ, Kauppi MJ. Acromioclavicular joint subluxation is rare in rheumatoid arthritis. A radiographic 15-year study. Rev Rhum Engl Ed. 1999;66(10):462–6.
6. Sadeghi N, Haen PS, Onstenk R. Atraumatic acromioclavicular dislocation: a case report and review of the literature. Case Rep Orthop. 2017;2017:8450538. https://doi.org/10.1155/2017/8450538.
7. Rockwood CA Jr. Fractures and dislocations of the shoulder. In: Rockwood Jr CA, Green DP, editors. Fractures in adults. Philadelphia, PA: Lippincott; 1984. p. 860–910.
8. Zanca P. Shoulder pain: involvement of the acromioclavicular joint. (Analysis of 1,000 cases). Am J Roentgenol Radium Therapy, Nucl Med. 1971;112:493–506.
9. Ibrahim EF, Forrest NP, Forester A. Bilateral weighted radiographs are required for accurate classification of acromioclavicular separation: an observational study of 59 cases. Injury. 2015;46(10):1900–5.
10. Pauly S, Kraus N, Greiner S, Scheibel M. Prevalence and pattern of glenohumeral injuries among acute high-grade acromioclavicular joint instabilities. J Shoulder Elb Surg. 2013;22(6):760–6. https://doi.org/10.1016/j.jse.2012.08.016.
11. Tang G, Zhang Y, Liu Y, Qin X, Hu J, Li X. Comparison of surgical and conservative treatment of Rockwood type-III acromioclavicular dislocation: a meta-analysis. Medicine (Baltimore). 2018;97(4):e9690. https://doi.org/10.1097/MD.0000000000009690.
12. Chang N, Furey A, Kurdin A. Operative versus nonoperative management of acute high-grade acromioclavicular dislocations: a systematic review and meta-analysis. J Orthop Trauma. 2018;32(1):1–9.
13. Moatshe G, Kruckeberg BM, Chahla J, Godin JA, Cinque ME, Provencher MT, LaPrade RF. Acromioclavicular and coracoclavicular ligament reconstruction for acromioclavicular joint instability: a systematic review of clinical and radiographic outcomes. Arthroscopy. 2018;34(6):1979–95.e8. https://doi.org/10.1016/j.arthro.2018.01.016.
14. Taranu R, Rushton PR, Serrano-Pedraza I, Holder L, Wallace WA, Candal-Couto JJ. Acromioclavicular joint reconstruction using the LockDown synthetic implant: a study with cadavers. Bone Joint J. 2015;97-B(12):1657–61.

15. Wood TA, Rosell PA, Clasper JC. Preliminary results of the 'Surgilig' synthetic ligament in the management of chronic acromioclavicular joint disruption. J R Army Med Corps. 2009;155(3):191–3.
16. Weaver JK, Dunn HK. Treatment of acromioclavicular injuries, especially complete acromioclavicular separation. J Bone Joint Surg Am. 1972;54(6):1187–94.
17. Guy DK, Wirth MA, Griffin JL, Rockwood CA Jr. Reconstruction of chronic and complete dislocations of the acromioclavicular joint. Clin Orthop Relat Res. 1998;347:138–49.
18. Weinstein DM, McCann PD, McIlveen SJ, Flatow EL, Bigliani LU. Surgical treatment of complete acromioclavicular dislocations. Am J Sports Med. 1995;23(3):324–31.

Chapter 40
Sterno-clavicular Joint Instability

A condition whereby there is abnormal displacement of the medial end of the clavicle in relation to the sternum at the sterno-clavicular joint. In most cases the clavicle displaces anteriorly and in a smaller proportion posteriorly.

40.1 Spectrum of Sterno-clavicular Joint Instability

Onset of symptoms may be [1–5]:

- Atraumatic or precipitated by minor trauma (which involves much lower forces that those required under normal conditions to cause sterno-clavicular dislocation)
- Precipitated by substantial trauma to the shoulder that causes extensive disruption to the sterno-clavicular joint stabilisers

Anterior dislocations tend not to be harmful, whereas posterior dislocations may result in compression of vital mediastinal structures (trachea, oesophagus, arteries) and could be life-threatening [6–12].

May be described as:

- First-time dislocation
- Recurrent instability

At the initial dislocation, the sterno-clavicular joint may spontaneously relocate, or the patient may manage to reduce it themselves, and this is often the case in those with atraumatic or minor injury first-time dislocations. Hence, it is important to get a clear history and define the mechanism of the first dislocation, even if seeing the patient many years after that initial event.

© Springer Nature Switzerland AG 2019

C. Panayiotou Charalambous, *The Shoulder Made Easy*,
https://doi.org/10.1007/978-3-319-98908-2_40

Sterno-clavicular joint – (a) intact, (b) anterior and (c) posterior dislocation right sterno-clavicular joint

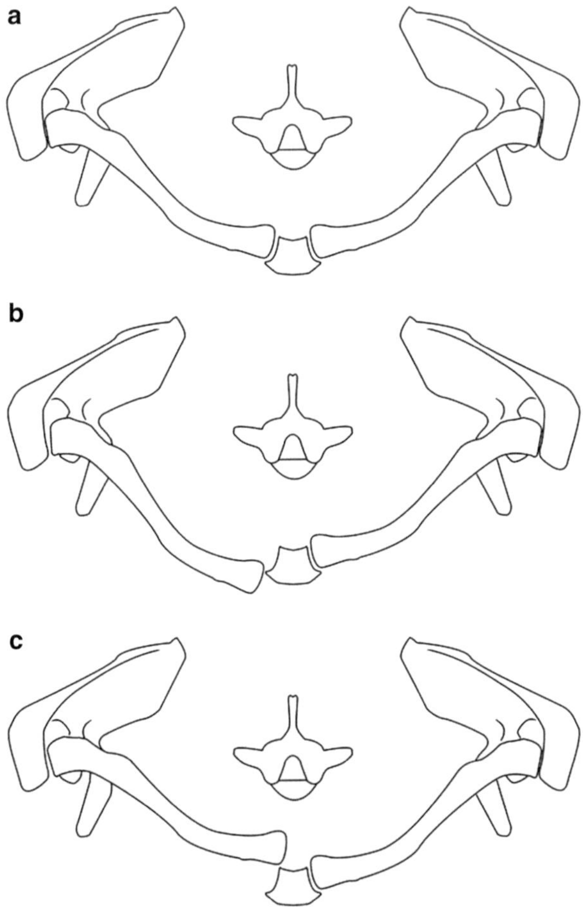

40.2 Classification of Sterno-clavicular Joint Instability

Classified according to the Stanmore triangle [13, 14] that takes into consideration the underlying pathological findings:

- Structural but with no trauma – such as in hyper-laxity, Marfan's, Ehler-Danlos syndrome
- Nonstructural – abnormal muscle patterning
- Structural – secondary to substantial trauma
- Combination of the above

40.3 Clinical Symptoms of Sterno-clavicular Joint Instability

- Pain
- Clicking
- Prominent swelling
- Change in contour
- Dyspnoea and dysphagia
- Upper limb paraesthesia if brachial plexus compression/stretching

40.4 Clinical Signs of Sterno-clavicular Joint Instability

- Clinical deformity
- Palpable step
- Visible recurrent translation of the clavicle with arm movement

40.5 Investigations for Sterno-clavicular Joint Instability

- Plain radiographs
  - AP view – to exclude a medial end of clavicle fracture or physeal injury
  - Serendipity view [15] – AP view with 40° cephalic angulation with the patient supine. With the sterno-clavicular joint in situ, the clavicle will be in line with the manubrium of the sternum, but this relation is altered in joint dislocation:

    In anterior dislocation, the medial end of the clavicle lies superior to the manubrium

    In posterior dislocation, the medial end of the clavicle lies inferior to the manubrium
- CT scan [16, 17] – gold standard – confirms dislocation and demonstrates relation of the displaced clavicle to mediastinal structures
- CT angiography to determine if there is vascular obstruction in posterior dislocations [18]

40.6 Management of Sterno-clavicular Joint Instability

40.6.1 Anterior Sterno-clavicular Joint Dislocation

In those presenting with an acute traumatic anterior dislocation, the initial decision is whether to:

- Accept
- Attempt closed reduction

Closed reduction may be achieved:

- Under sedation or general anaesthetic
- By placing a bolster between the shoulders and applying traction to the arm at 90° of abduction, whilst direct pressure is applied to the medial clavicle [19]

If the dislocation cannot be reduced by closed means, or if joint reduction cannot be maintained or if recurrent dislocations develop, the options are to:

- Accept the dislocated position
- Observe – especially in young patients in whom the physes have not fused as the joint may still stabilise with time
- Proceed with open reduction and stabilisation surgery

In those presenting with atraumatic recurrent dislocation due to ligamentous deficiency, non-surgical treatment is the management choice, as surgery is associated with unsatisfactory results. Activity modification and physiotherapy to address posture and restore muscle strength may be utilised. Steroid injections into the sterno-clavicular joint may improve associated pain.

Similarly, in those presenting with abnormal muscle patterning, biofeedback is the management choice, and surgery is to be avoided.

40.6.2 Posterior Sterno-clavicular Joint Dislocation

- Reduce unless no evidence of pressure effects and patient not candidate for reduction
- Reduction is achieved [1, 15, 20]:
  - Under sedation or general anaesthetic
  - With cardiothoracic cover unless emergency situation
  - By applying traction to the arm, abduction of the shoulder to 90° and hyperextension of the arm
  - With the arms in adduction, bolster between scapulae, applying arm traction and posterior force to both shoulders
  - Under aseptic conditions, holding the clavicle percutaneously with reduction forceps and pulling it forwards
  - Open reduction

Following reduction, if the reduction cannot be maintained, consider bracing with the arms in a figure of eight strap for 4–6 weeks [19, 21–23]. If, however, reduction cannot be maintained with bracing or if the patient continues with recurrent posterior instability, then it is advisable to offer surgical stabilisation due to the risk of compression of vital structures. Various techniques have been described for sterno-clavicular joint stabilisation [24–34] utilising:

- Local tendon
- Free tendon
  - Autograft
  - Allograft
- Synthetic ligament/anchor sutures
- Plating

Learning Pearls

- Pins should not be used for stabilising the sterno-clavicular joint [35–39] due to risk of migration, cardiovascular damage and death

References

1. Buckerfield CT, Castle ME. Acute traumatic retrosternal dislocation of the clavicle. J Bone Joint Surg Am. 1984;66(3):379–85.
2. Rockwood CA Jr, Odor JM. Spontaneous atraumatic anterior subluxation of the sternoclavicular joint. J Bone Joint Surg Am. 1989;71(9):1280–8.
3. Kumar Digge V, Meena S, Khan SA, Mittal R. Spontaneous atraumatic dislocation of sternoclavicular joint in Reiter syndrome. Chin J Traumatol. 2012;15(4):251–3.
4. Kayias EH, Drosos GI, Anagnostopoulou GA. Atraumatic retrosternal dislocation of the clavicle. Acta Orthop Belg. 2004;70(3):273–5.
5. Martin SD, Altchek D, Erlanger S. Atraumatic posterior dislocation of the sternoclavicular joint. A case report and literature review. Clin Orthop Relat Res. 1993;292:159–64.
6. Sykes JA, Ezetendu C, Sivitz A, Lee J Jr, Desai H, Norton K, Daly RA, Kalyanaraman M. Posterior dislocation of sternoclavicular joint encroaching on ipsilateral vessels in 2 pediatric patients. Pediatr Emerg Care. 2011;27(4):327–30.
7. Noda M, Shiraishi H, Mizuno K. Chronic posterior sternoclavicular dislocation causing compression of a subclavian artery. J Shoulder Elb Surg. 1997;6(6):564–9.
8. Rodríguez Suárez PM, Hussein Serhal M, Freixinet Gilart JL. Tracheal compression secondary to posterior sternoclavicular dislocation. Arch Bronconeumol. 2014;50(7):306–7.
9. Laffosse JM, Espié A, Bonnevialle N, Mansat P, Tricoire JL, Bonnevialle P, Chiron P, Puget J. Posterior dislocation of the sternoclavicular joint and epiphyseal disruption of the medial clavicle with posterior displacement in sports participants. J Bone Joint Surg Br. 2010;92(1):103–9.
10. Aure A, Hetland KR, Rokkum M. Chronic posterior sternoclavicular dislocation. J Orthop Trauma. 2012;26(4):e33–5.
11. Jougon JB, Lepront DJ, Dromer CE. Posterior dislocation of the sternoclavicular joint leading to mediastinal compression. Ann Thorac Surg. 1996;61(2):711–3.
12. Gangahar DM, Flogaites T. Retrosternal dislocation of the clavicle producing thoracic outlet syndrome. J Trauma. 1978;18(5):369–72.
13. Sewell MD, Al-Hadithy N, Le Leu A, Lambert SM. Instability of the sternoclavicular joint: current concepts in classification, treatment and outcomes. Bone Joint J. 2013;95-B(6):721–31.
14. Lewis A, Kitamura T, Bayley JIL. The classification of shoulder instability: new light through old windows! Curr Orthop. 2004;18:97–108.
15. Rockwood CA Jr, Wirth MA, Gilot GJ. Injuries to the sternoclavicular joint. Rockwood and Green's fractures in adults. 6th ed. Philadelphia, PA: Lippincott Williams & Wilkins; 2006.

16. Thomas DP, Davies A, Hoddinott HC. Posterior sternoclavicular dislocations--a diagnosis easily missed. Ann R Coll Surg Engl. 1999;81(3):201–4.
17. Levinsohn EM, et al. Computed tomography in the diagnosis of dislocations of the sternoclavicular joint. Clin Orthop. 1979;140:12–6.
18. Garretson RB 3rd, Williams GR Jr. Clinical evaluation of injuries to the acromioclavicular and sternoclavicular joints. Clin Sports Med. 2003;22(2):239–54.
19. Morell DJ, Thyagarajan DS. Sternoclavicular joint dislocation and its management: a review of the literature. World J Orthop. 2016;7(4):244–50.
20. Rockwood CA. Dislocations of the sternoclavicular joint. In: Evans E, editor. American academy of orthopaedic surgeons instructional course lectures: volume XXIV. St. Louis: CV Mosby; 1975. p. 144–59.
21. Groh GI, Wirth MA, Rockwood CA Jr. Treatment of traumatic posterior sternoclavicular dislocations. J Shoulder Elb Surg. 2011;20(1):107–13.
22. Kirby JC, Edwards E, Kamali Moaveni A. Management and functional outcomes following sternoclavicular joint dislocation. Injury. 2015;46(10):1906–13.
23. Yeh GL, Williams GR Jr. Conservative management of sternoclavicular injuries. Orthop Clin North Am. 2000;31(2):189–203.
24. Panzica M, Zeichen J, Hankemeier S, Gaulke R, Krettek C, Jagodzinski M. Long-term outcome after joint reconstruction or medial resection arthroplasty for anterior SCJ instability. Arch Orthop Trauma Surg. 2010;130(5):657–65.
25. Petri M, Greenspoon JA, Horan MP, Martetschläger F, Warth RJ, Millett PJ. Clinical outcomes after autograft reconstruction for sternoclavicular joint instability. J Shoulder Elb Surg. 2016;25(3):435–41.
26. Willinger L, Schanda J, Herbst E, Imhoff AB, Martetschläger F. Outcomes and complications following graft reconstruction for anterior sternoclavicular joint instability. Knee Surg Sports Traumatol Arthrosc. 2016;24(12):3863–9.
27. Armstrong AL, Dias JJ. Reconstruction for instability of the sternoclavicular joint using the tendon of the sternocleidomastoid muscle. J Bone Joint Surg Br. 2008;90(5):610–3.
28. Sabatini JB, Shung JR, Clay TB, Oladeji LO, Minnich DJ, Ponce BA. Outcomes of augmented allograft figure-of-eight sternoclavicular joint reconstruction. J Shoulder Elb Surg. 2015;24(6):902–7.
29. Kawaguchi K, Tanaka S, Yoshitomi H, Nagai I, Sato W, Karita T, Kondo T. Double figure-of-eight reconstruction technique for chronic anterior sternoclavicular joint dislocation. Knee Surg Sports Traumatol Arthrosc. 2015;23(5):1559–62.
30. Quayle JM, Arnander MW, Pennington RG, Rosell LP. Artificial ligament reconstruction of sternoclavicular joint instability: report of a novel surgical technique with early results. Tech Hand Up Extrem Surg. 2014;18(1):31–5.
31. Quispe JC, Herbert B, Chadayammuri VP, Kim JW, Hao J, Hake M, Hak DJ, Stahel PF, Mauffrey C. Transarticular plating for acute posterior sternoclavicular joint dislocations: a valid treatment option? Int Orthop. 2016;40(7):1503–8.
32. Hwang WJ, Lee Y, Yoon YS, Kim YJ, Ryu HY. Surgical treatment of sternoclavicular joint dislocation using a T-plate. Korean J Thorac Cardiovasc Surg. 2016;49(3):221–3.
33. Uri O, Barmpagiannis K, Higgs D, Falworth M, Alexander S, Lambert SM. Clinical outcome after reconstruction for sternoclavicular joint instability using a sternocleidomastoid tendon graft. J Bone Joint Surg Am. 2014;96(5):417–22.
34. Bae DS, Kocher MS, Waters PM, Micheli LM, Griffey M, Dichtel L. Chronic recurrent anterior sternoclavicular joint instability: results of surgical management. J Pediatr Orthop. 2006;26(1):71–4.
35. Durpekt R, Vojácek J, Lischke R, Burkert J, Spatenka J. Kirschner wire migration from the right sternoclavicular joint to the heart: a case report. Heart Surg Forum. 2006;9(6):E840–2.
36. Lyons FA, Rockwood CA Jr. Migration of pins used in operations on the shoulder. J Bone Joint Surg Am. 1990;72(8):1262–7.

37. Tubbax H, Hendzel P, Sergeant P. Cardiac perforation after Kirschner wire migration. Acta Chir Belg. 1989;89(6):309–11.
38. Fowler AW. Migration of a wire from the sternoclavicular joint to the pericardial cavity. Injury. 1981;13(3):261–2.
39. Clark RL, Milgram JW, Yawn DH. Fatal aortic perforation and cardiac tamponade due to a Kirschner wire migrating from the right sternoclavicular joint. South Med J. 1974;67(3):316–8.

Chapter 41
Thoracic Outlet Syndrome

Thoracic outlet syndrome is a condition whereby there is compression of the nerves or vascular structures as they pass through the thoracic outlet.

41.1 Spectrum of Thoracic Outlet Syndrome

Thoracic outlet syndrome (TOS) may be described according to the site of main compression, the structures compressed or the cause of compression [1–21].

Obstruction may occur at one or more of the following spaces:

1. Inter-scalene
2. Costo-clavicular
3. Sub-pectoralis minor

It may be described according to the main structures compressed as:

- Neurogenic
  - True
  - Disputed
- Vascular
  - Arterial
  - Venous
- Combined neurogenic and vascular

Most cases of thoracic outlet syndrome (TOS) are due to neurogenic (95%) rather than vascular compromise. Disputed neurogenic TOS is much more common than true TOS. Clinical symptoms and signs may be similar in true and disputed neurogenic TOS, but objective investigations are positive only in the true neurogenic TOS. Venous TOS is more common (4%) than arterial TOS (1%). Overall, TOS is more common in young and middle-aged females, but venous TOS is commoner in young athletic males.

© Springer Nature Switzerland AG 2019

C. Panayiotou Charalambous, *The Shoulder Made Easy*,
https://doi.org/10.1007/978-3-319-98908-2_41

41.2 Causes of Obstruction in TOS

41.2.1 Functional

- Abnormal posture
  - Thoracic spine kyphosis
  - Drooped shoulders
- Large breasts
- Abnormal scapular motion in glenohumeral instability
- Repeated overhead activities

41.2.2 Bony

- Prominent transverse process of C7
  - Isolated
  - Giving rise to a fibrous band that attaches to the first rib
- Accessory rib articulating with the first rib
  - Complete
  - Incomplete
  - Incomplete giving rise to a fibrous band that attaches to the first rib
- Clavicular
  - Fracture non-union with mobile segments
  - Fracture mal-union
  - Excessive fracture callus
  - Clavicle fracture fixation implants
  - Abnormal clavicular mobility due to dysfunction of the sterno-clavicular or acromio-clavicular joints
- Rib
  - Fracture non-union with mobile segments
  - Fracture mal-union
  - Excessive fracture callus

Fibrous bands or accessory ribs cause compression from below, with the neurovascular bundle arching suddenly over them to reach the arm.

41.2.3 Soft Tissue

- Fibrous bands
- Scalene muscle

  - Hypertrophy
  - Spasm
  - Fibrosis

- Mass lesions
- Neoplastic
- Infective
- Vascular

41.3 Onset of TOS

- No precipitating factor
- Traumatic
  - Post-acute trauma
  - Repetitive trauma
    - Abnormal posture
    - Repeated overhead activities

It is of note that TOS may be seen in:

- Individuals with low resting tone, drooping shoulders or dragging arms, which produce traction on the brachial plexus
- Highly competitive athletes in whom hypertrophy of the scalene muscles and fibrosis due to repeated micro trauma lead to compression
- Overhead activities – painting, window cleaning, overhead sports
- Forward posture activities – computer based
- Neck muscle strenuous activities – weightlifting, swimming
- Post soft tissue or bony neck injury

41.4 True Neurogenic TOS

In true neurogenic TOS:

- Lower plexus (C8/T1) involvement is most common
- Upper plexus (C5, C6, C7) involvement is less common

41.4.1 Clinical Symptoms of True Neurogenic TOS

- Pain over the shoulder, trapezius, neck, supraclavicular fossa, upper limb and chest
  - Ache or heaviness rather than sharp radicular pain
  - Pain may involve most of the arm or be localised to the ulnar part of arm, forearm and hand

- Pain over the mandible, ear or face if the upper plexus (C5, C6, C7) is involved
- Chest pain (especially if associated vascular TOS)
- Occipital headache, migraines
- Paraesthesia in the upper limb (not single dermatome)
  - May involve most of the arm or be more localised
  - Hand paraesthesia involvement:
    - All fingers > little and ring > thumb and index and middle
- Upper limb weakness/hand clumsiness (not single myotome)
- Raynaud vascular symptoms (hand coldness, redness, pallor, cyanosis) due to involvement of sympathetic nerves that travel on the surface of C8 and T1
- Symptoms may be worse at night or during daytime overhead activities

41.4.2 Clinical Signs of True Neurogenic TOS [22]

- Upper limb altered sensation (test medial border of the forearm)
- Upper limb weakness (in a non-peripheral nerve pattern)
- Atrophy of thenar and hypo-thenar eminence of the hand
- Supraclavicular fossa
  - Tenderness
  - Tinel's test positive
- Roos test – positive with reproduction of symptoms

41.5 Disputed Neurogenic TOS

In this condition, there are symptoms of upper limb pain, altered sensation and weakness as well as positive clinical signs as in the true neurogenic TOS. However, all objective investigations (neurophysiological tests, radiological imaging) are negative and fail to confirm the presence of neurological dysfunction.

41.6 Venous TOS

Venous TOS [12, 13] may present with:

- Chronic intermittent obstruction
- Acute thrombosis which may be precipitated by an episode of excessive overhead upper limb activity (effort thrombosis)

41.6.1 Clinical Symptoms of Venous TOS

- Pain/heaviness over shoulder, upper limb, chest
- Swelling

- Oedema
- Cyanosis

41.6.2 Clinical Signs of Venous TOS

Upper limb

- Swelling
- Oedema
- Dilated superficial veins on the upper limb, neck and chest

41.7 Arterial TOS

In this condition, there is compression of the subclavian artery with stenosis or aneurysm formation [11]. This is the rarest form of TOS. It may present with:

- Chronic intermittent obstruction
- Acute embolic event causing obstruction of distal arteries (brachial, digital)
- Post-stenosis arterial aneurysm formation

41.7.1 Clinical Symptoms of Arterial TOS

- Intermittent
  - Pallor
  - Claudication
  - Pain in the hand
  - Coldness
  - Paraesthesia
- Acute presentation if embolism or complete obstruction occurs
- Arm, neck and chest pain
- Neck mass – may fluctuate in size
- No symptoms – incidental finding

41.7.2 Clinical Signs of Arterial TOS [22]

- Weak distal pulses
- Audible bruit over thoracic outlet
- Adson's test positive – pulse obliteration and reproduction of symptoms
- Wright's test positive – pulse obliteration and reproduction of symptoms
- Blood pressure difference between arms (reduction in affected arm greater than 20 mmHg)

- Neck mass – pulsatile, compressible
- In acute ischemia – cold, pale arm

41.8 Investigations for TOS [1–3, 15]

- Plain radiographs of cervical spine to look for:
  - Elongated C7 transverse process
  - Accessory cervical rib
  - Cervical spondylosis
- MRI thoracic outlet to look for:
  - Abnormal masses causing compression
  - Vascular obstruction
- MRI cervical spine to assess:
  - Cervical nerve root entrapment
  - Spinal cord lesions
- Duplex ultrasound – to evaluate vascular obstruction
- Angiography/venography – to evaluate vascular obstruction
- Nerve conduction and EMG studies – to determine pattern of neurological compromise
- Diagnostic local anaesthetic injections into scalene muscles or pectoralis minor – temporary improvement of symptoms is suggestive of entrapment at those sides

41.9 Management of TOS

Non-surgical management to address the obstruction is preferred in chronic cases especially those of disputed neurogenic TOS. It is believed that the natural history of disputed neurogenic TOS is one of improvement, and surgery has not shown to confer any substantial advantage over non-surgical management in this group of patients.

Surgical decompression of the thoracic outlet is considered in those with true neurogenic or vascular TOS that fail non-surgical treatment.

In addition, early surgery is needed in cases of acute vascular compromise to re-establish the circulation followed by decompression of the thoracic outlet.

- Non-surgical [2, 10, 11, 16]
  - Leave alone
  - Pain control
  - Activity modification
  - Physiotherapy
    - Posture improvement
    - Scalene muscle and pectoralis minor muscle stretching

- Training to use diaphragmatic breathing to reduce scalene muscle activity
- First rib mobilisation
- Scapular muscle strengthening and coordination to address muscle dyskinesia
- Rotator cuff muscle strengthening
- Glenohumeral joint mobilisation to reduce stiffness
- Neural mobilisation

- Surgical or invasive [10–13, 16–21]
  This aims to reduce compression of the neurovascular structures and can be achieved directly by excising or removing the structure causing the compression or indirectly by excising the first rib. In cases where there is acute vascular compromise to the limb, intervention also aims to establish the circulation and reconstruct the vascular tree to ensure smooth blood flow. Interventions include:

  - First rib excision
  - Excision of accessory rib/fibrous bands
  - Release of constriction bands
  - Release of scalene muscles
  - Excision of clavicle non-union, excessive callus or compressive mass
  - Release of pectoralis minor
  - Removal of compressive fixation implants
  - Neurolysis to free the brachial plexus nerves

If vascular compromise [11–13]:

- Anticoagulation/thrombolysis for acute vascular obstruction due to thrombosis
- Venoplasty/embolectomy
- Arterial/venous reconstruction/bypass
- Thoracic outlet decompression

41.10 Distinguishing Between a Proximal Nerve Lesion vs. Ulnar Nerve Lesion

It is often necessary to distinguish neurogenic TOS from a peripheral ulnar nerve lesion or a cervical nerve root lesion. The following may assist in that:

The ulnar nerve provides sensation to the medial half of the ring finger and the whole of the little finger, as well as ulnar border of the hand, dorsal and palmar.

The ulnar nerve innervates all intrinsic hand muscles (flexor digiti minimi brevis, abductor digiti minimi, adductor pollicis, opponens digiti minimi, medial lumbricals, dorsal and palmar interossei) apart from the *LOAF* muscles:

- *L*ateral two lumbricals
- *O*pponens pollicis
- *A*bductor pollicis brevis
- *F*lexor pollicis brevis

which are supplied by C8 and T1 via the median nerve.

The medial antebrachial nerve (C8/T1) arises from the brachial plexus in the neck and supplies sensation to medial border of the forearm.

Clinical findings to help distinguish between an ulnar nerve lesion and a more proximal nerve root lesion

Ulnar nerve	Proximal C8/T1 lesion
• Weakness of intrinsic hand muscles except LOAF • Reduced sensation medial half of ring finger and whole of little finger • Intact sensation medial border of forearm	• Weakness of all intrinsic hand muscles including LOAF • Reduced sensation medial border of forearm

Hence, consider C8/T1 lesion rather than ulnar nerve lesion if:

- Flexor pollicis brevis is weak
- There is loss of sensation in the medial border of the forearm

41.11 Distinguishing Between a Cervical Nerve Root Lesion vs. Thoracic Outlet Lesion [14]

Certain clinical and radiological parameters may help distinguish between a cervical nerve root lesion and a thoracic lesion as described below:

Clinical findings to help distinguish between a cervical root lesion and a thoracic outlet lesion

Cervical root lesion

- Cervical spine pain
- Radicular pain – passing from neck to the distribution of the involved nerve root
- Spurling test positive
- Cervical spine extension increases pain
- Placing hand on top of head improves pain
- Muscle weakness is myotomal – but incomplete due to overlap of nerve roots
- Denervation of ipsilateral paraspinal muscles – supplied by the dorsal ramus of the spinal nerve that arises from the cervical nerve roots prior to the formation of the brachial plexus
- Reduced sensation in the midline skin of the back innervated by the dorsal ramus of the cervical nerve roots
- Cervical nerve root compression on cervical spine MRI

Thoracic outlet lesion

- Minimal or no cervical spine pain
- Absence of radicular pain
- Spurling test negative
- Tenderness suraclavicular fossa
- Tinel's test positive supraclavicular fossa
- Altered sensation medial forearm
- Radiological findings of possible thoracic outlet compression sites
- Intact pasaspinal muscles
- Intact sensation midline back

Learning Pearls

- The diagnosis of TOS is highly clinical
- Negative investigations do not exclude the presence of TOS
- Vascular symptoms do not necessarily signify vascular TOS – they may be encountered in neurogenic TOS due to sympathetic nerve involvement
- Non-surgical treatment is effective in most cases of TOS with surgery utilised in a minority

References

1. Sanders RJ, Hammond SL, Rao NM. Diagnosis of thoracic outlet syndrome. J Vasc Surg. 2007;46(3):601–4.
2. Micev AJ, Abzug JM, Osterman AL. Thoracic outlet syndrome: getting it right so you Don't have to do it again. Instr Course Lect. 2017;66:103–13.
3. Hooper TL, Denton J, McGalliard MK, Brismée JM, Sizer PS Jr. Thoracic outlet syndrome: a controversial clinical condition. Part 1: anatomy, and clinical examination/diagnosis. J Man Manip Ther. 2010;18(2):74–83.
4. Roos DB. Congenital anomalies associated with thoracic outlet syndrome. Anatomy, symptoms, diagnosis, and treatment. Am J Surg. 1976;132(6):771–8.
5. Leffert RD, Gumley G. The relationship between dead arm syndrome and thoracic outlet syndrome. Clin Orthop Relat Res. 1987;223:20–31.
6. Wright IS. The neurovascular syndrome produced by hyperabduction of the arms. Am Heart J. 1945;29(1):1–19.
7. Clein LJ. The droopy shoulder syndrome. Can Med Assoc J. 1976;114(4):343–4.
8. Bottros MM, AuBuchon JD, McLaughlin LN, Altchek DW, Illig KA, Thompson RW. Exercise-enhanced, ultrasound-guided anterior scalene muscle/Pectoralis minor muscle blocks can facilitate the diagnosis of neurogenic thoracic outlet syndrome in the high-performance overhead athlete. Am J Sports Med. 2017;45(1):189–94.
9. Balderman J, Holzem K, Field BJ, Bottros MM, Abuirqeba AA, Vemuri C, Thompson RW. Associations between clinical diagnostic criteria and pretreatment patient-reported outcomes measures in a prospective observational cohort of patients with neurogenic thoracic outlet syndrome. J Vasc Surg. 2017;66(2):533–44.
10. Hooper TL, Denton J, McGalliard MK, Brismée JM, Sizer PS Jr. Thoracic outlet syndrome: a controversial clinical condition. Part 2: non-surgical and surgical management. J Man Manip Ther. 2010;18(3):132–8.
11. Vemuri C, McLaughlin LN, Abuirqeba AA, Thompson RW. Clinical presentation and management of arterial thoracic outlet syndrome. J Vasc Surg. 2017;65(5):1429–39.
12. Vemuri C, Salehi P, Benarroch-Gampel J, McLaughlin LN, Thompson RW. Diagnosis and treatment of effort-induced thrombosis of the axillary subclavian vein due to venous thoracic outlet syndrome. J Vasc Surg Venous Lymphat Disord. 2016;4(4):485–500.
13. Illig KA, Doyle AJ. A comprehensive review of Paget-Schroetter syndrome. J Vasc Surg. 2010;51(6):1538–47.
14. McGillicuddy JE. Cervical radiculopathy, entrapment neuropathy, and thoracic outlet syndrome: how to differentiate? J Neurosurg Spine. 2004;1(2):179–87.
15. Rempel D, Dahlin L, Lundborg G. Pathophysiology of nerve compression syndromes: response of peripheral nerves to loading. J Bone Joint Surg Am. 1999;81(11):1600–10.
16. Landry GJ, Moneta GL, Taylor LM Jr, Edwards JM, Porter JM. Long-term functional outcome of neurogenic thoracic outlet syndrome in surgically and conservatively treated patients. J Vasc Surg. 2001;33(2):312–7.
17. Vemuri C, Wittenberg AM, Caputo FJ, Earley JA, Driskill MR, Rastogi R, Emery VB, Thompson RW. Early effectiveness of isolated pectoralis minor tenotomy in selected patients with neurogenic thoracic outlet syndrome. J Vasc Surg. 2013;57(5):1345–52.
18. Roos DB. Experience with first rib resection for thoracic outlet syndrome. Ann Surg. 1971;173(3):429–42.
19. Roos DB. Thoracic outlet syndrome. Rocky Mt Med J. 1967;64(2):49–55.
20. Roos DB. Transaxillary approach for first rib resection to relieve thoracic outlet syndrome. Ann Surg. 1966;163(3):354–8.
21. Adson AW. Surgical treatment for symptoms produced by cervical ribs and the scalenus anticus muscle. Surg Gynecol Obstet. 1947;85(6):687–700.
22. Charalambous CP. Clinical examination of the shoulder. In: Charalambous CP, editor. The shoulder made easy. Springer; 2019. pp. 77–122.

Chapter 42
Neuralgic Amyotrophy: Parsonage Turner Syndrome

This is a condition of the peripheral nervous system whereby there is dysfunction of one or more of the branches of the brachial plexus. It is characterised by episodes of extreme neuropathic pain, rapid onset weakness and atrophy of the involved muscles in the upper limbs. Both idiopathic and hereditary forms are described [1–3].

42.1 Causes of Neuralgic Amyotrophy [4–10]

Several causes have been proposed including:

- Immune-mediated response to the brachial plexus
  - Often occurring after a viral infection or immunisation (influenza)
- Genetic predisposition with susceptibility to mechanical injury of the brachial plexus
  - Hereditary – neuralgic amyotrophy can be an autosomal dominant disorder presenting as recurrent, episodic, painful brachial neuropathies
- Postsurgery
  - Coronary artery bypass
  - Oral surgery

42.2 Demographics of Neuralgic Amyotrophy [1–3]

- 30 to 70 years old
- Thirty-three percent bilateral involvement

© Springer Nature Switzerland AG 2019

C. Panayiotou Charalambous, *The Shoulder Made Easy*,
https://doi.org/10.1007/978-3-319-98908-2_42

42.3 Nerves Involved in Neuralgic Amyotrophy

Although any nerve can be affected some of the most commonly involved are:

- Suprascapular
- Long thoracic
- Axillary
- Anterior interosseous

42.4 Clinical Symptoms of Neuralgic Amyotrophy

Symptoms may be described in three phases as below.

- Painful phase
  - May last from few hours to several weeks
  - Constant pain
  - Severe – patient may present to accident and emergency department with severe pain
  - May involve any part of the arm
  - Not influenced by arm position
  - Worse at night
  - Reluctant to use the arm
- Weakness phase
  - Mild to almost complete paralysis and muscle wasting
  - Associated sensory abnormalities
- Recovering phase
  - Improving muscle strength and function

Hence, clinical symptoms and signs may vary depending on the phase at which the patient presents [1–3]:

Phases of neuralgic amyotrophy

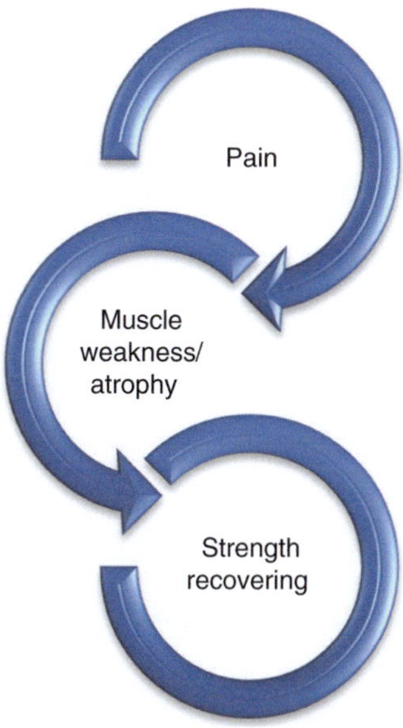

42.5 Clinical Signs of Neuralgic Amyotrophy

These will depend on the muscles affected

- Muscle weakness
- Muscle atrophy
- Impaired muscle function
  - Long thoracic nerve – scapular dyskinesia
  - Phrenic nerve – sudden-onset dyspnoea
  - Recurrent nerve – dysphonia

42.6 Investigations for Neuralgic Amyotrophy

- Nerve conduction studies and electromyography [11–13]
  - Impairment of axonal function – spontaneous fibrillations, positive sharp waves
  - Conduction velocities are usually normal
- Ultrasound – nerve appearance [14–16]
  - Focal or diffuse nerve enlargement
  - Incomplete nerve constriction
  - Complete nerve constriction and torsion (hourglass appearance)
  - Fascicle entwinement
- MRI – nerve thickening, muscle oedema and atrophy [17, 18]

42.7 Differential Diagnosis of Neuralgic Amyotrophy

Any condition that causes neuralgic pain, muscle weakness and atrophy. Such conditions include:

- Cervical radiculopathy
- Other causes of brachial plexus dysfunction (e.g. thoracic outlet syndrome)
- Mono-neuritis multiplex

In cases where weakness is severe there is a need to exclude:

- Cerebrovascular event
- Massive rotator cuff rupture

Hence, clinical history taking, clinical examination and investigations also aim to exclude these alternative possible diagnoses.

42.8 Management of Neuralgic Amyotrophy

- Non-surgical [19–21]
  - Expectant
    - Leave alone
    - Analgesia – control pain
    - Maintain motion, avoid contractures
    - Strengthen muscles

- Oral prednisolone given in the first month after onset of symptoms may shorten the duration of the initial painful phase and lead to earlier recovery, but evidence for its effectiveness is very limited

- Surgery (very rarely indicated) [22, 23]
  - Nerve decompression and neurolysis
  - Muscle transfer for weakness

42.9 Prognosis of Neuralgic Amyotrophy [24, 25]

- About 90% of patients show full recovery (pain, strength, function) by 3 years, but in some, this may take much longer, or they may not fully recover
- Recurrent episodes may occur

References

1. Seror P. Neuralgic amyotrophy. An update. Joint Bone Spine. 2017;84(2):153–8.
2. Van Eijk JJ, Groothuis JT, Van Alfen N. Neuralgic amyotrophy: an update on diagnosis, pathophysiology, and treatment. Muscle Nerve. 2016;53(3):337–50.
3. Gupta A, Winalski CS, Sundaram M. Neuralgic amyotrophy (Parsonage Turner syndrome). Orthopedics. 2014;37(2):75. 130–133
4. Sánchez Azofra M, Romero Portales M, Tortajada Laureiro L, García-Samaniego J, Mora Sanz P. Hepatitis E virus in neurological disorders: a case of Parsonage-Turner syndrome. Rev Esp Enferm Dig. 2018;110(6):402–3.
5. Shaikh MF, Baqai TJ, Tahir H. Acute brachial neuritis following influenza vaccination. BMJ Case Rep. 2012;28:bcr2012007673. https://doi.org/10.1136/bcr-2012-007673.
6. Reutens DC, Dunne JW, Leather H. Neuralgic amyotrophy following recombinant DNA hepatitis B vaccination. Muscle Nerve. 1990;13(5):461.
7. van Alfen N, Hannibal MC, Chance PF, van Engelen BGM. Hereditary neuralgic amyotrophy. In: Adam MP, Ardinger HH, Pagon RA, Wallace SE, Bean LJH, Stephens K, Amemiya A, editors. GeneReviews® [Internet]. Seattle: University of Washington; 2008.
8. Geiger LR, Mancall EL, Penn AS, Tucker SH. Familial neuralgic amyotrophy. Report of three families with review of the literature. Brain. 1974;97(1):87–102.
9. Klein CJ, Barbara DW, Sprung J, Dyck PJ, Weingarten TN. Surgical and postpartum hereditary brachial plexus attacks and prophylactic immunotherapy. Muscle Nerve. 2013;47(1):23–7.
10. Verhasselt S, Schelfaut S, Bataillie F, Moke L. Postsurgical Parsonage-Turner syndrome: a challenging diagnosis. Acta Orthop Belg. 2013;79(1):20–4.
11. Merino-Ramírez MÁ, Bolton CF. Electrodiagnostic studies for neuralgic amyotrophy. Muscle Nerve. 2016;54(2):341–2.
12. van Alfen N, Huisman WJ, Overeem S, van Engelen BG, Zwarts MJ. Sensory nerve conduction studies in neuralgic amyotrophy. Am J Phys Med Rehabil. 2009;88(11):941–6.
13. Feinberg JH, Nguyen ET, Boachie-Adjei K, Gribbin C, Lee SK, Daluiski A, Wolfe SW. The electrodiagnostic natural history of Parsonage-Turner syndrome. Muscle Nerve. 2017;56(4):737–43.

14. van Rosmalen M, Lieba-Samal D, Pillen S, van Alfen N. Ultrasound of peripheral nerves in neuralgic amyotrophy. Muscle Nerve. 2019;59(1):55–9.
15. Arányi Z, Csillik A, Dévay K, Rosero M, Barsi P, Böhm J, Schelle T. Ultrasonographic identification of nerve pathology in neuralgic amyotrophy: enlargement, constriction, fascicular entwinement, and torsion. Muscle Nerve. 2015;52(4):503–11.
16. ArÁnyi Z, Csillik A, DéVay K, Rosero M, Barsi P, BÖhm J, Schelle T. Ultrasonography in neuralgic amyotrophy: sensitivity, spectrum of findings, and clinical correlations. Muscle Nerve. 2017;56(6):1054–62.
17. Sneag DB, Rancy SK, Wolfe SW, Lee SC, Kalia V, Lee SK, Feinberg JH. Brachial plexitis or neuritis? MRI features of lesion distribution in Parsonage-Turner syndrome. Muscle Nerve. 2018;58(3):359–66.
18. Lieba-Samal D, Jengojan S, Kasprian G, Wöber C, Bodner G. Neuroimaging of classic neuralgic amyotrophy. Muscle Nerve. 2016;54(6):1079–85.
19. Tsairis P, Dyck PJ, Mulder DW. Natural history of brachial plexus neuropathy. Report on 99 patients. Arch Neurol. 1972;27(2):109–17.
20. van Eijk JJ, van Alfen N, Berrevoets M, van der Wilt GJ, Pillen S, van Engelen BG. Evaluation of prednisolone treatment in the acute phase of neuralgic amyotrophy: an observational study. J Neurol Neurosurg Psychiatry. 2009;80(10):1120–4.
21. Johnson NE, Petraglia AL, Huang JH, Logigian EL. Rapid resolution of severe neuralgic amyotrophy after treatment with corticosteroids and intravenous immunoglobulin. Muscle Nerve. 2011;44(2):304–5.
22. Akane M, Iwatsuki K, Tatebe M, Nishizuka T, Kurimoto S, Yamamoto M, Hirata H. Anterior interosseous nerve and posterior interosseous nerve involvement in neuralgic amyotrophy. Clin Neurol Neurosurg. 2016;151:108–12.
23. Steinmann SP, Wood MB. Pectoralis major transfer for serratus anterior paralysis. J Shoulder Elbow Surg. 2003;12(6):555–60.
24. Cup EH, Ijspeert J, Janssen RJ, Bussemaker-Beumer C, Jacobs J, Pieterse AJ, van der Linde H, van Alfen N. Residual complaints after neuralgic amyotrophy. Arch Phys Med Rehabil. 2013;94(1):67–73.
25. van Alfen N, van der Werf SP, van Engelen BG. Long-term pain, fatigue, and impairment in neuralgic amyotrophy. Arch Phys Med Rehabil. 2009;90(3):435–9.

Chapter 43
Axillary Nerve Dysfunction

This is a condition whereby there is impairment in the function of the axillary nerve, involving its motor component, sensory component or both. This may be complete involving the whole of the axillary nerve or partial involving one or more of its branches. Recognition of the anatomy of the axillary nerve is essential in explaining the clinical findings in axillary nerve dysfunction, as well as in minimising the risk of damage to the nerve during surgical interventions of the shoulder.

43.1 Causes of Axillary Nerve Dysfunction

Lesions of the axillary nerve may be defined as intrinsic or extrinsic [1–20]:

- Intrinsic
  1. Brachial neuritis
  2. Systemic disorders (e.g. diabetes)
  3. Neoplastic
- Extrinsic
  1. Compression
  2. Traction
  3. Laceration

  Causes of extrinsic lesions include:

43.1.1 Compression

- Quadrilateral space syndrome
- Displaced scapular fractures

© Springer Nature Switzerland AG 2019

C. Panayiotou Charalambous, *The Shoulder Made Easy*,
https://doi.org/10.1007/978-3-319-98908-2_43

43.1.2 *Traction*

- By dislocated glenohumeral joint

43.1.3 *Laceration*

- Penetrating trauma – stab wounds
- Surgery – open or arthroscopic
- Shoulder arthroscopy (adhesive capsulitis release, thermal shrinkage for instability)
- Plate fixation of proximal humeral fractures
- Deltoid intramuscular injections
- Glenohumeral and subacromial bursa steroid injections

43.2 Clinical Symptoms of Axillary Nerve Dysfunction

- Neurogenic pain in the shoulder area
- Arm weakness
- Altered shoulder contour due to deltoid weakness and muscle wasting

43.3 Clinical Signs of Axillary Nerve Dysfunction

- Weakness of deltoid and teres minor
- Muscle wasting, loss of shoulder contour
- Sensory disturbance around the shoulder – regimental patch sensory loss

43.4 Investigations for Axillary Nerve Dysfunction

- Plain radiographs
- MRI
  - Evaluate other causes of weakness such as rotator cuff tears or atrophy
  - Evaluate deltoid atrophy and fat infiltration
  - Look for compressive cause for the nerve due to a space occupying lesions
- Electromyography looking for muscle denervation
- Nerve conduction studies

43.5 Management of Axillary Nerve Dysfunction [21–23]

- Expectant, await recovery
- Control pain and maintain passive motion
- Surgical exploration if recovery does not occur within about 3 months:
  - Nerve decompression
  - Nerve repair, cable grafting, nerve transfer

References

1. Gurushantappa PK, Kuppasad S. Anatomy of axillary nerve and its clinical importance: a cadaveric study. J Clin Diagn Res. 2015;9(3):AC13–7.
2. Leechavengvongs S, Teerawutthichaikit T, Witoonchart K, Uerpairojkit C, Malungpaishrope K, Suppauksorn S, Chareonwat B. Surgical anatomy of the axillary nerve branches to the deltoid muscle. Clin Anat. 2015;28(1):118–22.
3. Tubbs RS, Tyler-Kabara EC, Aikens AC, Martin JP, Weed LL, Salter EG, Oakes WJ. Surgical anatomy of the axillary nerve within the quadrangular space. J Neurosurg. 2005;102(5):912–4.
4. Ball CM, Steger T, Galatz LM, Yamaguchi K. The posterior branch of the axillary nerve: an anatomic study. J Bone Joint Surg Am. 2003;85-A(8):1497–501.
5. Price MR, Tillett ED, Acland RD, Nettleton GS. Determining the relationship of the axillary nerve to the shoulder joint capsule from an arthroscopic perspective. J Bone Joint Surg Am. 2004;86-A(10):2135–42.
6. Beals TC, Harryman DT 2nd, Lazarus MD. Useful boundaries of the subacromial bursa. Arthroscopy. 1998;14(5):465–70.
7. Atef A, El-Tantawy A, Gad H, Hefeda M. Prevalence of associated injuries after anterior shoulder dislocation: a prospective study. Int Orthop. 2016;40(3):519–24.
8. Robinson CM, Shur N, Sharpe T, Ray A, Murray IR. Injuries associated with traumatic anterior glenohumeral dislocations. J Bone Joint Surg Am. 2012;94(1):18–26.
9. Blom S, Dahlbäck LO. Nerve injuries in dislocations of the shoulder joint and fractures of the neck of the humerus. A clinical and electromyographical study. Acta Chir Scand. 1970;136:461–6.
10. Berry H, Bril V. Axillary nerve palsy following blunt trauma to the shoulder region: a clinical and electrophysiological review. J Neurol Neurosurg Psychiatry. 1982;45:1027–32.
11. Westphal T, Woischnik S, Adolf D, Feistner H, Piatek S. Axillary nerve lesions after open reduction and internal fixation of proximal humeral fractures through an extended lateral deltoid-split approach: electrophysiological findings. J Shoulder Elb Surg. 2017;26(3):464–71.
12. Lenoir H, Dagneaux L, Canovas F, Waitzenegger T, Pham TT, Chammas M. Nerve stress during reverse total shoulder arthroplasty: a cadaveric study. J Shoulder Elb Surg. 2017;26(2):323–30.
13. Cetik O, Uslu M, Acar HI, Comert A, Tekdemir I, Cift H. Is there a safe area for the axillary nerve in the deltoid muscle? A cadaveric study. J Bone Joint Surg Am. 2006;88(11):2395–9.
14. Yung SW, Lazarus MD, Harryman DT 2nd. Practical guidelines to safe surgery about the subscapularis. J Shoulder Elb Surg. 1996;5(6):467–70.
15. Zanotti RM, Kuhn JE. Arthroscopic capsular release for the stiff shoulder. Description of technique and anatomic considerations. Am J Sports Med. 1997;25(3):294–8.
16. Eakin CL, Dvirnak P, Miller CM, Hawkins RJ. The relationship of the axillary nerve to arthroscopically placed capsulolabral sutures. An anatomic study. Am J Sports Med. 1998;26(4):505–9.

17. Gryler EC, Greis PE, Burks RT, West J. Axillary nerve temperatures during radiofrequency capsulorrhaphy of the shoulder. Arthroscopy. 2001;17(6):567–72.
18. Brown SA, Doolittle DA, Bohanon CJ, Jayaraj A, Naidu SG, Huettl EA, Renfree KJ, Oderich GS, Bjarnason H, Gloviczki P, Wysokinski WE, McPhail IR. Quadrilateral space syndrome: the Mayo Clinic experience with a new classification system and case series. Mayo Clin Proc. 2015;90(3):382–94.
19. Sanders TG, Tirman PF. Paralabral cyst: an unusual cause of quadrilateral space syndrome. Arthroscopy. 1999;15:632–7.
20. Turker H, Sarica M, Bilgici A, Cengiz N, Onar MK, Us O. Axillary neuropathy mimicking quadrilateral space syndrome and its follow up for one year. Neurosciences (Riyadh). 2008;13(1):79–83.
21. Visser CP, Coene LN, Brand R, Tavy DL. The incidence of nerve injury in anterior dislocation of the shoulder and its influence on functional recovery. A prospective clinical and EMG study. J Bone Joint Surg (Br). 1999;81:679–85.
22. Kostas-Agnantis I, Korompilias A, Vekris M, Lykissas M, Gkiatas I, Mitsionis G, Beris A. Shoulder abduction and external rotation restoration with nerve transfer. Injury. 2013;44(3):299–304. https://doi.org/10.1016/j.injury.2013.01.005.
23. Koshy JC, Agrawal NA, Seruya M. Nerve transfer versus interpositional nerve graft reconstruction for posttraumatic, isolated axillary nerve injuries: a systematic review. Plast Reconstr Surg. 2017;140(5):953–60.

Chapter 44
Suprascapular Nerve Dysfunction

The suprascapular nerve arises from the upper trunk of the brachial plexus and passes across the posterior triangle of the neck deep to the trapezius muscle to the superior border of the scapula. It then passes through the suprascapular notch of the scapula under the superior transverse scapular ligament to enter the supraspinous fossa. It passes underneath supraspinatus curving around the lateral border of the spine of the scapula under the spino-glenoid ligament to enter the infraspinous fossa [1–3].

It supplies the supraspinatus and infraspinatus muscles and gives sensory innervation to the acromio-clavicular and glenohumeral joints. Suprascapular nerve dysfunction can thus give rise to combined supra- and/or infraspinatus weakness depending on the cause of the palsy and the origin of the lesion.

The suprascapular nerve may have a cutaneous sensory branch, and hence patients with suprascapular nerve dysfunction may complain of sensory disturbance around the shoulder [1–3].

44.1 Causes of Suprascapular Nerve Dysfunction

Lesions of the suprascapular nerve may be defined as intrinsic or extrinsic [3–33]:

- Intrinsic
  1. Brachial neuritis
  2. Systemic disorder (diabetes)
  3. Neoplastic
- Extrinsic
  1. Compression
  2. Traction
  3. Laceration
  4. Radiation

© Springer Nature Switzerland AG 2019

C. Panayiotou Charalambous, *The Shoulder Made Easy*,
https://doi.org/10.1007/978-3-319-98908-2_44

Causes of extrinsic lesions include:

44.1.1 Compression

- Due to a hypertrophied or ossified ligament (transverse scapular ligament or spino-glenoid) ligament
- Narrow suprascapular notch
- Para-labrum cysts
- Displaced scapular fractures

44.1.2 Traction

- By a retracted superior-posterior rotator cuff tear (the most common)
- Excessive lateral advancement of a retracted rotator cuff tear, during repair (more than 3 cm)
- Repetitive overhead activity such as overhead throwing
- Shoulder dislocations

44.1.3 Laceration

- Penetrating trauma – stab wounds
- Surgery – open or arthroscopic

44.2 Clinical Symptoms of Suprascapular Nerve Dysfunction [34–40]

- Pain in the posterior-superior part of the shoulder
- Weakness of supraspinatus and infraspinatus
- Altered shoulder contour due to muscle wasting with scapular bony prominence

44.3 Clinical Signs of Suprascapular Nerve Dysfunction [36–40]

- Weakness of supraspinatus and/or infraspinatus
- Muscle wasting
- Sensory disturbance around the shoulder

44.4 Investigations for Suprascapular Nerve Dysfunction

- Plain radiographs
- MRI to:
  - Evaluate the continuity of the muscle tendon complex
  - Evaluate the rotator cuff muscles looking for atrophy and fat infiltration
  - Look for compressive cause for the nerve due to space occupying lesions
- Electromyography looking for muscle denervation
- Nerve conduction studies

44.5 Management of Suprascapular Nerve Dysfunction [41–49]

- Non-surgical
  - Leave alone
  - Activity modification
  - Non-steroidal anti-inflammatories
- Surgical
  - Nerve decompression – open or arthroscopic
  - Release of the transverse scapular ligament – arthroscopic or open
  - Release of the spino-glenoid ligament
  - Decompression/excision of para-labrum cysts
  - Repair of labrum or rotator cuff tears

44.6 Prognosis of Suprascapular Nerve Dysfunction

Pain and muscle strength tend to improve but muscle atrophy may not.

Learning Pearls
Suprascapular nerve palsy should be considered in a younger patient where a rotator tendon tear is not expected:

- The back packer's shoulder is a variant of suprascapular nerve entrapment thought to be caused by pressure from the shoulder straps of a backpack on the suprascapular nerve [50]
- Repetitive overhead activities – volleyball players, throwing athletes, baseball pitchers and weight lifters [51–55]

References

1. Warner JP, Krushell RJ, Masquelet A, Gerber C. Anatomy and relationships of the suprascapular nerve: anatomical constraints to mobilization of the supraspinatus and infraspinatus muscles in the management of massive rotator-cuff tears. J Bone Joint Surg Am. 1992;74(1):36–45.
2. Bigliani LU, Dalsey RM, McCann PD, April EW. An anatomical study of the suprascapular nerve. Arthroscopy. 1990;6(4):301–5.
3. Demirhan M, Imhoff AB, Debski RE, Patel PR, Fu FH, Woo SL. The spinoglenoid ligament and its relationship to the suprascapular nerve. J Shoulder Elb Surg. 1998;7(3):238–43.
4. Bruce J, Dorizas J. Suprascapular nerve entrapment due to a stenotic foramen: a variant of the suprascapular notch. Sports Health. 2013;5(4):363–6.
5. Polguj M, Sibiński M, Grzegorzewski A, Grzelak P, Majos A, Topol M. Variation in morphology of suprascapular notch as a factor of suprascapular nerve entrapment. Int Orthop. 2013;37(11):2185–92.
6. Boykin RE, Friedman DJ, Zimmer ZR, Oaklander AL, Higgins LD, Warner JJ. Suprascapular neuropathy in a shoulder referral practice. J Shoulder Elb Surg. 2011;20(6):983–8.
7. Houtz C, McCulloch PC. Suprascapular vascular anomalies as a cause of suprascapular nerve compression. Orthopedics. 2013;36(1):42–5.
8. Koh KH, Park WH, Lim TK, Yoo JC. Medial perforation of the glenoid neck following SLAP repair places the suprascapular nerve at risk: a cadaveric study. J Shoulder Elb Surg. 2011;20(2):245–50.
9. Kim SH, Koh YG, Sung CH, Moon HK, Park YS. Iatrogenic suprascapular nerve injury after repair of type II SLAP lesion. Arthroscopy. 2010;26(7):1005–8.
10. Bouliane M, Beaupre L, Ashworth N, Lambert R, Silveira A, Sheps DM. Suprascapular nerve injury during arthroscopic superior labral repair: a prospective evaluation. Knee Surg Sports Traumatol Arthrosc. 2015;23(2):517–22.
11. Maquieira GJ, Gerber C, Schneeberger AG. Suprascapular nerve palsy after the Latarjet procedure. J Shoulder Elb Surg. 2007;16(2):e13–5.
12. Sastre S, Peidro L, Méndez A, Calvo E. Suprascapular nerve palsy after arthroscopic Latarjet procedure: a case report and review of literature. Knee Surg Sports Traumatol Arthrosc. 2016;24(2):601–3.
13. Leschinger T, Hackl M, Buess E, Lappen S, Scaal M, Müller LP, Wegmann K. The risk of suprascapular and axillary nerve injury in reverse total shoulder arthroplasty: an anatomic study. Injury. 2017;48(10):2042–9.
14. Lopiz Y, Rodriguez-González A, Martín-Albarrán S, Marcelo H, García-Fernández C, Marco F. Injury to the axillary and suprascapular nerves in rotator cuff arthropathy and after reverse shoulder arthroplasty: a prospective electromyographic analysis. J Shoulder Elb Surg. 2018;27(7):1275–82.
15. Draeger RW, Messer TM. Suprascapular nerve palsy following supraclavicular block for upper extremity surgery: report of 3 cases. J Hand Surg Am. 2012;37(12):2576–9.
16. Ishimaru D, Nagano A, Terabayashi N, Nishimoto Y, Akiyama H. Suprascapular nerve entrapment caused by protrusion of an intraosseous ganglion of the glenoid into the spinoglenoid notch: a rare cause of posterior shoulder pain. Case Rep Orthop. 2017;2017:1704697. https://doi.org/10.1155/2017/1704697.
17. Lee BC, Yegappan M, Thiagarajan P. Suprascapular nerve neuropathy secondary to spinoglenoid notch ganglion cyst: case reports and review of literature. Ann Acad Med Singap. 2007;36(12):1032–5.
18. Semmler A, von Falkenhausen M, Schröder R. Suprascapular nerve entrapment by a spinoglenoid cyst. Neurology. 2008;70(11):890. https://doi.org/10.1212/01.wnl.0000304748.02041.cd.
19. Yi JW, Cho NS, Rhee YG. Intraosseous ganglion of the glenoid causing suprascapular nerve entrapment syndrome: a case report. J Shoulder Elb Surg. 2009;18(3):e25–7.

20. Kang SH, Park IJ, Jeong C. Suprascapular neuropathy caused by heterotopic ossification after clavicle shaft fracture: a case report. Eur J Orthop Surg Traumatol. 2012;22(Suppl 1):63–6.
21. Edeland HG, Zachrisson BE. Fracture of the scapular notch associated with lesion of the suprascapular nerve. Acta Orthop Scand. 1975;46(5):758–63.
22. Boerger TO, Limb D. Suprascapular nerve injury at the spinoglenoid notch after glenoid neck fracture. J Shoulder Elb Surg. 2000;9(3):236–7.
23. Hazrati Y, Miller S, Moore S, Hausman M, Flatow E. Suprascapular nerve entrapment secondary to a lipoma. Clin Orthop Relat Res. 2003;411:124–8.
24. Savoie FH 3rd, Zunkiewicz M, Field LD, Replogle WH, O'Brien MJ. A comparison of functional outcomes in patients undergoing revision arthroscopic repair of massive rotator cuff tears with and without arthroscopic suprascapular nerve release. Open Access J Sports Med. 2016;7:129–34.
25. Spinner RJ, Amrami KK. Intraneural ganglion of the suprascapular nerve: case report. J Hand Surg Am. 2006;31(10):1698–9.
26. Sanger J, Cortes W, Yan JG. Intraneural ganglion of the suprascapular nerve: case report. J Hand Surg Am. 2006;31(1):40–4.
27. Rozental TD, Donthineni-Rao R, Beredjiklian PK. Schwannoma of the suprascapular nerve: a case report. J Shoulder Elb Surg. 2006;15(1):127–9.
28. Economides CP, Christodoulou L, Kyriakides T, Soteriades ES. An unusual case of suprascapular nerve neuropathy: a case report. J Med Case Rep. 2011;5:419.
29. Kowalczuk M, Lin A. Isolated suprascapular mononeuropathy following nondisplaced scapular fracture. J Shoulder Elb Surg. 2018;27(2):e50–3.
30. Vigasio A, Marcoccio I. Hourglass-like constriction of the suprascapular nerve: a contraindication for minimally invasive surgery. J Shoulder Elb Surg. 2018;27(2):e29–37.
31. Van Meir N, Fourneau I, Debeer P. Varicose veins at the spinoglenoidal notch: an unusual cause of suprascapular nerve compression. J Shoulder Elb Surg. 2011;20(7):e21–4.
32. Podgórski M, Sibiński M, Majos A, Stefańczyk L, Topol M, Polguj M. The suprascapular vein: a possible etiology for suprascapular nerve entrapment and risk of complication during procedures around the suprascapular foramen region. Orthop Traumatol Surg Res. 2014;100(5):515–9.
33. Tubbs RS, Nechtman C, D'Antoni AV, Shoja MM, Mortazavi MM, Loukas M, Rozzelle CJ, Spinner RJ. Ossification of the suprascapular ligament: a risk factor for suprascapular nerve compression? Int J Shoulder Surg. 2013;7(1):19–22.
34. Banskota B, Bijukachhe B, Limbu H, Shrestha BK, Banskota AK. Refractory shoulder pain due to entrapment neuropathy of the suprascapular nerve: a case report. Kathmandu Univ Med J (KUMJ). 2004;2(4):364–6.
35. Plancher KD, Luke TA, Peterson RK, Yacoubian SV. Posterior shoulder pain: a dynamic study of the spinoglenoid ligament and treatment with arthroscopic release of the scapular tunnel. Arthroscopy. 2007;23(9):991–8.
36. Harbaugh KS, Swenson R, Saunders RL. Shoulder numbness in a patient with suprascapular nerve entrapment syndrome: cutaneous branch of the suprascapular nerve: case report. Neurosurgery. 2000;47(6):1452–5.
37. Yoshioka C, Suenaga N, Oizumi N, Yamane S. Association of the area of sensory disturbance with the area of suprascapular nerve palsy. J Orthop Surg (Hong Kong). 2015;23(3):304–8.
38. Ebraheim NA, Whitehead JL, Alla SR, Moral MZ, Castillo S, McCollough AL, Yeasting RA, Liu J. The suprascapular nerve and its articular branch to the acromioclavicular joint: an anatomic study. J Shoulder Elb Surg. 2011;20(2):e13–7.
39. Horiguchi M. The cutaneous branch of some human suprascapular nerves. J Anat. 1980;130(Pt 1):191–5.
40. Hill LJ, Jelsing EJ, Terry MJ, Strommen JA. Evaluation, treatment, and outcomes of suprascapular neuropathy: a 5-year review. PM R. 2014;6(9):774–80.
41. Momaya AM, Kwapisz A, Choate WS, Kissenberth MJ, Tolan SJ, Lonergan KT, Hawkins RJ, Tokish JM. Clinical outcomes of suprascapular nerve decompression: a systematic review. J Shoulder Elb Surg. 2018;27(1):172–80.

42. Radic RR, Wallace A. Arthroscopic release and labral repair for bifocal compression of the suprascapular nerve. Shoulder Elbow. 2016;8(1):32–6.
43. Lafosse L, Tomasi A, Corbett S, Baier G, Willems K, Gobezie R. Arthroscopic release of suprascapular nerve entrapment at the suprascapular notch: technique and preliminary results. Arthroscopy. 2007;23(1):34–42.
44. Kim SH, Kim SJ, Sung CH, Koh YG, Kim YC, Park YS. Arthroscopic suprascapular nerve decompression at the suprascapular notch. Knee Surg Sports Traumatol Arthrosc. 2009;17(12):1504–7.
45. Shah AA, Butler RB, Sung SY, Wells JH, Higgins LD, Warner JJ. Clinical outcomes of suprascapular nerve decompression. J Shoulder Elb Surg. 2011;20(6):975–82.
46. Dietrich LN, Bentley A, Savage JA, Momaya AM, Larrison MC, McGwin G, Ponce BA. Arthroscopic decompression at the suprascapular notch: a radiographic and anatomic roadmap. J Shoulder Elb Surg. 2015;24(3):433–8.
47. Gupta R, Kapoor L, Shagotar S. Arthroscopic decompression of paralabral cyst around suprascapular notch causing suprascapular neuropathy. J Clin Orthop Trauma. 2015;6(3):184–6.
48. Mall NA, Hammond JE, Lenart BA, Enriquez DJ, Twigg SL, Nicholson GP. Suprascapular nerve entrapment isolated to the spinoglenoid notch: surgical technique and results of open decompression. J Shoulder Elb Surg. 2013;22(11):e1–8.
49. Westerheide KJ, Dopirak RM, Karzel RP, Snyder SJ. Suprascapular nerve palsy secondary to spinoglenoid cysts: results of arthroscopic treatment. Arthroscopy. 2006;22(7):721–7.
50. Mäkelä JP, Ramstad R, Mattila V, Pihlajamäki H. Brachial plexus lesions after backpack carriage in young adults. Clin Orthop Relat Res. 2006;452:205–9.
51. Witvrouw E, Cools A, Lysens R, Cambier D, Vanderstraeten G, Victor J, Sneyers C, Walravens M. Suprascapular neuropathy in volleyball players. Br J Sports Med. 2000;34(3):174–80.
52. Cummins CA, Bowen M, Anderson K, Messer T. Suprascapular nerve entrapment at the spinoglenoid notch in a professional baseball pitcher. Am J Sports Med. 1999;27(6):810–2.
53. Ferretti A, De Carli A, Fontana M. Injury of the suprascapular nerve at the spinoglenoid notch. The natural history of infraspinatus atrophy in volleyball players. Am J Sports Med. 1998;26(6):759–63.
54. Sandow MJ, Ilic J. Suprascapular nerve rotator cuff compression syndrome in volleyball players. J Shoulder Elb Surg. 1998;7(5):516–21.
55. Ringel SP, Treihaft M, Carry M, Fisher R, Jacobs P. Suprascapular neuropathy in pitchers. Am J Sports Med. 1990;18(1):80–6.

Chapter 45
Long Thoracic Nerve Dysfunction

The long thoracic nerve arises from the fifth, sixth and seventh cervical spine nerve roots. It is a long, slender nerve, surrounded by minimal connective tissue, characteristics which make it prone to injury. It is a purely motor nerve and innervates the serratus anterior muscle. Its dysfunction may lead to serratus anterior nerve weakness with resultant winging of the scapula [1–3].

45.1 Causes of Long Thoracic Nerve Dysfunction

Lesions of the long thoracic nerve may be defined as intrinsic or extrinsic [4–17].

- Intrinsic
  1. Brachial neuritis
  2. Systemic disorder (e.g. diabetes)
  3. Neoplastic
- Extrinsic
  1. Compression
  2. Traction
  3. Laceration
  4. Radiation

  Causes of extrinsic lesions include:

Compression

- Fibrous fascial or muscular bands
- Crossing vessels
- Heavy weights carried over shoulder
- Blunt chest wall trauma

© Springer Nature Switzerland AG 2019

C. Panayiotou Charalambous, *The Shoulder Made Easy*,
https://doi.org/10.1007/978-3-319-98908-2_45

Traction

- Repetitive overhead activity such as overhead throwing

Laceration

- Penetrating trauma – stab wounds
- Surgery – open

Radiation

- Radiation therapy for cancer

45.2 Clinical Symptoms of Long Thoracic Nerve Dysfunction

- Pain in the scapular area
- Weakness of serratus anterior
- Prominent scapula
- Shoulder/arm weakness, limited motion

45.3 Clinical Signs of Long Thoracic Nerve Dysfunction

- Weakness of serratus anterior
- Scapular winging

45.4 Investigations for Long Thoracic Nerve Dysfunction

- MRI to evaluate structural causes of scapular winging
- Electromyography looking for muscle denervation
- Nerve conduction studies

45.5 Management of Long Thoracic Nerve Dysfunction

- Non-surgical [17–19]
  - Leave alone
  - Expectant – await recovery
  - Activity modification
  - Non-steroidal anti-inflammatories

- Surgical [19–27]
  - Surgical decompression of the long thoracic nerve
  - Tendon transfer (sternal head of pectoralis major to inferior angle of scapula – direct or indirect with interpositional graft)
  - Scapulo-thoracic fusion

References

1. Bertelli JA, Ghizoni MF. Long thoracic nerve: anatomy and functional assessment. J Bone Joint Surg Am. 2005;87(5):993–8.
2. Wang JF, Dang RS, Wang D, Zhang ZY, Liu Z, Huang HL, Wu AQ, Zhang CS, Chen EY. Observation and measurements of long thoracic nerve: a cadaver study and clinical consideration. Surg Radiol Anat. 2008;30(7):569–73.
3. Kauppila LI. The long thoracic nerve: possible mechanisms of injury based on autopsy study. J Shoulder Elb Surg. 1993;2(5):244–8.
4. Packer GJ, McLatchie GR, Bowden W. Scapula winging in a sports injury clinic. Br J Sports Med. 1993;27(2):90–1.
5. Sahin F, Yilmaz F, Esit N, Aysal F, Kuran B. Compressive neuropathy of long thoracic nerve and accessory nerve secondary to heavy load bearing. A case report. Eura Medicophys. 2007;43(1):71–4.
6. Schultz JS, Leonard JA Jr. Long thoracic neuropathy from athletic activity. Arch Phys Med Rehabil. 1992;73(1):87–90.
7. Safran MR. Nerve injury about the shoulder in athletes, part 2: long thoracic nerve, spinal accessory nerve, burners/stingers, thoracic outlet syndrome. Am J Sports Med. 2004;32(4):1063–76.
8. Berthold JB, Burg TM, Nussbaum RP. Long thoracic nerve injury caused by overhead weight lifting leading to scapular dyskinesis and medial scapular winging. J Am Osteopath Assoc. 2017;117(2):133–7.
9. Oakes MJ, Sherwood DL. An isolated long thoracic nerve injury in a navy airman. Mil Med. 2004;169(9):713–5.
10. Aycock RD, Kass D, Hahn B. Young man with stab wound to the neck. Winged scapula as a result of long thoracic nerve injury. Ann Emerg Med. 2012;59(1):81, 85. https://doi.org/10.1016/j.annemergmed.2011.04.015.
11. Hankins CL. Injury to the long thoracic nerve as a complication of neck dissection: a case report. Br J Oral Maxillofac Surg. 2005;43(6):526–7.
12. Krasna MJ, Forti G. Nerve injury: injury to the recurrent laryngeal, phrenic, vagus, long thoracic, and sympathetic nerves during thoracic surgery. Thorac Surg Clin. 2006;16(3):267–75.
13. Thomas SE, Winchester JB, Hickman G, DeBusk E. A confirmed case of injury to the long thoracic nerve following a posterior approach to an interscalene nerve block. Reg Anesth Pain Med. 2013;38(4):370. https://doi.org/10.1097/AAP.0b013e3182905b98.
14. Omar N, Alvi F, Srinivasan MS. An unusual presentation of whiplash injury: long thoracic and spinal accessory nerve injury. Eur Spine J. 2007;16(Suppl 3):275–7.
15. Nawa S. Scapular winging secondary to apparent long thoracic nerve palsy in a young female swimmer. J Brachial Plex Peripher Nerve Inj. 2015;10(1):e57–61.

16. Pugliese GN, Green RF, Antonacci A. Radiation-induced long thoracic nerve palsy. Cancer. 1987;60(6):1247–8.
17. Belmonte R, Monleon S, Bofill N, Alvarado ML, Espadaler J, Royo I. Long thoracic nerve injury in breast cancer patients treated with axillary lymph node dissection. Support Care Cancer. 2015;23(1):169–75.
18. Friedenberg SM, Zimprich T, Harper CM. The natural history of long thoracic and spinal accessory neuropathies. Muscle Nerve. 2002;25(4):535–9.
19. Galano GJ, Bigliani LU, Ahmad CS, Levine WN. Surgical treatment of winged scapula. Clin Orthop Relat Res. 2008;466(3):652–60.
20. Nath RK, Lyons AB, Bietz G. Microneurolysis and decompression of long thoracic nerve injury are effective in reversing scapular winging: long-term results in 50 cases. BMC Musculoskelet Disord. 2007;8:25.
21. Le Nail LR, Bacle G, Marteau E, Corcia P, Favard L, Laulan J. Isolated paralysis of the serratus anterior muscle: surgical release of the distal segment of the long thoracic nerve in 52 patients. Orthop Traumatol Surg Res. 2014;100(4 Suppl):S243–8.
22. Disa JJ, Wang B, Dellon AL. Correction of scapular winging by supraclavicular neurolysis of the long thoracic nerve. J Reconstr Microsurg. 2001;17(2):79–84.
23. Chalmers PN, Saltzman BM, Feldheim TF, Mascarenhas R, Mellano C, Cole BJ, Romeo AA, Nicholson GP. A comprehensive analysis of pectoralis major transfer for long thoracic nerve palsy. J Shoulder Elb Surg. 2015;24(7):1028–35.
24. Elhassan BT, Wagner ER. Outcome of transfer of the sternal head of the pectoralis major with its bone insertion to the scapula to manage scapular winging. J Shoulder Elb Surg. 2015;24(5):733–40.
25. Connor PM, Yamaguchi K, Manifold SG, Pollock RG, Flatow EL, Bigliani LU. Split pectoralis major transfer for serratus anterior palsy. Clin Orthop Relat Res. 1997;341:134–42.
26. Atasoy E, Majd M. Scapulothoracic stabilisation for winging of the scapula using strips of autogenous fascia lata. J Bone Joint Surg Br. 2000;82(6):813–7.
27. Bizot P, Teboul F, Nizard R, Sedel L. Scapulothoracic fusion for serratus anterior paralysis. J Shoulder Elb Surg. 2003;12(6):561–5.

Chapter 46
Dorsal Scapular Nerve Dysfunction

The dorsal scapular nerve arises from the C5 root (with occasional contribution from C6) and is the most proximal branch of the brachial plexus. It enters the inter-scalene triangle, pierces the scalene medius and passes downwards deep to levator scapulae, eventually piercing the deep surface of the rhomboid major and minor. It is a motor nerve and supplies [1–3]:

- Rhomboid major
- Rhomboid minor
- Levator scapulae

46.1 Causes of Dorsal Scapular Nerve Dysfunction

Lesions of the dorsal-scapular nerve may be defined as intrinsic or extrinsic [4–12]:

- Intrinsic
  1. Brachial neuritis
  2. Systemic disorder (diabetes)
  3. Neoplastic
- Extrinsic
  1. Compression
  2. Traction
  3. Laceration
  4. Radiation

  Causes of extrinsic lesions include:

© Springer Nature Switzerland AG 2019

C. Panayiotou Charalambous, *The Shoulder Made Easy*,
https://doi.org/10.1007/978-3-319-98908-2_46

Compression

- Between the anterior and middle scalene muscles
- Elongated C7 process
- Hypertrophied rhomboids in those with repetitive overhead activities (weight lifting or athletics – volleyball, basketball)

Traction

- Repetitive overhead activity such as overhead throwing

Laceration

- Penetrating trauma – stab wounds
- Surgery

46.2 Clinical Symptoms of Dorsal Scapular Nerve Dysfunction

- Pain along the medial border of the scapula (between spine and scapula) which may radiate to the posterolateral part of the shoulder and down the arm in the C5/C6 distribution. Pain may be:
  - Nerve trunk pain – neuropathic due to activation of nociceptors in nerve sheaths activated by compression or stretch – this is usually not associated with any innervation changes
  - Due to scapular winging which stretches the dorsal primary rami of the thoracic spinal nerves
- Scapular winging
- Reduced shoulder motion/strength

46.3 Clinical Signs of Dorsal Scapular Nerve Dysfunction

- Peri-scapular tenderness
- Rhomboid muscle wasting
- Scapular winging
- Limitation of shoulder movements
- Rhomboid weakness
- Hypertrophied, contracted trapezius

46.4 Investigations for Dorsal Scapular Nerve Dysfunction

- Plain radiographs
- MRI to:
  - Evaluate the rotator cuff muscles and tendons
  - Look for compressive cause due to space-occupying lesions
- Electromyography looking for muscle denervation
- Nerve conduction studies

46.5 Management of Dorsal Scapular Nerve Dysfunction

This aims to reduce pain and improve scapular winging

- *Non-surgical*
  - Leave alone
  - Activity modification
  - Non-steroidal anti-inflammatories
  - Physiotherapy:
    - Relax and stretch trapezius
    - Regain passive movements
    - Regain shoulder movements
    - Strengthen deltoid and rotator cuff
  - Injection around the dorsal scapular nerve (local anaesthetic + steroid)
  - Radiofrequency nerve lesioning for pain
- *Surgical* [12]
  - Surgical decompression – open

Learning Pearls
- In those with pain, there may not be any obvious clinical signs, with neurophysiological abnormalities being the only detectable positive finding

References

1. Tubbs RS, Tyler-Kabara EC, Aikens AC, Martin JP, Weed LL, Salter EG, Oakes WJ. Surgical anatomy of the dorsal scapular nerve. J Neurosurg. 2005;102(5):910–1.
2. Nguyen VH, Liu HH, Rosales A, Reeves R. A cadaveric investigation of the dorsal scapular nerve. Anat Res Int. 2016;2016:4106981. https://doi.org/10.1155/2016/4106981.

3. Argyriou AA, Karanasios P, Makridou A, Makris N. Dorsal scapular neuropathy causing rhomboids palsy and scapular winging. J Back Musculoskelet Rehabil. 2015;28(4):883–5.
4. Sultan HE, Younis El-Tantawi GA. Role of dorsal scapular nerve entrapment in unilateral interscapular pain. Arch Phys Med Rehabil. 2013;94(6):1118–25.
5. Muir B. Dorsal scapular nerve neuropathy: a narrative review of the literature. J Can Chiropr Assoc. 2017;61(2):128–44.
6. Lee DG, Chang MC. Dorsal scapular nerve injury after trigger point injection into the rhomboid major muscle: a case report. J Back Musculoskelet Rehabil. 2018;31(1):211–4.
7. Saporito A. Dorsal scapular nerve injury: a complication of ultrasound-guided interscalene block. Br J Anaesth. 2013;111(5):840–1.
8. Jerosch J, Castro WH, Geske B. Damage of the long thoracic and dorsal scapular nerve after traumatic shoulder dislocation: case report and review of the literature. Acta Orthop Belg. 1990;56(3–4):625–7.
9. Benedetti MG, Zati A, Stagni SB, Fusaro I, Monesi R, Rotini R. Winged scapula caused by rhomboid paralysis: a case report. Joints. 2017;4(4):247–9.
10. Akgun K, Aktas I, Terzi Y. Winged scapula caused by a dorsal scapular nerve lesion: a case report. Arch Phys Med Rehabil. 2008;89(10):2017–20.
11. Trescot A. Dorsal scapular nerve entrapment. In: Peripheral nerve entrapments: clinical diagnosis and management. Berlin: Springer; 2016. p. 315–24.
12. Chen D, Gu Y, Lao J, Chen L. Dorsal scapular nerve compression. Atypical thoracic outlet syndrome. Chin Med J. 1995;108(8):582–5.

Chapter 47
Scapular Dyskinesis

This is a condition whereby there is abnormal scapular motion [1–10]. It may refer to:

- Abnormal static positioning – including prominence of its medial border or inferior angle
- Abnormal scapular movement – including early scapula elevation on arm elevation or rapid downward scapular rotation during arm descend

Scapular motion is very complex. However, in a simplified version, one may consider the effect of trapezius, rhomboids and serratus anterior (SA) upon the scapula:

- The trapezius and rhomboids elevate and retract the scapula, whereas SA protracts the scapula
- The trapezius and SA rotate the scapula upwards. The rhomboids rotate the scapula downwards

Hence, if one of the above muscles is dysfunctional, the clinical picture may reflect the consequence of its loss in activity.

Winging of the scapula is used to describe prominence of the medial border of the scapula along with medial or lateral translation of the scapula due to the action of unopposed muscles. This may occur at rest, during movement or both.

Winging due to SA palsy is known as medial winging, whereas winging due to trapezius or rhomboid palsy is known as lateral winging, a description based on the position of the scapula in relation to the spine.

© Springer Nature Switzerland AG 2019

C. Panayiotou Charalambous, *The Shoulder Made Easy*,
https://doi.org/10.1007/978-3-319-98908-2_47

Medial (a) and lateral (b) scapular winging

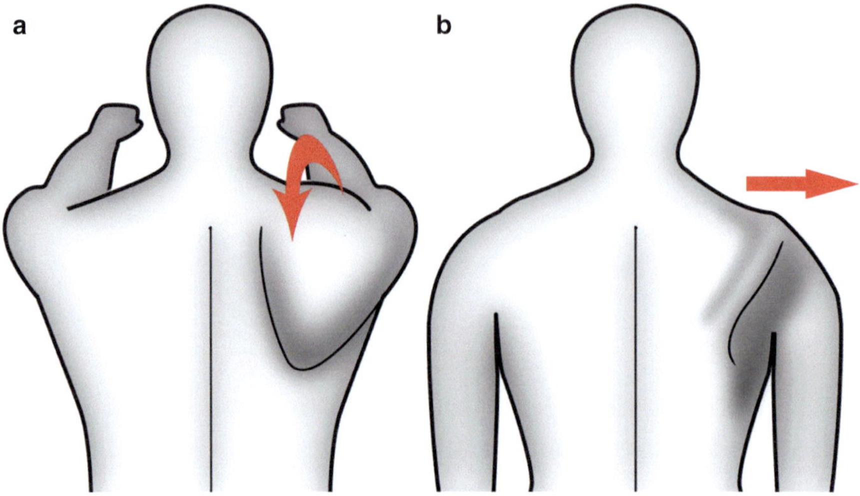

47.1 Causes of Scapular Dyskinesis

Abnormal scapular motion may be either primary or secondary [1–29] (compensating for shoulder pathology).

47.1.1 Primary

Due to abnormalities arising in the scapulo-thoracic articulation, peri-scapular muscles and nerves:

- Neurological dysfunction due to intrinsic or extrinsic nerve lesion. Nerves involved in decreasing frequency:
  - Long thoracic nerve
  - Spinal accessory nerve
  - Dorsal scapular nerve
- Osseous
  - Osteochondromas arising from the scapula or the ribs can cause pseudo-winging. There may be associated crepitus on arm movement, and the winging may be static (not changing with the position of the arm unlike true winging)
  - Fractures – ribs, scapula
  - Thoracic spine – scoliosis, kyphosis

- Soft tissue
  - Congenital absence of muscles (SA, trapezius, rhomboids)
  - Muscle avulsion due to trauma (SA)
  - Scapulo-thoracic bursitis causing pain
- Voluntary

47.1.2 *Secondary*

Arises as a response to abnormalities in the shoulder:

- Shoulder pain – causing reflex spasm of peri-scapular muscles
- Glenohumeral stiffness – causing abnormal scapular motion in an attempt to maintain overall motion
- Deltoid fibrosis (congenital, secondary to intramuscular injections)

The scapula may try to compensate for limited movement in the glenohumeral joint by increasing scapulo-thoracic motion, leading to scapular muscle fatigue and winging.

Similarly, in response to shoulder pain, the patient may adjust the glenohumeral motion, which then leads to an attempted compensation by scapulo-thoracic motion.

47.2 Clinical Symptoms of Scapular Dyskinesis

- Shoulder weakness, especially on arm abduction
- Reduced functional performance, especially in athletes or high-demand labourers
- Abnormal prominence of the scapula noticed by the patient or others
- Reduced shoulder motion
- Dull ache, heaviness and burning pain in the area of the scapula, neck and arm
- Muscle pain due to over compensating muscles causing muscle spasm
- Drooping of the affected shoulder (in trapezius dysfunction) and shoulder asymmetry
- Feeling of abnormal movement in the shoulder
- Wasting of peri-scapular muscles

The clinical history enquires about the onset of symptoms, severity of pain (which if sudden onset and severe may point to neuritis as the underlying cause), history of trauma and history of surgery to the neck, shoulder, thorax or axilla.

47.3 Clinical Signs of Scapular Dyskinesis

- Surgical scars suggestive of iatrogenic course
- Muscle wasting

- Muscular, bursa or bony tenderness
- Abnormal scapular posture – static and/or dynamic
- Winging
  - Static (pseudo-winging):

    Present at rest with arm by the side
    Does not increase on forward elevation of the arm against resistance
    Due to structural abnormalities of scapula or ribs

  - Dynamic (true-winging):

    Increases on forward flexion of the arm against resistance
    Due to muscle imbalance

Pressing on the wall with arms to assess scapular winging

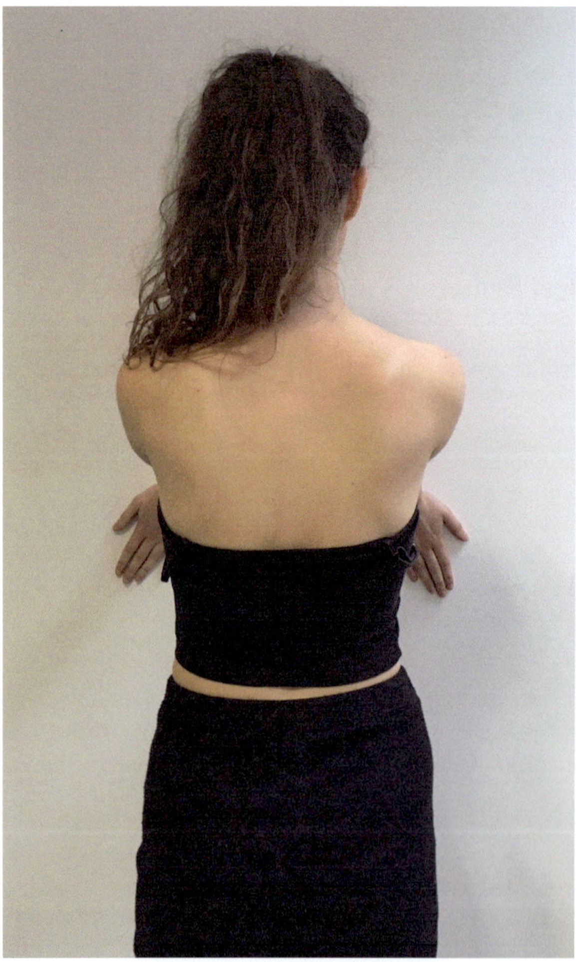

Pressing on the wall with arms in forward flexion, to assess scapular winging

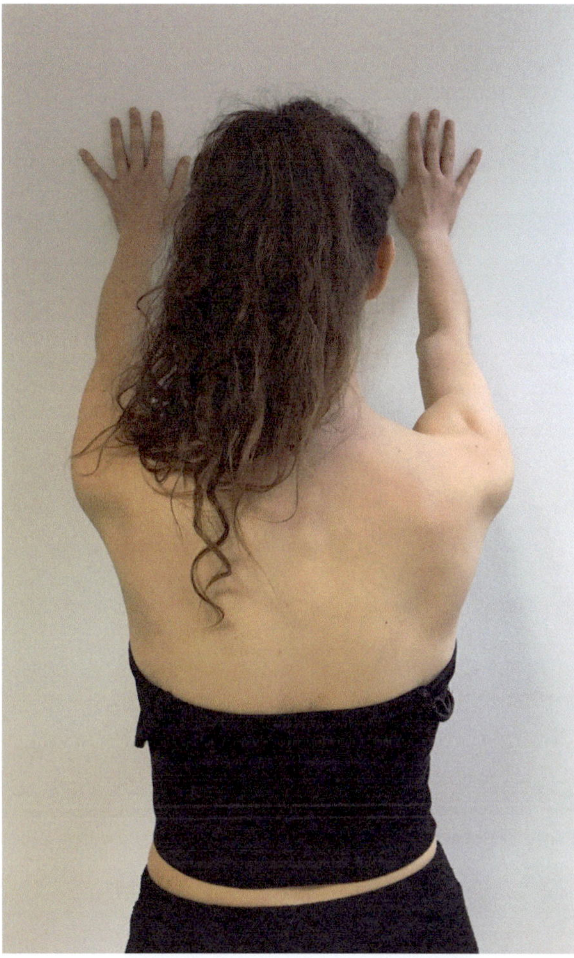

- Palpable crepitus
  - Detected by palpation
  - Pressing the scapula onto the chest wall during arm movement may aggravate crepitus
- Painful or limited shoulder movements

  In evaluating the possible causes of abnormal scapular motion, consider:

  - Is there muscle wasting?
  - Is the medial border of the scapula lifting off the chest wall?

- Is the scapula translated medially or laterally?
  - Medially – in SA palsy
  - Laterally – in trapezius or rhomboids palsy
- What aggravates winging?

Clinical findings to help determine the muscle contributing to scapular winging

Serratus anterior palsy (long thoracic nerve)

- Scapula translated medially
- Inferior scapular angle translated medially
- Medial scapular border lifting off the chest wall
- Winging
  - at rest
  - worse on forward arm elevation
  - worse on wall pressing

Trapezius palsy (spinal accessory nerve)

- Trapezius wasting
- Shoulder depressed
- Scapula translated laterally
- Inferior scapular angle translated laterally
- Inability to shrug the shoulder
- Winging
  - minimal
  - worse on arm abduction
  - less on forward arm elevation

Rhomboids palsy (dorsal scapular nerve)

- Rhomboid wasting
- Shoulder depressed
- Scapula translated laterally
- Inferior scapular angle translated laterally
- Winging
  - worse on arm extension from full forward elevation

Lateral winging of the scapula due to trapezius weakness secondary to iatrogenic injury of the spinal accessory nerve sustained in neck dissection surgery for throat cancer

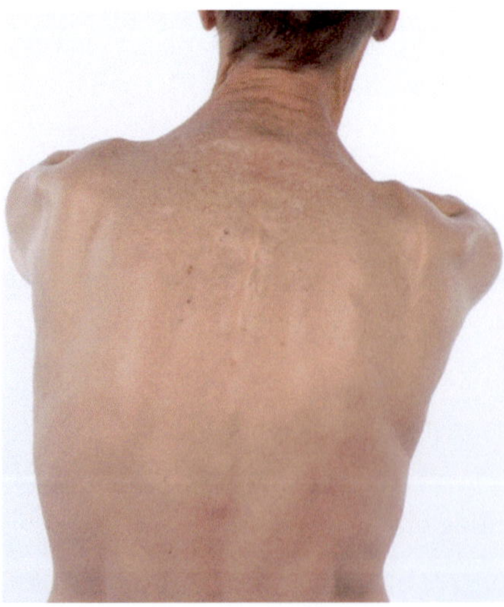

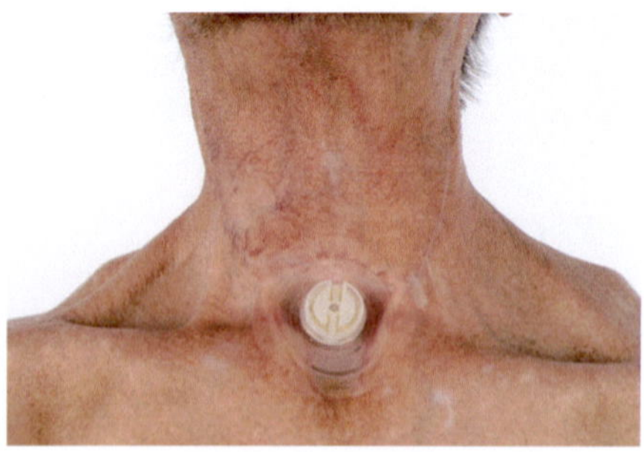

Scapular winging due to serratus anterior palsy

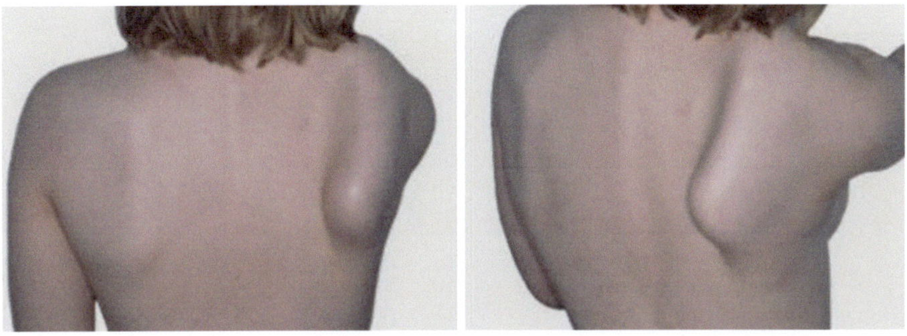

47.4 Investigations for Scapular Dyskinesis

- Radiological
  - Plain radiographs, CT scans – look for osseous causes
  - MRI – looking for osseous bursitis and soft tissue lesions
- Nerve conduction studies
- Electromyography

CT scan showing large exostosis arising from the anterior surface of the scapula (red arrow) causing static winging

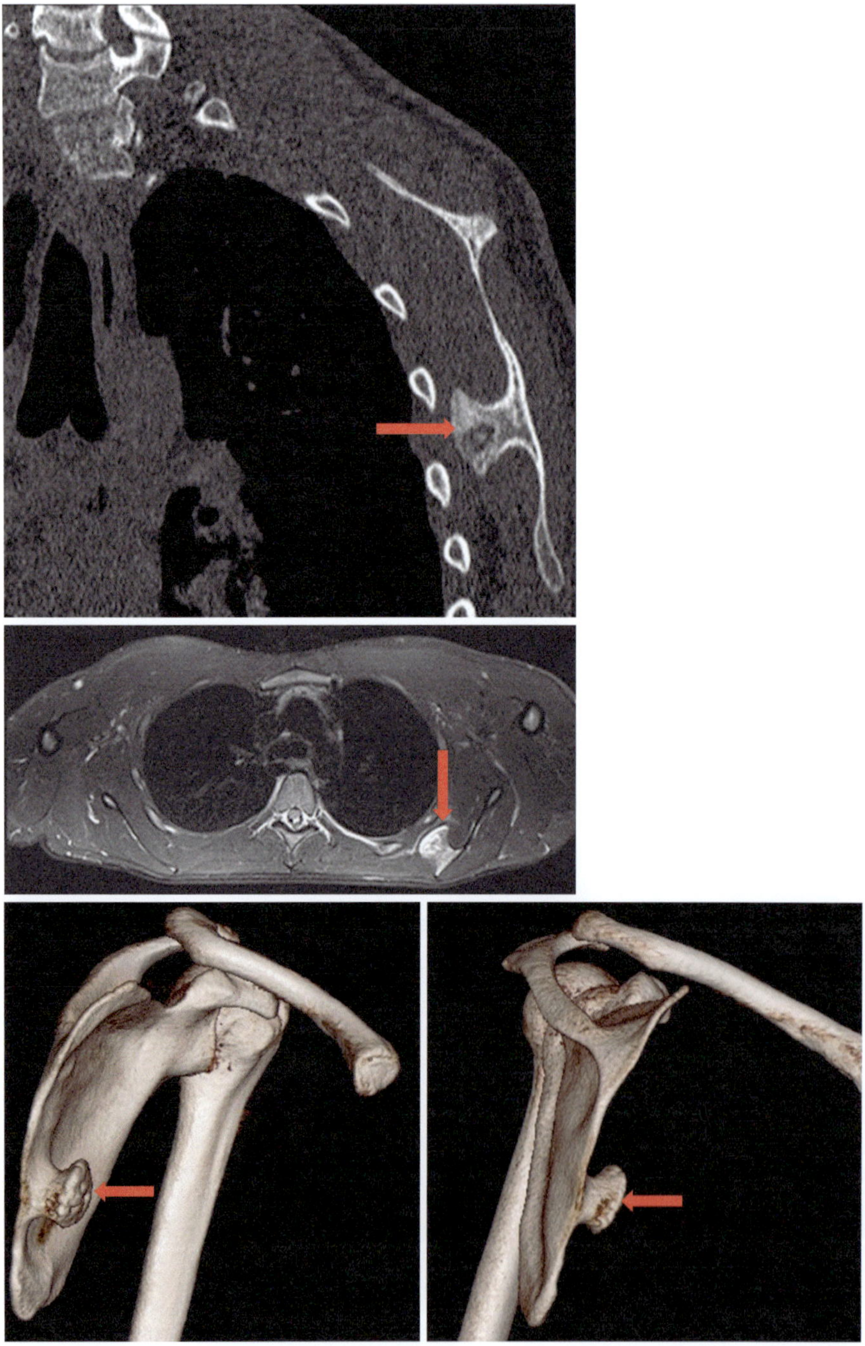

47.5 Management of Scapular Dyskinesis

This will depend on underlying cause and clinical symptoms.

- Scapular dyskinesis secondary to a shoulder disorder – address the primary shoulder disorder
- Primary scapular dyskinesis – address scapula per se as below

Non-surgical [29–36]

- Leave alone
- Analgesia
- Steroid injections of bursae in scapulo-thoracic bursitis
- Physiotherapy
  - Maintain glenohumeral motion
  - Stretch stiff muscles
  - Improve posture
  - Strengthen weak or compensatory muscles
  - Correct muscle dis-coordination – biofeedback

Surgical [37–49]

- Nerve surgery
  - Neurolysis
  - Nerve grafting
- Muscle transfers – to improve pain and function and reduce winging.
  - Trapezius dysfunction – Eden-Lange procedure involves transfer of the levator scapulae to the acromion and the rhomboid muscles to the infraspinous fossa
  - SA dysfunction – transfer of the sternocostal head of pectoralis major with a graft extension (fascia lata, semitendinosus) – the sternocostal head of pectoralis major is released from its insertion on the bicipital groove of the humerus, and a graft of fascia lata is harvested from the lateral part of the thigh, or semitendinosus is harvested from the knee and together are sutured to the inferior angle of the scapula
- Osseous procedures
  - Osteochondromas – resection
  - Mal-unions of scapular fractures – osteotomy
  - Scapulothoracic fusion – fusion aims to improve pain but at the expense of arm motion

References

1. Kibler WB, Sciascia A. Current concepts: scapular dyskinesis. Br J Sports Med. 2010;44(5):300–5.
2. Martin RM, Fish DE. Scapular winging: anatomical review, diagnosis, and treatments. Curr Rev Musculoskelet Med. 2008;1(1):1–11.
3. Ludewig PM, Phadke V, Braman JP, Hassett DR, Cieminski CJ, LaPrade RF. Motion of the shoulder complex during multiplanar humeral elevation. J Bone Joint Surg Am. 2009;91(2):378–89.
4. Srikumaran U, Wells JH, Freehill MT, Tan EW, Higgins LD, Warner JJ. Scapular winging: a great masquerader of shoulder disorders: AAOS exhibit selection. J Bone Joint Surg Am. 2014;96(14):e122.
5. Ludewig PM, Reynolds JF. The association of scapular kinematics and glenohumeral joint pathologies. J Orthop Sports Phys Ther. 2009;39(2):90–104.
6. Preziosi Standoli J, Fratalocchi F, Candela V, Preziosi Standoli T, Giannicola G, Bonifazi M, Gumina S. Scapular dyskinesis in young, asymptomatic elite swimmers. Orthop J Sports Med. 2018;6(1) https://doi.org/10.1177/2325967117750814.
7. Littlewood C, Cools AMJ. Scapular dyskinesis and shoulder pain: the devil is in the detail. Br J Sports Med. 2018;52(2):72–3.
8. Huang TS, Lin JJ, Ou HL, Chen YT. Movement pattern of scapular dyskinesis in symptomatic overhead athletes. Sci Rep. 2017;7(1):6621. https://doi.org/10.1038/s41598-017-06779-8.
9. Huang TS, Huang CY, Ou HL, Lin JJ. Scapular dyskinesis: patterns, functional disability and associated factors in people with shoulder disorders. Man Ther. 2016;26:165–71.
10. Rossi DM, Pedroni CR, Martins J, de Oliveira AS. Intrarater and interrater reliability of three classifications for scapular dyskinesis in athletes. PLoS One. 2017;12(7):e0181518.
11. Nawa S. Scapular winging secondary to apparent long thoracic nerve palsy in a young female swimmer. J Brachial Plex Peripher Nerve Inj. 2015;10(1):e57–61.
12. Benedetti MG, Zati A, Stagni SB, Fusaro I, Monesi R, Rotini R. Winged scapula caused by rhomboid paralysis: a case report. Joints. 2017;4(4):247–9.
13. Kibler WB, Sciascia A, Uhl T. Medial scapular muscle detachment: clinical presentation and surgical treatment. J Shoulder Elb Surg. 2014;23(1):58–67.
14. Berthold JB, Burg TM, Nussbaum RP. Long thoracic nerve injury caused by overhead weight lifting leading to scapular dyskinesis and medial scapular winging. J Am Osteopath Assoc. 2017;117(2):133–7.
15. Burn MB, McCulloch PC, Lintner DM, Liberman SR, Harris JD. Prevalence of scapular dyskinesis in overhead and nonoverhead athletes: a systematic review. Orthop J Sports Med. 2016;4(2):2325967115627608. https://doi.org/10.1177/2325967115627608.
16. Carbone S, Moroder P, Runer A, Resch H, Gumina S, Hertel R. Scapular dyskinesis after Latarjet procedure. J Shoulder Elb Surg. 2016;25(3):422–7.
17. Shields E, Behrend C, Beiswenger T, Strong B, English C, Maloney M, Voloshin I. Scapular dyskinesis following displaced fractures of the middle clavicle. J Shoulder Elb Surg. 2015;24(12):e331–6.
18. Carbone S, Postacchini R, Gumina S. Scapular dyskinesis and SICK syndrome in patients with a chronic type III acromioclavicular dislocation. Results of rehabilitation. Knee Surg Sports Traumatol Arthrosc. 2015;23(5):1473–80.
19. Huang TS, Ou HL, Huang CY, Lin JJ. Specific kinematics and associated muscle activation in individuals with scapular dyskinesis. J Shoulder Elb Surg. 2015;24(8):1227–34.
20. Lazar MA, Kwon YW, Rokito AS. Snapping scapula syndrome. J Bone Joint Surg Am. 2009;91(9):2251–62.
21. Gaskill T, Millett PJ. Snapping scapula syndrome: diagnosis and management. J Am Acad Orthop Surg. 2013;21(4):214–24.
22. Charalambous CP. Long thoracic nerve dysfunction. In: Charalambous CP, editor. The shoulder made easy. Springer; 2019. pp. 569–71.

23. Charalambous CP. Dorsal scapular nerve dysfunction. In: Charalambous CP, editor. The shoulder made easy. Springer; 2019. pp. 573–75.
24. Hannah DC, Scibek JS, Carcia CR. Strength profiles in healthy individuals profiles in healthy individuals with and without scapular dyskinesis. Int J Sports Phys Ther. 2017;12(3): 305–13.
25. Uga D, Nakazawa R, Sakamoto M. Strength and muscle activity of shoulder external rotation of subjects with and without scapular dyskinesis. J Phys Ther Sci. 2016;28(4):1100–5.
26. Merolla G, De Santis E, Campi F, Paladini P, Porcellini G. Supraspinatus and infraspinatus weakness in overhead athletes with scapular dyskinesis: strength assessment before and after restoration of scapular musculature balance. Musculoskelet Surg. 2010;94(3): 119–25.
27. Lopes AD, Timmons MK, Grover M, Ciconelli RM, Michener LA. Visual scapular dyskinesis: kinematics and muscle activity alterations in patients with subacromial impingement syndrome. Arch Phys Med Rehabil. 2015;96(2):298–306.
28. Alibazi RJ, Moghadam AN, Cools AM, Bakhshi E, Ahari AA. The effect of shoulder muscle fatigue on acromiohumeral distance and scapular dyskinesis in women with generalized joint hypermobility. J Appl Biomech. 2017;33(6):424–30.
29. Seitz AL, McClure PW, Lynch SS, Ketchum JM, Michener LA. Effects of scapular dyskinesis and scapular assistance test on subacromial space during static arm elevation. J Shoulder Elb Surg. 2012;21(5):631–40.
30. Turgut E, Duzgun I, Baltaci G. Effects of scapular stabilization exercise training on scapular kinematics, disability, and pain in subacromial impingement: a randomized controlled trial. Arch Phys Med Rehabil. 2017;98(10):1915–23.
31. Moura KF, Monteiro RL, Lucareli PR, Fukuda TY. Rehabilitation of subacromial pain syndrome emphasizing scapular dyskinesis in amateur athletes: a case series. Int J Sports Phys Ther. 2016;11(4):552–63.
32. Hickey D, Solvig V, Cavalheri V, Harrold M, Mckenna L. Scapular dyskinesis increases the risk of future shoulder pain by 43% in asymptomatic athletes: a systematic review and meta-analysis. Br J Sports Med. 2018;52(2):102–10.
33. Sanchez HM, Sanchez EG, Tavares LI. Association between scapular dyskinesia and shoulder pain in young adults. Acta Ortop Bras. 2016;24(5):243–8.
34. Intelangelo L, Bordachar D, Barbosa AW. Effects of scapular taping in young adults with shoulder pain and scapular dyskinesis. J Bodyw Mov Ther. 2016;20(3):525–32.
35. Holtermann A, Mork PJ, Andersen LL, Olsen HB, Søgaard K. The use of EMG biofeedback for learning of selective activation of intra-muscular parts within the serratus anterior muscle: a novel approach for rehabilitation of scapular muscle imbalance. J Electromyogr Kinesiol. 2010;20(2):359–65.
36. Weon JH, Kwon OY, Cynn HS, Lee WH, Kim TH, Yi CH. Real-time visual feedback can be used to activate scapular upward rotators in people with scapular winging: an experimental study. J Physiother. 2011;57(2):101–7.
37. Novak CB, Mackinnon SE. Surgical treatment of a long thoracic nerve palsy. Ann Thorac Surg. 2002;73:1643–5.
38. Tomaino MM. Neurophysiologic and clinical outcome following medial pectoral to long thoracic nerve transfer for scapular winging: a case report. Microsurgery. 2002;22:254–7.
39. Vetter M, Charran O, Yilmaz E, Edwards B, Muhleman MA, Oskouian RJ, Tubbs RS, Loukas M. Winged scapula: a comprehensive review of surgical treatment. Cureus. 2017;9(12):e1923. https://doi.org/10.7759/cureus.1923.
40. Romero J, Gerber C. Levator scapulae and rhomboid transfer for paralysis of trapezius. J Bone Joint Surg. 2003;85:1141–5.
41. Galano GJ, Bigliani LU, Ahmad CS, Levine WN. Surgical treatment of winged scapula. Clin Orthop Relat Res. 2008;466(3):652–60.
42. Chalmers PN, Saltzman BM, Feldheim TF, Mascarenhas R, Mellano C, Cole BJ, Romeo AA, Nicholson GP. A comprehensive analysis of pectoralis major transfer for long thoracic nerve palsy. J Shoulder Elb Surg. 2015;24(7):1028–35.

43. Streit JJ, Lenarz CJ, Shishani Y, McCrum C, Wanner JP, Nowinski RJ, Warner JJ, Gobezie R. Pectoralis major tendon transfer for the treatment of scapular winging due to long thoracic nerve palsy. J Shoulder Elb Surg. 2012;21(5):685–90.
44. Tauber M, Moursy M, Koller H, Schwartz M, Resch H. Direct pectoralis major muscle transfer for dynamic stabilization of scapular winging. J Shoulder Elb Surg. 2008;17(1 Suppl):29S–34S.
45. Iceton J, Harris WR. Treatment of winged scapula by pectoralis major transfer. J Bone Joint Surg. 1987;69:108–10.
46. Li T, Yang ZZ, Deng Y, Xiao M, Jiang C, Wang JW. Indirect transfer of the sternal head of the pectoralis major with autogenous semitendinosus augmentation to treat scapular winging secondary to long thoracic nerve palsy. J Shoulder Elb Surg. 2017;26(11):1970–7.
47. Krishnan SG, Hawkins RJ, Michelotti JD, et al. Scapulothoracic arthrodesis: indication, technique, and results. Clin Orthop Relat Res. 2005;435:126–33.
48. Sewell MD, Higgs DS, Al-Hadithy N, Falworth M, Bayley I, Lambert SM. The outcome of scapulothoracic fusion for painful winging of the scapula in dystrophic and non-dystrophic conditions. J Bone Joint Surg Br. 2012;94(9):1253–9.
49. Bizot P, Teboul F, Nizard R, Sedel L. Scapulothoracic fusion for serratus anterior paralysis. J Shoulder Elb Surg. 2003;12(6):561–5.

Chapter 48
Snapping Scapula

This is a condition whereby there is clicking or snapping during movement between the scapula and underlying chest wall. This may be painful or painless.

48.1 Causes of Snapping Scapula [1–13]

Scapula snapping may be due to bony abnormalities of the scapula or rib cage or due to changes in the muscles and bursae that are located between the scapula and chest wall. These include:

- Bursal inflammation and fibrosis following trauma or chronic overuse
- Muscle fibrosis
- Bony
  - Superior medial and inferior medial scapula angles may be thickened, hooked or angulated or may have an associated bony protuberance
- Scapular or rib fractures
  - Mal-union
  - Excessive callus formation
- Spinal abnormalities – kyphosis/scoliosis
- Mass lesions located between the scapula and the rib cage such as osteochondromas, chondro-sarcomas and elastofibroma dorsi (found near the inferior medial angle of the scapula)

© Springer Nature Switzerland AG 2019

C. Panayiotou Charalambous, *The Shoulder Made Easy*,
https://doi.org/10.1007/978-3-319-98908-2_48

48.2 Classification of Snapping Scapula

Scapulo-thoracic crepitus has been classified into three types by Mauclaire [14] as:

- Froissement – a gentle friction sound – may be physiological
- Frottement – loud sound with grating – likely to be related to a pathological condition
- Craquement – loud, snapping sound – pathological

48.3 Clinical Symptoms of Snapping Scapula

- Pain (but snapping may also be painless)
  - At superior medial angle – infra-serratus or supra-serratus bursae
  - At inferior medial angle – infra-serratus bursa
  - Near the base of the scapular spine – scapulo-trapezial bursa (located deep to the trapezius and superficial to the scapular spine)
- Audible and palpable crepitus with scapular movements

48.4 Clinical Signs of Snapping Scapula

- Palpable crepitus
- Audible snapping – the crepitus may be made more pronounced by pressing the superior angle of the scapula against the chest wall during arm elevation
- Pain and snapping may decrease when crossing the arm forwards which lifts the scapula off the ribcage
- Tenderness over the medial border of the scapula or over the peri-scapular muscles due to abnormal contracture or spasm
- Scapular winging
- Peri-scapular and scapular muscle weakness
- Trigger points of inflamed bursa
  - Superior medial angle of the scapula
  - Inferior angle of the scapula
  - Medial base of the spine of the scapula underlying the trapezius muscle

48.5 Investigations for Snapping Scapula

- Radiological
  - Plain radiographs and CT scans looking for osseous causes or bursitis
  - MRI and ultrasound to identify inflamed bursal tissue and soft tissue lesions

- Nerve conduction studies
- Electromyography

48.6 Management of Snapping Scapula

Non-surgical [15–19]: Successful in Most Cases

- Leave alone
- Analgesia
- Activity modification
- Extracorporeal shock wave therapy
- Steroid injections of the bursae – the bursae are accessed by cross adduction of the arm (to elevate the medial border of the scapula off the chest wall). The needle is inserted towards the point of maximum tenderness ensuring that it is parallel between the scapular border and the posterior chest wall to avoid intra-thoracic penetration and pneumothorax [13]

Surgical (Open or Arthroscopic) [15, 17, 20–25]

- Bursectomy
- Partial resection of the involved scapular angle or any associated bony prominence (open or arthroscopic)
- Resection of other osseous lesions

References

1. Kuhn JE, Plancher KD, Hawkins RJ. Symptomatic scapulothoracic crepitus and bursitis. J Am Acad Orthop Surg. 1998;6(5):267–73.
2. Warth RJ, Spiegl UJ, Millett PJ. Scapulothoracic bursitis and snapping scapula syndrome: a critical review of current evidence. Am J Sports Med. 2015;43(1):236–45.
3. Lazar MA, Kwon YW, Rokito AS. Snapping scapula syndrome. J Bone Joint Surg Am. 2009;91(9):2251–62.
4. Gaskill T, Millett PJ. Snapping scapula syndrome: diagnosis and management. J Am Acad Orthop Surg. 2013;21(4):214–24.
5. Frank RM, Ramirez J, Chalmers PN, McCormick FM, Romeo AA. Scapulothoracic anatomy and snapping scapula syndrome. Anat Res Int. 2013;2013:635628. https://doi.org/10.1155/2013/635628.
6. Spiegl UJ, Petri M, Smith SW, Ho CP, Millett PJ. Association between scapula bony morphology and snapping scapula syndrome. J Shoulder Elb Surg. 2015;24(8):1289–95.
7. Boyle MJ, Misur P, Youn SM, Ball CM. The superomedial bare area of the costal scapula surface: a possible cause of snapping scapula syndrome. Surg Radiol Anat. 2013;35(2):95–8.
8. Totlis T, Konstantinidis GA, Karanassos MT, Sofidis G, Anastasopoulos N, Natsis K. Bony structures related to snapping scapula: correlation to gender, side and age. Surg Radiol Anat. 2014;36(1):3–9. https://doi.org/10.1007/s00276-013-1130-4.
9. Dharmadhikari RP. Painful snapping and pseudo-winging scapula due to a large scapular osteochondroma. J Orthop Case Rep. 2012;2(2):10–3.

10. Zaidenberg EE, Rossi LA, Bongiovanni SL, Tanoira I, Maignon G, Ranalletta M. Snapping scapular syndrome secondary to rib intramedullary fixation device. Int J Surg Case Rep. 2015;17:158–60.
11. Patzkowski JC, Owens BD, Burns TC. Snapping scapula syndrome in the military. Clin Sports Med. 2014;33(4):757–66.
12. Tittal P, Pawar I, Kapoor SK. Pseudo-winging of scapula due to benign lesions of ventral surface of scapula - two unusual causes. J Clin Orthop Trauma. 2015;6(1):30–5.
13. Deveci MA, Özbarlas HS, Erdoğan KE, Biçer ÖS, Tekin M, Özkan C. Elastofibroma dorsi: clinical evaluation of 61 cases and review of the literature. Acta Orthop Traumatol Turc. 2017;51(1):7–11.
14. Mauclaire M. Craquements sous-scapulaires pathologiques traits par l'interposition musculaire interscapuothoracique. Bull Mem Soc Chir Paris. 1904;30:164–8.
15. Merolla G, Cerciello S, Paladini P, Porcellini G. Snapping scapula syndrome: current concepts review in conservative and surgical treatment. Muscles Ligaments Tendons J. 2013;3(2):80–90. https://doi.org/10.11138/mltj/2013.3.2.080.
16. Manske RC, Reiman MP, Stovak ML. Nonoperative and operative management of snapping scapula. Am J Sports Med. 2004;32(6):1554–65.
17. Warme WJ. Open surgical treatment for snapping scapula provides durable pain relief, but so does nonsurgical treatment. Clin Orthop Relat Res. 2016;474(3):806–7.
18. Acar N. Low-energy versus middle-energy extracorporeal shockwave therapy for the treatment of snapping scapula bursitis. Pak J Med Sci. 2017;33(2):335–40.
19. Acar N, Karaarslan AA, Karakasli A. The effectiveness of extracorporeal shock wave therapy in snapping scapula. J Orthop Surg (Hong Kong). 2017;25(1):2309499016684723.
20. Vastamäki M, Vastamäki H. Open surgical treatment for snapping scapula provides durable pain relief, but so does nonsurgical treatment. Clin Orthop Relat Res. 2016;474(3):799–805.
21. Conduah AH, Baker CL 3rd, Baker CL Jr. Clinical management of scapulothoracic bursitis and the snapping scapula. Sports Health. 2010;2(2):147–55.
22. Tahal DS, Katthagen JC, Marchetti DC, Mikula JD, Montgomery SR, Brady A, Dornan GJ, Millett PJ. A cadaveric model evaluating the influence of bony anatomy and the effectiveness of partial scapulectomy on decompression of the scapulothoracic space in snapping scapula syndrome. Am J Sports Med. 2017;45(6):1276–82.
23. Ten Duis K, IJpma FF. Surgical treatment of snapping scapula syndrome due to malunion of rib fractures. Ann Thorac Surg. 2017;103(2):e143–4.
24. Ross AE, Owens BD, DeBerardino TM. Open scapula resection in beach-chair position for treatment of snapping scapula. Am J Orthop (Belle Mead NJ). 2009;38(5):249–51.
25. Menge TJ, Horan MP, Tahal DS, Mitchell JJ, Katthagen JC, Millett PJ. Arthroscopic treatment of snapping scapula syndrome: outcomes at minimum of 2 years. Arthroscopy. 2017;33(4):726–32.

Chapter 49
Myofascial Trigger Points

A condition whereby there are spots of discreet bands of taut skeletal muscle or fascia that produce clinical symptoms and are tender on palpation. These often involve the trapezius and other paraspinal muscles. Tender spots may reflect hypersensitive areas within the muscle secondary to muscle overload (overuse, abnormal posture or trauma) [1–3].

49.1 Clinical Symptoms of Myofascial Trigger Points

- Localised muscle pain, exacerbated by movements of the cervical spine and shoulder
- Referred pain distant from the tender spot (may mimic neurological pain, radiculopathies) – its distribution does not follow a specific nerve pattern but is constant
- Arm weakness
- Autonomic phenomena – sweating, erythema
- Altered sensation, increased sensitivity to pain (hyperalgesia)

49.2 Clinical Signs of Myofascial Trigger Points

- Tender muscular spots that on palpation cause pain reproducing the clinical symptoms including referred pain
- Apparent muscle weakness due to pain
- Pain worsened by stretching

© Springer Nature Switzerland AG 2019
C. Panayiotou Charalambous, *The Shoulder Made Easy*,
https://doi.org/10.1007/978-3-319-98908-2_49

49.3 Management of Myofascial Trigger Points [4–14]

- Leave alone
- Inactivate tender points and eliminate causative factors
- Physiotherapy:
  - Manual techniques (compression on the trigger point or massage)
  - Stretching of the involved muscle
  - Postural correction
  - Relaxation
- Injection
  - Dry needling acupuncture
  - Normal saline
  - Local anaesthetic
  - Steroid
  - Botulinum toxin
- Ultrasound
- TENS
- Skin cooling
- Local heat treatment

Learning Pearls
- The diagnosis of myofascial trigger points is clinical and must be considered when dealing with the painful shoulder, especially in the presence of normal radiological investigations
- Referred pain may have a neurological source but may also originate from trigger points

References

1. Lavelle ED, Lavelle W, Smith HS. Myofascial trigger points. Med Clin North Am. 2007;91(2):229–39.
2. Fernández-de-Las-Peñas C, Dommerholt J. International consensus on diagnostic criteria and clinical considerations of myofascial trigger points: a Delphi study. Pain Med. 2018;19(1):142–50.
3. Money S. Pathophysiology of trigger points in myofascial pain syndrome. J Pain Palliat Care Pharmacother. 2017;31(2):158–9.
4. Moraska AF, Schmiege SJ, Mann JD, Butryn N, Krutsch JP. Responsiveness of myofascial trigger points to single and multiple trigger point release massages: a randomized, placebo controlled trial. Am J Phys Med Rehabil. 2017;96(9):639–45.
5. Kalichman L, Ben David C. Effect of self-myofascial release on myofascial pain, muscle flexibility, and strength: a narrative review. J Bodyw Mov Ther. 2017;21(2):446–51.

6. Vernon H, Schneider M. Chiropractic management of myofascial trigger points and myofascial pain syndrome: a systematic review of the literature. J Manip Physiol Ther. 2009;32(1):14–24.
7. Li X, Wang R, Xing X, Shi X, Tian J, Zhang J, Ge L, Zhang J, Li L, Yang K. Acupuncture for myofascial pain syndrome: a network meta-analysis of 33 randomized controlled trials. Pain Physician. 2017;20(6):E883–902.
8. Hall ML, Mackie AC, Ribeiro DC. Effects of dry needling trigger point therapy in the shoulder region on patients with upper extremity pain and dysfunction: a systematic review with meta-analysis. Physiotherapy. 2017;104:167–77. pii: S0031-9406.
9. Espejo-Antúnez L, Tejeda JF, Albornoz-Cabello M, Rodríguez-Mansilla J, de la Cruz-Torres B, Ribeiro F, Silva AG. Dry needling in the management of myofascial trigger points: a systematic review of randomized controlled trials. Complement Ther Med. 2017;33:46–57.
10. Ong J, Claydon LS. The effect of dry needling for myofascial trigger points in the neck and shoulders: a systematic review and meta-analysis. J Bodyw Mov Ther. 2014;18(3):390–8.
11. Kwanchuay P, Petchnumsin T, Yiemsiri P, Pasuk N, Srikanok W, Efficacy HC. Safety of single botulinum toxin type A (Botox®) injection for relief of upper trapezius myofascial trigger point: a randomized, double-blind, placebo-controlled study. J Med Assoc Thail. 2015;98(12):1231–6.
12. Borg-Stein J, Iaccarino MA. Myofascial pain syndrome treatments. Phys Med Rehabil Clin N Am. 2014;25(2):357–74.
13. Gemmell H, Hilland A. Immediate effect of electric point stimulation (TENS) in treating latent upper trapezius trigger points: a double blind randomised placebo-controlled trial. J Bodyw Mov Ther. 2011;15(3):348–54.
14. Dissanayaka TD, Pallegama RW, Suraweera HJ, Johnson MI, Kariyawasam AP. Comparison of the effectiveness of transcutaneous electrical nerve stimulation and interferential therapy on the upper trapezius in myofascial pain syndrome: a randomized controlled study. Am J Phys Med Rehabil. 2016;95(9):663–72.

Index

© Springer Nature Switzerland AG 2019

C. Panayiotou Charalambous, *The Shoulder Made Easy*,
https://doi.org/10.1007/978-3-319-98908-2

MIX
Papier aus verantwortungsvollen Quellen
Paper from responsible sources
FSC® C105338

If you have any concerns about our products, you can contact us on
ProductSafety@springernature.com

In case Publisher is established outside the EU, the EU authorized representative is:
Springer Nature Customer Service Center GmbH
Europaplatz 3, 69115 Heidelberg, Germany

Printed by Libri Plureos GmbH
in Hamburg, Germany